COMMON PROBLEMS IN PEDIATRIC PATHOLOGY

COMMON PROBLEMS IN PEDIATRIC PATHOLOGY

Vijay V. Joshi, M.D., Ph.D., F.R.C.Path.
Professor and Director of Pediatric Pathology
and Clinical Professor of Pediatrics
East Carolina University School of Medicine
Greenville, North Carolina
and
Consultant in Pediatric Pathology
Beth Israel Medical Center
New York, New York

IGAKU-SHOIN 1944

IGAKU-SHOIN NEW YORK • TOKYO

Published and distributed by

IGAKU-SHOIN Medical Publishers, Inc.
One Madison Avenue, New York, New York 10010

IGAKU-SHOIN Ltd.,
5-24-3 Hongo, Bunkyo-ku, Tokyo 113-91.

Library of Congress Cataloging-in-Publication Data

Joshi, Vijay V., 1936–
Common problems in pediatric pathology / Vijay V. Joshi.
p. cm.
Includes bibliographical references and index.
1. Pediatric pathology. I. Title.
[DNLM: 1. Pediatrics. 2. Pathology. WS 200 J83c 1994]
RJ49.J67 1994
618.92'007—dc20
DNLM/DLC
for Library of Congress 93-38969
CIP

ISBN: 0-89640-242-8 (New York)
ISBN: 4-260-14242-9 (Tokyo)

Printed and bound in the U.S.A.
10 9 8 7 6 5 4 3 2 1

DEDICATION

Dedicated with love and gratitude to my wife, Jayashree, and our sons, Abhijit and Jitendra; to my mother, Aai, and the memory of my late father, Baba; and to the memory of my grandparents, Kakasaheb and Kaku.

PREFACE

न चोरहार्यं न च राजहार्यं
न भ्रातृभाज्यं न च भारकारि ।
व्यये कृते वर्धत एव नित्यं
विद्याधनं सर्वधन-प्रधानम् ॥

(Na chorhārya na cha rājahāryam
Na bhrātrubhājyam na cha bhārakāri
Vyaye krute vardhata eva nityam
Vidyādhanam sarvadhana pradhānam)

The essential principle enunciated in the aforementioned Sanskrit maxim can be liberally translated as follows: The wealth of knowledge cannot be stolen by thieves, confiscated by the king, or divided among brothers. The more one "spends" it, the more it grows.

The seeds of this book were sown when I started giving short courses on "Essentials of Neonatal Pathology" and "Pediatric Surgical Pathology" at the American Society of Clinical Pathologists' conferences. My main objective in teaching these courses was to share my experiences in pediatric pathology with general pathologists and trainees in general pathology and pediatric pathology. My belief that their knowledge of pediatric pathology needed updating was strengthened by three observations: (1) Pediatric pathology is not and cannot be adequately covered during the residency program in most institutions; (2) A significant amount of pediatric pathology material in the areas of both perinatal autopsy pathology and pediatric surgical pathology is seen and signed out by general pathologists because pediatrics in the United States is practiced not only in children's hospitals but also in "general" hospitals; and (3) In recent years, pediatric pathology has become more complex and more involved than in the past. The explosion of knowledge in neonatal pathology and pediatric tumor pathology, as well as the increasing use of therapeutic termination of pregnancy for fetal abnormalities, requires the surgical pathologist to deal with various congenital anomalies and fetal disorders.

I cover more than 20 different topics in my courses. It was not possible to include all of these in a moderate sized book in which I wished to give broad and in-depth coverage of topics of practical importance to the pathologist. Therefore, I decided to include important lesions and diseases which are representative of principal categories in pediatric autopsy and surgical pathology. Thus, after the first chapter which gives an overview of principal disease processes in perinatal pathology, the subsequent chapters represent the following topics: (a) immunologic disorders, (b) diseases of the respiratory system and gastrointestinal tract which are unique to the neonatal age group, (c) perinatal ischemic and traumatic lesions of the brain, (d) iatrogenic lesions, (e) congenital anomalies, (f) metabolic disorders, and (g) general and specific aspects of tumors in children.

Although my basic approach in writing these chapters has been to cover the morphologic diagnostic characteristics, I feel strongly that even in our rather restricted role as diagnosticians, familiarity with clinical features, pathogenesis, and tumor biology is essential. Hence the chapters include coverage of not only the morphologic aspects but also the "nonmorphologic" aspects of the various lesions and disease processes.

I feel that the success of this book can be measured in terms of the number of pathology trainees and pathologists whose practice of pediatric pathology is significantly influenced by it and who develop a special interest in the broad specialty of pediatric pathology as a result of this book. The specialty of pediatric pathology is at a critical juncture and needs major reinforcements in its ranks at various levels.

Vijay V. Joshi, M.D., Ph.D., F.R.C.Path.
Greenville, North Carolina

ACKNOWLEDGMENTS

Although the writing of this book took about two years, it has actually been in preparation for many more years. It would not have been possible without the guidance and knowledge imparted by my teachers and mentors since the beginning of my career and during my formative years as a pathologist, as well as the help and encouragement for the actual preparation of the book provided by many individuals. I have benefited from many teachers, including Professor R. K. Gadgil and the late Professor P. V. Gharpuray of Grant Medical College, Bombay; Professor Fairfield Goodale and Professor Saul Kay of the Medical College of Virginia, Richmond; and Professor John Frei of the University of Western Ontario, London, Canada. I have been lucky to have stellar physicians such as Professor M. Daria Haust of the University of Western Ontario and Professor Richard H. Rapkin of Childrens' Hospital of New Jersey, Newark, NJ, as my mentors. Professor J. Bruce Beckwith and Professor Costan Berard have provided inspiration and opportunities for carrying out work on the pathology of tumors in children. I have had the good fortune to work closely with many clinical colleagues, including the late Professor Leo Stern, Professor Omkar Bhakoo, Professor R. K. Gandhi, Dean Lata Deshmukh, Dean Bill Laupus, Professor Tate Holbrook, and Professor Jim Oleske. These and other colleagues have provided the impetus for maintaining a clinical orientation in my work. I would especially like to mention Dr. Harry F. Hoke and Dr. Gladstone E. Smith, whose invaluable support at a critical stage made continuation of my academic career possible. Many other colleagues—clinicians, pathologists, and pathology trainees too numerous to mention—have shared their insights and provided encouragement over the years.

Some of the illustrations were very kindly lent to me by colleagues including Professor J. Bruce Beckwith, Professor Robert Bolande, Dr. Alexander Knisely, Dr. Gary Mierau, Dr. Timothy Benning, Professor Stan Harris, Professor Jim Finley, Professor Jan Silverman, Dr. John Fisher, Dr. Stephen Qualman, and Dr. Greg Gagnon. Dr. Gagnon also was helpful in offering constructive comments regarding portions of the chapter on Pathology of Tumors in Children—General Aspects. I have been at the East Carolina University School of Medicine in Greenville, North Carolina during the preparation of this (and my previous) book. The chairman of my department, Professor H. Thomas Norris, has given his unstinting support and encouragement. Dean James Hallock of the School of Medicine has provided invaluable advice and understanding. Ms. Tricia Robbins through her expertise and indefatigable enthusiasm accomplished the tremendous task of typing numerous drafts of the chapters. Ms. Pauline Hardee typed one of the chapters and along with Ms. Wendy Johnson contributed to the organization of the book. John Artois and his staff put in a great deal of effort and expertise in the preparation of the photographs. Alan Branigan and his staff used their artistic talents in preparing the diagrams included in various chapters. Lila Maron and the production staff of Igaku-Shoin provided support during the preparation of the book.

I gratefully acknowledge my debt and express my most sincere thanks to all these individuals who have acted as teachers, mentors, helpful colleagues, and coworkers.

Writing a book has proven to be far more strenuous and time-consuming than I had anticipated. It involves not only spending time away from the family but also being preoccupied with ideas, thoughts, and concerns about the book even when one is with them. My wife, Jayashree, and our sons Abhijit and Jitendra showed patience and understanding and gave their full cooperation while I was preparing this book.

CONTENTS

1 ANALYSIS OF AUTOPSY FINDINGS: FACTORS RELATED TO DEATH OF THE FETUS AND NEWBORN

INTRODUCTION

In the final analysis, the major consideration for the parents and the clinicians in a case of stillbirth or neonatal death is *the* cause of death found at perinatal autopsy. However, it appears to me that undue emphasis is placed on *the* cause of death. In many instances the death is multifactorial. Thus the "causes" of death can be divided into primary or basic cause and secondary (or immediate, or terminal) cause. I prefer to consider these "causes" as primary and secondary factors related to death. Associated maternal conditions, placental abnormalities, and abnormalities of labor and delivery may also play a contributing role. The following example illustrates the futility of assessing *the* cause of death: a low-birth-weight (1750-g) infant born at 31 weeks' gestation to 15-year-old single mother died at the age of 68 hours. The major findings at autopsy were as follows: Acute stage of idiopathic respiratory distress syndrome (IRDS), mild focal superimposed bronchopneumonia, and massive bilateral intraventricular hemorrhage (IVH) of the brain. The placenta examined by the surgical pathologist showed acute chorioamnionitis. Bronchopneumonia, which was mild and focal, cannot be considered as the cause of death. Is *the* cause of death IVH or IRDS? I would consider massive IVH as the secondary cause and IRDS as the primary cause. If one stretches the argument further, prematurity could be considered as the basic or primary cause. Most cases of perinatal mortality involve premature newborn infants. Therefore, in all such cases the primary cause of death could be considered as prematurity. Going one step further, one would like to ask if there is a demonstrable cause of premature onset of labor. It is likely that acute chorionamnionitis found in the example given above may have initiated the premature labor, resulting in premature delivery. Young age and single status of the mother can be considered in the epidemiologic sense as factors contributing to prematurity. Thus the analysis becomes complex, revealing the multifactorial nature of the fatal outcome.

I have used the following approach to the analysis of factors related to death in a fetus or newborn infant. There are four types of factors: (1) primary or basic factors, (2) secondary (or immediate) factors, (3) obstetric and/or maternal factors, and (4) epidemiologic factors. Thus in the example given above: (1) IRDS is the primary factor, (2) IVH is the secondary factor, (3) premature labor and delivery probably initiated by acute chorioamnionitis are the obstetric factors, and (4) young age and single status of the mother are the epidemiologic factors. The epidemiologic factors need not be considered in routine hospital autopsy cases unless there is an ongoing special prospective study of perinatal mortality.

The major primary (or basic) factor related to death can be defined as the basic pathologic or pathophysiologic disease process responsible for the major presenting clinical and biochemical manifestations seen in the infant. Examples include congenital anomalies and IRDS. The secondary factor related to death can be defined as a severe complication of the basic disease process or (rarely) of its therapy.

In occasional cases there may be two major primary factors related to death, e.g., IRDS and erythroblastosis fetalis. Some factors can be considered primary or secondary depending on the type of case. For example, severe intrauterine pneumonia is a primary factor in a stillbirth, whereas it is a secondary factor in an infant with IRDS. The various primary and secondary factors [1–6] related to perinatal mortality are listed in Tables 1-1 and 1-4 and discussed below.

PRIMARY FACTORS RELATED TO PERINATAL DEATHS

Many of the lists of causes of perinatal mortality published in the literature include secondary causes, and show overlap of different entities, but do not show breakdown of extrinsic perinatal asphyxia according to different associated conditions, and exclude certain important primary factors. All the entities included in the modified list devised by the Perinatal Mortality Committee of Province of Quebec, Canada[3–6] are described to obviate these criticisms.

TABLE 1-1 Primary Factors Related to Perinatal Death[a]

Idiopathic respiratory distress syndrome and its sequelae
Congenital anomalies
Extrinsic perinatal asphyxia associated with placental abnormalities, umbilical cord abnormalities, labor and delivery abnormalities, maternal disorders, unknown factors
Infection (pulmonary, extrapulmonary, and systemic infection without localization)
Neonatal necrotizing enterocolitis
Intrauterine growth retardation
Birth trauma
Isoimmunization related to blood group incompatibility
Other specific causes[b]
Extreme prematurity
Undetermined

[a] All these conditions except idiopathic respiratory distress syndrome, neonatal necrotizing enterocolitis and extreme prematurity can be primary factors in both antepartum and intrapartum intrauterine death.

[b] These include a variety of conditions such as twin transfusion syndrome, idiopathic massive pulmonary hemorrhage, maternal abdominal trauma, congenital malignancy, massive fetomaternal hemorrhage, and possibly sudden infant death syndrome.

TABLE 1-2 Birth Weight by Gestational Age for non-Spanish California White Singleton Infants

Gestational age (completed week)	10th percentile		50th percentile		90th percentile	
	Male	Female	Male	Female	Male	Female
22	326	314	530	496	736	755
23	376	354	609	569	852	869
24	433	400	699	651	982	996
25	499	454	800	745	1127	1136
26	574	518	913	850	1288	1290
27	662	591	1041	969	1466	1460
28	762	678	1184	1102	1661	1645
29	878	780	1343	1252	1873	1845
30	1007	902	1537	1430	2159	2113
31	1159	1041	1752	1637	2439	2364
32	1348	1219	1979	1861	2727	2619
33	1561	1436	2220	2090	2972	2847
34	1787	1668	2459	2329	3205	3058
35	2030	1918	2694	2562	3415	3250
36	2278	2169	2910	2788	3591	3450
37	2499	2410	3112	2992	3765	3646
38	2696	2587	3292	3161	3931	3802
39	2849	2730	3434	3294	4064	3923
40	2944	2817	3534	3389	4154	4005
41	3018	2873	3598	3450	4214	4040
42	3086	2936	3665	3513	4276	4094
43	3120	2967	3703	3548	4315	4126
44	3120	2966	3712	3554	4330	4136
45	3085	2932	3691	3531	4321	4126
46	3016	2866	3641	3479	4288	4093
47	2916	2771	3563	3400	4231	4040
48	2789	2650	3459	3295	4152	3966

Adapted from Williams RL et al: *Obstet Gynecol* 59:624, 1982.

CONGENITAL ANOMALIES

The term "anomaly" is used to include congenital structural, cytogenetic, functional, and metabolic abnormalities. Cases are assigned to this category when specific congenital anomaly or anomalies are a primary factor related to death directly (e.g., hypoplastic left heart syndrome, renal agenesis) or indirectly (e.g., death in postoperative period of corrective surgery). Needless to say, cases with minor congenital anomaly or anomalies that are present incidentally and do not play a major role in the death of the infant are not included in this category.

Multiple congenital anomalies present in a particular case may be characteristic of a well-established syndrome with or without chromosomal abnormalities. The diagnosis of a particular syndrome requires collation of not only the pathologic findings in the internal organs but also of external abnormalities (facial features, etc.). Radiologic features may also have to be considered in some syndromes. In most cases, a diagnosis of a particular syndrome can be readily made on the basis of the clinical, external, internal, radiologic, and chromosomal abnormalities. Careful dissection and study of appropriate sections of the organs affected by anomaly or anomalies for histologic confirmation are of critical importance. Dissecting microscope may have to be used in small fetuses. The pathologic findings are an essential component of the diagnosis of fatal cases of a particular syndrome, and I recognize the confirmatory and definitive nature of pathologic findings at autopsy. However, in poorly delineated or rare syndromes, input from the geneticist and radiologist is advisable in order to arrive at the correct or the most plausible diagnosis. A joint effort and consensus are in the best interest of the parents of the infant who are concerned about the risk of recurrence in subsequent pregnancies. In such cases, I consult the geneticist (dysmorphologist) and radiologist freely and take their findings for granted when I cannot verify their findings because of limitations of an autopsy examination. The best single readily available source of data for diagnosis of the syndromes is Smith's monograph on patterns of human malformation.[7] A more exhaustive computer database[8] usually available with the geneticist may have to be consulted in rare instances. As indicated above, the term "anomalies" includes all types of anomalies, i.e., of structural, biochemical, chromosomal and functional origin. The structural anomalies are of the following four types: malformation, disruption, deformation, and dysplasia.[9]

Malformation. A "malformation" is a morphologic defect of an organ, part of an organ, or larger region of the body resulting from an intrinsically abnormal developmental process. The term "intrinsic" indicates that the anlage or primordium of the organ was abnormal or absent. Renal agenesis and ventricular septal defect of the heart are examples of malformation.

Disruption. A "disruption" is a morphologic defect of an organ, or a larger region of the body resulting from the extrinsic breakdown of, or an interference with, an originally normal developmental process. The term "disruption" implies that the anlage (primordium) of the organ was intrinsically normal. The anomaly results from an extrinsic factor such as infection, teratogen, trauma, or vascular accidents interfering with further development of the organ. The amputation of a limb seen in amniotic band syndrome and intestinal atresia resulting from vascular accident are examples of disruption.

Deformation. A deformation is an abnormal form, shape or position of a part of body caused by extrinsic mechanical forces acting on intrinsically normal tissues. (see section of sequence below).

Dysplasia. A "dysplasia" is an abnormal organization of cells into tissue(s) and its morphologic result(s). It has also been called "dyshistogenesis." Osteogenesis imperfecta and connective tissue abnormality in Marfan's syndrome serve as examples of dysplasia. (In surgical pathology the term "dysplasia" is used to connote a cellular abnormality with neoplastic potential.)

The other terms such as "hyperplasia," "hypertrophy," and "atrophy" retain the original connotation. The terms "agenesis" and "aplasia" have been defined specifically. Agenesis represents the absence of an organ due to absence of anlage of the organ, whereas aplasia represents total failure of the anlage (which is present) to develop.

The foregoing terms define individual structural anomalies. Multiple structural anomalies are present in certain cases. Many of these follow certain patterns; thus they may be etiopathogenetically related or they may occur together on a statistical basis or by chance. The following terms define these various types of relationship between multiple structural anomalies present in an individual case.

Polytopic field defect. This connotes multiple anomalies resulting from a single developmental field disturbance. For example, defective mesodermal migration to the area anterior to the notochord leads to defects in the field of forebrain and midfacial structures. The result is alobar holoprosencephaly (cyclopia, proboscis, absence of olfactory lobes and optic nerves, etc.).

Sequence. A "sequence" is a pattern of multiple anomalies derived from a single known or presumed prior anomaly or mechanical factor. The initiating anomaly in the sequence may be a malformation, disruption, or mechanical factor. Anomalies seen in Potter's syndrome associated with renal agenesis or urethral obstruction or chronic leakage of amniotic fluid are considered as a sequence by this definition. Renal anomalies such as renal agenesis result in oligohydramnios, which, in turn as a result of a mechanical factor (compression of fetal structures against the uterine wall), will lead to deformations such as facial and limb anomalies, pulmonary hypoplasia and amnion nodosum. The Potter sequence can be described in the following order: renal agenesis–oligohydramnios–pulmonary hypoplasia and facial and limb abnormalities.

Syndrome. A "syndrome" is a pattern of multiple anomalies thought to be pathogenetically related and not known to represent a single sequence or a polytopic field defect. "Syndrome" implies a single cause. Down's syndrome and Marfan's syndrome serve as examples of the category of syndrome.

Association. An "association" is a nonrandom occurrence in two or more individuals or multiple anomalies not known to be a polytopic field defect, sequence, or syndrome. The term "association" refers to statistically related anomalies. Etiologic or pathogenetic relationship is not implied. Presence of vertebral defects, anal atresia, tracheoesophageal fistula, and radial and renal dysplasia in an infant serves as example of VATER association.

IDIOPATHIC RESPIRATORY DISTRESS SYNDROME (IRDS)

The diagnosis of IRDS and the stage to which the lesion belongs are determined on the basis of clinical, radiologic, and pathologic findings. The findings and the stages in the natural history of IRDS are described in detail in the chapter on IRDS.

EXTRINSIC PERINATAL ASPHYXIA

"Asphyxia" is defined as a combination of hypoxemia, hypercapnia, and metabolic acidemia. McPherson prefers the term "uteroplacental circulation disorder" to extrinsic perinatal asphyxia (EPA).[5] Apgar scores based on heart rate, respiratory effort, color, muscle tone, and reflex irritability assessed at 1, 5, and 10 minutes were considered indicators of asphyxia. However, it has been shown that Apgar score alone does not necessarily correlate with asphyxia. Therefore, the diagnosis of asphyxia based on Apgar score of <7 alone is not recommended.[10,11] The neurologic features (hypotonia, apnea, etc.) and biochemical parameters ($\downarrow P_{O_2}$, $\uparrow P_{CO_2}$, and base deficit) should be taken into consideration. Other systemic features of EPA include dysrhythmia, myocardial and valvular insufficiency, persistent fetal circulation, shock lung, pulmonary hemorrhage, disseminated intravascular coagulation, renal failure, adrenal hemorrhage, pancreatic insufficiency, and subcutaneous fat necrosis. In the fetus, the abnormalities of heart rate measured by continuous electronic monitoring along with those of blood gases of the capillary blood collected from the scalp if inidicated are considered in the diagnosis of EPA. I would recommend that the neonatologist and obstetrician be consulted if the clinical and biochemical data as recorded in the chart are not clear. The diagnosis of EPA may have medicolegal implications. Therefore, the diagnosis should be made when the clinical and biochemical criteria are met. The pathologic findings listed below support the diagnosis made on the basis of clinical and biochemical data. If the clinical or biochemical data are not available or were not obtained, pathologic findings alone will have to be considered for diagnosis.

The terms "extrinsic" and "perinatal" indicate that the cause of asphyxia is outside the fetus (maternal and obstetric factors) and that it occurs around the time of birth (i.e., shortly before, during, and shortly after delivery). The factors associated with EPA are divided into four subgroups: (1) placental abnormalities (e.g., placenta previa, abruptio placentae); (2) umbilical cord abnormalities (e.g., prolapse, knots), (3) labor and delivery abnormalities (e.g., unduly prolonged labor, obstructed labor, abnormal presentation, and (4) maternal disorders (e.g., preeclampsia, hypertension). The known associated factor(s) should be stated in the final autopsy diagnosis (FAD). In cases in which the factors associated with EPA are unclear or unknown, a statement to that effect should be included in the FAD.

The pathologic findings in cases of EPA are as follow:

1. *Visceral congestion with or without hemorrhage.* The most characteristic site for congestion is the corticomedullary junction of the kidneys (Figure 1-1). The hemorrhages, which vary in severity, include petechiae over the thymus, pleura (Figure 1-2), and pericardium; pulmonary hemorrhage; and subependymal, germinal matrix hemorrhage of the brain with or without intraventricular; and/or intracerebral extension.
2. *Aspiration of amniotic debris.* As a result of the normal intrauterine fetal respiratory movements there is a minimal to small amount of amniotic debris in the lower respiratory tract and even alveoli. However, in asphyxia large amounts of amniotic debris are aspirated into the bronchioles and alveoli. The bronchioles are distended due to plugs of amniotic debris (Figure 1-3), and even the peripheral subpleural alveoli contain moderate to large amounts of it. It should be emphasized that the presence of a severe degree of amniotic aspiration is indicative of asphyxia but its absence does not rule it out. The absence of massive aspiration of amniotic debris in EPA may be related to the

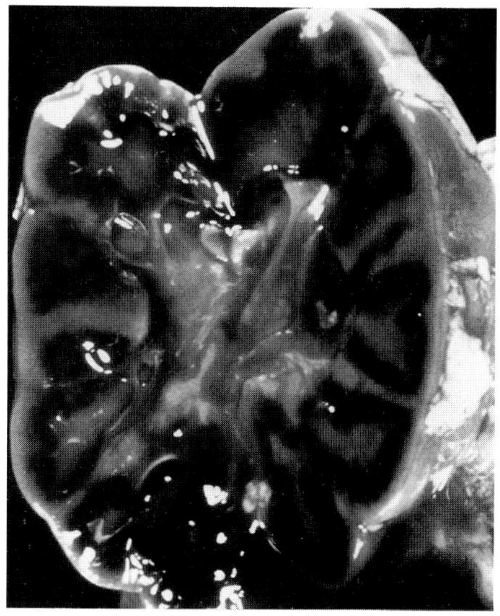

FIGURE 1-1. Marked congestion of the corticomedullary junction of the kidney in a newborn infant with extrinsic perinatal asphyxia.

timing and duration of EPA. If EPA occurs after rupture of the amniotic sac or if EPA is shortly followed by delivery, aspiration is absent or not excessive.

3. *Meconium aspiration.* When a relatively mature fetus (>34 weeks' gestation) is asphyxiated it may discharge meconium. However, it should be noted that the fetus may pass meconium in the absence of distress or conversely, a distressed fetus may not always pass meconium. However, only a distressed fetus would make gasping efforts in utero. Meconium can be aspirated into

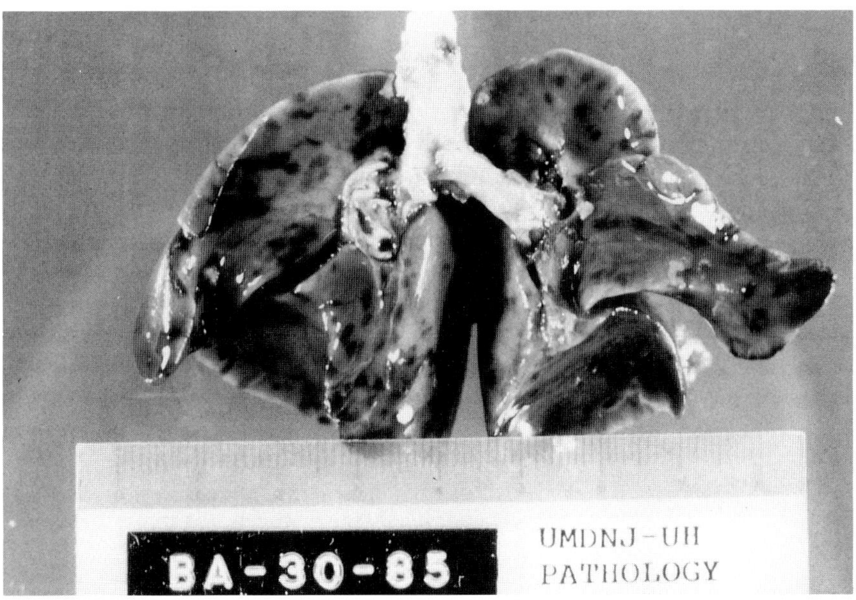

FIGURE 1-2. Subpleural petechial hemorrhages in an infant with asphyxia neonatorum.

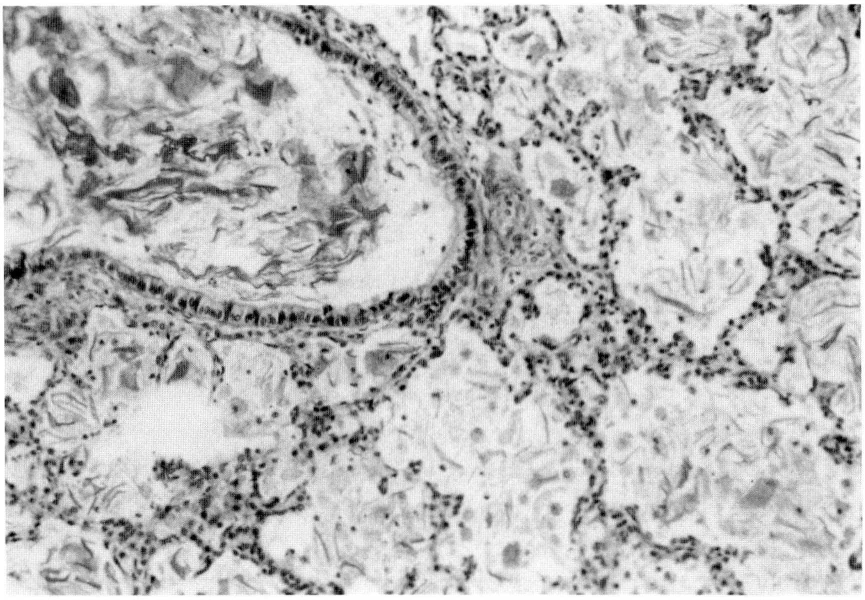

FIGURE 1-3. Note the distension of the bronchioles and alveoli due to aspiration of large amounts of amniotic debris in any asphyxiated newborn infant (H&E, ×250).

the airway either from these gasping efforts of the asphyxiated fetus or with the first breaths of life. Meconium aspiration syndrome is diagnosed when there is presence of meconium in the trachea, clinical signs of respiratory distress, and a characteristic chest x-ray finding of fluffy infiltrates. However, meconium may be thin and evenly mixed with amniotic fluid. In such instances a meconium plug as such may not be found clinically in the upper respiratory tract since the thin, evenly dispersed meconium is aspirated into the lower respiratory tract and alveoli. Respiratory insufficiency can occur with aspiration of both types of meconium. Because of suctioning of the upper respiratory tract done during life, a meconium plug is virtually never found on gross examination at autopsy. In these cases meconium may not be found also on histologic examination of lungs. However, if the thin, evenly dispersed meconium has been aspirated deep into the lower airways, it can be detected on histologic examination of the lungs (Figure 1-4). The remaining histologic findings in the lungs in the cases of meconium aspiration syndrome depend upon the time of death (Joshi, VV: Unpublished data, 1975). If the infant dies within a short time after birth, the only findings will be those of meconium aspiration, irregular hyperinflation of lung due to vigorous resuscitative efforts, and petechial hemorrhages. If the infant dies after a few to several days, the lesions of oxygen toxicity and effects of mechanical ventilation will be present. Meconium may not be found at this stage since it may be cleared by the macrophages. Focal pneumonia may be present due to superimposed infection. Meconium itself is sterile and nonirritant, but it promotes bacterial growth if it is contaminated.[12] Therefore, meconium does

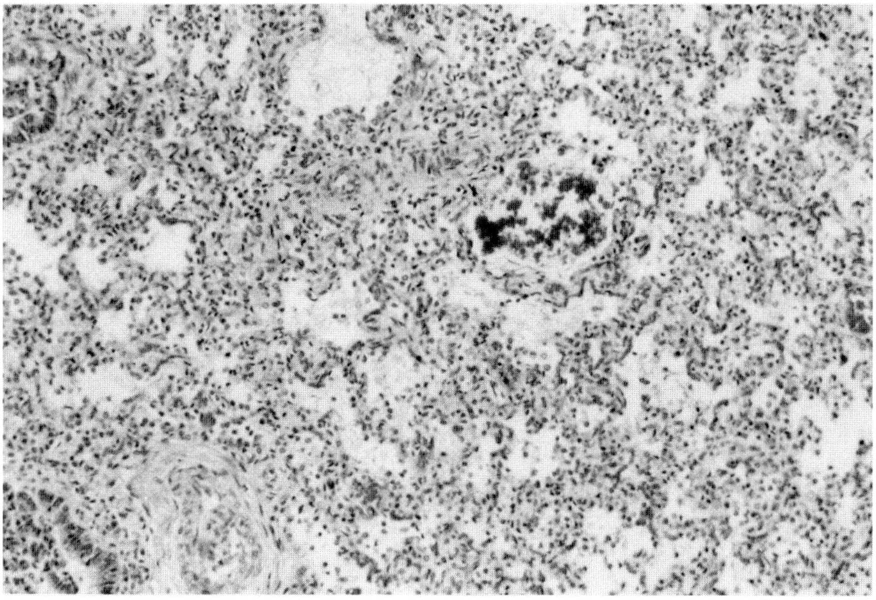

FIGURE 1-4. Aspiration of meconium is an alveolus in an asphyxiated newborn infant. Note the absence of inflammatory reaction (H&E, ×100).

not cause inflammatory reaction unless it is contaminated with bacteria.[13] In late deaths due to meconium aspiration syndrome, lungs show bronchopulmonary dysplasia associated with prolonged mechanical ventilation and oxygen therapy. In my opinion, meconium aspiration syndrome is a manifestation of EPA in most cases. It also perpetuates asphyxia. It should be considered as a consequence and manifestation of EPA and not a primary factor related to death. In cases in which there is no evidence of fetal distress noted on fetal monitoring and in which meconium aspiration occurs while taking first breaths after birth, it may be considered as a primary factor related to death.

4. *Hypoxic ischemic injury to various organs.* This may be seen in the form of an adult respiratory distress syndrome in the term infant,[14] tubular necrosis of the kidneys, necrosis of papillary muscles of the heart with or without calcification[15,16] (Figure 1-5) contraction band necrosis (CBN) of anterolateral costal diaphragm,[17] foci of contraction bands, wavy fibers, thick waves and coagulation necrosis in the smooth muscle of the intestine and urinary bladder,[18] and hypoxic ischemic encephalopathy (HIE) of the brain. Contraction bands appear as intensely eosinophilic transversely oriented bands along the longitudinal axis. Wavy fibers are characterized by regular periodic bending of densely eosinophilic fibers with pyknotic nuclei. Thick waves are broad, transversely oriented bands of densely eosinophilic portion of muscle fibers with pyknotic nuclei. HIE is described in the chapter on perinatal lesions of the head and brain (Chapter 5).

These lesions are associated with specific clinical manifestations. The neonatologists are interested in knowing the pathologic findings that correlate

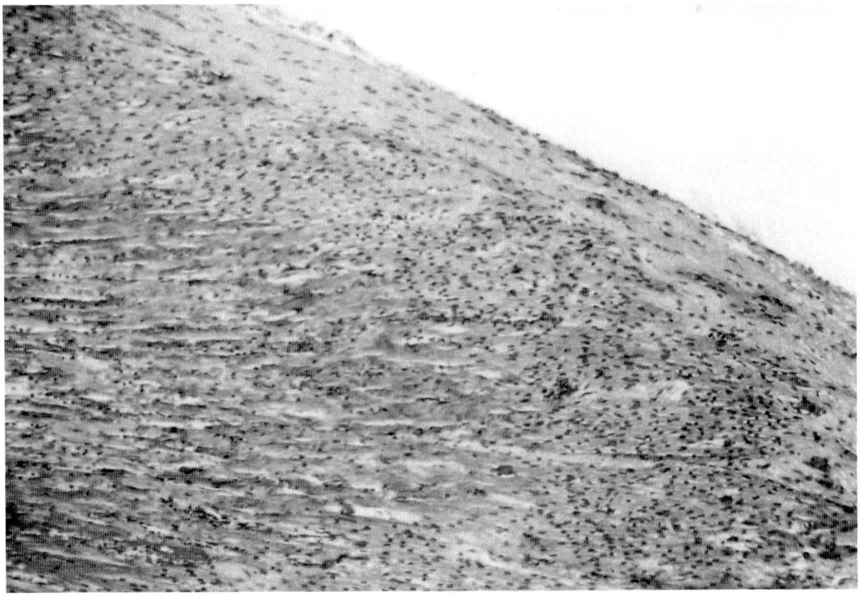

FIGURE 1-5. Necrosis of papillary muscle of the right ventricle in an asphyxiated infant (H&E, ×100).

with the clinical manifestations. For example, in a fatal case of EPA tricuspid or mitral valve insufficiency may have occurred during the clinical course. Papillary muscle necrosis with or without calcification will be found at autopsy if the infant dies shortly after the cardiac dysfunction. If the infant survives the episode and dies later (of some other terminal complication), there may be scarring of the papillary muscle. In the cases with renal tubular necrosis, there will be oliguria or anuria.

It should be noted that in the fatal cases of EPA, death may occur early or late. In the early fatal cases, the findings are of more acute nature such as visceral congestion with or without hemorrhage, aspiration of amniotic debris, tubular necrosis of kidneys, and meconium aspiration. In late fatal cases, findings of a chronic nature such as posthemorrhagic hydrocephalus and cystic encephalomalacia, and findings related to complications of therapy such as bronchopulmonary dysplasia, are noted. However, acute terminal events (lesions) such as pneumonia and papillary necrosis of the kidneys may also occur in these late deaths of infants with EPA.

INFECTION

Systemic and localized infections such as group B streptococcal sepsis or intrauterine pneumonia of sufficient severity are considered as major primary factors in the death of the infant when no predisposing factors for the infection are present. For example, pneumonia may be superimposed in infants with EPA, acute stage of IRDS, congenital heart disease, or bronchopulmonary dysplasia. In such cases infection is considered as a secondary factor related to the death.

Sufficient severity of localized infections is judged by clinical manifestations, laboratory data, and extent of severity of involvement of the organ. For example, in a case with pneumonia, the infection is considered significant if at least three of the five sections of the lungs (one from each lobe) show moderate to severe pneumonia. Another criterion to determine the significance of pneumonia is the abnormally heavy weight of the lungs (beyond 1 standard deviation from the mean expected for the birth weight of the infant).

Presence of infection should be documented by at least two of the following:

1. *Morphologic demonstration of organisms by routine or special stains.* Besides the conventional special stains (Gram stain, etc.) (Figure 1-6), specific immunoperoxidase stains for viruses (herpes simplex, cytomegalovirus, etc), and parasites (*Toxoplasma gondii*) are now available (Figure 1-7). Viral structure is fairly well preserved in the autopsy specimens, and electron microscopy may be used for demonstration of the viruses (Figure 1-8). The viral inclusions are not present in some viral infections (e.g., coxsackie viruses) or may be subtle (e.g., in human parvovirus) and may require confirmation by culture and electron microscopy (Figures 1-9, 1-10).[19,20]
2. *Foci of necrosis with or without inflammatory reaction.* The fetus or premature infant may not be able to mount an inflammatory reaction to an overwhelming infection, and only foci of hemorrhagic necrosis in various organs with organisms present in the parenchymal cells may be seen (e.g., disseminated herpes simplex infection) (Figure 1-11). In certain infections such as enteroviral infection, foci of necrosis in the liver and adrenal do not

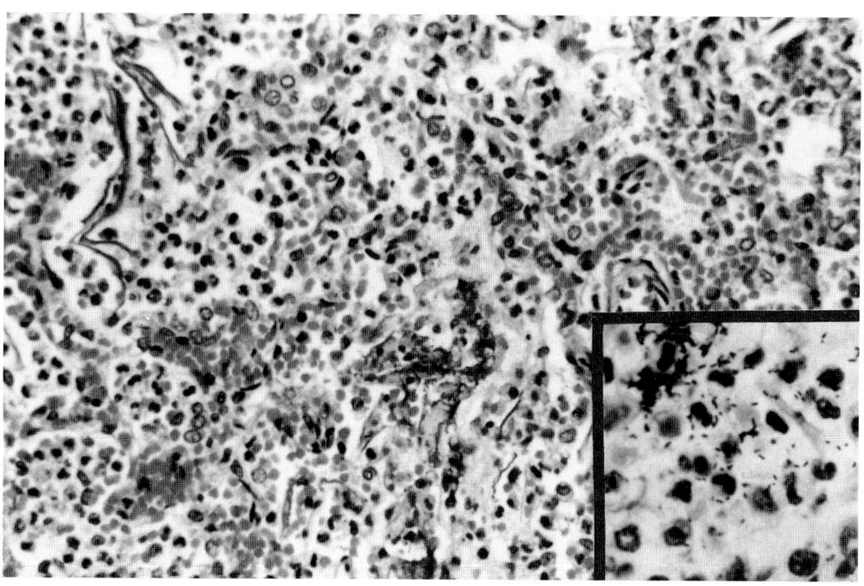

FIGURE 1-6. Lung showing pneumonia due to listeria monocytogenes (H&E, ×400). Inset: note the Gram-positive organisms.

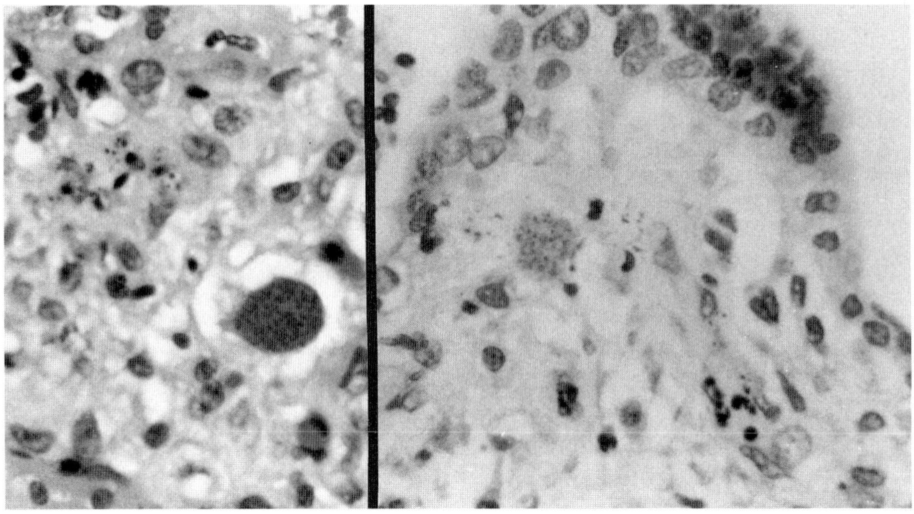

FIGURE 1-7. *Toxoplasma gondii* cyst containing trophozoites in a section of placenta (left panel: H&E, ×400; right panel, immunoperoxidase stain, ×400).

contain morphologically demonstrable organisms. In such instances, the infectious etiology can be proved only by culture.

3. Miscellaneous pathologic lesions that are known to be associated with certain types of infection; such as (a) in congenital rubella, malformations of various

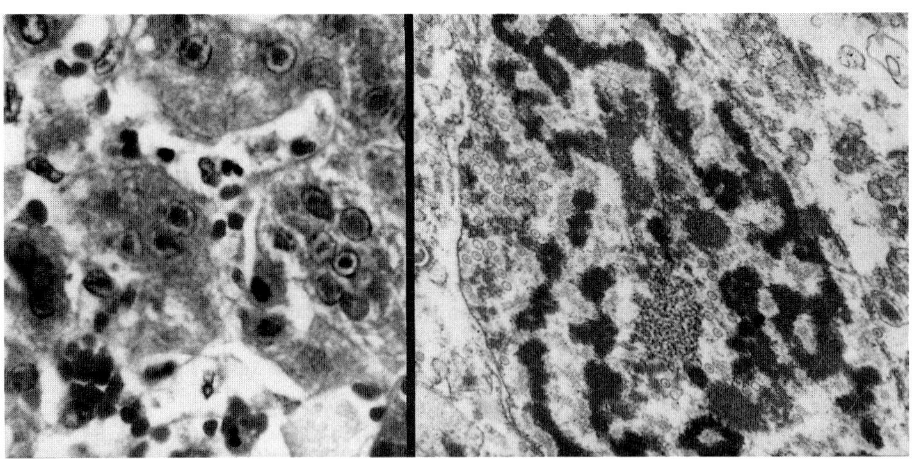

FIGURE 1-8. Left panel: degenerating and necrotic liver cells containing characteristic intranuclear viral inclusions (H&E, ×400); right panel: electron micrograph from an autopsy specimen of liver from a newborn infant with disseminated herpes simplex infection. Note the well-preserved intranuclear viral particles. (Uranyl acetate and lead citrate, ×22,000.)

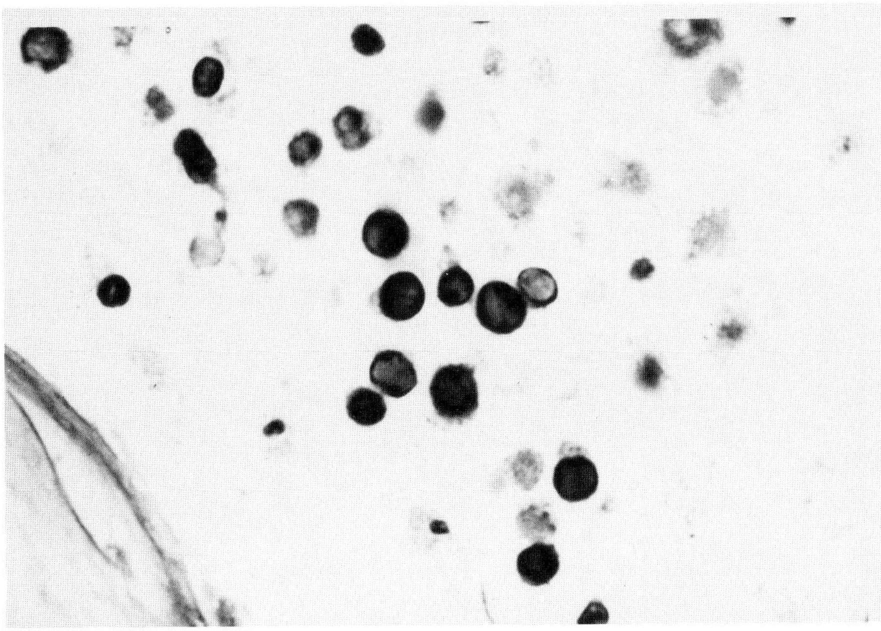

FIGURE 1-9. Bone marrow showing intranuclear eosinophilic inclusions in the normoblasts (H&E, 400).

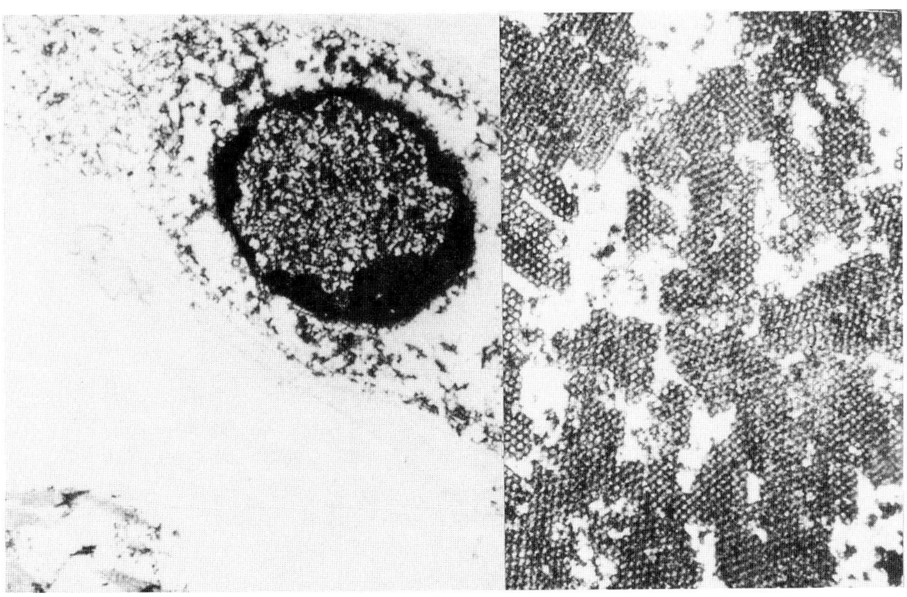

FIGURE 1-10. Left panel: electron micrograph of normoblast showing intranuclear viral inclusion (uranyl acetate and lead citrate, ×10,000); right panel: parvovirus showing its crystalline structure (×58,000) (Courtesy of Dr. Alexander S. Knisely).

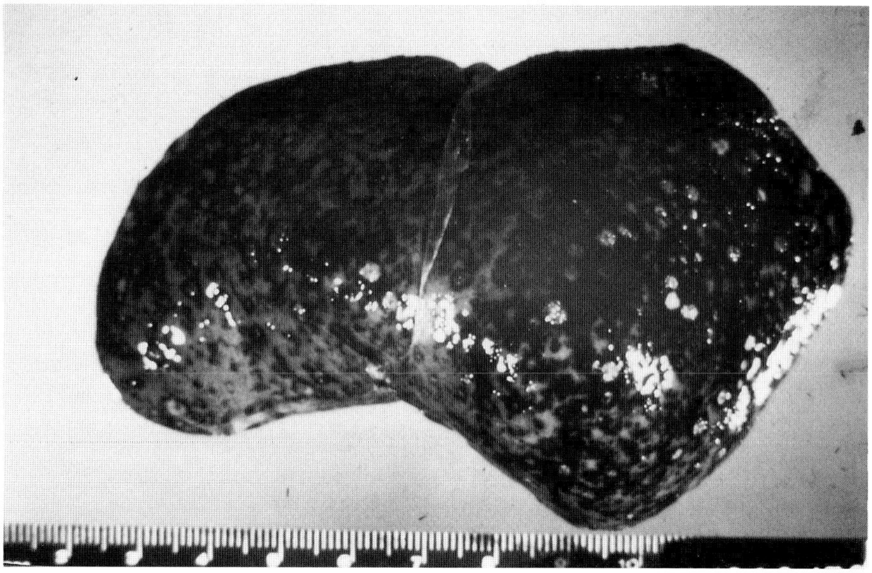

FIGURE 1-11. Liver showing characteristic yellowish nodular and hemorrhagic necrotic foci in newborn infant with disseminated herpes simplex infection.

organs, sclerotic and calcific lesions in the blood vessels of various organs, and/or desquamative interstitial pneumonia like reaction in the lungs may be present[21,22] (Figures 1-12 and 1-13); (b) in group B streptococcal (GBS) infection[23,24] resulting in early death, only pulmonary edema and congestion with virtually no inflammatory reaction may be present (Figure 1-14). Gram-positive organisms can be cultured and demonstrated morphologically in the sections. GBS infection of the lungs may also simulate IRDS because of the presence of hyaline membranes (organisms can be demonstrated in the membranes) (Figure 1-15).

4. *Positive culture by routine or rapid (DNA or RNA hybridization)* methods of material obtained during the clinical course and/or at autopsy.
5. Serologic evidence of infection.

Although clinical diagnosis is made or suspected in most fatal cases of infections, the etiologic agent may not have been clearly identified. Thus the overwhelming hepatic necrosis in enteroviral infection may be suspected to be of infectious origin, but the organism may not have been identified. In some instances the infection may not have been suspected (e.g., in intrapartum stillbirth due to intrauterine pneumonia or listeriosis). In GBS infection the clinical features can simulate IRDS or persistent fetal circulation, and the diagnosis of GBS infection can be made at autopsy.

A variety of factors (delay in autopsy, antibiotic therapy during the clinical course, or faulty technique of collection of material) can reduce the chances of getting meaningful positive cultures at autopsy. Despite these limitations, it is

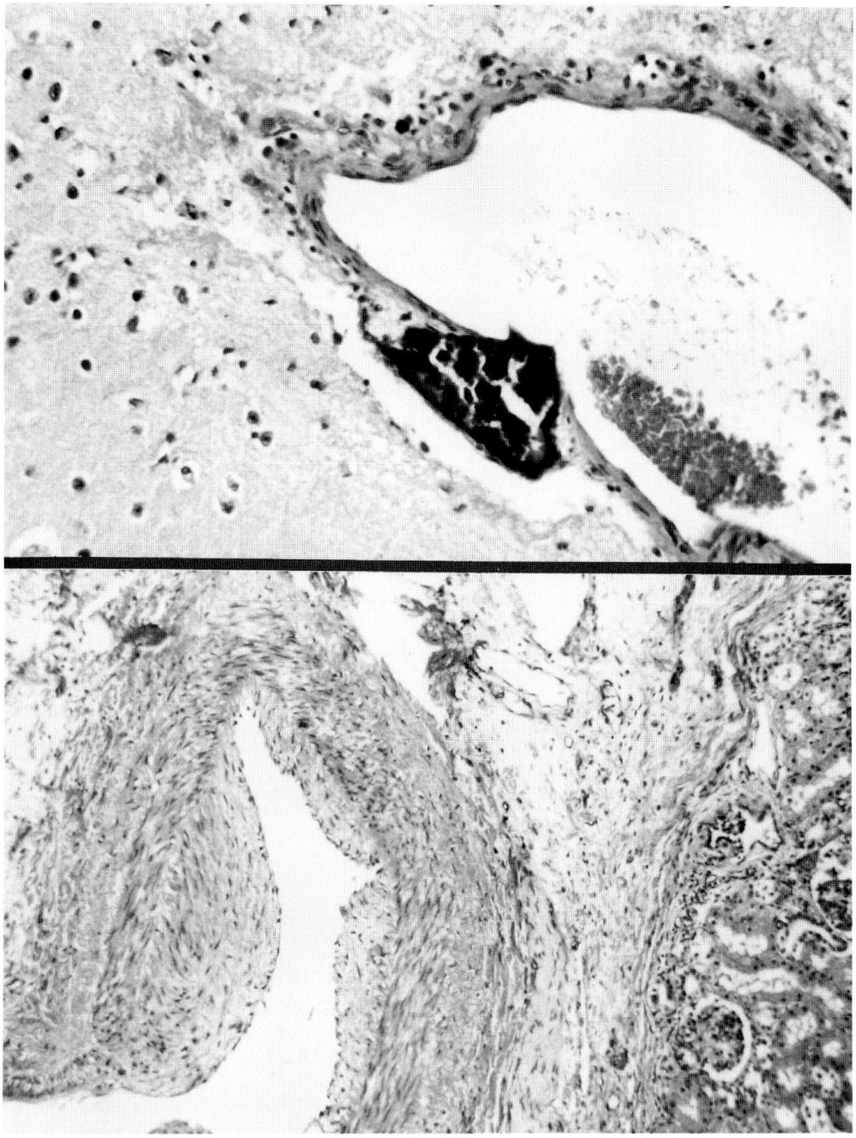

FIGURE 1-12. Upper panel: calcification of the wall of a blood vessel in the brain; lower panel: intimal fibrosis of a branch of renal artery from an infant with congenital rubella (H&E, ×100).

advisable to obtain cultures from blood and lungs in all perinatal autopsy cases in which there is no clinical explanation for the death or in which there is the slightest possibility of an infection, and in all stillbirths. Such a routine practice will detect unsuspected cases of listeriosis, GBS infection and rare etiologic agents of pneumonia such as *Citrobacter freundii*.[25]

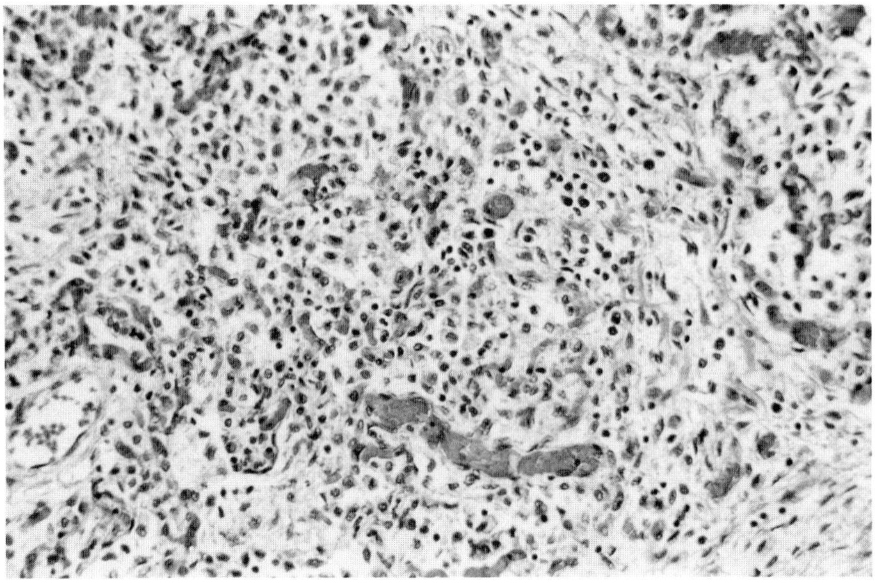

FIGURE 1-13. Desquamative interstitial pneumonia-like reaction in an infant with congenital rubella (H&E, ×100).

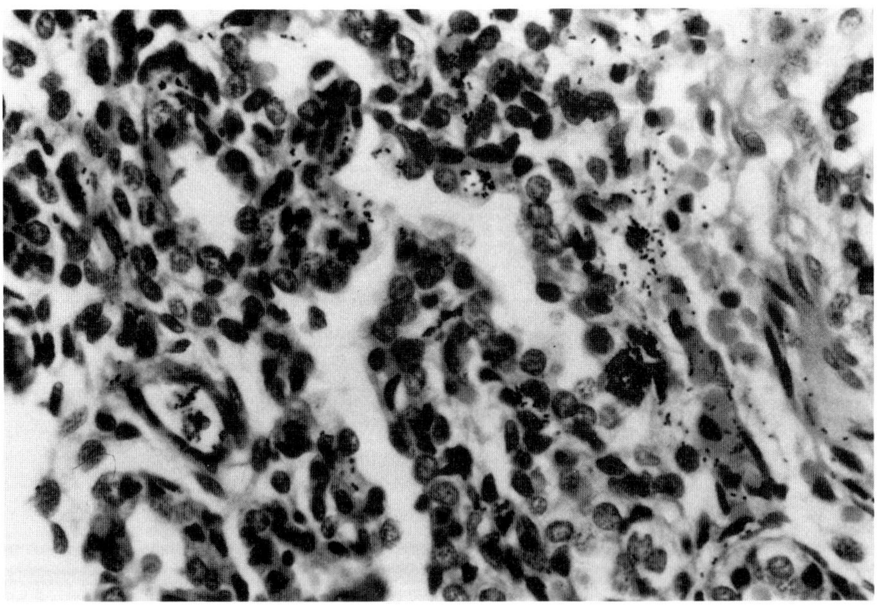

FIGURE 1-14. Gram-positive cocci in the alveolar septa of lungs in a newborn infant with group B streptococcal pneumonia. Minimal acute inflammatory reaction (not seen in this field) was present focally. (Gram stain, ×400.)

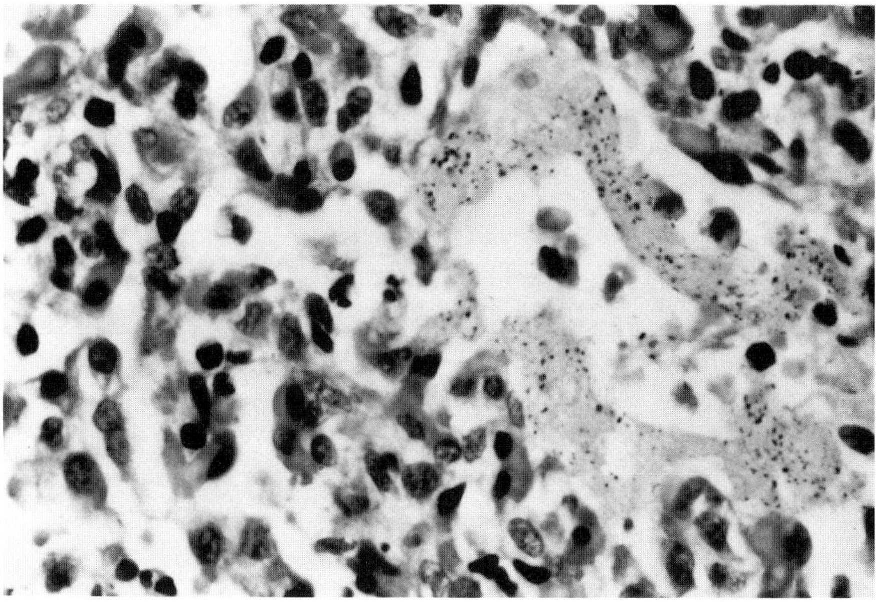

FIGURE 1-15. Gram-positive cocci in a hyaline membrane in group B streptococcal pneumonia. Minimal acute inflammatory reaction (not seen in this field) was present focally. (Gram stain, ×400.)

NEONATAL NECROTIZING ENTEROCOLITIS (NEC)

This is considered to be the major primary factor related to death in the cases in which medical management has failed or in the cases in which surgical resection was done and the death occurred in the postoperative period. In both operated and unoperated cases perforation with peritonitis, septicemia, DIC (disseminated intravascular coagulation), etc. may be the secondary factor related to death. The clinical, radiologic and pathologic features of NEC are described in the chapter on that disease.

INTRAUTERINE GROWTH RETARDATION (IUGR)

Infants with IUGR are also referred to as small for gestational age (SGA) babies. Birth weight less than 10th percentile for the gestational age is considered as IUGR (Table 1-2).[26–28] IUGR is of two types: (1) *symmetric (hypoplastic)* IUGR—the overall growth of the infant is reduced because the fetal insult acting in the first 16 weeks of gestation results in generalized reduced cell number; and (2) *asymmetric IUGR*—there is wasting, absence of or reduction in subcutaneous fat (Figure 1-16) and reduced body weight with normal head circumference and normal body length.[28] Fetal insult acting in the third trimester leads to these changes.

In most cases IUGR is an associated finding rather than primary factor in relation to death of newborn infants. However, in rare instances, IUGR may be

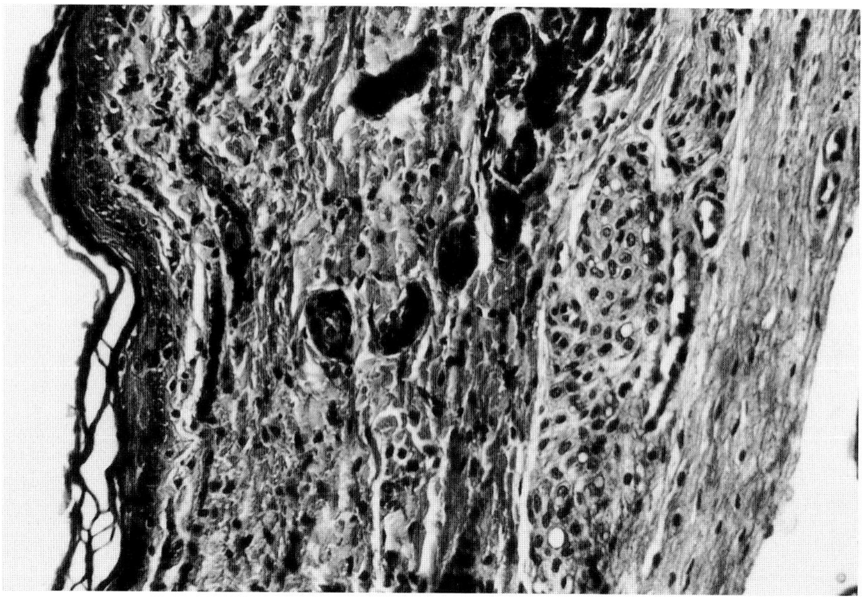

FIGURE 1-16. Fat cells with virtual absence of fat in the subcutaneous tissue of a newborn infant with asymmetric intrauterine growth retardation (H&E, ×100).

the major primary factor. Infants with asymmetric IUGR have certain metabolic and immunologic abnormalities. The infants with IUGR tend to have fetal heart rate decelerations, fetal acidosis, and low Apgar scores. Chronic hypoxia, hypercapnia, acidosis, hyperlacticemia, hypoglycemia, hyperviscosity, hypothermia, and disseminated intravascular coagulation occur more frequently in infants with IUGR than in normal-growth infants.[29–31] Low immunoglobulin levels and impairment of cellular immunity have also been described.[32,33] Delayed development of thymus has been reported in association with IUGR in experimental animals.[34] Severe lymphocytic depletion of the thymus is seen at autopsy in infants with IUGR (Joshi VV: Unpublished data, 1980). The immunologic deficiency may make these infants more susceptible to infection. In rare instances these factors may play a major role in the death of the infant.

Some babies have intermediate or combined type of IUGR, while others are healthy babies who are SGA because of genetic and constitutional factors (short parents with small body stature). Etiologic classification of IUGR has also been proposed.[35] The etiology is intrinsic in the fetus (chromosomal abnormalities, intrauterine infections, toxic effects of drugs and radiation) or extrinsic (utero-placental insufficiency due to maternal disease such as preeclampsia and chronic hypertension leading to placental infarcts and/or abruption or due to abnormal placentation).

In about 5–10% of cases both extrinsic (placental infarcts, partial abruption, multiple gestation etc.) and intrinsic (severe maternal malnutrition, smoking, alcohol and drug abuse) etiologic factors are involved. In 40–60% of the cases of IUGR, the etiology remains undetermined. The IUGR due to intrinsic factors is of symmetric type, that due to extrinsic and unknown factors is asymmetric, and that due to combined (intrinsic and extrinsic) factors is of intermediate type. In about 40% of cases IUGR, in which etiologic factor(s) cannot be detected, the IUGR is of asymmetric type. The salient features of the two main types of IUGR are summarized in Table 1-3.

BIRTH TRAUMA

This is considered as the primary cause of death only when the trauma is sufficiently severe such as tear of the tentorium cerebelli with severe subdural hemorrhage (Figure 1-17), spinal cord avulsion (Figure 1-18), bilateral adrenal hemorrhages (in breech delivery) (Figure 1-19), or multiple fractures. Cases with minor trauma such as bruises or mild cephalhematoma, are not included in this category.

I have not seen cases of fatal birth injury of the type listed above in the last 15 years. This low incidence in recent years is probably attributable to the liberal use of cesarean section as a substitute for midforceps and vaginal breech deliveries. Nonfatal birth injuries such as brachial plexus or facial nerve injury and fractured clavicle continue to occur in neonates.[36]

Newborn infants with severe birth injury such as intracranial or adrenal hemorrhage may also have suffered from severe intrauterine asphyxia. In such cases, both factors—viz., birth trauma and asphyxia—will have to be considered as primary factors related to death.

ISOIMMUNIZATION

Rh isoimmunization has become vanishingly rare in recent years, which is attributable to the widespread use of Rhogam (anti-D immunoglobulin given to

TABLE 1-3 Salient Features of Two Types of Intrauterine Growth Retardation (IUGR)

Type of IUGR	Features
Asymmetric IUGR	More common (75%), timing of insult >28 weeks, normal head and brain size, decreased liver and thymus size, (brain liver weight ratio >6, normal up to 4.5) normal body length, wasting (loss of muscle and subcutaneous fat) present, good postnatal catch-up growth, congenital anomalies rare, associated with uteroplacental insufficiency (toxemia, chronic hypertension, congenital heart disease etc in the mother); unknown etiology in ~40%
Symmetric IUGR (hypoplastic IUGR)	Uncommon (25%), timing of insult <28 weeks, microcephaly, decreased liver and thymus size, normal brain liver weight ratio, reduced body length, wasting absent, congenital anomalies frequent, associated with congenital anomalies and intrauterine infections, poor postnatal catch-up growth

Adapted from Brar HS et al: *Sem Perinatol* 12:2–10, 1988.

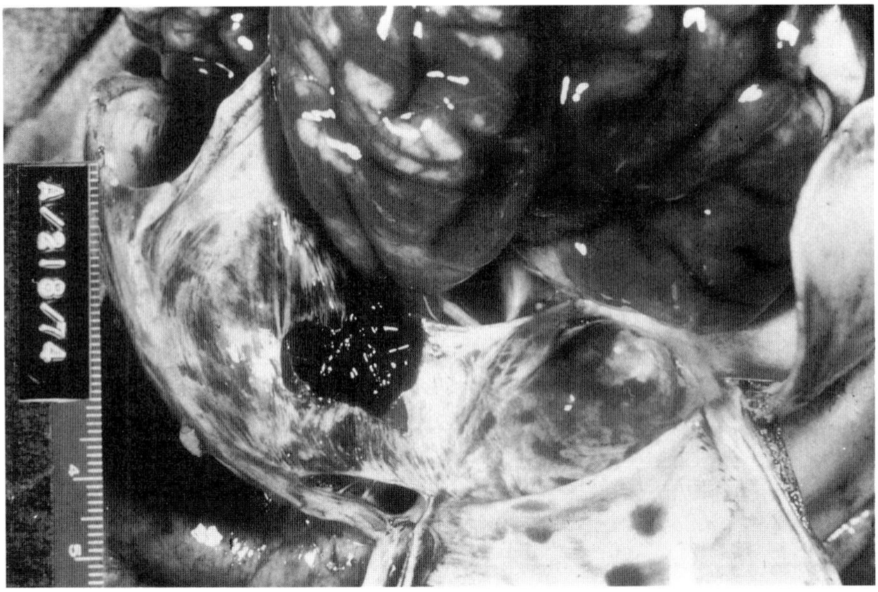

FIGURE 1-17. Subdural hemorrhages due to tear of tentorium cerebelli. The torn portion of the tentorium is almost completely covered by the supratentorial blood clot. There was more severe diffuse infratentorial hemorrhage, parts of which are seen as dark areas through the intact portion of the tentorium cerebelli.

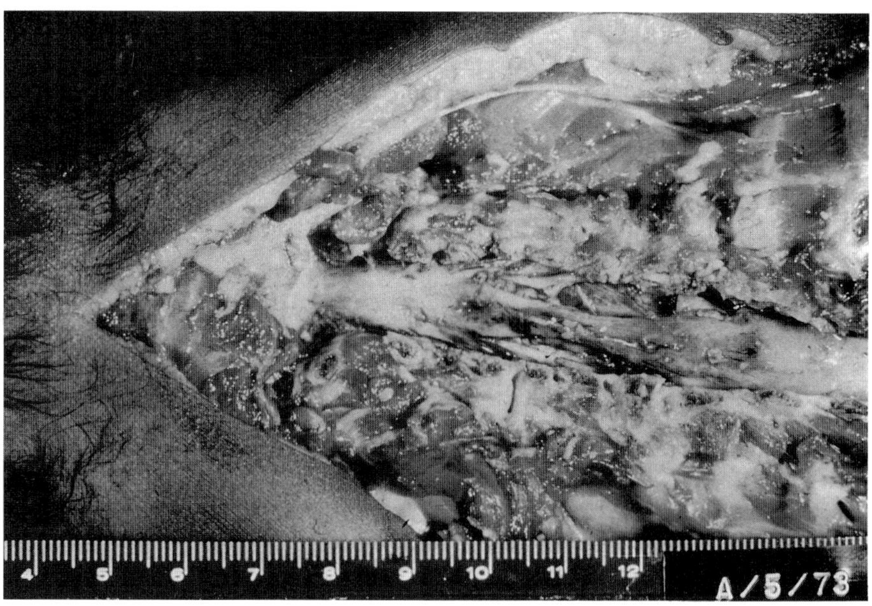

FIGURE 1-18. Spinal cord avulsion in a newborn infant born by breech delivery.

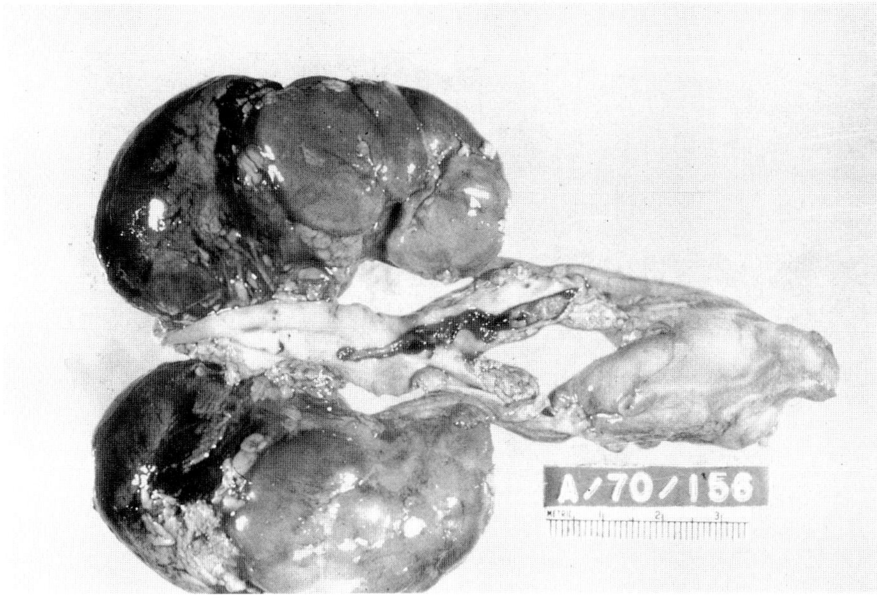

FIGURE 1-19. Massive bilateral adrenal hemorrhages in a newborn infant born by breech delivery. Note also the mural thrombus in the aorta associated with umbilical arterial catheterization.

Rh (D) negative mothers of Rh (D)-positive babies) for prevention of disease related to Rh incompatibility. However, sensitization in mothers with missed abortions or inadequate dosage of Rhogam continues to occur and isolated cases of Rh isoimmunization are still seen in neonates.[37] Fatal outcome in such cases is extremely rare. ABO incompatibility results in mild to moderately severe disease. However, fatal cases of ABO incompatibility or incompatibility due to rare blood group such as Kell group may rarely be seen.[38]

Hydrops fetalis, hepatosplenomegaly with increased extramedullary hematopoiesis, and hemosiderin deposition in reticuloendothelial system are the major pathologic findings in isoimmunization.

OTHER SPECIFIC CAUSES

These are too numerous to enlist. The following are a few important examples: twin transfusion syndrome, idiopathic massive pulmonary hemorrhage, fetal death due to maternal abdominal trauma, congenital malignancy, massive fetomaternal hemorrhage, idiopathic persistent pulmonary hypertension of the newborn (PPHN), and sudden infant death syndrome.[39–51]

Twin Transfusion Syndrome

Twin transfusion syndrome can be fatal in both or one of the twins.[39,40] Discrepancy of >20% in the birth weights and difference in the hemoglobin of

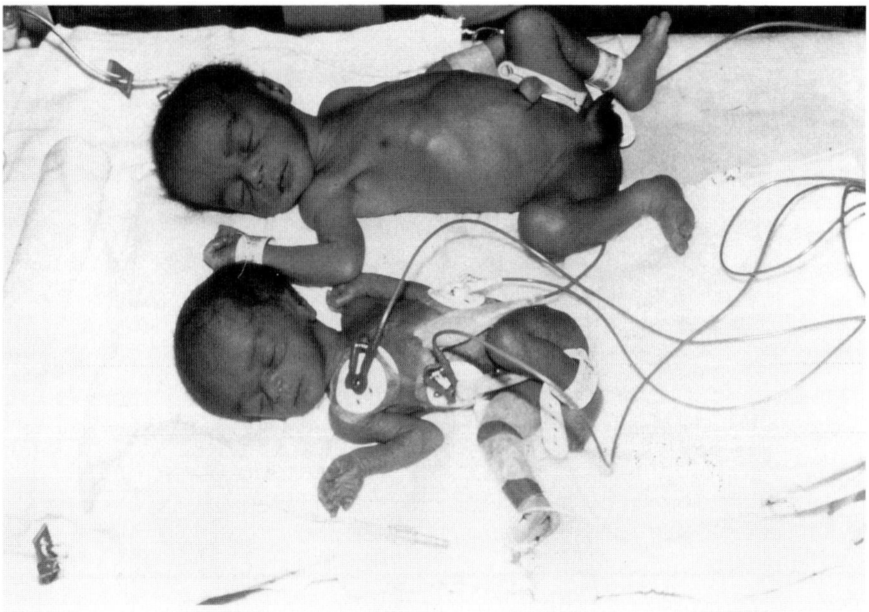

FIGURE 1-20. Note the difference in the size (and weight) of the twins, the smaller twin being the donor and the larger the recipient in twin transfusion syndrome (courtesy of Dr. Shyan Sun).

>5 g are considered as criteria for the diagnosis (Figure 1-20). Hydrops in the donor twin may obscure the difference in the birth weights. The placenta is monochorionic. Deep vascular anastomoses between artery of the donor and the vein of the recipient via shared placental lobules are the most significant vascular communications through which twin transfusion occurs (Figure 1-21). The recipient twin, which is hypervolemic, shows cardiomegaly, glomerular enlargement, and medial hypertrophy of the pulmonary and systemic arteries[39] (Figure 1-22). Disseminated intravascular coagulation allegedly occur in the surviving twin as a result of release of thromboplastic substances from the circulation of the dead fetus into the circulation of the surviving fetus via the vascular anastomoses. Examination of the placenta for demonstration of vascular anastomoses is an integral part of the autopsy on the cases of twin transfusion syndrome. It should be noted that discrepancy in birth weight of monochorionic twins may be related to factors other than twin transfusion syndrome such as velamentous insertion of the cord of one of the fetuses.

Idiopathic Massive Pulmonary Hemorrhage

Interstitial and intraalveolar pulmonary hemorrhage is a common finding in perinatal autopsies. The hemorrhage is mild to moderate in most of these cases. In occasional cases the hemorrhage is massive (involving all lobes with increase in weight of the lungs by more than 1 standard deviation from the mean).[3,4,41] In overwhelming majority of the cases one or more of the following predisposing factors are present: EPA, IUGR, hypothermia, generalized or pulmonary infec-

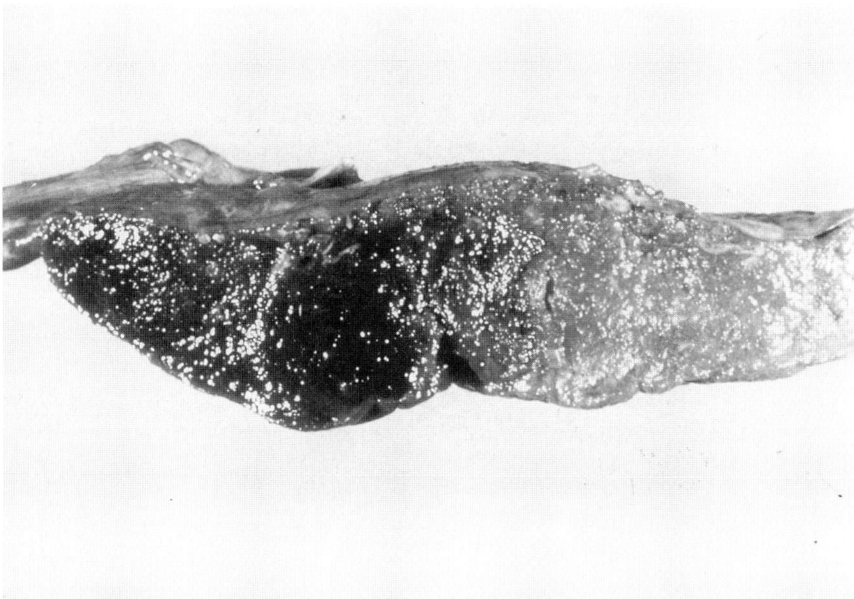

FIGURE 1-21. Cut surface of monochorionic diamniotic placenta showing congestion of the territory belonging to the recipient twin and pallor of the territory of the donor twin in twin transfusion syndrome.

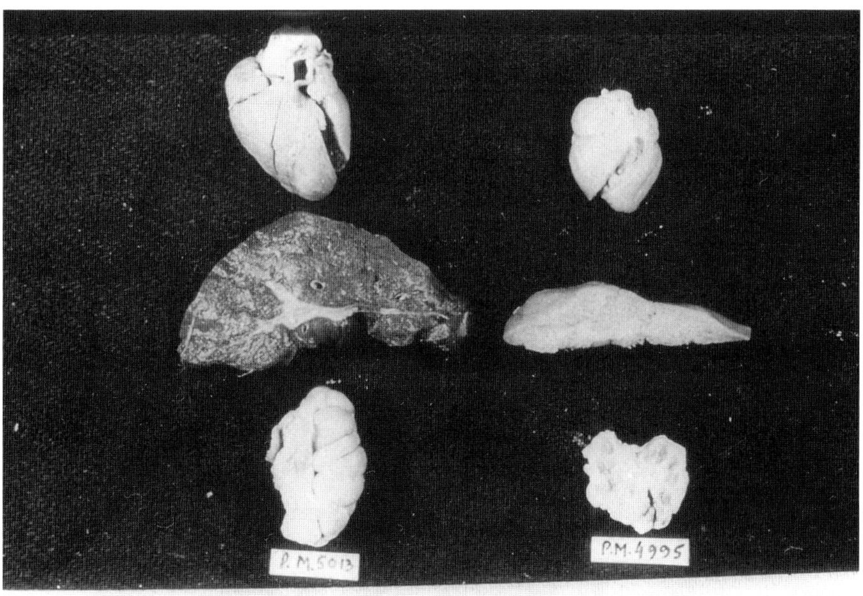

FIGURE 1-22. Smaller heart and pale and smaller liver and smaller kidney of the donor twin compared to the larger heart, larger and conjested liver, and larger kidney of the recipient twin in twin transfusion syndrome in which both the donor and the recipient twin died.

tion, congenital heart disease, and IRDS. Disseminated intravascular coagulation leading to bleeding diathesis or acute left ventricular failure are the two mechanisms related to pulmonary hemorrhage.[42] In all such cases pulmonary hemorrhage is considered as a secondary factor related to death. In rare instances no predisposing factor can be demonstrated. Such cases are labeled as idiopathic massive pulmonary hemorrhage, which is considered as a primary factor related to death.[3,4]

Maternal Trauma

Maternal trauma leading to fetal death involves most commonly automobile accidents.[43] Performance of autopsy in such fetal deaths is within the jurisdiction of a forensic pathologist. There may be traumatic intracranial hemorrhage in the fetus, or the death may be related to intrauterine asphyxia associated with placental abruption due to maternal trauma. The pediatric pathologist may be consulted about the interpretation and significance of the findings at autopsy and the findings in the placenta.

Malignancy

Malignant neoplastic disorder (leukemia, neuroblastoma, teratoma, Wilms' tumor, retinoblastoma, melanoma, etc.) may be present in the neonate.[44] Death may occur during the neonatal period.

Fetomaternal Hemorrhage[45]

Some degree of fetomaternal hemorrhage occurs in about 50% of the pregnancies. If >150 ml is lost, it is considered as a potentially fatal massive hemorrhage. The infant looks pale. Shock and hypotension may be present. The peripheral smear of the infant shows microcytic hypochromic anemia in chronic hemorrhage. Amniocentesis, external version, placenta previa, and abruptio placentae may be associated with the fetomaternal hemorrhage. Fetomaternal bleeding resulting in perinatal death is rare. Severe anemia may be associated with hydropic changes in the neonate. The diagnosis is made by acid elution technique of Kleihauer–Betke to demonstrate fetal RBCs in the maternal peripheral smear. The amount of fetal blood is assessed on the basis of percentage of fetal cells in the maternal peripheral smear and maternal blood volume.

Idiopathic Persistent Pulmonary Hypertension of the Newborn (PPHN)

PPHN[46] can occur as a result of maladaptation of the pulmonary vascular bed at birth, hypoplasia of the pulmonary vascular bed due to interference with lung development (congenital diaphragmatic hernia, renal malformation, etc.), hemodynamic disturbances associated with congenital heart disease, hypoxia, hyperoxia,[47] and thromboembolic occlusion as a result of nonbacterial thrombotic endocarditis[48] (Figures 1-23, 1-24). A large proportion of the cardiac output in the fetus enters the systemic circulation via the ductus arteriosus. In the newborn the cardiac output must enter the pulmonary circulation. For this change to occur the pulmonary vascular resistance in the fetus, related to pulmonary vasoconstriction and to the presence of thick muscle layer in the

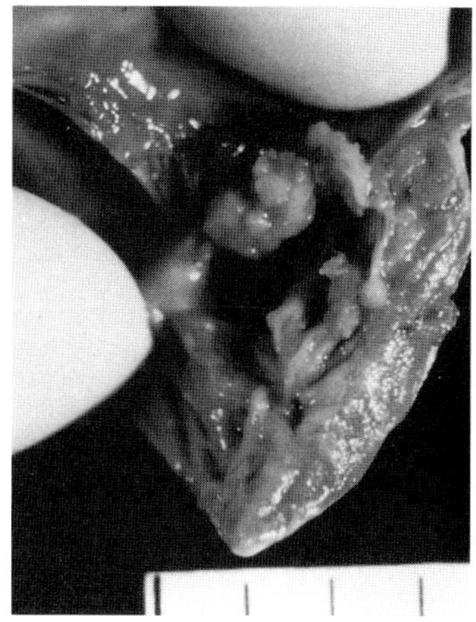

FIGURE 1-23. Nonbacterial thrombotic endocarditis. Note the vegetation on the tricuspid valve.

small pulmonary artery must diminish.[46] Idiopathic PPHN occurs when the vascular resistance does not fall because of the abnormal structure of the pulmonary vasculature at the acinar level.[47] Clinically the infants have central cyanosis. Idiopathic PPHN does not respond to the vasodilator drugs (tolazoline) and carries a high mortality rate.

Ideally the demonstration of excessive muscularization of the intraacinar arteries requires vascular injection of barium gelatin suspension at a pressure of

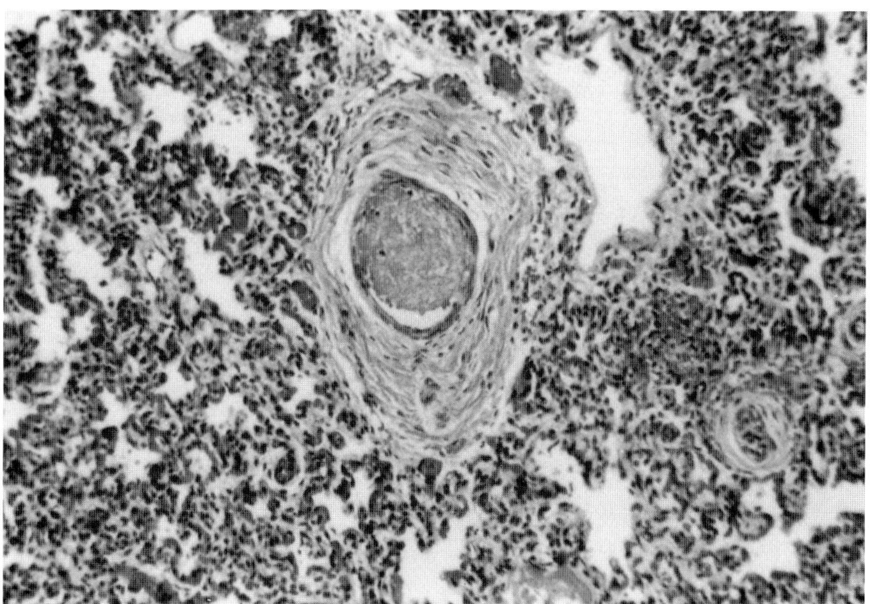

FIGURE 1-24. Thromboembolus from nonbacterial thrombotic endocarditis in a newborn infant with persistent pulmonary hypertension (H&E, ×100).

about 76 mmHg at 60°C. The lungs are inflated and fixed in formalin.[49] Pulmonary arteries <150 μm are of three types: muscular, partially muscular, and nonmuscular. In the adult there are numerous muscular arteries even in the septa of the distal alveoli of the acinus. In the fetus, the muscular arteries reach only up to the preacinar level. (Acinus includes respiratory bronchiole, alveolar duct, and alveoli.) There are only nonmuscular arteries in the acini of the fetus. These intraacinar arteries (Figure 1-25) measuring ≤75 μm are larger than capillaries and consist of a single endothelial cell lining surrounded by a thin layer of connective tissue. Ultrastructural studies have demonstrated pericyte in the wall of these nonmuscular arteries.[49] Muscularization of these arteries occurs during childhood and adulthood, when it reaches the distal alveolar level. In idiopathic PPHN precocious muscularization of intraacinar arteries has its onset in the fetus. These arteries have abnormally thick walls and narrowed lumen (Figure 1-26). Marked proliferation of adventitial connective tissue was also present. Muscularization can be better visualized by trichome stain and stain for elastic tissue. Processing of the lungs as described above is essential for proper evaluation of arterial changes. Erroneous impression of presence of muscularized arteries may be obtained by examination of lung in which vascular injection has not been done.[46]

Sudden Infant Death Syndrome

In extremely rare cases the factor(s) related to death of a neonate cannot be found. An apparently healthy neonate dies suddenly and unexpectedly. The

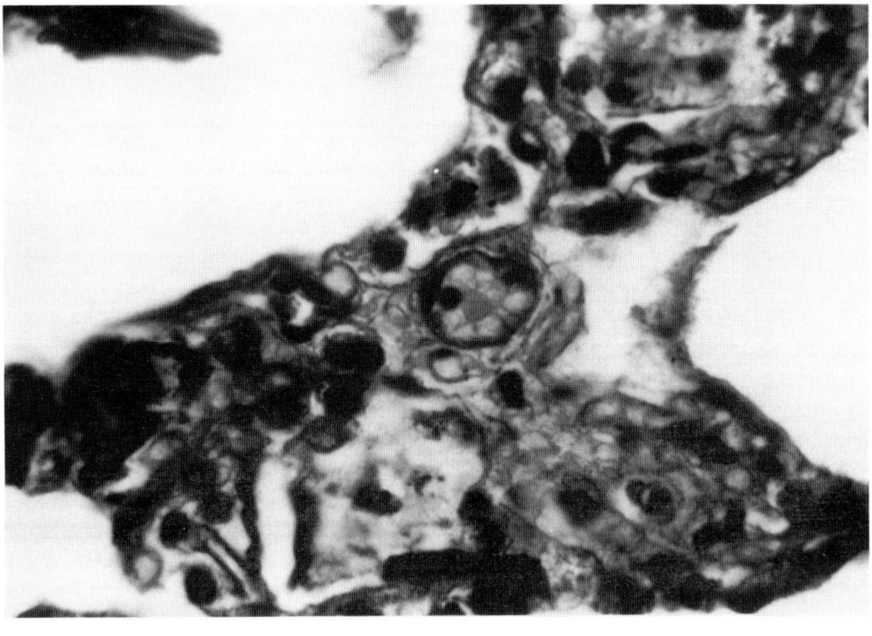

FIGURE 1-25. Nonmuscularged intraacinar artery in a normal newborn infant (H&E, ×400).

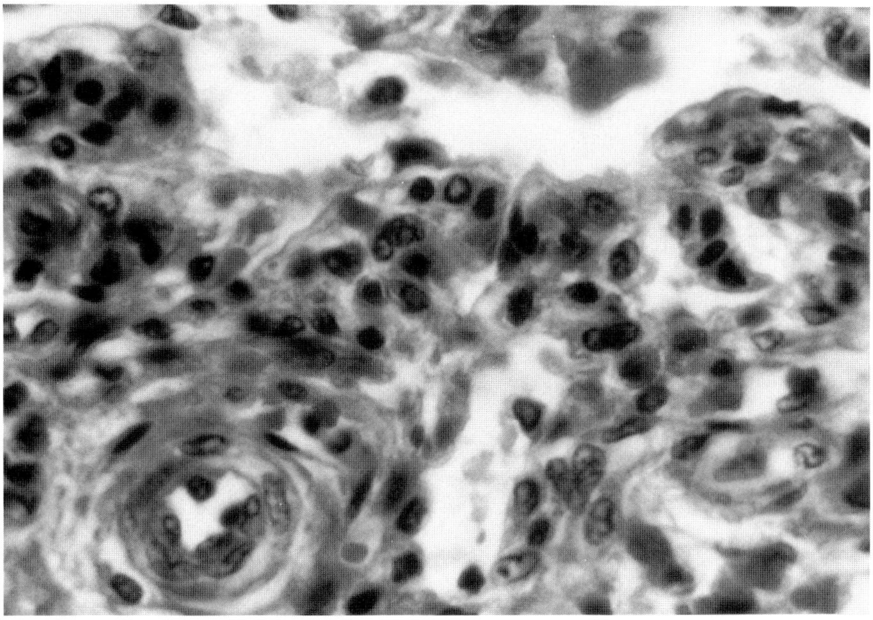

FIGURE 1-26. Muscularized intraacinar artery in a newborn infant with idiopathic persistent pulmonary hypertension (trichrome stain, ×400).

possibility of SIDS occurring in the neonatal period should be considered in such cases.[3,51] A failure to find the primary factor related to death despite a detailed autopsy is not uncommon in macerated antepartum intrauterine deaths.

EXTREME PREMATURITY

Extreme prematurity is considered as a primary factor related to death when in a newborn infant of <28 weeks' gestation or <1000 g, no other primary factor such as IRDS, infection, or any other specific disease process can be found after a detailed autopsy examination.

SECONDARY OR IMMEDIATE FACTORS RELATED TO PERINATAL DEATHS

As indicated above, some of the primary factors can also act as secondary factors in certain situations. Thus severe pneumonia may be a secondary factor when it develops as a complication in an infant with IRDS or with congenital heart disease. The various secondary factors are listed in Table 1-4.

In the majority of cases hydrops fetalis is secondary to other primary factors such as Rh isoimmunization, congenital anomalies (hypoplastic left heart syndrome, congenital cystic adenomatoid malformation of the lung, etc.),

TABLE 1-4 Secondary Factors Related to Perinatal Death

Infections: pneumonia, septicemia, etc.
Circulatory disturbances: congestive heart failure, severe edema and serous effusions (hydrops fetalis), persistent fetal circulation, etc.
Hemorrhagic phenomena: pulmonary hemorrhage, nontraumatic intracranial hemorrhages of various types, etc.
Iatrogenic complications: severe airleak phenomenon, severe liver disease associated with total parenteral nutrition, catheter-related complications, etc.
Miscellaneous factors: IUGR and its metabolic complications, etc.

intrauterine infection, hematologic disorders (e.g., thalassemia), chromosomal abnormalities, twin transfusion syndrome, or metabolic diseases. In about 20% of the cases hydrops fetalis is idiopathic.[52] In such cases it may be considered as a primary factor.

METHOD OF REPORTING THE FINAL AUTOPSY DIAGNOSIS (FAD)

I have followed the following method over the years. The first item on the FAD is a short clinical summary. The pertinent clinical features included in item 1 of FAD (Figure 1-27) focus attention on the major pathologic findings that can be expected and also on the presence or absence of clinicopathologic correlation. The importance of mentioning gestational age, and birth weights (observed and expected for the gestational age) in item 1 relates to the diagnosis of IUGR that may otherwise be overlooked. The second item is the basic pathologic or pathophysiologic process, which was a primary factor related to the death. The next item is the secondary factor related to death. There may be more than one secondary factors, or even primary factors. These are listed in order of their severity or clinicopathologic significance. The remaining findings, which represent complications of the primary factor(s) or that may be incidental or iatrogenic, are listed at the end. A note or summary giving a brief review of the clinical and pathologic findings, clinicopathologic correlation, and unexpected or unexplained findings, if any, should be written at the end of the main text of the autopsy protocol or at the end of FAD. I prefer the latter. Undue speculation should be avoided in these notes or summaries. Also, passing definitive judgments regarding clinical (mis)interpretation or therapy may not be appropriate if the pathologist does not have sufficient current knowledge regarding therapeutic measures indicated in specific individual situations. Lack of clinicopathologic correlation or presence of clinically undiagnosed complication or even of primary disease process should be simply stated in the note without embellishment. References to articles in the literature are indicated when unusual or recently described findings are detected in a particular case. Maternal and obstetric factors related to the death of the infant should also be mentioned in the note.

COMMENT

Of the various primary factors listed and discussed above, congenital anomalies, IRDS, extrinsic perinatal hypoxia, and infection account for >85% of

FINAL AUTOPSY DIAGNOSIS

PATIENTS'NAME:______________________Autopsy NO.________________________

1. 23 day old low birth weight (820 g), male infant of 28 wks' gestation (normal range of birth weight: 1020 ± 340 g), born to a fifteen year old single mother with apparently uneventful pregnancy, onset of premature labor, vaginal delivery, Apgar core 6,6 at 1,5 minutes, respiratory distress noted after birth.

2. Idiopathic respiratory distress syndrome, transitional stage.

3. Old intraventricular hemorrhage with extension to basal subarachnoid space.

   a) Chronic arachnoiditis with posthemorrhagic hydrocephalus.

4. Persistent interstitial pulmonary emphysema with multiple cyst formation and giant cell reaction in the wall of the cysts.

5. Focal pulmonary hemorrhage and bronchopneumonia (combined wt: 42 g, N: 18 ± 6 g).

6. Perforation (1 mm) of left main stem bronchus (H/O endotracheal intubation).

7. Cholestasis of liver with distension of gallbladder.
   a) Normal extrahepatic biliary tract
   b) S/P parenteral nutrition

8. Lymphocytic depletion of thymus (wt: 1 g, N: 3.0 ± 2.3 g)

REFERENCES:

1. Stocker JT, Madewell JE: Persistent interstitial pulmonary emphysema: Another complication of respiratory distress syndrome: Pediatr 1977, 59, 847-857.

2. Saldhana RL, Stein CA, Kopleman AE: Gallbladder distension in ill preterm infants: Am J Dis Child 1983, 137, 1179 - 1180.

3. Anderson KD, Chandra R: Pneumothorax secondary to perforation of segmental bronchi by suction catheters: J Pediatr Surg 1976, 11, 687-693.

____
Attending Pathologist

FIGURE 1-27. Format of writing final autopsy diagnosis. Other items such as medical record number, time of death, time of autopsy, restrictions and names of the clinicians in charge and the prosector are also included on the FAD sheet.

the cases.[3,4] In my experience, there has been a decline in recent years in EPA and acute-stage IRDS as primary factors related to death in the early neonatal period (7 days of age) and a relative rise in congenital anomalies as primary factors. These changes are at least partly due to better and longer survival in infants with EPA and IRDS. Increased rate of ultrasonographic detection of "fetal" congenital anomalies incompatible with life, leading to the medical termination of pregnancy, also contributes to these changes in frequency, although strictly speaking these autopsies fall under the category of abortions.

The approach to determination of primary and secondary factors related to perinatal death described in this chapter is useful not only for collection of data for epidemiologic purposes but also for a consistent clinicopathologic analysis leading to better understanding of the autopsy findings by the clinicians and the parents. It is advisable to prepare lists of primary and secondary factors and to define the criteria for the diagnosis of the different conditions in the lists. The terminology and criteria should preferably be prepared in consultation with the obstetricians and neonatologists involved with the case so that there is consistency in the interpretation of findings and diagnostic labels used. It is the regular practice in many teaching institutions to review perinatal mortality data periodically. The approach described in this chapter will be helpful in making this review process consistent and comparable for different time periods. It will also be useful in explaining to the parents in simple terms the different factors involved in the morbidity and mortality of the infant. I have used this approach over the last 20 years not only for the perinatal autopsies but also for autopsies of older infants and children. The clinicians have appreciated such an approach.

The inclusion of the same conditions in the lists of both primary and secondary factors should not create confusion if it is understood that the interpretation of the role of a particular condition is individualized according to the totality of the circumstances of a given case and concurrent or sequential presence or absence of other conditions. It should be noted that many of the conditions that appear in both lists are related far more frequently as secondary factors than as primary ones. Thus IUGR, massive pulmonary hemorrhage, and similar conditions are related to perinatal death as secondary factors far more frequently than as primary factors. It is also important to bear in mind that some of the conditions, such as IVH, considered as a primary factor by some investigators,[5,53] are in fact secondary factors.

REFERENCES

1. Cole SK, Hey EN, Thomas AM: Classifying perinatal death: an obstetric approach. *Br J Ob Gyn* 93:1204–1212, 1986.
2. Hey EN, Lloyd DJ, Wigglesworth JS: Classifying perinatal death: Fetal and neonatal factors. *Bri J Ob Gyn* 93:1213–1223, 1986.
3. Joshi VV: Primary of perinatal mortality. Autopsy study of 100 cases. *Arch Pathol Lab Med* 100:106–109.
4. Joshi VV, Bhakoo ON, Gopalan S, et al: Primary causes of perinatal mortality—autopsy study of 134 cases. *Indian J Med Res* 69:963–971, 1979.
5. McPherson TA: Categorization of perinatal deaths—USA. *Pediatr Pathol* 10:v–viii, 1990.
6. Perinatal Mortality Committee of the Province of Quebec, Canada, Quebec City: *A guide for study of perinatal mortality*, 1967, pp. 16–20.
7. Jones KL: *Smith's recognizable patterns of human malformation*, 4th ed. Saunders, Philadelphia, 1988.
8. Murdock Institute for Research into Birth Defects: *Pictures of Standard Syndromes and Undiagnosed Malformations*, Version 2.5, 3rd ed., 1990.
9. Spranger J, Benirschke K, Hall JG, et al: Errors in morphogenesis: Concepts and terms—recommendations of an international working group. *J Pediatr* 100:160–165, 1982.
10. Morrison M, Paes BA: Birth asphyxia: Does Apgar score have prognostic value. *Obstet Gynecol* 72:120–123, 1988.

11. Sykes GS, Johnson P, Ashworth F, et al: Do Apgar scores indicate asphyxia? *Lancet* 1:494–496, 1982.
12. Florman AL, Teubner D: Enhancement of bacterial growth in amniotic fluid by meconium. *J Pediatr* 74:111–114, 1969.
13. Lauweryns J, Bernat R, Lerut A, et al: Intrauterine pneumonia. An experimental study. *Biol Neonate* 22:301–318, 1973.
14. Pfenniger J, Tschaeppeler H, Wagner BP, et al: The paradox of adult respiratory distress syndrome in neonates. *Pediatr Pulmonol* 10:18–24, 1991.
15. Donnelly WH, Bucciarelli RL, Nelson RM: Ischemic papillary muscle necrosis in stressed infants. *J Pediatr* 96:295–300, 1980.
16. DeSa DJ, Donnelly WH: Myocardial necrosis in the newborn. *Persp Pediatr Pathol* 8:295–311, 1984.
17. Silver MM, Smith CR: Diaphragmatic contraction band necrosis in a perinatal and infantile autopsy population. *Hum Pathol* 23: 817–827, 1992.
18. Salinas-Madrigal L, Bruk A, DeMello DE: Myofibrillar degeneration and necrosis of the visceral smooth musculature: An ischemic visceral myopathy. *Hum Pathol* 18:815–823, 1987.
19. Berry PJ, Gray ES, Porter HJ, et al: Parvovirus infection of the human fetus and newborn. *Sem Diag Pathol* 9:4–12, 1992.
20. Knisely AS, O'Shea P, McMillan P, et al: Electron microscopic identification of parvovirus virions in erythroid-line cells in fatal hydrops fetalis. *Pediatr Pathol* 8:163–170, 1988.
21. Rosenberg HS, Oppenheimer EH, Esterly JR: Congenital rubella syndrome. The late effects and their relation to early lesions. *Persp Pediatr Pathol* 6:183–202, 1981.
22. Boner A, Wilmott R, Dinwiddie R, et al: Desquamative interstitial pneumonia and antigen-antibody complexes in two infants with congenital rubella. *Pediatrics* 72:835–838, 1982.
23. Albow RC, Driscoll SG, Effman EL, et al: A comparison of early onset Group B streptococcal neonatal infection and the respiratory distress syndrome of the newborn. *N Engl J Med* 294:65–70, 1976.
24. Payne NR, Burke BA, Day DL, et al: Correlation of clinical and pathologic findings in early onset neonatal group B streptococcal infection with disease severity and prediction of outcome. *Pediatr Inf Dis* 7:836–847, 1988.
25. Imaizumi SO, Balsara GR: Sudden unexpected death in a neonate. *Am J Perinatol* 6:281–283, 1989.
26. Lubchenco LC, Hansman C, Boyd E: Intrauterine growth in length and head circumference as estimated from live births at gestational ages from 26 to 42 weeks. *Pediatrics* 37:403–408, 1966.
27. Battaglia FC, Lubchenco LC: A practical classification of newborn infants by weight and gestational age. *J Pediatr* 71:159–163, 1967.
28. Williams RL, Creasy RK, Cunningham GC, et al: Fetal growth and perinatal viability. *Obstet Gynecol* 59:624–632, 1982.
29. Low JA, Galbsmith RS, Muir D, et al: Intrauterine Growth Retardation: A study of long-term morbidity. *Am J Obstet Gynecol* 142:670–677, 1982.
30. Gross GP, Hathaway WE, McGaughey HR: Hyperviscosity in the neonate. *J Pediatr* 82:1004–1006, 1973.
31. Soothill PW, Nicolaides KU, Campbell S: Prenatal asphyxia, hyperlacticemia, hypoglycemia and erythroblastosis in growth retarded fetuses. *Br Med J* 294:1051–1053, 1987.
32. Yang SL, Lin CC, River P, et al: Immunoglobulin concentrations in newborn infants associated with intrauterine growth retardation. *Obstet Gynecol* 62:561–564, 1983.
33. Ferguson AC: Prolonged impairment of cellular immunity in children with intrauterine growth retardation. *J Pediatr* 93:52–56, 1978.

34. Lansdown ABG, Histological observations in thymic development in fetal and newborn mammals subject to intrauterine growth retardation. *Biol Neonate* 31:252–259, 1977.
35. Brar HS, Rutherford SE: Classification of intrauterine growth retardation. *Sem Perinatol* 12:2–10, 1988.
36. Levine MG, Holroyde J, Woods JR, et al: Birth trauma: Incidence and predisposing factors. *Obstet Gynecol* 63:792–795, 1984.
37. Anonymous. Hemolytic disease of the newborn. *Lancet* 1:361–362, 1989.
38. Miser A, Geraci TK, Wennberg RP: Fatal erythroblastosis fetalis due to anti-Kell isoimmune disease. *J Pediatr* 86:567–569, 1975.
39. Blickstein I: The twin-twin transfusion syndrome. *Obstet Gynecol* 76:714–722, 1990.
40. Naeye RL: Human intrauterine parabiotic syndrome and its complications. *N Engl J Med* 268:804–809, 1963.
41. Fedrick J, Butler NR: Certain causes of neonatal death: IV. Massive pulmonary hemorrhage. *Biol Neonate* 18:243–262, 1971.
42. Cole VA, Normand ICS, Reynolds EOR, et al: Pathogenesis of hemorrhagic pulmonary edema and massive pulmonary hemorrhage in the newborn. *Pediatrics* 51:175–187, 1973.
43. Lifschult BD, Donoghue ER: Fetal death following maternal trauma. Two case reports and a survey of the literature. *J Forens Sci* 36:1740–1744, 1991.
44. Crom DB, Wilimus JA, Green AA, et al: Malignancy in the neonate. *Med Ped Oncol* 17:101–104, 1989.
45. Laube DW, Schauberger CW: Fetomaternal bleeding as a cause for "unexplained fetal death." *Obstet Gynecol* 60:649–651, 1982.
46. Patterson K, Kapur SP, Chandra RS: Persistent pulmonary hypertension of the newborn: Pulmonary pathologic aspects. *Persp Pediatr Pathol* 12:139–154, 1988.
47. Reid LM: Constrictive and restrictive pulmonary hypertension in the newborn and infant. *Am J Cardiovasc Pathol* 1:287–299, 1987.
48. Morrow WR, Haas JE, Benjamin DR: Nonbacterial endocardial thrombosis in neonates: Relationship to persistent fetal circulation. *J Pediatr* 100:117–122, 1982.
49. Murphy JD, Rabinovitch M, Goldstein JD, et al: The structural basis of persistent pulmonary hypertension of the newborn infant. *J Pediatr* 98:962–967, 1981.
50. Haworth SG, Hislop AA: Pulmonary vascular development: Normal values of peripheral vascular structure. *Am J Cardiol* 52:578–583, 1985.
51. Burchfield DJ, Rawlings J: Sudden deaths and apparent life-threatening events in hospitalized neonates presumed to be healthy. *Am J Dis Child* 145:1319–1322, 1991.
52. Machin GA: Hydrops revisited, Literature review of 1414 cases published in the 1980s. *Am J Med Genet* 34:366–390, 1989.
53. Butler NR, Bonham DG: *Perinatal mortality. The first report of the British perinatal mortality survey.* Livingstone, London, 1963, Section I, pp 202–224.

2 PATHOLOGY OF ACQUIRED IMMUNODEFICIENCY SYNDROME IN CHILDREN

INTRODUCTION

Human immunodeficiency virus (HIV) infection in children resulting in acquired immunodeficiency syndrome (AIDS) is a multisystem disease. We have noted in the autopsy material from 25 cases and biopsy material of various tissues from 45 cases a variety of pathologic lesions of infectious, degenerative, proliferative, and vascular types in the tissues and organs of the different systems. More studies are needed to confirm and extend the description of pathologic lesions available in the literature. However, on the basis of the data currently available, a classification of these numerous systemic lesions based on known, presumptive, or undetermined pathogenesis can be formulated (Table 2-1). Thus the primary lesions are due to HIV infection of tissues or organs. Associated lesions are those that are associated with direct or indirect sequelae of HIV infection or its treatment such as immunodeficiency or iatrogenic lesions. The third category comprises lesions of undetermined pathogenesis. The fourth category consists of lesions of multifactorial pathogenesis. Tentative as the classification may be, the available data are reasonably supportive of its basic framework. Modification and additions can be made without altering its basic framework as more data related to pathogenesis becomes available. For example, HIV enteropathy may be added to the category of primary lesions. Certain preliminary recent observations made in relation to lesions of undetermined pathogenesis (e.g., cardiomyopathy) contribute to understanding the possible pathogenesis of these lesions, and eventually some of the lesions in this category may be classified under other categories in Table 2-1. We feel that a classification of the lesions would lead to better understanding of the multisystem disease process of HIV infection and its numerous sequelae. It should be noted that some of the lesions may be related to more than one pathogenetic mechanism.

In this chapter clinical implications of the pathologic studies are discussed. Processing of the tissue specimens and autopsy protocol for current and possible future studies are briefly described. Finally the pathologic lesions according to the classification in Table 2-1, perinatal pathology, and future direction of pathologic studies of HIV infection will be described and discussed.

DEFINITION OF AIDS IN CHILDREN

The three essential criteria of the Centers for Disease Control (CDC) definition[1] are (1) presence of diseases at least moderately indicative of cellular

TABLE 2-1 Scheme of Pathogenesis of Lesions in Children with AIDS

- Primary lesions of HIV infection
  - Lymphoreticular system
    - Thymus
    - Lymph nodes
  - Brain
  - Other organs (?HIV enteropathy)
- Associated lesions due to direct or indirect sequela(e) of HIV infection
  - Lesions associated with immunodeficiency
    - Opportunistic infections
    - Repeated pathogenic bacterial infections
  - Lesions associated with Epstein–Barr virus
    - Pulmonary lymphoid hyperplasia/lymphoid interstitial pneumonitis (PLH/LIP) complex
    - Nodal and extranodal lymphoid hyperplasia
    - Lymphoproliferative disorder
    - Malignant lymphoma
  - Lesions associated with chronic debilitating disease process
    - Inanition (failure to thrive) and its sequelae
  - Lesions associated with iatrogenic injury related to
    - Total parenteral nutrition (liver disease)
    - Mechanical ventilation and oxygen therapy (lung injury)
    - Zidovudine and other retroviral agents (bone marrow, liver, and CNS toxicity and myopathy)
    - Other
- Lesions of undetermined pathogenesis
  - Arteriopathy
  - Cardiomyopathy
  - Nephropathy
  - Neoplastic disorders
  - Thrombocytopenia
- Lesions of multifactorial pathogenesis
  - Villous atrophy of small intestine
  - Precocious involution and dysinvolution of thymus
  - Wasting of tissues and organs

immunodeficiency (Table 2-2), (2) laboratory evidence of HIV infection, and (3) absence of any cause of immunodeficiency other than HIV infection. The indicator diseases can be divided into opportunistic and pathogenic bacterial infections, malignancies, and a miscellaneous category (HIV encephalopathy, wasting syndrome, etc.). The indicator diseases are listed in Table 2-2. A presumptive diagnosis of certain indicator diseases may be acceptable if laboratory evidence of HIV infection is present. A definitive diagnosis of indicator diseases is essential if laboratory evidence of HIV infection is lacking. There is also a CDC classification system of HIV infection in children (Table 2-3).[2] Many of the diseases in Class P-2 (Table 2-3) are indicator diseases for diagnosis of AIDS. Laboratory evidence of HIV infection includes demonstration of HIV antibodies detected by ELISA (enzyme-linked immunosorbent assay) and confirmed by Western blot techniques. Demonstration HIV antigens or culture of

TABLE 2-2 AIDS Indicator Diseases

- Laboratory evidence of HIV infection required
  - Multiple and recent bacterial infection (subclass D-1 of class P-2[a])
  - Extrapulmonary or disseminated coccidioidomycosis (subclass D-1 of class P-2)
  - HIV encephalopathy (subclass B of class P-2)
  - Extrapulmonary or disseminated histoplasmosis (subclass D-1 of class P-2)
  - Chronic intestinal isosporiosis
  - Primary malignant lymphoma, Burkitt's or immunoblastic type
  - Extrapulmonary or disseminated tuberculosis
  - Wasting syndrome due to HIV
- Definitive diagnosis of the disease required if laboratory evidence of HIV is not available
  - Candidiasis of trachea, bronchi, lungs, or esophagus
  - Extrapulmonary cryptococcosis
  - Chronic intestinal cryptosphoridiosis
  - CMV infection (other than liver, spleen, lymph nodes) with onset at >1 month of age
  - CMV retinitis (with loss of vision)
  - Chronic herpes simplex ulcer (>1 month's duration) or HSV pneumonitis or esophagitis with onset at >1 month of age
  - Kaposi's sarcoma
  - Lymphoid interstitial pneumonitis (subclass C of class P-2)
  - Primary lymphoma of brain
  - Extrapulmonary or disseminated MAI or *M. kansasii* infection
  - *Pneumocystis carinii* pneumonia
  - Progressive multifocal leukoencephalopathy
  - Toxoplasmosis of brain with onset at >1 month of age
- Presumptive diagnosis accepted when laboratory evidence of HIV is available
  - Candidiasis of esophagus
  - CMV retinitis (with loss of vision)
  - Kaposi's sarcoma
  - Lymphoid interstitial pneumonitis (subclass C of class P-2)
  - *Pneumocystis carinii* pneumonia
  - Toxoplasmosis of brain with onset at >1 month of age

[a] See Table 2-3 for details of classes and subclasses of HIV infection.

HIV is also acceptable as laboratory evidence. The following causes of immunodeficiency should be excluded: high-dose or long-term systemic corticosteroid therapy or other immunosuppressive cytotoxic therapy ≤3 months before the onset of indicator disease; Hodgkin's disease, non-Hodgkin's lymphoma (other than occurring in the brain), lymphocytic leukemia, multiple myeloma, other malignancies of lymphoreticular system and angioimmunoblastic lymphadenopathy ≤3 months after diagnosis of the indicator disease; and a congenital immunodeficiency syndrome. The new modification of the CDC definition of AIDS in adolescents and adults includes[3] (1) CD4 count of <200/μl and (2) three indicator diseases: pulmonary tuberculosis, recurrent bacterial pneumonia, and carcinoma of cervix. The CD4 counts in children are age-dependent, and it is not clear whether a single fixed cutoff point can be used for children of all ages. Recurrent bacterial infection had been included in the CDC definition of

TABLE 2-3 CDC Classification System for HIV in Children

Class P-0. Indeterminate Infection		
Infants <15 months born to infected mothers but without definitive evidence of HIV infection or AIDS		
Class P-1. Asymptomatic Infection		
Subclass A.	Normal immune function	
Subclass B.	Abnormal immune function: hypergammaglobulinemia, T4 lymphopenia, decreased T4:T8 ratio, or absolute lymphopenia	
Subclass C.	Immune function not tested	
Class P-2. Symptomatic Infection		
Subclass A.	Nonspecific findings (⩾2 for ⩾2 months): unexplained fever, failure to thrive, generalized lymphadenopathy, hepatomegaly, splenomegaly, enlarged parotid glands, persistent or recurrent diarrhea	
Subclass B.	Progressive neurologic disease: loss of developmental milestones or intellectual ability, impaired brain growth, or progressive symmetrical motor deficits	
Subclass C.	Lymphoid interstitial pneumonitis (histologically confirmed or presumptive diagnosis by clinical and radiologic features)	
Subclass D.	Secondary infectious diseases	
	Category D-1.	Opportunistic infections in the CDC case definition
	Bacterial:	mycobacterial infection (noncutaneous, extrapulmonary, or disseminated); nocardiosis
	Fungal:	candidiasis (esophageal, bronchial, or pulmonary), extrapulmonary or disseminated coccidioidomycosis, disseminated histoplasmosis, extrapulmonary cryptococcosis
	Parasitic:	*Pneumocystis carinii* pneumonia, disseminated toxoplasmosis with onset ⩾1 month of age, chronic cryptosporidiosis or isosporiasis, extraintestinal strongyloidiasis
	Viral:	cytomegalovirus disease (onset ⩾1 month of age), chronic mucocutaneous or disseminated herpes (onset ⩾1 month age), progressive multifocal leukoencephalopathy
	Category D-2.	Unexplained, recurrent, serious bacterial infections (2 or more in a 2-year period): sepsis, meningitis, pneumonia, abscess of an internal organ, bone or joint infections
	Category D-3.	Other infectious diseases: including persistent oral candidiasis, recurrent herpes stromatitis (⩾2 episodes in 1 year), multidermatomal or disseminated herpes zoster
Subclass E.	Secondary cancers	
	Category E-1.	Cancers in the AIDS case definition: Kaposi's sarcoma, B-cell non-Hodgkin's lymphoma, or primary lymphoma of brain
	Category E-2.	Other malignancies possibly associated with HIV
Subclass F.	Other conditions possibly due to HIV infection: hepatitis, cardiomyopathy, nephropathy, hematologic disorders (anemia, thrombocytopenia), dermatologic diseases, etc.	

pediatric AIDS modified in 1987. Cervical carcinoma is unlikely to occur in children with AIDS. However, the precursor human papilloma-virus-related dysplastic cervical lesions do occur in older children, particularly in adolescent girls (see section on neoplastic disorders below).

The CDC definition is readily applicable for diagnosis of AIDS in children in the developed countries. Children with AIDS in developing and developed countries have similar clinical features. However, since laboratory facilities for making specific diagnoses of many infectious diseases are lacking in the developing countries, the World Health Organization (WHO) has recommended a provisional definition based on clinical findings (Table 2-4).[4] Pediatric AIDS is suspected when at least two major signs *and* at least two minor signs are present in the child who has no other known cause of immunodeficiency such as malignancy or severe malnutrition. Elimination of cases of severe malnutrition leads to underdiagnosis of AIDS. Lack of inclusion of LIP and HIV encephalopathy in the criteria is also likely to lead to underdiagnosis.

CLINICAL FEATURES AND IMMUNOLOGIC ABNORMALITIES

Failure to thrive, fever, lymphadenopathy, respiratory findings, and neurologic abnormalities are among the most common clinical features. Recurrent infections with common pathogenic bacteria or opportunistic organisms are seen at various times during the clinical course. Many of the children presenting with respiratory symptoms and signs with characteristic chest x-ray abnormalities have pulmonary lymphoid lesions on open-lung biopsy (see the section below on associated lesions). During the clinical course or in rare instances at the time presentation the patients may show symptoms and signs of cardiac failure, renal failure, and encephalopathy. The latter is characterized by loss of and delay in neurodevelopmental milestones, progressive motor dysfunction, and impaired brain growth determined by serial head circumference measurements or by neuroimaging studies. Hemorrhagic manifestations related to thrombocytopenia and local and systemic manifestations related to neoplastic disorders are also seen in some cases. Initially the majority of the children were less than 1

TABLE 2-4 Provisional WHO Definition of AIDS in Children

Major signs
Weight loss or failure to thrive
Chronic diarrhea >1 month
Chronic fever >1 month
Minor signs
Generalized lymphadenopathy
Oropharyngeal candidiasis
Persistent cough
Repeated chronic infections (otitis, pharyngitis, etc.)
Generalized dermatitis
Confirmed maternal HIV infection

year of age at presentation, but in recent years AIDS is being diagnosed in older children. HIV antibodies are present in the serum, but demonstration of antigen or HIV itself may be required for diagnosis of AIDS in children younger than 15 months. The immunologic disturbances include both T- and B-cell abnormalities such as cutaneous anergy, reversed T4/T8 ratio, lack of response to mitogen, and polyclonal hypergammaglobulinemia.

CLINICAL IMPLICATIONS OF PATHOLOGIC STUDIES

Besides providing material for virologic and immunologic studies, the pathologic examination of biopsy and autopsy specimens from children with a new disease such as AIDS has yielded valuable data with implications in diagnosis, prognosis, natural history, extension of the clinical spectrum, and management.[5] Thus pathologic study of thymic biopsies and thymus at autopsy enabled the differentiation of AIDS from certain congenital immune deficiency disorders when the etiology of AIDS was not yet known. Delineation of the pulmonary lymphoid lesions [pulmonary lymphoid hyperplasia/lymphoid interstitial pneumonitis complex (PLH/LIP complex)] has led to the inclusion of PLH/LIP complex in the criteria for the diagnosis of AIDS and also to the possibility of making the diagnosis of the PLH/LIP complex itself on the basis of clinical and radiologic features. The presence of the PLH/LIP complex in a child with AIDS indicates a relatively better prognosis,[6] but the possibility of progression to polyclonal polymorphic B-cell lymphoproliferative disorder (PBLD)[7] is to be taken into consideration. Pathologic study of pulmonary lymphoid lesions and thymic lesions in biopsy and autopsy specimens in the same patients has contributed to an understanding of the natural history of these lesions. Recognition at autopsy of lesions such as cardiomyopathy, arteriopathy, and PBLD that were not diagnosed clinically has extended the clinicopathologic spectrum of pediatric AIDS. Luminal narrowing due to arteriopathy may play a contributory role in the pathogenesis of atrophy, cell depletion, scarring, necrosis, or infarction in the organs and thus contribute to the failure to thrive seen frequently in children with AIDS. Thymic injury documented by pathologic[8,9] and functional studies[10] may be irreversible. This will have repercussions on the long-term management of children with AIDS after effective specific anti-HIV therapy becomes available. In the future, pathologic study of bone marrow and liver biopsy specimens may be helpful in assessing toxicity associated with AZT and other anti-HIV drugs.[11,12]

With accumulation of more clinical experience and familiarity with autopsy findings in fatal cases in their own institutions and as described in the literature, a learning curve has developed among the clinicians, and they have learned to diagnose lesions and the extent of disease processes associated with AIDS that were previously recognized only at autopsy. However, even in this relatively late phase of the learning curve of AIDS, biopsy and autopsy studies continue to provide data regarding both established and newer aspects of the disease. Thus, for example, we have seen a case of atypical PLH/LIP complex in a lung biopsy specimen (see below). Autopsy studies reveal unexpected lesions in tissues unreachable for biopsy, e.g., focal necrosis of adrenals and posterior pituitary in a disseminated CMV infection. Ongoing systematic autopsy studies in fatal cases of AIDS are part of what can be called "pathologic surveillance" (see below). In future pathologists may also be seeing material from adolescents with HIV infection. In one case of a 19-year-old homosexual male who we studied at autopsy, the findings of opportunistic infection consisting of disseminated cryptococcosis, *Pneumocystis carinii* pneumonia with hilar lymph node involvement and CMV pneumonitis, resembled opportunistic infections seen in sexually or parenterally transmitted adult AIDS.

PROCESSING OF BIOPSIES AND AUTOPSY TISSUES

Precautions

Biopsies of various tissues may be required for diagnosis of different types of lesions associated with AIDS. Each biopsy sample should be placed in a sterile container with a specific label to alert the pathologist that the biopsy was taken from a child with definitively diagnosed or suspected HIV infection. Most fixatives used in pathology laboratories such as neutral buffered formalin, glutaraldehyde, and ethanol inactivate HIV effectively at the concentrations recommended for adequate fixation.[13] Mask, double gloves, gowns, and protective eyewear should be used while handling the tissues. Cleaning of the surfaces of the dissection table by using 10% clorox is essential.

Routine and Special Studies of Biopsy Samples

The biopsies are processed for paraffin sections and ultrastructural studies. The following stains besides hematoxylin and eosin should be routinely done in every case: Ziehl–Neelsen stain for acid-fast mycobacterial organisms, Gomori's methenamine silver (GMS) stain for fungi and *Pneumocystis carinii*, and Gram's stain for bacteria. Immunoperoxidase stains for toxoplasma, cytomegalovirus (CMV), HIV antigen, etc. are becoming available and may be used when indicated. Electron microscopic examination is helpful in identification of certain organisms such as *Cryptosporidia* and *Isospora belli*. A portion of the biopsy should be sent for viral, bacterial (routine, mycobacterial, and anaerobic organisms), and fungal cultures. Depending on the size of the biopsy, portions of it may be snap-frozen for immediate or subsequent immunologic cell marker studies and molecular biologic analysis including demonstration of viral nucleic acids by in situ hybridization, Southern blot technique, polymerase chain reaction, and gene rearrangements for neoplastic disorders. Tissue samples collected at autopsy done within a few hours of death should also be processed in a similar manner.

Material for cytologic studies such as bronchoalveolar lavage (BAL) should be processed by taking universal precautions for handling infectious material such as using biologic hood, mask, gloves, gown, and shoe covers. Prefixation in 50% ethanol may be done to inactivate HIV. Same special stains as described above should be done on the cytologic material. Immunologic cell marker studies may be performed on BAL fluid.

Autopsy Protocol in Fatal Cases of Pediatric AIDS

If research protocols are being followed for these cases, it is imperative that the autopsy be done as early after death as possible for the collection of fresh specimens from tissues and organs for special microbiologic, immunologic, and molecular biologic studies. If there is delay in conducting an autopsy the neuropathologists have recommended wrapping ice-containing plastic bag around the head. Universal precautions recommended by CDC should be strictly observed. Special guidelines for conducting autopsies on AIDS patients include the presence of only the minimum number of personnel necessary for efficient and proper collection of samples in the autopsy room, avoidance of aerosol formation during opening of skull and cutting of tissues, and intensive decontamination of the surface after the autopsy. In my own practice, I have fixed at least for one week the entire eviscerated specimen in a large container of formalin after collection of fresh tissue samples for cultures and special studies. Several deep incisions are made in the organs before immersing the eviscerated specimen in formalin. The dissection of the organs and the histologic sections are the same as for any other pediatric autopsy. In addition, the following studies are recommended: (1) one section from each lobe of the lung since the lungs are a frequent site of pathology in these patients; (2) a separate section from the hilum of each organ to include the arteries for histologic assessment of arteriopathy; (3) sections of bone marrow, multiple lymph nodes, thymus, spleen, Peyer's patches of intestine, and appendix for assessment of changes in the lymphoreticular tissues; (4) detailed study of conduction system of the heart if the child had a history of arrhythmia or cardiomyopathy associated with AIDS; (5) examination of spinal cord; and (6) adequate histologic sampling of any grossly visible lesions.

PATHOLOGIC LESIONS

Primary Lesions

Lymphoreticular System

We have studied biopsy and/or autopsy specimens of the thymus, lymph nodes, spleen, Peyer's patches of the small intestine, and appendix.[5,9,14] Cell depletion or proliferation is noted in the lymphoid tissues of these organs. The evidence that the cell depletion in the lymph nodes and other organs is related to infection and consequent destruction of T helper (CD4) lymphocytes by HIV is well established.[15] We would like to suggest that the epithelial cells of the thymus are also the primary targets of HIV infection since HIV has been cultured from a thymic biopsy specimen[9] and from fetal thymus;[16] cultured thymic epithelial cells can be infected with HIV.[17] Simian T-cell lymphocytic virus type III (STLV-III) has been demonstrated by immunoperoxidase staining in the thymic epithelial cells in rhesus monkeys with AIDS-like disease complex,[18] and decreased levels of thymic hormones secreted by thymic epithelial cells are present in children with AIDS.[10] There are four types of thymic epithelial cell: subcapsular, cortical and medullary epithelial cells, and "nurse" cells. These epithelial cells provide the microenvironment for differentiation and maturation of thymic lymphocytes by secretion of hormones and by cell contact.

Thymus

Three types of lesions are noted:[5,8,9]

1. Precocious involution (Figure 2-1) defined as involution occurring prematurely and in excess of the amount of stress was characterized by marked depletion to virtual absence of lymphocytes, loss of corticomedullary differentiation, and microcystic dilatation of Hassall's corpuscles (HC), which were present in normal numbers. Hyalinization of cortex and medulla with calcification was noted in some cases. Configuration, location, and blood vessels of the thymus were normal. The weight was markedly decreased, often to <1 g.
2. Dysinvolution (Figure 2-2) defined as involution mimicking dysplasia seen in certain congenital immune deficiency disorders was characterized by the same features as above except for marked reduction in the number to virtual absence of HC.
3. Thymitis seen primarily in the thymic biopsies was characterized by presence of lymphoid follicles with germinal centers, multinucleated giant cells

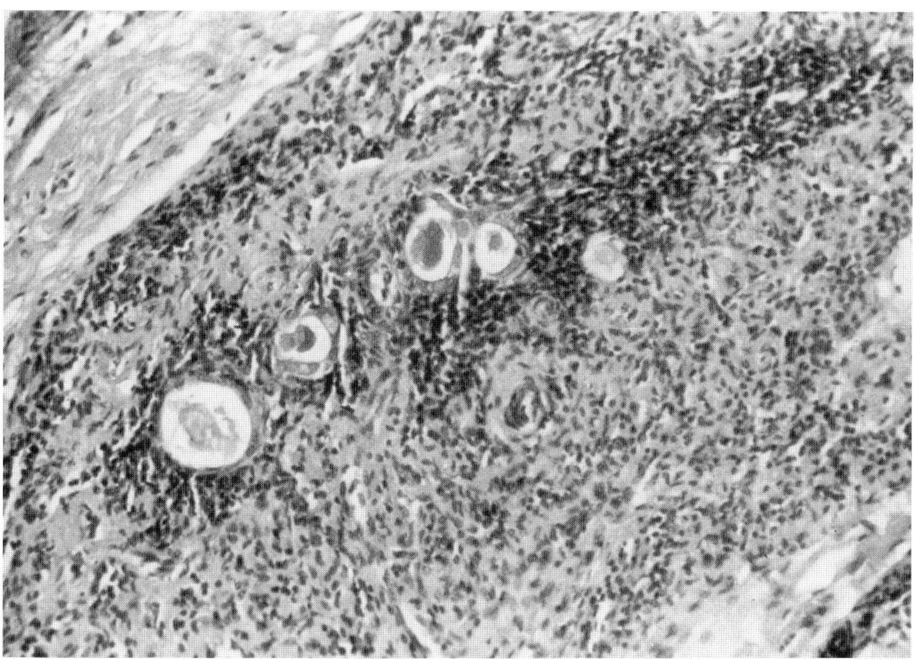

FIGURE 2-1. Precocious involution of thymus characterized by loss of corticomedullary demarcation, virtual absence of lymphocytes, particularly in the cortex, and microcystic dilatation of Hassall's corpuscles, which are present in normal numbers (H&E, ×100). (Reprinted with permission from Joshi VV et al, reference 14).

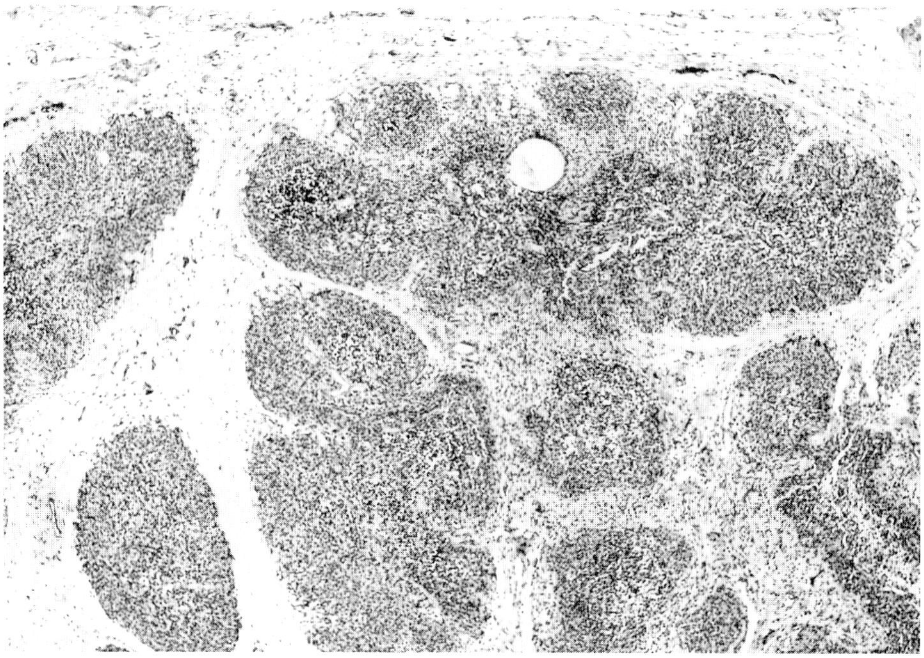

FIGURE 2-2. Dysinvolution of thymus characterized by the same features as shown in Figure 2-1 with the exception of marked reduction in the number of Hassall's corpuscles (HC). Only one microcystically dilated HC is seen (H&E, ×100). (Reprinted with permission from: Joshi VV, and Oleske, reference 8.)

in the medulla (Figures 2-3, 2-4), or diffuse lymphoplasmacytic or lymphomononuclear infiltrate of both the cortex and medulla.

In two cases the thymus at autopsy showed burned-out lymphoid follicles in the medulla and precocious involution. In some cases in which both the biopsy and autopsy material was available progression of thymitis to precocious involution or dysinvolution was noted. These findings suggest that thymitis may be the earliest lesions in children with AIDS. The severity of involutionary changes with or without hyalinization of the thymus suggests that the thymic changes may be irreversible. (In only 2 of the 25 autopsy cases studied by us was there partial reconstitution of the structure of the thymus.) In the event that specific curative anti-HIV therapy becomes available, the long-term prognosis in children with AIDS will still be affected by permanent immunodeficiency resulting from irreversible thymic injury. Thymic epithelial cell transplantation has been attempted in adults with AIDS.[19] Transient partial immunoreconstitution was observed in these patients. We are not aware of such attempts in children with AIDS.

Another thymic lesions that I have seen recently in two cases probably represents multilocular thymic cyst.[20] In both these cases the lesion presented as a mediastinal mass first detected on chest x-ray.

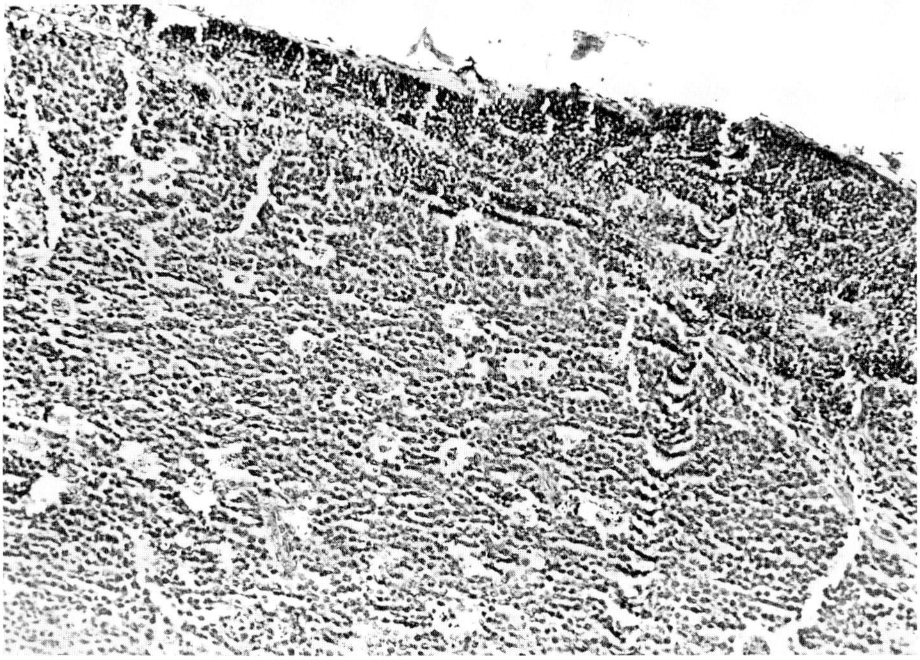

FIGURE 2-3. Thymic biopsy showing lymphoid follicle with prominent germinal center in the medulla; note the compression of the cortex by the lymphoid follicle (H&E, ×250). (Reprinted with permission from Joshi VV et al, reference 9.)

Lymph Nodes

Three different patterns were noted in the lymph nodes:[14] follicular hyperplasia with a normocellular paracortex, follicular hyperplasia with lymphocyte depletion of paracortex, and severe atrophy with marked lymphocytic depletion of the entire lymph node (Figure 2-5). The second and third types of lesion are related to cell depletion due to HIV infection. The follicular hyperplasia and other proliferative lesions are described under the category of associated lesions. The atrophic lymph nodes show marked attenuation of lymphoid follicles with absent or inactive germinal centers and narrowing and depletion of paracortical zone. Sinus histiocytosis may be present. Multinucleated giant cells, probably formed by fusion of HIV-infected lymphocytes, are seen in the atrophic follicles in some cases. (Similar giant cells are also seen in the lymph nodes showing follicular hyperplasia.) The atrophic changes are present in lymph nodes examined at autopsy and represent a terminal stage of the HIV-related lymphoid depletion. Other factors such as inanition and "immune exhaustion" probably also contribute to the pathogenesis of the lymph node atrophy.

Other Lymphoreticular Tissues

Similar atrophic changes characterized by profound cell depletion are also seen in the other lymphoreticular tissues such as spleen, appendix, and Peyer's patches of the small intestine at autopsy.[14]

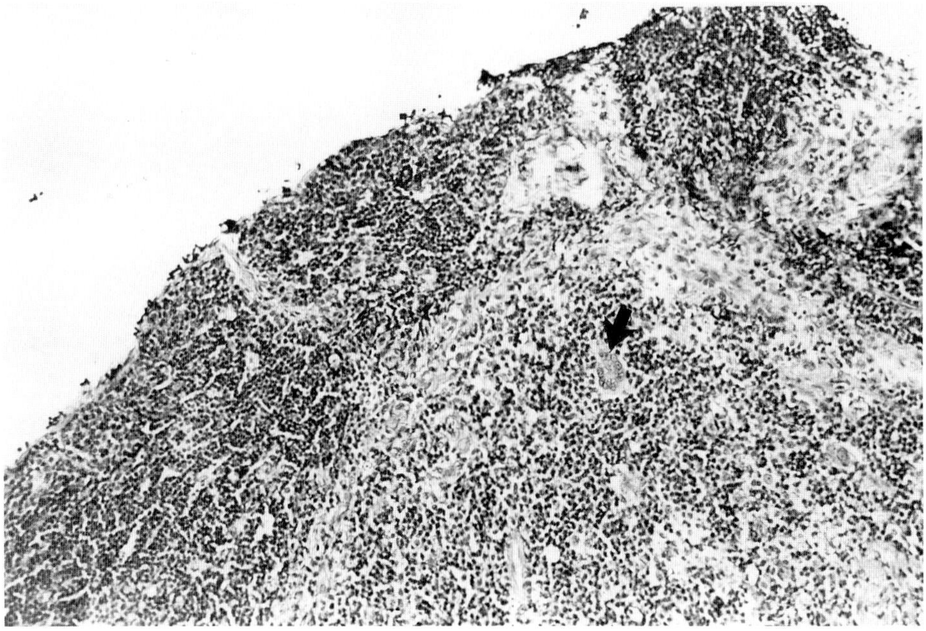

FIGURE 2-4. Thymic biopsy showing a multinucleated giant cell (arrow) in the medulla (H&E, ×250). (Reprinted with permission from Joshi VV et al, reference 9.)

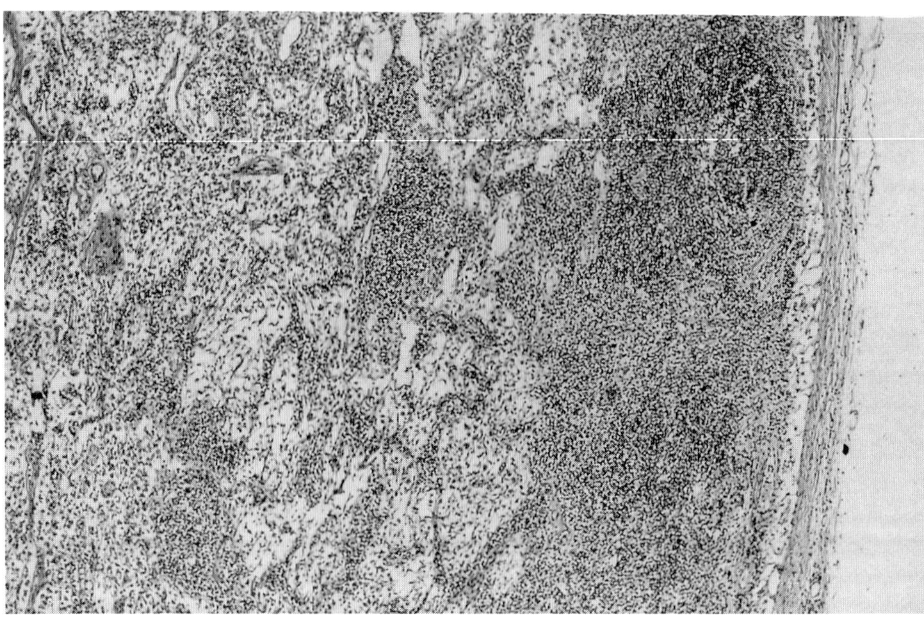

FIGURE 2-5. Lymph node showing poorly defined lymphoid follicles with vague to absent germinal centers in the cortex, depletion of cell content and narrowing of paracortical zone and sinus histiocytosis (H&E, ×100). (Reprinted with permission from Joshi VV et al, reference 14.)

Peripheral Blood and Bone Marrow

Anemia, lymphopenia, and reversal of T helper/suppressor cell ratio are characteristically found in children with AIDS.[14,21] Plasmacytosis and eosinophilia have been observed in children with pulmonary lymphoid lesions.[21] Thombocytopenia is being observed with increasing frequency in recent years. It is described in the section on lesions of undetermined pathogenesis. The bone marrow is slightly hypercellular to normocellular with normal to increased megakaryocytes. Lymphoid aggregates have been described in the bone marrow in some patients.[21] We have observed these lymphoid aggregates particularly in patients with lymphoproliferative disorder (see below).

Central Nervous System

In our series of pediatric AIDS case studies, 68% of the children have shown encephalopathy.[22] Progressive HIV encephalopathy is characterized by delayed development or loss of milestones, pyramidal or extrapyramidal signs, and microcephaly with cerebral calcification detected by computerized tomographic (CT) scan.[23]

Brain

The following pathological features have been noted:[24] atrophy, gliosis, microglial nodules, foci of necrosis with or without inflammatory cell infiltrate around them, loss of myelin, vasculitis and perivasculitis, vascular and parenchymal calcification, and characteristic multinucleated giant cells in the parenchyma and perivascular location (Figures 2-6–2-10). The multinucleated giant cells are probably derived from mononuclear cells.

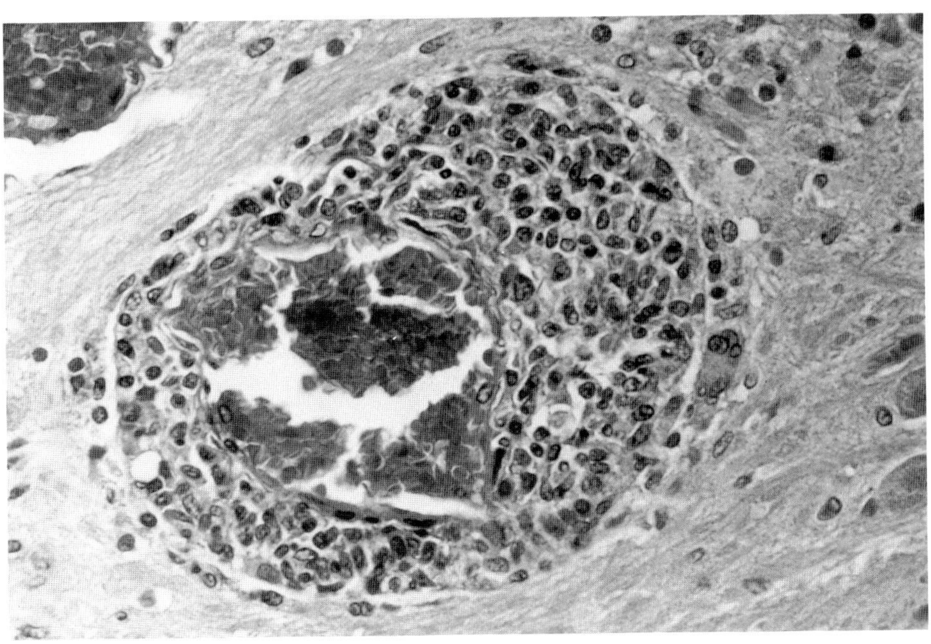

FIGURE 2-6. Perivascular inflammatory infiltrate in the brain; note the multinucleated giant cell (H&E, ×250). (Reprinted with permission from Joshi VV et al, reference 64.)

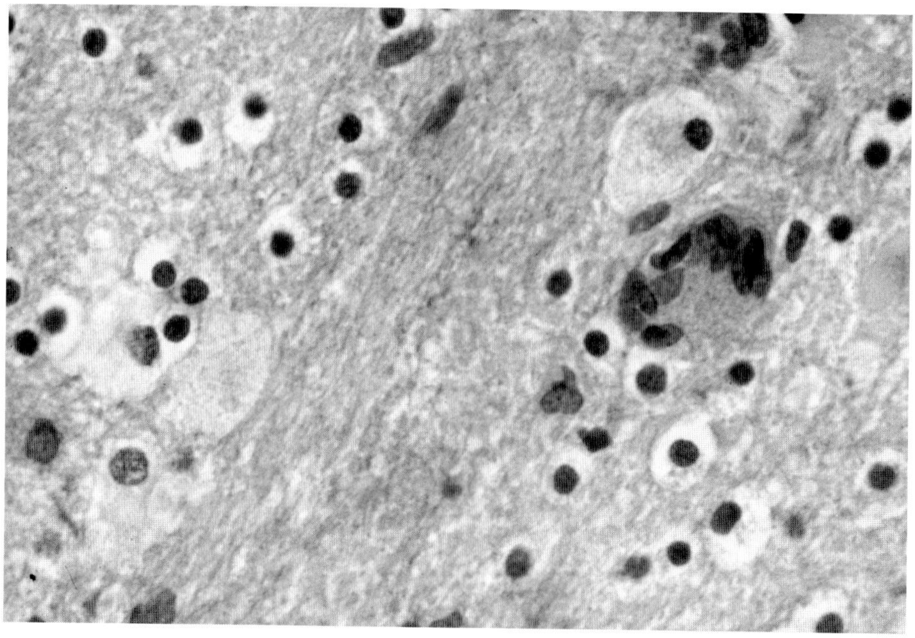

FIGURE 2-7. Multinucleated giant cell in the parenchyma of the brain (H&E, ×400).

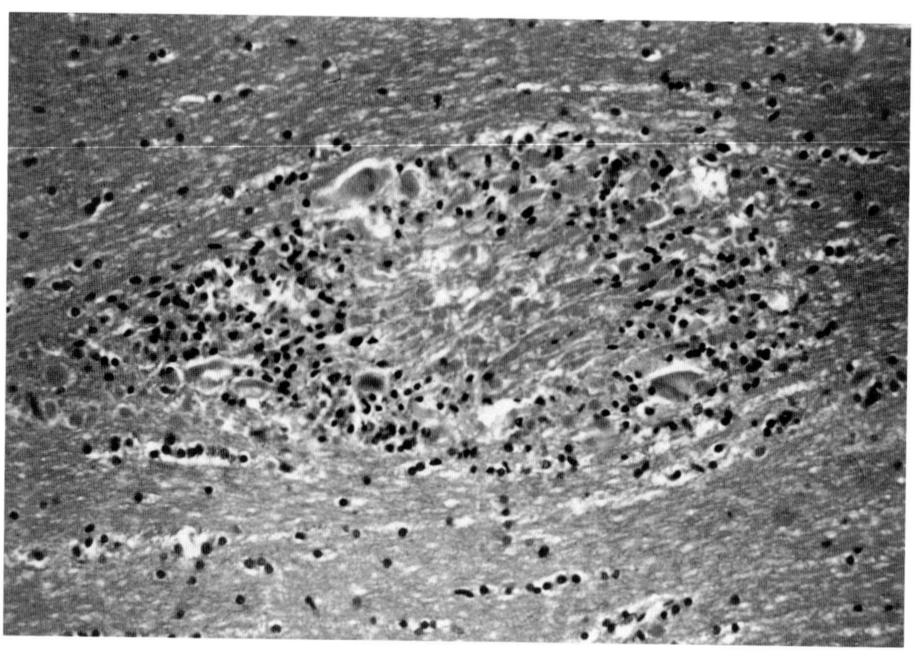

FIGURE 2-8. Focus of necrosis with inflammatory cell infiltrate around it in the brain (H&E, ×100).

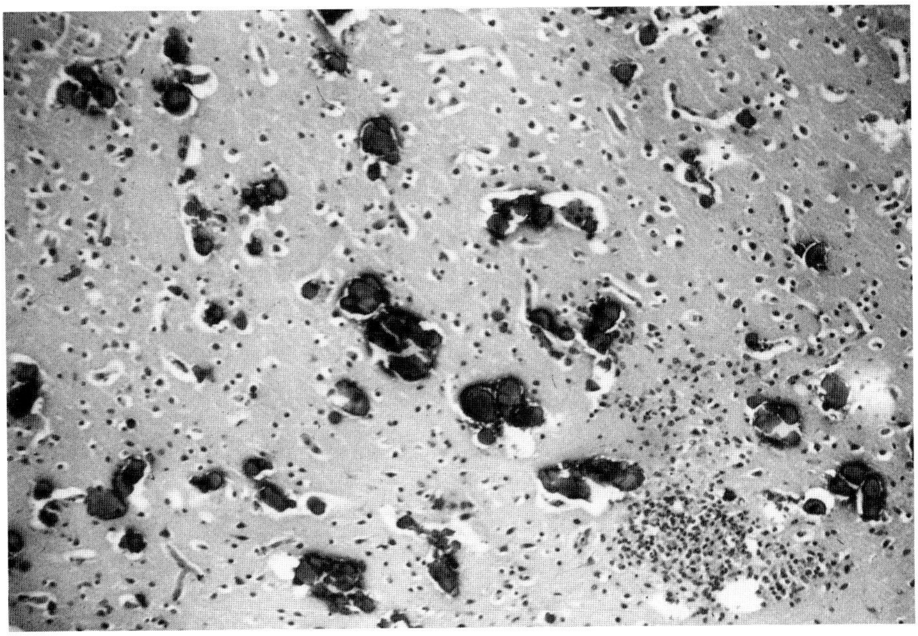

FIGURE 2-9. Microcalcification in the brain (H&E, ×100).

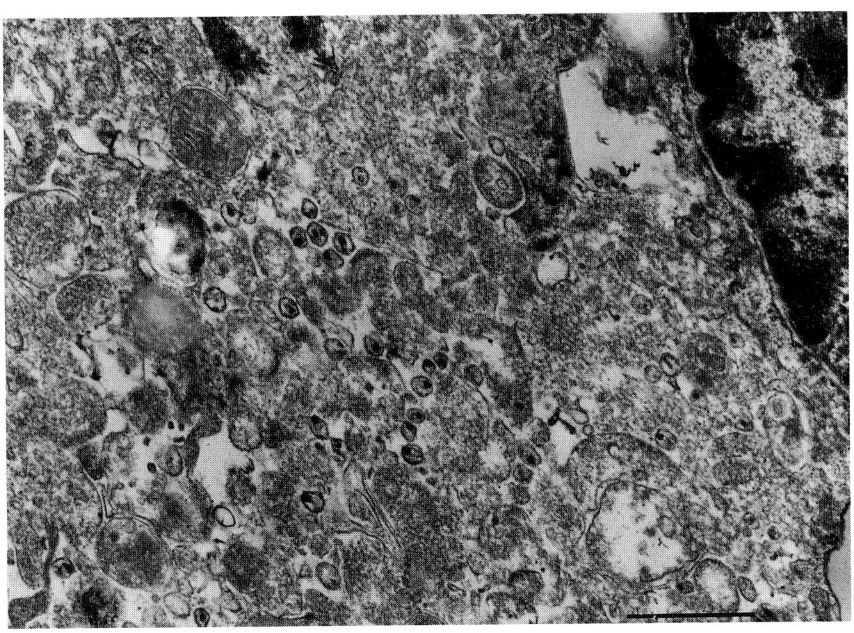

FIGURE 2-10. Electron micrograph of a giant cell of the type shown in Figures 2-6 and 2-7. Note in the cytoplasm the presence of HIV particles with eccentric and cylindrical nucleoids (formalin-fixed tissue, uranyl acetate and lead citrate; bar represents 500 nM). (Reprinted with permission from Sharer LR et al, reference 24.)

These lesions are related to HIV, which has been demonstrated in the brain by electron microscopy (Figure 2-10) and in situ hybridization.[25,26] Stoler and colleagues[27] have localized the virus by in situ hybridization to macrophages, microglia, giant cells, and less commonly to glial cells and neurons. The relationship between HIV infection of mononuclear cells in the brain and encephalopathy is not clear. Release of neurotoxic substances by the inflammatory cells may be one of the mechanisms of injury to the brain.[28,29] It is possible that the resultant damage and atrophy of the brain may not be completely repairable in terms of morphologic reconstitution even after anti-HIV therapy is given. Besides the primary lesions of HIV infection, lesions related to the other two categories (Table 2-1) such as involvement in opportunistic infections (OI) and foci of necrosis or infarction are also seen in the lymphoreticular system and brain.

Spinal Cord

Vacuolar myelopathy[30] due to swelling within myelin sheaths characterized by vacuolar degeneration and the presence of lipid-laden macrophages, particularly in the lateral and posterior columns of the thoracic spinal cord, has been observed in two children in our series (Figure 2-11). The pathogenesis of vacuolar myelopathy is not clear. It may be related directly to HIV and/or to sequelae of HIV infection such as metabolic abnormalities secondary to inanition associated with the chronic debilitating disease process of AIDS (Table 2-1).

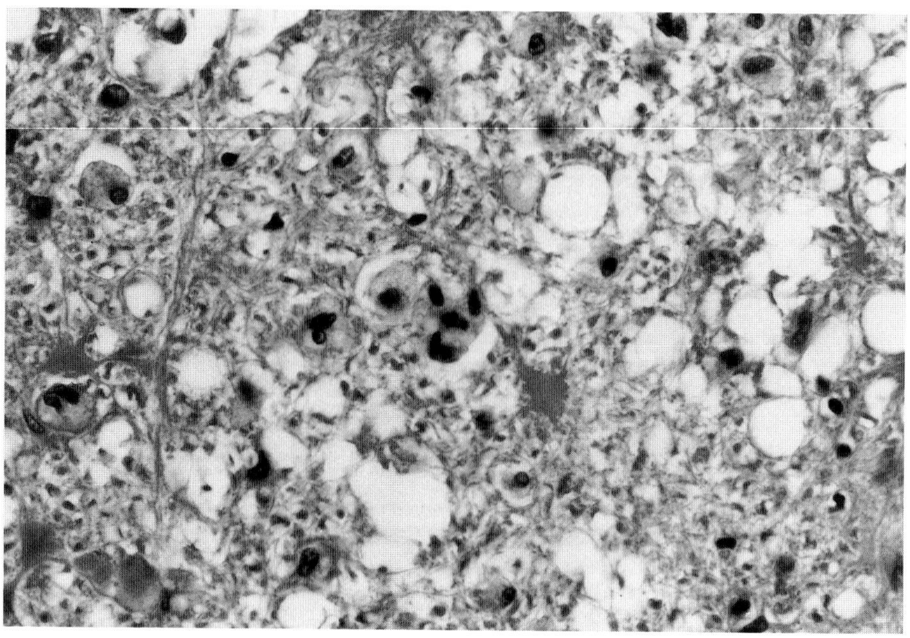

FIGURE 2-11. Vacuolar myelopathy; note that some of the vacuoles contain foamy lipid-laden macrophages (H&E, ×400).

HIV Enteropathy

To the category of primary lesions, HIV enteropathy may be added. This entity, described in adults with AIDS and characterized by diarrhea and malabsorption in the absence of known demonstrable specific gastrointestinal infections appears to be related to HIV.[31] HIV antigens (p24) and RNA have been demonstrated in the mononuclear cells, lymphocytes, enterocytes, and enterochromaffin cells in the biopsy specimens of duodenum and rectum by immunoperoxidase and in situ hybridization techniques.[31,32] These results, which cannot be considered as conclusive at this time, have not been confirmed in the biopsy material from children, although HIV-infected children with persistent diarrhea have been shown by polymerase chain reaction to shed HIV nucleic acid in the stool.[33] On histologic examination, the duodenal biopsy shows mucosal atrophy, normal crypt depth, reduced mitotic activity, and increased number of lymphocytes in the epithelium and in the lamina propria (Figure 2-12). These findings are non-specific and were initially considered by us as representative of an associated lesion related to chronic inanition due to AIDS and its complications.[34] It appears that investigation of intestinal mucosal biopsy specimens from children with AIDS having diarrhea should be undertaken for demonstration of HIV itself or its antigens.

Associated Lesions

Opportunistic and Repeated Bacterial Infections

These infections are the most frequent life-threatening sequelae of immunodeficiency associated with HIV infection. Opportunistic infections occurring in patients in our series[35] were caused by parasites (*Pneumocystis carinii*, *Toxoplasma gondii*, crystosporidia), fungi (*Candida* species, *Aspergillus* species), bacteria [*Mycobacterium avium–intracellulare* (MAI)] and viruses [CMV, herpes simplex virus (HSV)]. Viral infections due to varicella-zoster virus and HSV can be more severe, of longer duration and may show superimposed bacterial infection with fatal outcome.[36] Because cultures of these organisms are

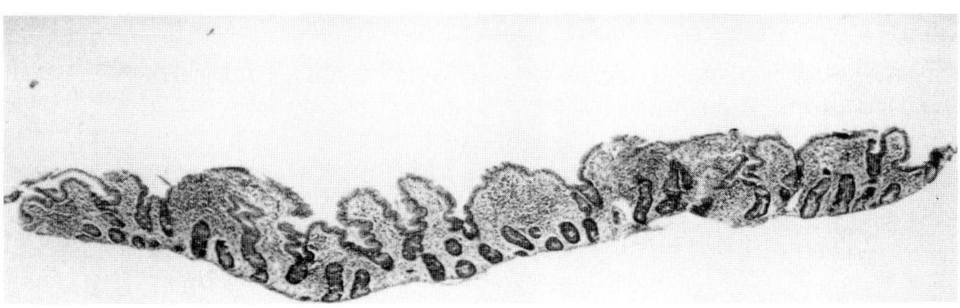

FIGURE 2-12. Jejunal biopsy showing nonspecific moderately severe villous atrophy of the mucosa (H&E, ×4). (Reprinted with permission from McLoughlin L et al, reference 85.)

time-consuming, rapid morphologic demonstration of the organisms is of practical importance (Table 2-5).

Open biopsy of the lungs has been used in our institution for the diagnosis of opportunistic infections and other pulmonary lesions. Minimal to mild morbidity and no mortality were seen in patients subjected to open-lung biopsy. Imprints of the biopsy specimen can be helpful in rapid diagnosis of *P. carinii* pneumonia. Special stains (Gomori's methenamine silver and Ziehl–Neelsen stains) for *Pneumocystis carinii*, fungi, and acid-fast organisms should be routinely carried out on lung biopsy specimens. A portion of the specimen should be submitted for bacterial, fungal, and viral cultures. Thorough examination of the biopsy specimen, carefully inflated by injecting formalin with minimal pressure via a butterfly needle, is essential since only rare small clusters of *P. carinii* organisms may be present in the sections.[35] BAL has also been used for the diagnosis of opportunistic infections.[37] Jejunal biopsy has been helpful in the diagnosis of MAI infections.[35] The diagnosis of cryptosporidiosis is best made by examination of stool or duodenal aspirate.

We have noted the following unusual types of lesions related to opportunistic infections in our patients:[35] (1) granulomatous and DIP-like reaction in *P. carinii* pneumonia (PCP); (2) locally invasive PCP with involvement of regional lymph nodes; (3) focal cavitation and calcification in PCP; (4) diffuse alveolar damage obscuring the features of PCP; (5) the presence of *P. carinii* and CMV pneumonitis in the same specimen (Figure 2-13); (6) MAI infection of the jejunum resembling Whipple's disease (Figures 2-14, 2-15);[38] (7) a histoid reaction in mesenteric lymph nodes showing MAI infection (this type of reaction may be confused with a soft tissue tumor such as fibrous histiocytoma or smooth muscle tumor) (Figure 2-16);[39] (8) foci of necrosis in adrenals and posterior pituitary in disseminated CMV infections; (9) CMV enteritis with CMV inclusions in the myenteric plexuses; (10) involvement of multiple groups of lymph nodes, spleen, and liver in MAI infection resembling malignant lymphoma on gross examination; (11) dissemination and fatal outcome in varicella infection; and (12) persistent chronic lesions of HSV skin infection. In addition to these opportunistic infections, repeated infections with common pathogenic bacteria (*Hemophilus influenzae*, *Staphylococcus aureus*, *Streptococcus pneumoniae*, and *salmonella*) are frequently seen in children with AIDS.[35]

Spectrum of Lymphoproliferation Probably Associated with Epstein–Barr Virus

The lymphoproliferative lesions form a broad spectrum extending from benign reactive hyperplasia, lymphoproliferative disorder intermediate between benign and malignant lymphoproliferation, and malignant lymphoma (Table 2-6).[40] A comparable spectrum of lymphoproliferation is seen in patients with congenital immunodeficiency syndromes. The lesions seen in pediatric AIDS involve various nodal and extranodal sites such as lungs, liver, brain, and gastrointestinal tract and overlap one another. The most characteristic example of this spectrum that illustrates the overlap between these lesions and is also considered as an indicator disease for diagnosis of AIDS is the pulmonary lymphoid hyperplasia/lymphoid interstitial pneumonitis complex (PLH/LIP complex). PLH is characterized by lymphoid follicles with germinal centers

TABLE 2-5 Opportunistic Infections in Children with AIDS

Organism	Predominant organs and tissues involved in infection	Morphologic method of diagnosis*	Other comments
Pneumocystis carinii	Lungs	Gomori's methenamine silver (GMS) stain for cyst wall, Giemsa for trophozoites in bronchoalveolar lavage or lung biopsy specimen	Rare extrapulmonary spread described in adults not reported in children; not infrequently associated with CMV pneumonitis; diffuse alveolar damage may obscure the true nature of the lesions in the biopsy specimen, atypical reactions include granulomatous and DIP-like reaction
Toxoplasma gondii	Brain	Routine H&E, immunoperoxidase stain	Uncommon in children; lesions outside CNS not reported
Cryptosporidium	GI tract	Ziehl–Neelsen (ZN) method for acid-fast organisms on concentrated stool specimen or routine H&E and electron microscopy on endoscopic biopsy of GI tract	Stool examination more convenient and rapid method of diagnosis; extraintestinal involvement (biliary tract, respiratory tract) nor reported in children

TABLE 2-5 Continued.

Organism	Predominant organs and tissues involved in infection	Morphologic method of diagnosis*	Other comments
Candida	Oral mucosa, esophagus, skin	GMS and periodic acid-Schiff (PAS) stains	Systemic candida infection rare
Aspergillus	Lungs	GMS and PAS	Usually found unexpectedly at autopsy
Mycobacterium avium–intracellulare	GI tract, liver, spleen, lymph nodes, lungs	PAS stain and ZN method for acid-fast bacteria	Histoid reaction in lymph nodes and intestinal lesion resembling Whipple's disease, infection may be found unexpectedly at autopsy, necrosis and granuloma formation usually absent
Cytomegalovirus	Lungs, GI tract, lymph nodes, heart, brain, adrenals, posterior pituitary	Routine H&E, immunoperoxidase stain, and in situ hybridization are available	Little inflammatory reaction may be seen; tissue necrosis may or may not be present
Herpes simplex	Skin	Tzanck smear or biopsy: H&E or immunoperoxidase method	Chronic lesions may be present

[a]Culture for definitive identification should be done for organisms that can be grown.

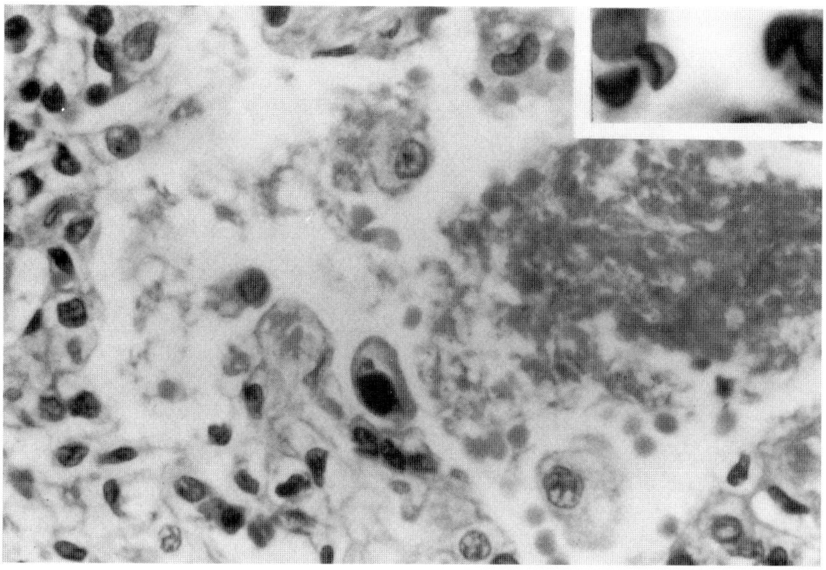

FIGURE 2-13. Pneumocystis carinii pneumonia characterized by characteristic foamy material in the alveolar lumen (inset shows organisms in the foamy material demonstrated by Gomori's methenamine silver stain). Note also the intranuclear inclusion of cytomegalovirus (H&E, ×250, inset: GMS ×400). (Reprinted with permission from: Joshi VV et al, reference 14.)

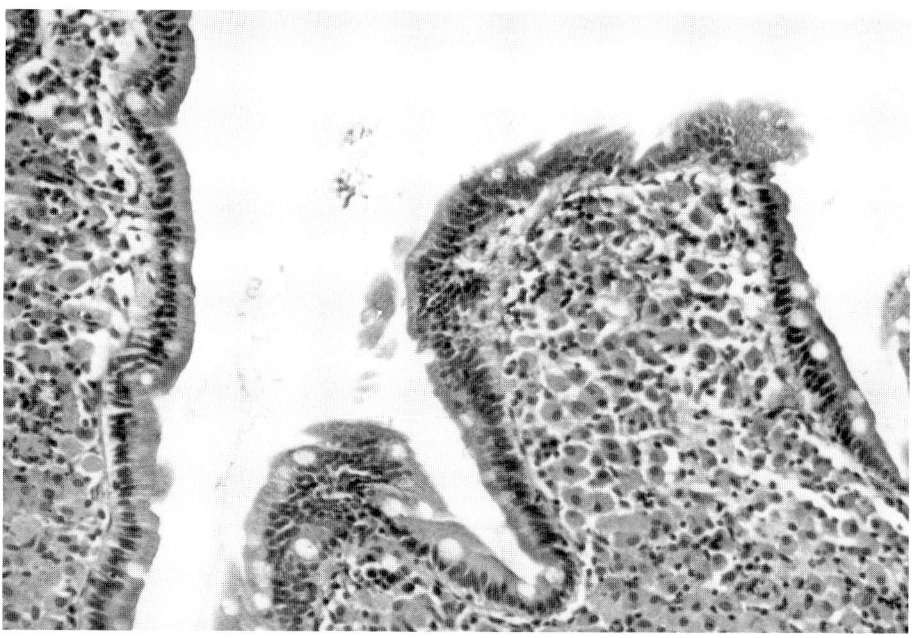

FIGURE 2-14. Jejunal biopsy showing diffuse dense infiltration of the lamina propria by pale staining mononuclear cells resembling the lesion of Whipple's disease (see Figure 2-15) (H&E, ×250).

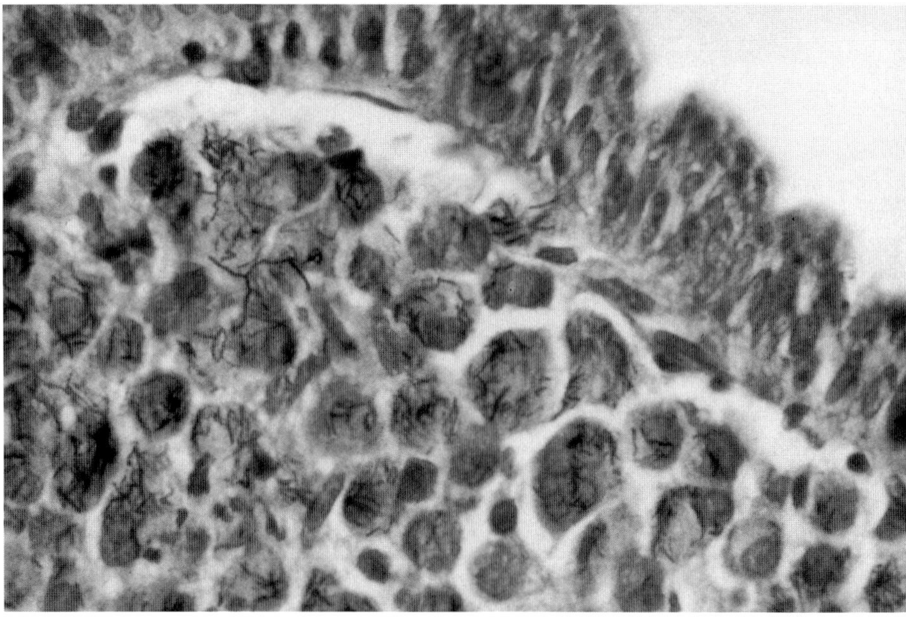

FIGURE 2-15. Jejunal biopsy showing numerous acid-fast bacilli in mononuclear cells in Figure 2-14 (Ziehl–Neelsen stain ×400). (Reprinted with permission from Joshi VV, Oleske JM: in *AIDS and other manifestations of HIV infection*, Noyes Publications, Park Ridge, NJ, 1987.)

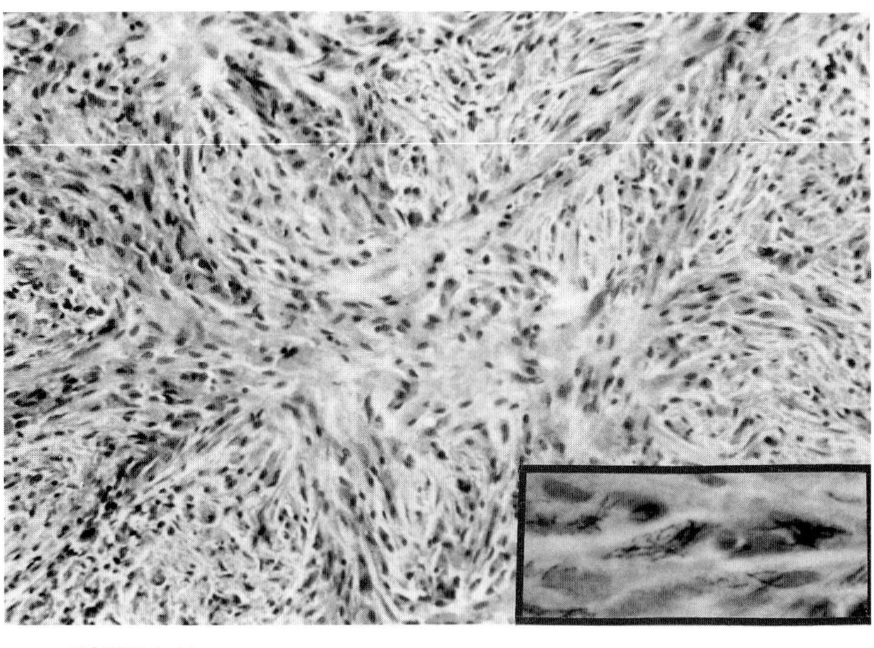

FIGURE 2-16. Histoid reaction in *Mycobacterium avium*–intracellulare infection; note the spindle-shaped and fusiform cells arranged in vague bundles reminiscent of a mesenchymal tumor (H&E, ×100). Inset shows acid-fast bacilli (Ziehl–Neelsen stain, ×400).

TABLE 2-6 Spectrum of Systemic Lymphoproliferative Lesions[a] in Children with AIDS

Hyperplasia involving
Lymph nodes
Peyer's patches of ileum
Lymphoic nodules in the esophagus and colon
Thymus (lymphoid follicles with germinal centers in the medulla)
Lungs [pulmonary lymphoid hyperplasia (PLH)][a]
Lymphoplasmacytic Infiltrates in
Lungs [lymphoid interstitial pneumonitis (LIP)][a]
Salivary glands
Liver
Overlapping lesions[a]
PLH/LIP complex involving lungs
Atypical PLH/LIP complex
Polyclonal polymorphic B-cell lymphoproliferative disorder (PBLD) involving
Lungs
Liver
Spleen
Kidneys
Salivary glands
Lymph nodes
Muscle
Periadrenal fat
Non-Hodgkin's malignant lymphoma (B cell) involving
Brain and other extranodal sites (lung, GI tract)
Lymph nodes
Hodgkin's lymphoma
B-cell acute lymphoblastic leukemia

[a] The lesions listed above may show overlap. Thus PLH and LIP are characteristically present in the same patient; hence the term "PLH/LIP complex."

around the bronchioles and LIP by diffuse alveolar septal infiltration by an admixture of lymphocytes, plasma cells, plasmacytoid lymphocytes, and a few immunoblasts (Figures 2-17–2-19).[41,42] These cells are polyclonal B lymphocytes as indicated by immunoperoxidase stains for kappa and lambda light chains of immunoglobulins. There is also an admixture of T cells, particularly T8 suppressor subtype, as shown by cell marker studies on BAL and lung biopsy specimens.[43,44] In most cases there is an overlap between PLH and LIP (Figures 2-17, 2-20). Hence the term PLH/LIP complex. In this lesion, there is no involvement of blood vessels or destruction of bronchi. Eosinophils are not present in the infiltrate. Special stains for fungi, acid-fast bacilli, and *Pneumocystis carinii* are negative. Viral inclusions are not seen. Interstitial pneumonitis with lymphoid infiltrate seen in CMV pneumonitis (Figure 2-21) should not be considered as PLH/LIP complex. Nonnecrotizing granulomas and multinucleated giant cells were seen in some cases. Sometimes there may be a marked intraalveolar accumulation of mononuclear cells (Figure 2-20). Initially this reaction, which obscured the lymphoid infiltrate in some cases, was interpreted as a distinctive type of interstitial pneumonitis, viz., desquamative interstitial pneumonitis (DIP).[46] However, later it became apparent that it merely represents

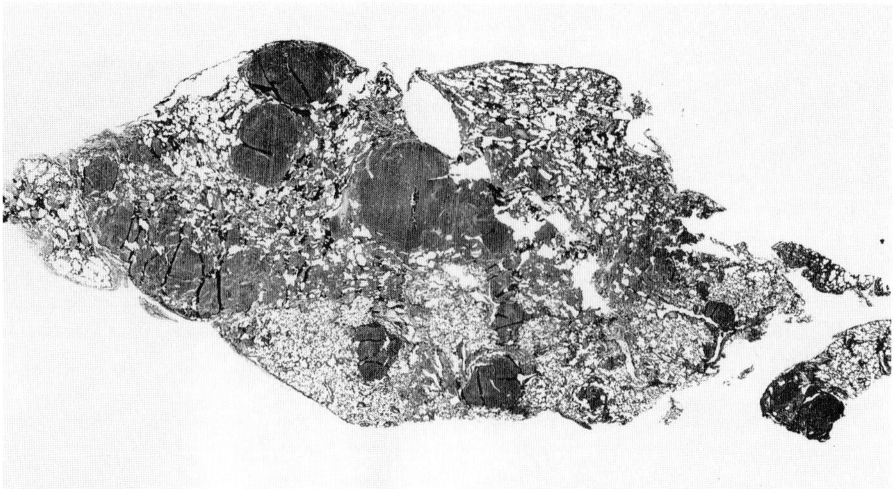

FIGURE 2-17. Lung biopsy showing pulmonary lymphoid hyperplasia characterized by peribronchiolar lymphoid nodules; note focal extension of lymphoid infiltrate to surrounding alveolar septa (H&E, ×40).

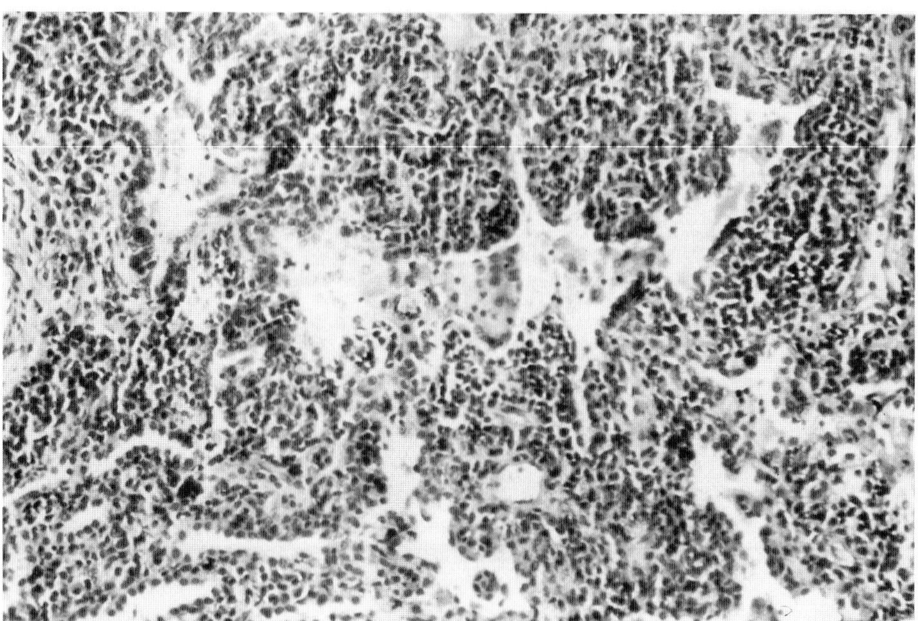

FIGURE 2-18. Lung biopsy showing lymphoid interstitial pneumonitis characterized by lymphoid infiltration of alveolar septa (H&E, ×250).

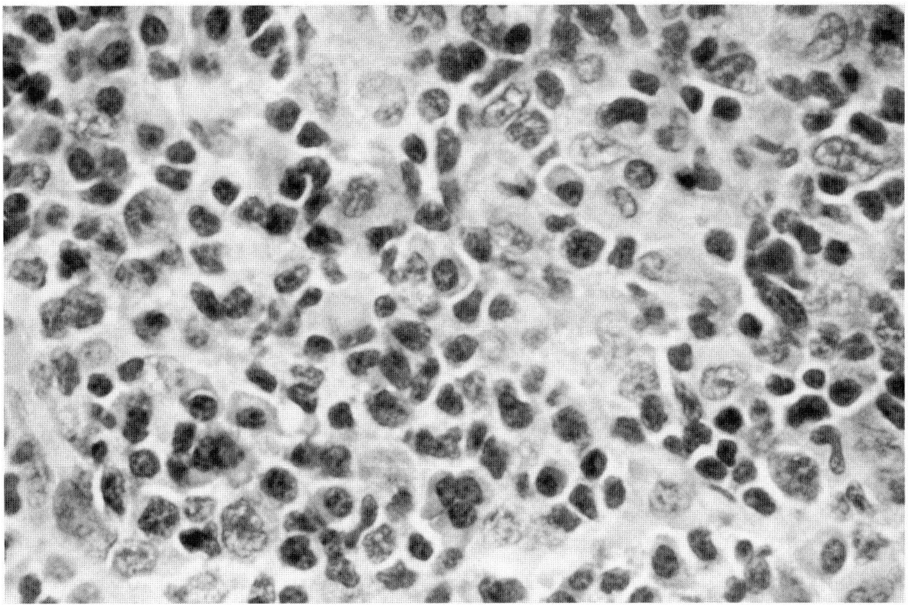

FIGURE 2-19. Lung biopsy showing the cell composition of the lymphoid infiltrate of PLH/LIP complex. Note the presence of polymorphic infiltrate composed of lymphocytes, plasma cells, plasmacytoid lymphocytes, and occasional large immunoblasts (H&E, ×400). (Reprinted with permission from Joshi VV et al, reference 14.)

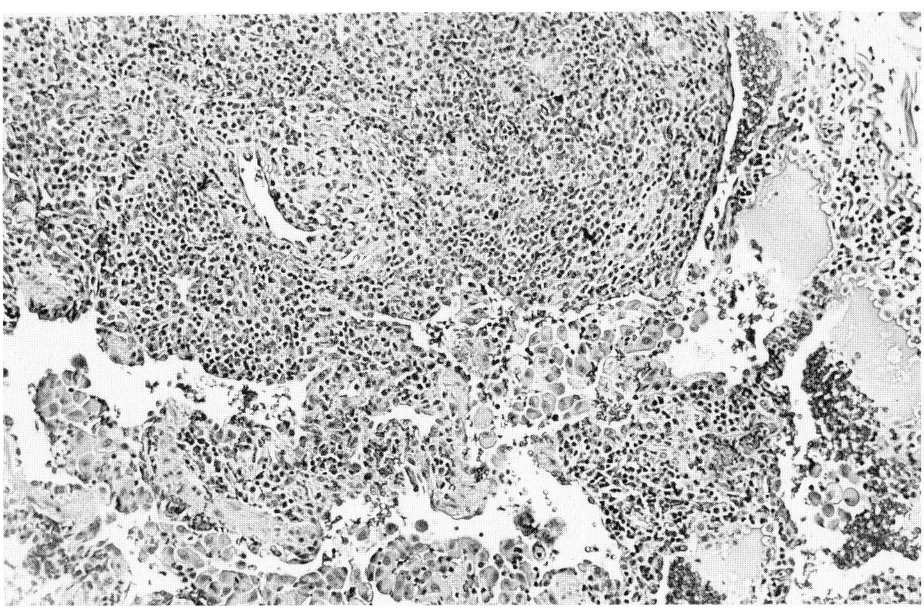

FIGURE 2-20. Lung biopsy showing PLH/LIP complex. Note the lymphoid nodule with extension of lymphoid infiltrate into the alveolar septa. Note also the presence of mononuclear cells in the alveoli representing desquamative interstitial pneumonitis-like reaction. (H&E, ×250.)

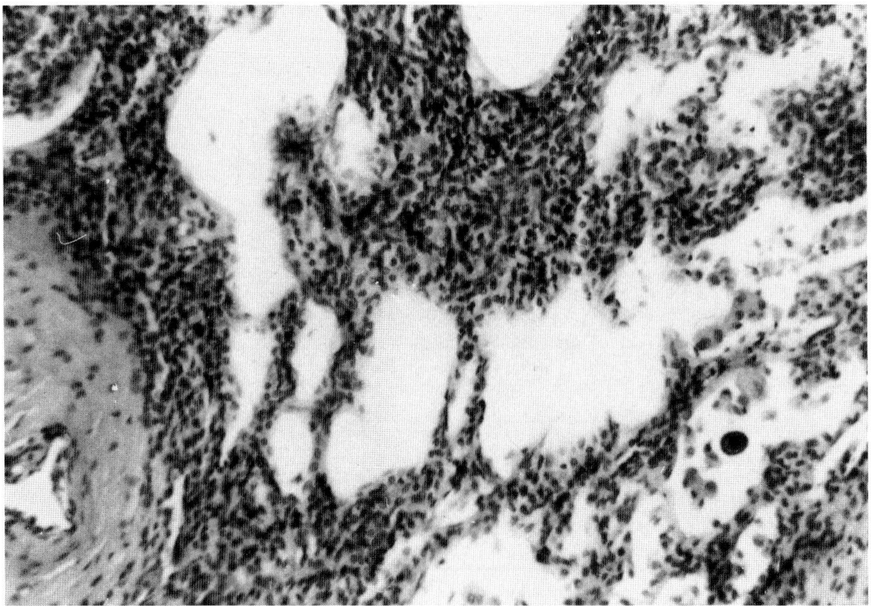

FIGURE 2-21. Lung biopsy showing dense interstitial lymphoid infiltrate; note the CMV inclusion (H&E, ×250).

a DIP-like mononuclear reaction occurring in association with PLH/LIP complex and rarely PCP.[42] PLH/LIP complex produces a characteristic nodular–linear infiltrative pattern on chest roentgenogram.[45]

Since the original description of PLH/LIP complex, we have seen a case with foci of atypical histologic features in the lung biopsy.[46] Besides the typical pathologic features of PLH/LIP complex as described above, the biopsy in this case showed foci of monomorphic infiltration by atypical lymphocytes (Figure 2-22). Occasional atypical mitotic figures were present. No definitive conclusions can be drawn from a single case. However, it is possible that atypical PLH/LIP complex belongs to the spectrum of systemic lymphoproliferation. It is suggested that lung biopsies showing PLH/LIP complex should be carefully examined for focal atypical features described above.

Follow-up on 19 cases of PLH/LIP complex showed that 11 children were alive with persistent but less severe disease 9 to 58 months after diagnosis.[47] Of the 8 patients who died, 4 had autopsies. In two of these autopsies, PLH/LIP complex progressed to a lymphoproliferative disorder[7] involving the lungs, liver, spleen, kidneys, and lymph nodes (Figures 2-23–2-26) with the formation of grossly demonstrable nodules. The cellular infiltrates in the different organs were qualitatively similar to that in PLH/LIP complex (Figure 2-19) except for focal prominence of immunoblasts. In the spleen and kidneys, vascular invasion by the cellular infiltrate was noted (Figure 2-24). The paraaortic and mediastinal lymph nodes were commonly involved by a diffuse polyclonal polymorphic lymphoid proliferation effacing the normal architecture (Figure 2-26). Fatal infectious mononucleosis, angioimmunoblastic lymphadenopathy, and periph-

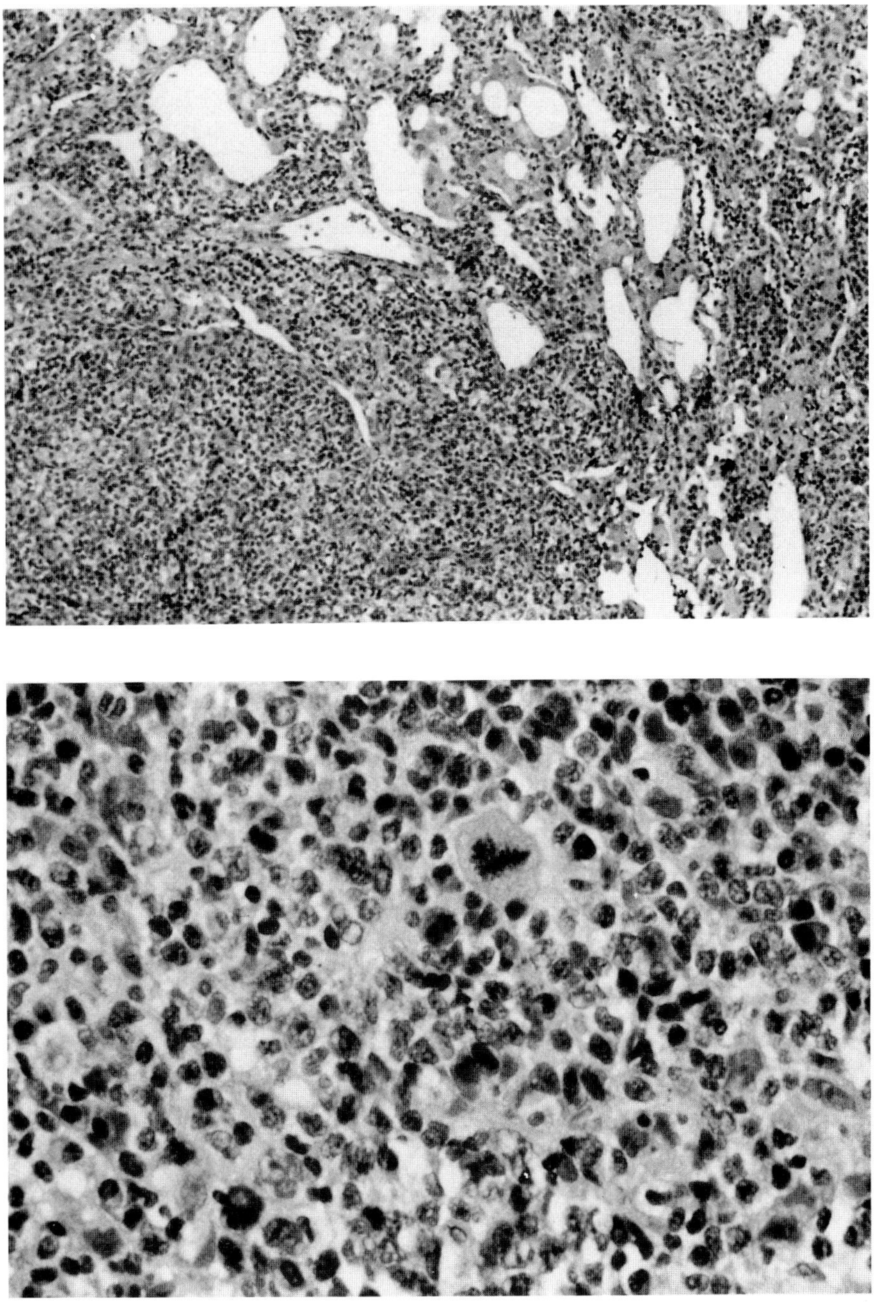

A

B

FIGURE 2-22. (A) Lung biopsy showing typical features of PLH/LIP complex (H&E, ×100); (B) focus of atypical feature in the biopsy characterized by monomorphic lymphocytic infiltrate and an atypical mitotic figure (H&E, ×400). (Reprinted with permission from Joshi VV, reference 77.)

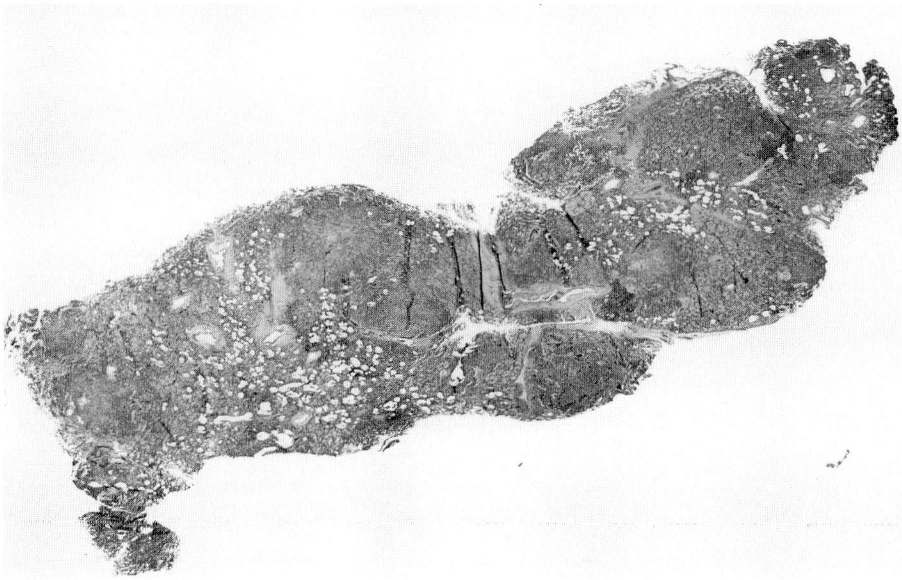

FIGURE 2-23. Whole mount of a section of lung at autopsy involved by polyclonal polymorphic B-cell lymphoproliferative disorder (PBLD). Note the prominent nodular involvement, which was grossly visible (H&E, ×4).

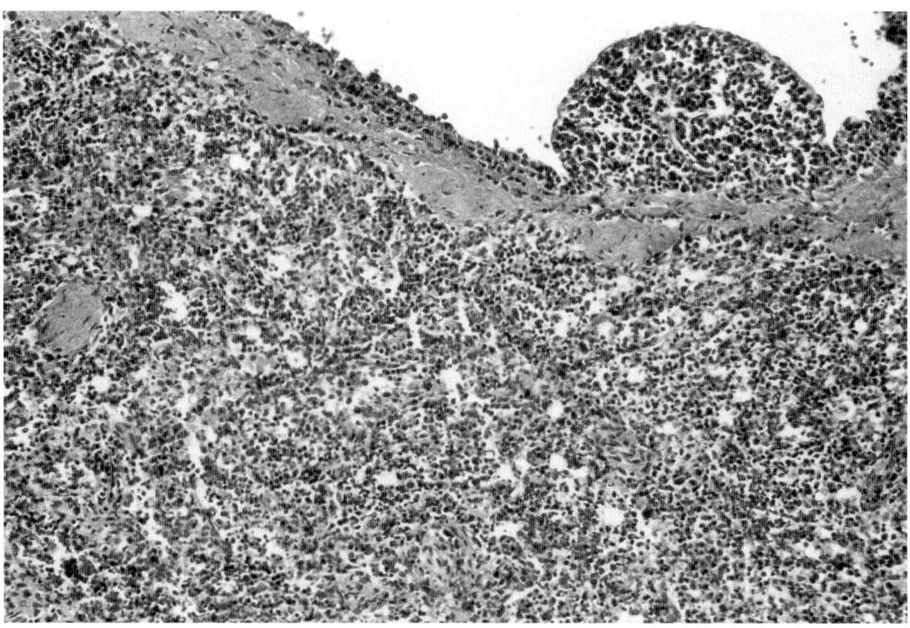

FIGURE 2-24. Involvement of spleen by PBLD; note the cellular infiltration of the wall of a trabecular vein with subendothelial micronodule formation (H&E, ×100). (Reprinted with permission from Joshi VV et al, reference 7).

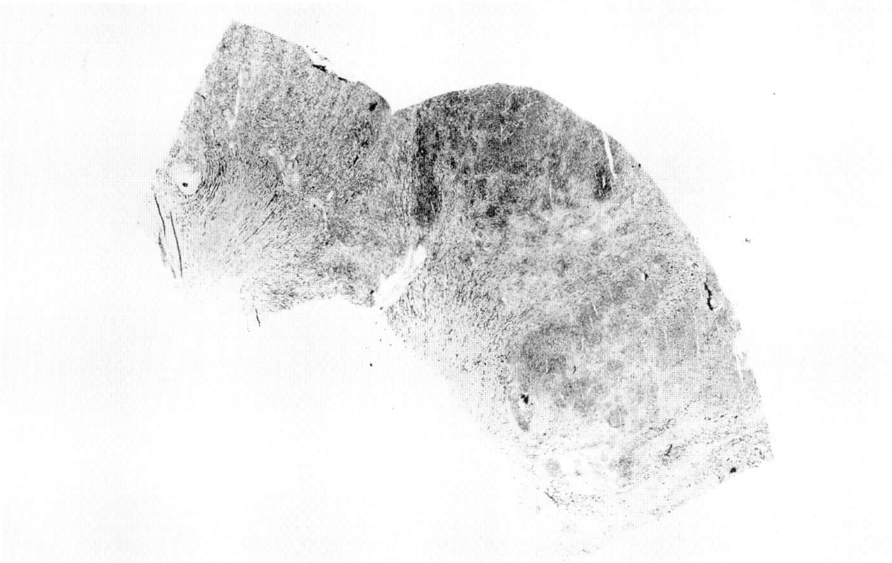

FIGURE 2-25. Whole mount of a kidney showing involvement by PBLD (H&E, ×4). (Reprinted with permission from Joshi VV et al, reference 7.)

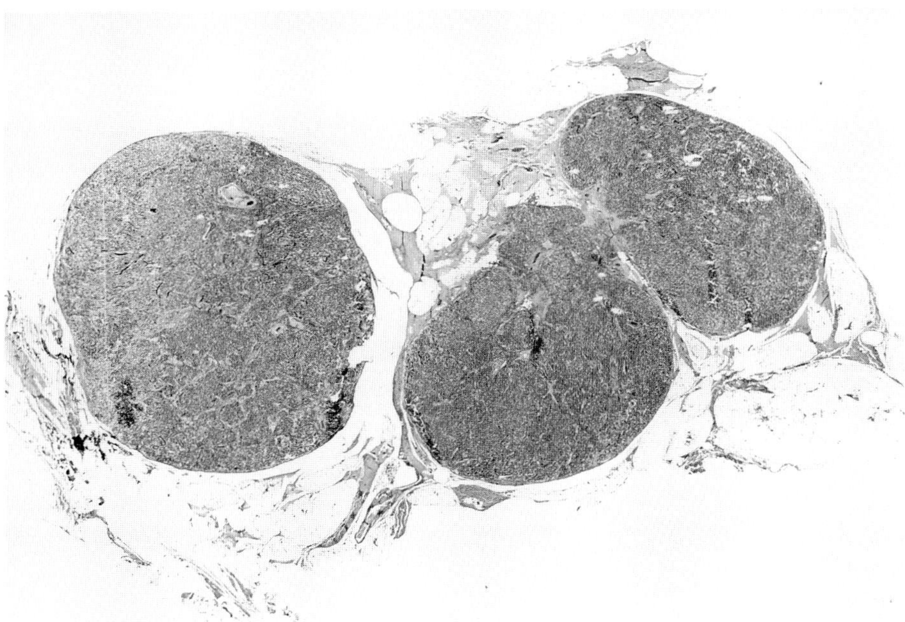

FIGURE 2-26. Involvement of para-aortic lymph nodes by PBLD. There is enlargement with effacement of normal lymph node architecture (H&E, ×4). [Reprinted with permission from Joshi VV et al: Pathology of AIDS in children. *Pathol Annu* 24 (part 1):355–381, 1989.]

eral T-cell lymphoma with a prominent B-cell reactive component were considered in the differential diagnosis but ruled out because of the absence of cellular atypia, atypical mitosis, necrosis, and perivascular eosinophilic smudgy material. It appears that this lymphoproliferative disorder is distinctive, and it has been referred to as the "polyclonal polymorphic B-cell lymphoproliferative disorder" (PBLD). It is considered to be intermediate between a benign and a full-fledged malignant lymphoproliferative disorder.[7] In three cases of primary malignant lymphoma of the brain seen in our series[48] the lesion was multifocal with rapid progression to fatal outcome. These tumors were B-cell-derived; two were large cell and one was small cell noncleaved (Burkitt-like) type (Table 2-6).

Pathogenesis of Systemic Lymphoproliferative Lesions

Many of these lesions may be related to EBV, since the EBV genome has been demonstrated in lung tissue showing the PLH/LIP complex and in tissue derived from primary malignant lymphoma of the brain in children with AIDS.[49] Synergism between HIV and EBV may also be involved in the pathogenesis of these lymphoid lesions, since HIV can replicate in EBV-transformed B cells[50] and in alveolar macrophages.[51] Macrophages are seen in association with PLH/LIP complex and multinucleated giant cells characteristic of HIV infection are seen in the proliferative lesions in the lymph nodes and other organs.[6,14] Ovine lentivirus belonging to the same subfamily of retroviruses as HIV induces the PLH/LIP complex-like lesions in neonatal lambs[52] and also lymphoproliferative disorder resembling PBLD.[53] An LIP-like lesion and a PBLD-like lymphoproliferative disorder have also been described in an simian immunodeficiency virus–infected rhesus monkey.[54,55]

Lesions Related to Inanition Resulting from the Chronic Debilitating Disease Process of AIDS

Although deficiency of specific nutritional factor(s) has not been documented, nutritional status as judged by the growth and development of these children remains subnormal, and failure to thrive continues despite adequate diet and nutritional support by hyperalimentation.[56] Growth retardation and wasting are commonly noted at autopsy. Fatty change of the liver, villus atrophy of the small intestine (Figure 2-12), and atrophic changes in the tissues of lymphoreticular system are partly related to inanition. Vacuolar myelopathy may also be related to metabolic abnormalities associated with inanition. Maturation delay of testes seen at autopsy in older children may be secondary to effects of inanition.

Iatrogenic Lesions

The following iatrogenic lesions have been noted in our patients who require intensive diagnostic and therapeutic intervention: (1) portal fibrosis with early cirrhosis of the liver associated with prolonged total parenteral nutrition (TPN) started during early infancy; (2) acute and chronic diffuse alveolar damage related to the administration of high concentration oxygen, particularly during the preterminal stage of the disease;[6] (3) thrombosis of the TPN catheter; and (4) vilus atrophy of the small intestine partly related to TPN. We have not yet seen any biopsy material from bone marrow or liver to assess the effects of toxicity of AZT or other antiretroviral drugs.[11,12]

Lesions of Undetermined Pathogenesis

Dilated Cardiomyopathy

In some of our patients, cardiovascular compromise or congestive heart failure evidenced by shortness of breath, fatigability, costal and subcostal retraction, sinus tachycardia with gallop rhythm, hepatomegaly, scattered rales, and weak peripheral arterial pulses was noted. Cardiomegaly was seen on chest roentgenograms. At autopsy, the heart was enlarged and overweight.[57] Biventricular dilatation was present (Figure 2-27). No gross abnormalities of the valves or coronary arteries were noted. None of the chambers or appendages contained mural thrombi. Hypertrophy of the ventricular walls was not appreciated because of the dilatation. Intramural fibrosis was not observed on gross examination. On microscopic examination, the following findings were noted: (1) hypertrophy as indicated by nuclear enlargement and increased diameter of myocardial fibers; (2) foci of vacuolation, probably related to hydropic or fatty change in the myocardium; (3) interstitial edema with or without foci of myxoid

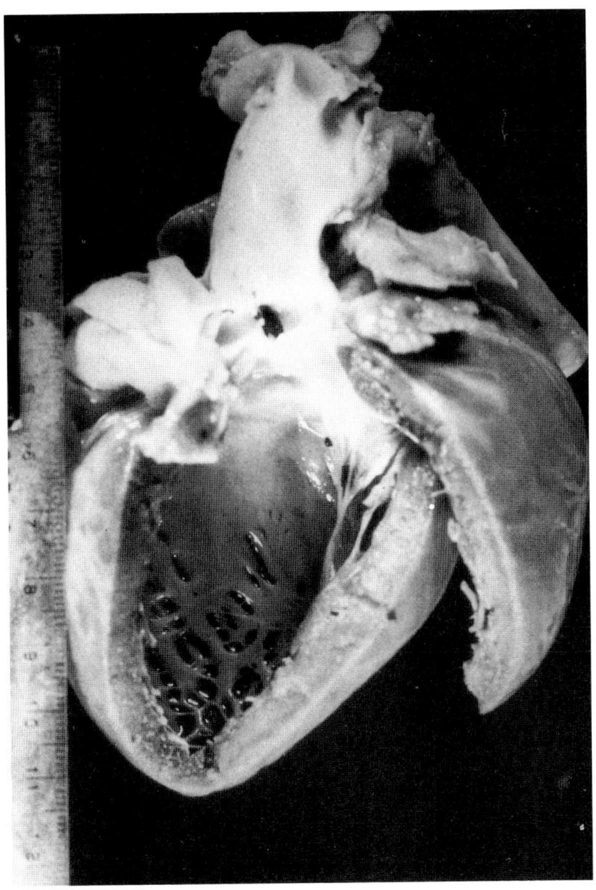

FIGURE 2-27. Cardiomyopathy with left ventricular dilatation. (Reprinted with permission from Joshi VV, et al, reference 57.)

change; (4) occasional small foci and myocardial fibrosis; and (5) endocardial thickening, particularly of the left ventricle. Autopsy findings related to cardiovascular compromise or congestive heart failure included serious effusions and visceral congestion. Florid congestive heart failure was the cause of death in one case.

In addition to these relatively readily demonstrable findings, rare focal cardiac changes included (1) myocarditis with sparse mononuclear and lymphocytic inflammatory infiltrates and myocyte necrosis (Figure 2-28), (2) rare intranuclear CMV inclusions in the endocardium and capillary endothelium without inflammatory reaction in one case, (3) slight focal intimal fibrosis or medial calcification of small branches of the coronary arteries without significant luminal narrowing, and (4) small chronic inflammatory infiltrates of the pericardium. Electron-microscopic examination of the myocardium in one case showed degenerative changes characterized by lipid droplets, swelling of mitochondria and of the sarcoplasmic reticulum, and cellular edema.

The pathogenesis of dilated cardiomyopathy is not known. Infection, immunologic factors, anemia, deficiency of nutritional factors, and longer survival due to early diagnosis of AIDS and aggressive antimicrobial and supportive therapy may be related to the pathogenesis. Cellular and humoral immunodeficiency in children with AIDS may be associated with more severe damage by infections with cardiotropic viruses or by the more frequent occurrence of myocardial damage in those viral infections (e.g., EBV or CMV) in which myocardial

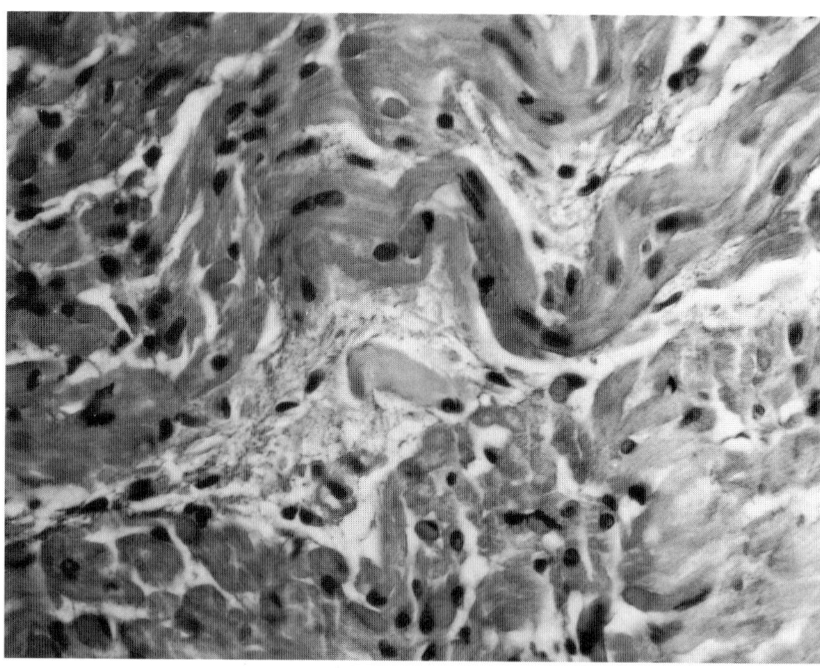

FIGURE 2-28. Myocardium showing focus of myocarditis characterized by myocardial necrosis and sparse inflammatory infiltrate (H&E, ×250). (Reprinted with permission from Joshi VV et al, reference 57.)

involvement occurs rarely in immunologically intact hosts. If viral infection is related to pathogenesis, the infection might have occurred as a remote event, with cardiomyopathy as its late sequela.[58] Increased titers of antiheart antibodies have been demonstrated in AIDS patients with myocarditis.[59] The immunopathologic findings of presence of T lymphocytes and absence of B cells, monocytes, and natural-killer cells have been considered as indicative of a cell mediated autoimmune injury to the myocardium.[60] HIV has been cultured from the endomyocardial biopsy of a 32-year-old man with AIDS-associated congestive cardiomyopathy.[61] Although culturing of HIV by itself does not prove conclusively its etiologic role in cardiomyopathy, the observation is certainly worthy of further investigation. Among the nutritional deficiencies related to nutritional cardiomyopathy, selenium deficiency is an important factor related to Keshan disease, which is characterized by cardiomyopathy and is endemic in mountainous areas of China. Selenium deficiency has also been associated with cardiomyopathy in patients with long-term total parental nutrition. Dworkin et al[62] have documented low selenium levels in the cardiac tissue removed at autopsy (0.327 ± 0.082 μg/g dry weight as compared with 0.534 ± 0.184 μg/g dry weight in control hearts; $p < .01$) from eight patients with AIDS.

Cardiac Conduction System

Bharati et al[63] have recently reported the findings of a detailed study of the conduction system in six children with AIDS. Fragmentation of the bundle of His with lobulation and fibrosis, vacuolation and fibrosis of the bundle branches, and inflammatory infiltration of the myocardium and vessels of the different parts of the conduction system were observed in a study involving detailed examination of 1000–2000 histologic sections of the conduction system in each case. In one of the children in the series there was left hemiblock on EKG that corresponded to pathologic abnormalities seen in the left bundle branch. The pathogenesis of the lesions of the conduction system is unclear.

Arteriopathy

The lesion designated as arteriopathy[64] is seen in small and medium-sized arteries of different organs (heart, lungs, kidneys, spleen, intestine, brain). It is characterized by intimal fibrosis, fragmentation of elastic tissue, fibrosis, and calcification of media with variable luminal narrowing (Figs 2-29, 2-30). (Vasculitis or perivasculitis, shown in Figure 2-6 and seen only in the brain in association with HIV encephalopathy, is not considered as part of the lesions of arteriopathy.)

In one case, aneurysms of the right coronary artery with thrombosis (Figure 2-31) and myocardial infarction were seen. Stroke associated with arteriopathy of meningocerebral arteries with or without aneurysm formation has also been described.[65] The nature of fibrocalcific arterial lesions is not clear. Atherosclerosis, Monckeberg's sclerosis, Takayasu's disease, giant cell arteritis, and fibromuscular dysplasia, which occur more commonly in adulthood and old age, can be ruled out in our cases on the basis of both intimal and medial involvement, prominence of calcification, and absence of lipid deposition and inflammatory changes including giant cells. Arterial lesions that occur primarily in the pediatric age group and that should be considered in the differential diagnosis are Kawasaki disease and idiopathic arterial calcification of infancy. These two

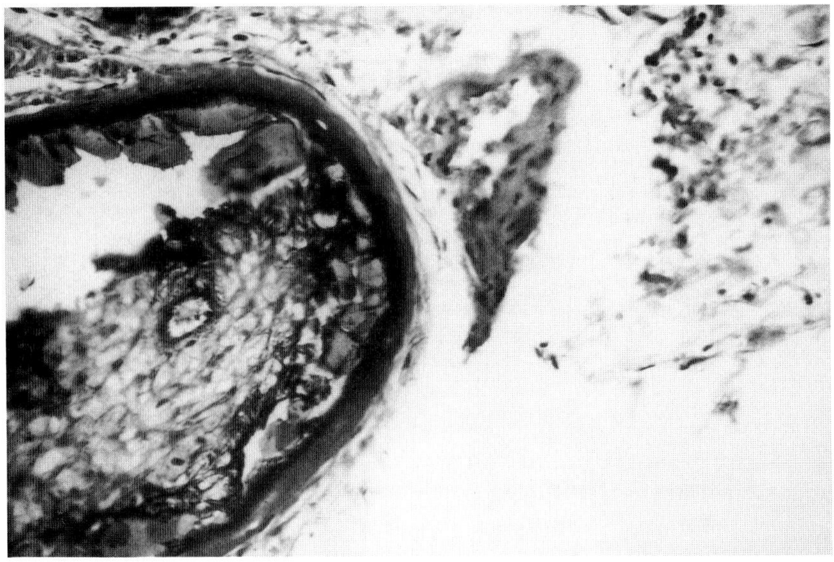

FIGURE 2-29. A medium sized artery showing marked luminal narrowing due to intimal and medial fibrosis with calcification (H&E, ×100). (Reprinted with permission from Joshi VV et al, reference 64.)

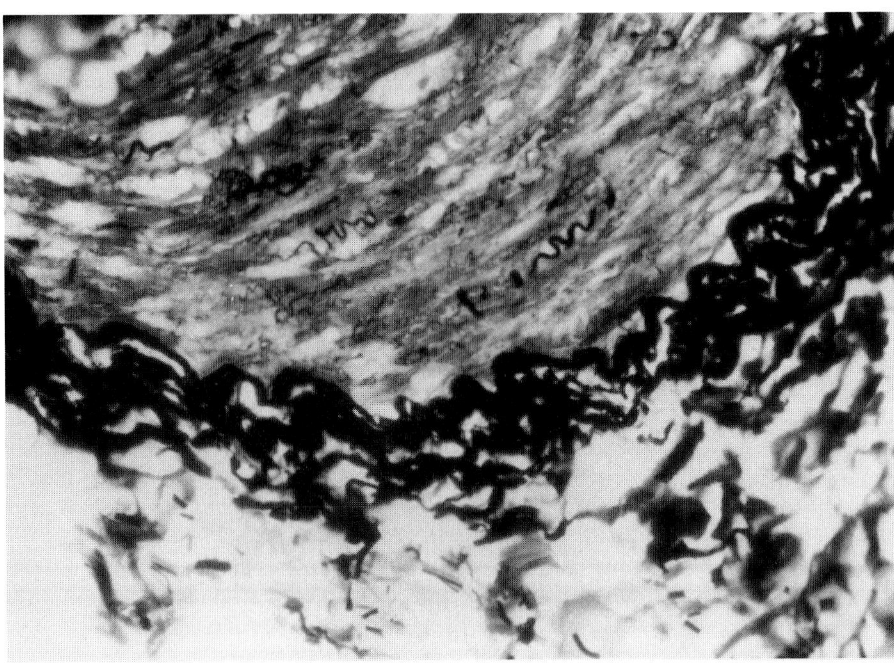

FIGURE 2-30. Media of a medium-sized artery showing fragmentation of elastic tissue (H&E, ×400). (Reprinted with permission from Joshi VV et al, reference 64.)

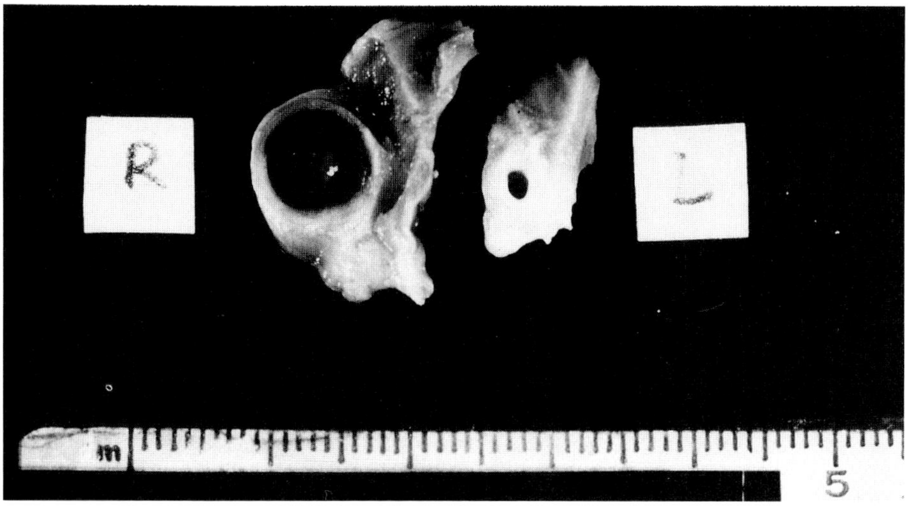

FIGURE 2-31. Aneurysm formation with thrombosis of right coronary artery; note the normal-sized left coronary artery for comparison.

conditions can be differentiated from the lesions seen in our cases on the basis of the size of the arteries involved, consistent involvement of coronary arteries, sparing of cerebral arteries, and absence of immunologic abnormalities in these two conditions. It was therefore suggested that the arterial lesions in pediatric AIDS constitute a distinctive arteriopathy.[64]

The pathogenesis of this arteriopathy is not clear. Elastic tissue injury may be the basic defect. Repeated infections secondary to immunodeficiency and resulting in increased exposure to endogenous and exogenous elastases may be contributory.[64] Recently Kure et al[65] demonstrated HIV antigens by immunocytochemical methods in aneurysmal cerebral arteries of a child with AIDS, suggesting the possibility of direct role of HIV in the pathogenesis of arteriopathy. Their observations need to be confirmed.

Renal Disease Associated with AIDS in Children

In some of our patients clinically significant renal disease was present.[66] These children had proteinuria, hypoalbuminemia, and edema. One patient had persistent azotemia. In two cases, renal disease was the first manifestation of HIV infection. Pathologic studies were performed on biopsy and autopsy specimens. Focal segmental glomerulosclerosis nad mesangial proliferative glomerulonephritis were demonstrated by light microscopy and confirmed by electron microscopy. Immunoglobulin and complement (C3) deposits were seen in all cases by immunofluorescent microscopy. Electron-dense material in mesangial, paramesangial, subendothelial, or intramembranous locations was present on electron microscopy. The glomerular endothelium and epithelium contained tubuloreticular structures in one case each. Similar clinicopathologic features have been described recently by Strauss et al[67] in 12 of 155 children with AIDS from Miami.

The pathogenesis of renal disease in children with AIDS is not known, but circulating immune complexes that are known to occur in these patients[68] may be involved. The recent demonstration of HIV antigen (p24) by monoclonal antibodies and HIV nucleic acid by in situ hybridization in the tubular and glomerular epithelial cells in renal biopsy specimens of adults with AIDS-associated renal disease indicates the possibility of a direct pathogenetic role of HIV.[69]

Neoplastic Disorders

Until 1990 we had seen 7 cases of neoplastic disorders (non-Hodgkin's malignant lymphoma of the brain, PBLD, Kaposi's sarcoma, and leiomyosarcomatosis of the GI tract) in a total of 102 consecutive cases of pediatric AIDS at Children's Hospital of New Jersey.[70,71] Since then two more cases of B-cell non-Hodgkin's lymphoma (NHL) (1 of kidney and 1 of lung) and a case of presacral leiomyosarcoma have been observed.[72] Mueller et al[73] have recently reviewed the various neoplastic disorders in children with AIDS reported in the literature and described three more cases of smooth muscle tumors. The precise incidence of neoplastic disorders in pediatric AIDS is not known. It appears to be less than that in adults with AIDS. However, it should be noted that the incidence in HIV infected children is much higher than in normal children. The total incidence of various types of neoplastic disorders was found to be 70,000 per million children with AIDS at Children's Hospital of New Jersey as compared with 124 per million normal children.[70] In the Italian multicenter study the incidence was found to be 1804 per million HIV-infected children.[74] Soft tissue sarcomas have an incidence of 8.4 per million children.[75,76] Leiomyosarcomas represent $<2\%$ of the soft tissue sarcomas in children.[71] The incidence of leiomyosarcoma is 3500 per million in HIV-infected children, compared to <0.16 per million in normal children.[71] The specific types of tumors known to occur in children with HIV infection and/or AIDS are given in Table 2-7.[77,78] It will be noted that B-cell lymphoproliferative disorders and smooth muscle tumors are the commonest in these children. Because of the occurrence of numerous cases of many of the neoplastic disorders listed in Table 2-7 in this selected population of children, it can be concluded that there is a true association between them and HIV infection. Those disorders (e.g., hepatoblastoma) (Table 2-7) of which only single cases have been reported may have occurred coincidentally in these children. Lymphoproliferative disorders have been described above in the section on associated lesions. Smooth muscle tumors, Kaposi's sarcoma and HPV-associated lesions are briefly discussed below.

Smooth Muscle Tumors. It is essential that the smooth muscle origin of the tumor be established by immunohistologic stain for muscle-specific actin and/or by ultrastructural features consisting of external lamina, abundant piocytotic vesicles, and intermediate filaments with dense bodies. Mitotic activity is used as a criterion for malignancy (Figure 2-32). Histoid reaction to *Mycobacterium avium*–intracellulare can produce a mass lesion consisting of fusiform to spindle-shaped cells and may be mistaken for a smooth muscle or other soft tissue neoplasm. Acid-fast stain for demonstration of the bacilli should be done in these cases (Figure 2-16).

Both leiomyoma and leiomyosarcomas have been described in children with AIDS (Table 2-7).[70–73,77] Most of the tumors arose in the viscera (Table 2-7). In

TABLE 2-7 Neoplastic Disorders in Children with AIDS

Type of disorder	No. of cases	Comment
Non-Hodgkin's malignant lymphoma	27	Extranodal sites (particularly brain) are more common; all lymphomas in which cell markers were done were B cell type; majority were Burkitt's lymphoma
Neoplastic angioendotheliomatosis (NAE)	1	NAE represents intravascular B cell lymphoma
Hodgkin's lymphoma	1	Hodgkin's lymphoma may be incidental
Acute lymphoblastic leukemia	5	These were of B-cell type
Polyclonal polymorphic B-cell lymphoproliferative disorder (PBLD)	4	In two of these cases PBLD represented progression of pulmonary lymphoid lesions, there was multiorgan involvement.
Leiomyoma/leiomyosarcoma	11	Mostly visceral sites (GI tract, lung, liver)
Kaposi's sarcoma (KS) of skin	6	KS is much less common in children than in adults with AIDS.
Kaposi's sarcoma, lymph node(s)	5	Many lymph node groups may be involved; most of these tumors have occurred in Haitian and African children
Condyloma acuminatum with or without dysplasia	3	Perianal and uterine cervix were sites of these human papilloma virus associated lesions
Fibrosarcoma of liver	1	Immunohistologic and ultrastructural studies to rule out smooth muscle origin of the tumor were not done
Embryonal rhabdomyosarcoma	1	Gallbladder was the probable site of origin
Hepatoblastoma	1	
Ewing's sarcoma of left fibula	1	Tumors occurring in single isolated cases may represent a coincidental occurrence
Total	67	

one of our cases[71] there were over 40 leiomyosarcomas involving the entire gastrointestinal tract from the stomach to the rectum. The original diagnosis was suspected in the endoscopic biopsy of the stomach (Figure 2-33). It appears that smooth muscle tumors (SMTs) are the second commonest neoplastic disorder in pediatric AIDS. SMTs have not been reported in adults with AIDS except for one case in a 23-year-old hemophiliac in whom the diagnosis of HIV infection was first made at the age of 15 years.[77] Leiomyosarcoma has been reported in renal transplant patients given immunosuppressive therapy.[77]

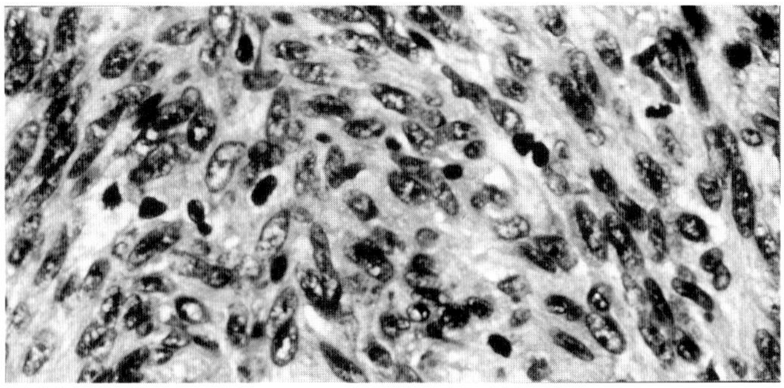

FIGURE 2-32. Leiomyosarcoma composed of fusiform cells arranged in vague bundles; note the mitotic figures (H&E, ×400).

Kaposi's Sarcoma (KS). The reported cases have occurred primarily in two sites: the skin and lymph nodes. The lymphadenopathic form was seen mostly in children born to Haitian parents and African children (Table 2-7) and probably represents the epidemic form of Kaposi's sarcoma unrelated to AIDS. The cutaneous form is a true indicator of disease related to AIDS. KS has also been reported in the liver, spleen, thymus, lung, and myocardium. Focus or foci of increased vascularity as part of reactive process in response to a variety of factors or apparent prominence of vascularity in the lymph nodes, thymus, and spleen due to marked cell depletion may be mistaken for KS.

HPV-Related Genital Lesions. Only three cases of HPV associated condylomatous lesions with or without dysplasia have been reported in children and adolescents with AIDS[79–81] (Table 2-7). In one of these cases (an 18-year-old female), the uterine cervix was the site of the lesion. The incidence of HPV in the

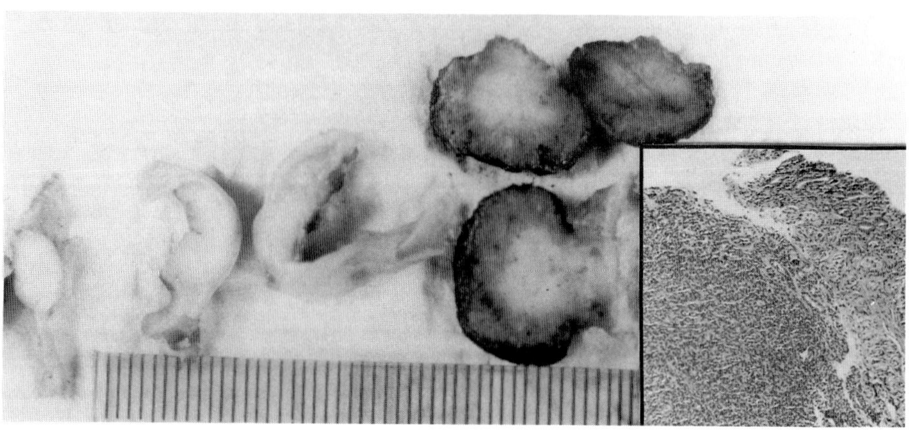

FIGURE 2-33. Multiple leiomyosarcomas of the gastrointestinal tract; inset shows the endoscopic gastric biopsy in which the presence of leiomyosarcoma was suspected (H&E, ×100).

genital tract of urban female adolescents is high.[82] With increasing incidence of HIV infection in adolescents in recent years and the possibility of HIV transmission via sexual abuse in children,[83] HPV related uterine cervical epithelial lesions are likely to become more prevalent in older children and adolescents.

Pathologic Features of HPV-Related Lesions and Their Progression. These lesions constitute a spectrum extending from condyloma acuminatum with minimal, mild, moderate, or severe dysplasia to cervical intraepithelial neoplasia (CIN). The progression of the dysplastic lesions and CIN eventually to invasive carcinoma, which occurs over a period of many years may be accelerated in immunosuppressed individuals. HPV-related cervical neoplasia is unlikely to be seen in pediatric AIDS but may be seen in young women with AIDS. However, the precursor lesions as described above are likely to be more prevalent in adolescent females with HIV infection and should be looked for and treated promptly, if diagnosed, so that their progression to malignancy is prevented.

Diagnosis of HPV-Related Genital Lesions. These lesions may be flat or papillary. Colposcopic magnification with application of acetic acid is necessary for the diagnosis of flat condylomas. On application of acetic acid, the flat lesions stand out as white slightly raised plaques. Cytologic examination and biopsy of the lesion establish the diagnosis. The morphologic hallmark of HPV-related genital lesions in the presence of koilocytotic atypia (Koilos = hollow or empty). Over 60 types of HPV have been delineated on the basis of DNA homology. Immunoperoxidase stains and in situ hybridization methods for detection of specific types of HPV (6/11 vs. 16/18) are available and are widely used. The types 6/11 are more often associated with benign and low-grade dysplastic lesions and 16/18 with higher-grade dysplastic and malignant lesions.

Thrombocytopenia

Thrombocytopenia has been observed in some of our recent cases of AIDS. Severe and rarely even fatal GI bleeding was seen in a few of these children. The pathogenesis of thrombocytopenia is not clear. Bone marrow examined in the biopsy and autopsy specimens shows an adequate to increased number of megakaryocytes. Hypersplenism and autoimmune mechanisms have been implicated. Platelet-associated antibodies were elevated in all pediatric AIDS cases with thrombocytopenia reported by Sandhaus and Scudder.[21] Zucker-Franklin et al[84] have shown structural damage of megakaryocytes characterized by an increased number of denuded nuclei and peripheral cytoplasmic blebbing seen on ultrastructural examination. The pathogenesis of the structural damage is not clear but the authors raised the possibility of HIV infection of megakaryocytes.

Lesions of Multifactorial Pathogenesis

Some of the lesions described above may have multifactorial pathogenesis. For example, villous atrophy of small intestine may be due to a combination of HIV enteropathy, inanition, and disuse atrophy. Thymic involution and dysinvolution may have added elements of stress as a pathogenetic factor. Wasting of tissues and organs may be due to inanition and occlusive arteriopathy.

Gastrointestinal and Hepatic Lesions

Besides the lesions mentioned above, several gastrointestinal and hepatic lesions deserve separate mention since they belong to several of the pathogenetic categories. These include severe gastrointestinal and hepatic involvement in opportunistic infections (e.g., CMV, MAI), segmental necrotizing jejunitis of undetermined pathogenesis,[85] massive GI bleeding related to thrombocytopenia, microscopic lymphoid infiltrates in the portal triads of the liver and submucosa of the intestines related to extranodal lymphoid hyperplasia, liver cirrhosis associated with TPN, fatty change, centrilobular necrosis of the liver related to heart failure associated with cardiomyopathy, and hepatitis B seen in biopsy, autopsy, and surgically resected specimens in our series. In addition, giant cell transformation, portal fibrosis, Kaposi's sarcoma, and chronic active hepatitis with predominance of T8 lymphocytes have been noted by other authors.[86–88]

Miscellaneous Lesions

The pathology of HIV-associated myopathy (HIVM) and AZT myopathy has been described adequately in the adults.[89] Inflammatory, degenerative and mitochondrial myopathic changes can occur in these patients. There is only one case report of AZT myopathy in a child with HIV infection.[90] In one of our cases we have seen involvement of the muscle in the lymphoproliferative disorder (PBLD), which may be mistaken for inflammatory HIVM. Pulmonary hypertension with plexiform arterial lesions has been reported in adults with AIDS.[91] We are not aware of any reports of pulmonary hypertension in pediatric AIDS. Further pathologic studies of the muscle and lungs would provide data that would be useful in increasing the awareness of the presence of these lesions in children with AIDS and in improving the understanding of their pathogenesis.

Besides systematic description of histologic features, pathologic studies should also include special procedures such as immunoperoxidase stains and in situ hybridization for components of HIV and other viruses. There is a tendency to implicate HIV in the pathogenesis of many of the lesions seen in the patients with AIDS. Such speculation is best avoided unless there are appropriate controls, thorough evaluations for other pathogens and substantial evidence for the implication.[92]

PERINATAL PATHOLOGY

Maternal Genital Tract

Pomerantz et al[93] studied cervical tissue from HIV-infected women. They found chronic cervicitis characterized by mononuclear cell infiltration and lymphoid aggregates in the mucosa and/or submucosa. HIV was isolated from these biopsy specimens, and HIV antigens were demonstrated in the mononuclear cells, endothelial cells, and lymphocytes. HIV has also been isolated from vaginal and cervical secretions of HIV-infected women.[94]

Placenta

Jauniaux and coworkers[95] studied 49 placentas, seven fetuses, and two stillbirths from central African and European HIV-positive women with or without full-blown AIDS. No villitis was noted in the placenta, but irrespective of gestational age, the villi were coarse, cellular, and hypovascularized. There was a high incidence of chorioamnionitis (42%). Ultrastructural studies revealed isolated retrovirus like particles with some morphologic similarities to HIV (100 n*M* in size, dense central or eccentric core) in the syncytiotrophoblast, fibroblasts, and endothelial cells of villous capillaries and free membranes in 5 of the 13 of the placentas. The authors pointed out that the viral particles seen in their cases also resembled the type c viral particles described in the syncytiotrophoblast of normal human term placenta. More recently Chandwani et al[96] have demonstrated HIV p24 antigen and nucleic acids in the trophoblast by immunoperoxidase method and in situ hybridization in 2 of 20 (10%) term placentas from HIV-infected mothers. Chorioamnionitis was seen in 60% of the 43 placentas examined histologically. Martin et al[97] found positive staining for p24 by immunoperoxidase method in the Hofbauer cells, vascular endothelium, and intermediate trophoblast in 4 of 9 (44%) placentas from HIV-positive women. Receptors for HIV, viz., CD4, are present on the trophoblastic and stromal cells of the chorionic villi and endothelial cells of the placental blood vessels.[98] HIV infection of first trimester placental tissue has been shown in the organ culture.[98] In contrast to these positive findings, Peuchmauer et al[99] failed to find HIV proteins by immunohistochemical method and nucleic acids by in situ hybridization in any of the 75 placentas from HIV-positive women. There is one report of culturing HIV from the placenta from an asymptomatic HIV-positive mother.[100] The details of how contamination with material blood was avoided at the time of obtaining placental material was not given, and the authors commented that the positive culture was probably the result of positive maternal blood culture.

Amniotic Fluid

There is one case report in which HIV has been cultured from and HIV antigens have been demonstrated in the amniotic fluid and amniotic cells.[101]

Fetal Tissues

Sprecher et al[102] and Jovaisas et al[16] found presence of HIV reverse transcriptase activity and antigens in various organs (thymus, brain, lung, and spleen) from a 15- and a 20-week-old fetus. These findings have been confirmed by Lyman et al,[103] Papiernik et al,[104] and Gourgnaud et al.[105] In situ hybridization, immunofluorescence, and polymerase chain reaction (PCR) techniques were used by these investigators. Viral DNA could be demonstrated in fetal tissues (thymus and spleen) in about 75% of the cases even when attempts at viral cultures from these tissues were unsuccessful.[105] Attempts at culturing HIV cord blood from fetuses of HIV-positive mothers have been unsuccessful.[106]

Pathologic Features of HIV-Positive Fetal Tissues

There is either absence of any pathologic findings or of any mention of pathologic study of the fetal tissues in most of the reports discussed above.[95,16,103] Focal lymphocytic depletion, infiltration by CD4 positive macrophages, increased density of epithelial cells, and thickening of lobular septa were found in the HIV-positive fetal thymuses by Papiernik et al.[104]

Mechanism and Timing of Fetal Infection

The results described above indicate that there are HIV receptors on the cells in the normal placentas (trophoblast, endothelium, stromal cells) and these cells are infectable by HIV. The frequency of HIV "infection" of the placenta varied from 0 to 44% in the different series.[95,96,99,105] The presence of HIV in the fetal tissues has been shown after 15 weeks of gestation. Fetal specimens from earlier gestations have not been tested. The brain and CD4 lymphocytes in the thymus and the spleen have been the primary sites of localization of HIV in the fetus. Cells expressing CD4 marker are detected in the thymus by 11 weeks' gestation.[107] Therefore, infection of fetal tissues is unlikely before 11 weeks' gestation.

Besides the infection of the placenta followed by that of the fetal tissues, other mechanisms of HIV transmission to the fetus include passive transfer during the maternal viremic phase, passage of infected CD4 lymphocytes from the mother, and active transport of HIV–immunoglobulin G complex.[99] It should be noted that in none of the known fetal infections (CMV, toxoplasmosis, syphilis, rubella, etc.) does passive transfer without infection of the placenta occur.

The low frequency of the localization of the virus in the placenta and the fetal tissues in some of the series[95,96,103,104] may be due to the low frequency of intrauterine transplacental maternofetal transmission of HIV in early pregnancy or to low sensitivity of the techniques other than PCR. The presence of HIV in the secretions and tissues of the maternal genital tract and the exposure of fetus to the maternal blood during delivery would support the intrapartum transmission of HIV. The failure of localization of HIV by in situ hybridization and PCR in 10 of 12 fetuses of HIV-positive mothers reported recently by Ehrnst et al[108] supports perinatal (i.e., at the time of delivery) HIV transmission as the more frequent mode.

Placental barrier may be effective in preventing viral transmission. But concurrent placental inflammation may compromise the integrity of the placental barrier.[109] Thus presence of other placental infections such as chorioamnionitis, which is commonly present in placentas from HIV-positive mothers or syphilis, may enhance the perinatal transmission of HIV. It is of interest to note that maternal–fetal transmission of HIV has been observed in a chimpanzee.[110]

Importance of Timing of HIV Maternal–Fetal Transmission

The transmission of HIV can occur (1) transplacentally during intrauterine life, (2) at the time of delivery, and (3) in the postpartum period (mainly via breast feeding). The timing is of importance from embryologic considerations.

The morphogenesis of various organs takes place between 4th and 8th or 9th weeks of gestation, which is referred to as the "embryonic period." Exposure to noxious influences (infection, nutritional deficiency, drugs, etc.) during the embryonic period may interfere with normal development of the organs.

The time sequence of the development of the thymus and HIV transmission is of interest from this point of view. As indicated above, HIV has been localized in the fetal thymus in isolated cases and morphologic abnormalities of the fetal thymus have been described.[102,104] Up to 8th week of gestation the thymic primordium is primarily epithelial. During the 9th week hematopoietic stem cells and lymphoid cells appear in the thymus. The differentiation into cortex and medulla start at 14 weeks and is complete by 17 weeks of gestation.[111] The observations on the thymic involvement in HIV infection have been made after 15 weeks of gestation. It will be of great importance to study the thymus in the abortuses during the embryonic period. If indeed the thymic injury occurs during the period of morphogenesis, there may be defective thymic development. Pathologic features which resemble thymic dysplasia are seen in some of the children with AIDS. This lesion, labeled as "thymic dysinvolution," suggests that the thymic injury may have occurred during the embryonic period.[5] If HIV transmission occurs during the perinatal period, the thymic injury would be of an acquired type, i.e., precocious involution, which is also seen in children with AIDS.[8,9]

The timing of HIV transmission and localization of HIV in different organs is also pertinent in the consideration of the pathologic lesions in the brain, lungs, and heart in children with AIDS. HIV has been localized in the fetal brain and lungs but not the heart.[16,102] Microcephaly in children with AIDS has been described by Marion et al,[112] although their findings were not confirmed by others.[113] Vogel and coauthors[114] observed congenital heart disease (valvular stenosis or atresia and septal defects) in 5 of a total of 175 children with HIV infection (2.8% incidence vs. 0.8% in general population, $p < .04$), raising the question of whether congenital infection contributed to these cardiac abnormalities. The localization of HIV in the fetal lung may be of significance in the consideration of pathogenesis of pulmonary lymphoid lesions in children.[34]

Another important aspect of perinatal pathology is the possible toxic effects of embryonic and fetal exposure to Zidovudine (AZT) given to HIV-infected mothers. To the best of my knowledge, no data regarding possible embryonic toxicity in man has been published. Toltzis et al have presented preliminary evidence of direct toxic effect of AZT on developing mouse embryo.[115] AZT given to pregnant mice was associated with significantly higher fetal wastage (abortions and resorption of fetus) ($p = .003$). The adult animals themselves did not show any toxic effects of AZT with respect to growth, appetite, activity, or ovarian histology. In vitro studies on fertilized oocytes demonstrated failure to develop to the blastocyst stage in increasing concentrations of AZT.

PATHOLOGY OF AIDS IN CHILDREN VERSUS THAT IN ADULTS

Certain differences emerge when the pathologic findings in children are compared with those in adults with AIDS. The thymic lesions are more severe and show a wider spectrum in children. The involvement of central nervous system (CNS) in children is more commonly due to HIV encephalopathy than to opportunistic infection (OI) of CNS. In contrast to children, adults show PLH/LIP complex rarely. The spectrum of neoplastic disorders is different in children. Lymphoproliferative disorders and SMTs constitute the more common neoplastic disorders in them; cutaneous Kaposi's sarcoma is extremely rare. Cardiomyopathy occurs in both children and adults, but arteriopathy has not been reported in adults. The spectrum of organisms producing OI is wider in adults than in children. Failure to thrive, progressive neurologic disease, and infection by pathogenic bacteria are more common in children. Certain differences in clinical and immunologic features are also notable. Peripheral lymphopenia is less common, whereas polyclonal hypergammaglobulinemia is more consistently present in children.

It is of interest to note that hemophiliac children who acquire HIV infection via transfusion differ from children with perinatally acquired HIV infection and also from hemophiliac adults with HIV infection.[116] PLH/LIP complex is much less common in hemophiliac children (5 vs. 48%), and lymphopenia and hypergammaglobulinemia are not as marked as in children with perinatally acquired HIV infection. PCP is less common in hemophiliac children than in hemophiliac adults with AIDS.

These differences may be related to the dose and timing of HIV infection, frequency of certain risk factors in the mother, the fact that the host is a developing and growing individual, environment and lifestyle of children, relatively greater chronicity of the disease process of AIDS, and sequence of HIV and certain other infections occurring in children (e.g., HIV followed by EBV infection in children in contrast to EBV followed by HIV infection in adults).

FUTURE DIRECTION OF PATHOLOGIC STUDY OF PEDIATRIC AIDS

Pathologic "Surveillance" of Pediatric AIDS

Although systematic and detailed pathologic study of every biopsy and autopsy in pediatric AIDS may not reveal any new features, rare cases may show atypical features of a previously described lesion, may shed light on the relationship between different lesions, or may show previously unreported lesions. Thus, for example, we have seen a case of atypical PLH/LIP as described above.

We have called the ongoing pathologic study of AIDS in children "pathologic surveillance,"[117] which should be continued in future. Pathologic surveillance enlarges the pathologic database of initial observations.[118,119] For example, arteriopathy, cardiomyopathy, and two of the three cases of SMTs described by Mueller et al[73] were detected at autopsy as unexpected findings.

Pathologic Study of Placentas, Abortions, and Fetal Deaths

As indicated above in the section on perinatal pathology, there is paucity of systematic pathologic study of perinatal material from abortions and fetal deaths. Multiinstitutional cooperative studies for collection of adequate number of cases should be conducted in future. Some of the ongoing prospective national studies on HIV infection in women and children have incorporated this aspect.

Pathologic Study of Neoplastic Disorders

Horowitz and Pizzo[120] recommended establishing a central registry of all neoplastic disorders in children with AIDS. A prospective multiinstitutional, multidisciplinary study of neoplastic disorders with emphasis on malignant lymphomas in children with AIDS [Pediatric AIDS Lymphoma Network (PALN)] is now in progress.* A central registry of histologic slides of the neoplastic disorders has also been started as part of the study. We urge all the pediatricians taking care of children with AIDS to participate fully in PALN.

It is estimated that there will be 6000–20,000 cases of pediatric AIDS in the next several years. The risk of developing NHL is considered to be about 5%. Thus 300–1000 cases of NHL are expected to occur within the next several years. The antiretroviral and anticancer treatments will be integrated in this prospective study.

CD-8 Lymphocytosis in Adults

The lymphoreticular neoplastic disorders occurring in adults with AIDS have also been described in children with AIDS. However, the diffuse infiltrative CD8 lymphocytosis syndrome characterized by parotid gland enlargement, sicca symptoms, and LIP described by Itescu et al[121] in adults has not been reported in children. The lymphoid infiltrates in PLH/LIP complex and PBLD consist predominantly of B cells. Predominance of CD8 lymphocytes among the T cells present in the bronchoalveolar lavage in children with PLH/LIP complex has been reported.[43] Detailed and systematic in situ and flow cytometric immunophenotyping of the lymphocytic infiltrates in various organs in the lymphoproliferative lesions need to be done in future.

Causes of Death in Children with AIDS

Kline et al[122] have recently analyzed their data on mortality in 21 cases of pediatric AIDS. Over 75% of their patients died of infections. *Pneumocystis carinii* was the cause of infection in half of these cases. In the remaining cases *Mycobacterium avium*–intracellulare, histoplasma, cryptococcus, cytomegalovirus, and streptococci were the causative organisms. Cardiomyopathy, renal failure, and GI hemorrhage were responsible in one case each (4.7%). In addition to the infections, we have seen neoplastic disorders (malignant lymphoma, disseminated Kaposi's sarcoma, and leiomyosarcomatosis) and GI hemorrhage due to probable GI involvement by Kaposi's sarcoma or to idiopathic thrombocytopenia as causes of death in our experience. Cardiomyopathy was responsi-

*Dr. Sharon B. Murphy, Director of Hematology/Oncology Division of the Children's Memorial Hospital in Chicago, is the Principal investigator of PALN. Her office will be able to provide all the information regarding registration of patients on Pediatric Oncology Group Protocol #9182 and the various types of samples (blood, tissue) to be sent and the methods of sending the samples.

ble for death in some of our patients. Arteriopathy was the cause of death in one case. Systematic analysis of causes of death in children with AIDS needs to be done.

Collection of Tissues for Special Studies

It is of great importance that samples (blood, tissue) be collected for appropriate molecular biologic and virologic studies related to HIV and other viruses and cell marker studies and be sent to appropriate laboratories if such studies cannot be done in the local institutions. Appropriate investigations conducted on these samples would be helpful in understanding the pathogenesis of previously described lesions and of new lesions. The requirements of the protocols of various ongoing national multiinstitutional studies on various aspects of pediatric AIDS would also be satisfied.

REFERENCES

1. Centers for Disease Control: Revision of the CDC surveillance case definition for AIDS. *MMWR* 36:1S–15S, 1987.
2. Centers for Disease Control: Classification system for HIV infection in children under 13 years of age. *MMWR* 36:225–236, 1987.
3. Centers for Disease Control: Revised classification system for HIV infection and expanded surveillance case definition for AIDS among adolescents and adults. *MMWR* 41:1–19, 1992.
4. World Health Organization. Provisional WHO clinical case definition for AIDS. *Wkly Epidemiol Rec* 10:72–73, 1986.
5. Joshi VV, Oleske JM, Connor EM: Morphologic findings in children with AIDS. Pathogenesis and clinical implications. *Pediatr Pathol* 10:155–165, 1990.
6. Joshi VV, Oleske JM, Minnefor AB, et al: Pathologic pulmonary findings in children with the acquired immunodeficiency syndrome: A study of ten cases. *Hum Pathol* 16:241–246, 1985.
7. Joshi VV, Kauffman S, Oleske JM, et al: Polyclonal polymorphic B-cell lymphoproliferative disorder with prominent pulmonary involvement in children with acquired immune deficiency syndrome. *Cancer* 59:1455–1462, 1987.
8. Joshi VV, Oleske JM: Pathologic appraisal of the thymus gland in acquired immunodeficiency syndrome in children. A study of four cases and a review of the literature. *Arch Pathol Lab Med* 109:142–146, 1985.
9. Joshi VV, Oleske JM, Saad S, et al: Thymus biopsy in children with acquired immunodeficiency syndrome. *Arch Pathol Lab Med* 110:837–842, 1986.
10. Rubinstein A, Novick BE, Sicklick MJ, et al: Circulating thymulin and thymosin-alpha 1 activity in pediatric acquired immune deficiency syndrome: In vivo and in vitro studies. *J Pediatr* 109:422–427, 1986.
11. Pizzo PA, Eddy J, Falloon J, et al: Effect of continuous intravenous infusion of zidovudine (AZT) in children with symptomatic HIV infection. *N Engl J Med* 319:889–896, 1988.
12. Dubin G, Braffman MN: Zidovudine-induced hepatotoxicity. *Ann Intern Med* 1989;110:85–86.
13. Martin LS, Loskoski SL, McDougal JS: Inactivation of human T-lymphotropic virus type III/lymphadenopathy-associated virus by formaldehyde-based reagents. *Appl Environ Microbiol* 53:708–709, 1987.

14. Joshi VV, Oleske JM, Minnefor AB, et al: Pathology of suspected acquired immune deficiency syndrome in children: A study of eight cases. *Pediatr Pathol* 2:71–87, 1984.
15. Gallo RC, Salahuddin SZ, Popovic M, et al: Frequent detection and isolation of cytopathic retroviruses (HTLV-III) from patients with AIDS and at risk for AIDS. *Science* 224:500–503, 1984.
16. Jovaisas E, Koch MA, Schafer A, et al: LAV/HTLV-III in 20-week fetus [letter]. *Lancet* 2:1129, 1985.
17. Numazaki K, Bai XQ, Goldman H, et al: Infection of cultured human thymic epithelial cells by human immunodeficiency virus. *Clin Immunol Immunopathol* 51:185–195, 1989.
18. Ward JM, OLery TJ, Baskin GB, et al: Immunohistochemical localization of human and simian immunodeficiency viral antigens in fixed tissue sections. *Am J Pathol* 127:199–205, 1987.
19. Dupuy JM, Gilmore N, Goldman HY, et al: Thymic epithelial cell transplantation in patients with AIDS: Evidence for infection by HIV-1 of newly differentiated T cells at the site of transplantation. *Thymus* 17:205–218, 1991.
20. Suster S, Rosai J: Multilocular thymic cyst: An acquired reactive process. *Am J Surg Pathol* 15:388–398, 1991.
21. Sandhaus LM, Scudder R: Hematologic and bone marrow abnormalities in pediatric patients with human immunodeficiency (HIV) infection. *Pediatr Pathol* 9:277–288, 1989.
22. Connor E, Morrison S, Boland M, et al: Children's Hospital AIDS program (CHAP): 1. Demographic and clinical data 1984–1986. In *Proceedings of the Third International Conference on AIDS* (Washington, DC, June 1987) (abstract), p 37.
23. Epstein LG, Sharer LR, Joshi VV, et al: Progressive encephalopathy in children with acquired immune deficiency syndrome. *Ann Neurol* 17:488–496, 1985.
24. Sharer LR, Epstein LG, Cho ES, et al: Pathologic features of AIDS encephalopathy in children: Evidence for LAV/HTLV-III infection of brain. *Hum Pathol* 17:271–284, 1986.
25. Sharer LR, Cho E, Epstein LG: Multinucleated giant cells and HTLV-III in AIDS encephalopathy. *Hum Pathol* 16:760, 1985.
26. Shaw GM, Harper ME, Hahn BH, et al: HTLV-III infection in brains of children and adults with AIDS encephalopathy. *Science* 227:177–182, 1985.
27. Stoler MH, Eskin TA, Benn S, et al: Human T cell lymphotropic virus type III infection of the central nervous system. A preliminary in situ analysis. *JAMA* 256:2360–2364, 1986.
28. Sharer LR: AIDS virus and the brain. *West J Med* 146:88, 1987.
29. Ho DD, Pomerantz RJ, Kaplan JC: Pathogenesis of infection with human immunodeficiency virus. *N Engl J Med* 317:278–286, 1987.
30. Petito CK, Navia BA, Cho ES, et al: Vacuolar myelopathy pathologically resembling subacute combined degeneration in patients with the acquired immunodeficiency syndrome. *N Engl J Med* 312:874–879, 1985.
31. Ullrich R, Zeitz M, Heise W, et al: Small intestinal structure and function in patients infected with human immunodeficiency virus (HIV). *Ann Intern Med* 111:15–21, 1989.
32. Nelson JA, Wiley CA, Reynolds-Kohler C, et al: Human immunodeficiency virus detected in epithelium from patients with gastrointestinal symptoms. *Lancet* 1:259–262, 1988.
33. Yolken RH, Li S, Perman J, et al: Persistent diarrhea and fecal shedding of retroviral nucleic acids in children infected with HIV. *J Inf Dis* 164:61–66, 1992.
34. Joshi VV: Pathologic findings associated with HIV infection in children. In *Pediatric*

AIDS—the challenge of HIV infection in infants, children and adolescents (Pizzo PA, Wilfert CM, Eds). Williams & Wilkins, Baltimore, 1991, Chap 8, pp 113–119.
35. Joshi VV, Oleske JM, Saad S, et al: Pathology of opportunistic infections in children with acquired immune deficiency syndrome. *Pediatr Pathol* 6:145–150, 1986.
36. Jura E, Chadwick EG, Josephs SH, et al: Varicella-zoster virus infections in children infected with human immunodeficiency virus. *Pediatr Infect Dis J* 8:586–590, 1989.
37. Bye MR, Bernstein L, Shah K, et al: Diagnostic bronchoalveolar lavage in children with AIDS. *Pediatr Pulmonol* 3:425–428, 1987.
38. Roth RI, Owen RL, Keren DF: AIDS with Mycobacterium avium-intracellulare lesions resembling those of Whipple's disease. *N Engl J Med* 309:1324, 1983.
39. Wood C, Nickoloff BJ, Todes-Taylor NR: Pseudotumor resulting from atypical mycobacterial infection: A "histoid" variety of Mycobacterium avium-intracellulare complex infection. *Am J Clin Pathol* 83:524–527, 1985.
40. Joshi VV: Systemic lymphoproliferative lesions in children with AIDS. *Pediatr AIDS HIV Inf Fet Adolesc* 1:44–48, 1990.
41. Joshi VV: Pathology of childhood AIDS. Ped Clin N Am 38:97–119, 1991.
42. Joshi VV, Oleske JM: Pulmonary lesions in children with the acquired immunodeficiency syndrome: A reappraisal based on data in additional cases and follow-up study of previously reported cases [letter]. *Hum Pathol* 17:641–642, 1986.
43. Boccon-Gibod L, Sacre JP, Just J, et al: Lymphoid interstitial pneumonia in children with AIDS or AIDS-related complex (ARC). *Pediatr Pathol* 5:238–239, 1986 (abstract).
44. Oleske JM, Denny T, Joshi VV: Unpublished data, 1985.
45. Morrison S, Connor E, Marquis J, et al: Predictive value of chest x-rays (CXR) for lymphocytic interstitial pneumonitis (LIP)/desquamative interstitial pneumonitis (DIP) in pediatric patients with AIDS. In *Proceedings of III International Conference on AIDS* (Washington, DC, June 1987) (abstract), p 108.
46. Joshi VV: Unpublished data, 1990.
47. Joshi VV, Morrison S, Connor EM, et al: Pulmonary pathology of AIDS in children. In *Pediatric Pulmonary disease* (Stocker JT, Ed). Hemisphere Publishing, New York, 1989, Chap 6, pp 181–206.
48. Epstein LG, DiCarlo FJ Jr, Joshi VV, et al: Primary lymphoma of the central nervous system in children with acquired immunodeficiency syndrome. *Pediatrics* 82:355–363, 1988.
49. Andiman WA, Eastman R, Martin K, et al: Opportunistic lymphoproliferations associated with Epstein-Barr viral DNA in infants and children with AIDS. *Lancet* 2:1390–1393, 1985.
50. Montagnier L, Gruest J, Chamaret S, et al: Adaptation of lymphadenopathy associated virus (LAV) to replication in EBV-transformed B lymphoblastoid cell lines. *Science* 225:63–66, 1984.
51. Salahuddin SZ, Rose RM, Groopman JE, et al: Human T lymphotropic virus type III infection of human alveolar macrophages. *Blood* 68:281–284, 1986.
52. Lairmore MD, Rosadio RH, DeMartini JC: Ovine lentivirus lymphoid interstitial pneumonia. Rapid induction in neonatal lambs. *Am J Pathol* 125:173–181, 1986.
53. Lairmore MD, Poulson JM, Adducci TA, et al: Lentivirus-induced lymphoproliferative disease. Comparative pathogenicity of phenotypically distinct ovine lentivirus strains. *Am J Pathol* 130:80–90, 1988.
54. Chalifoux LV, King NW, Daniel MD, et al: Lymphoproliferative syndrome in an immunodeficient rhesus monkey naturally infected with an HTLV-III-like virus (STLV-III). *Lab Invest* 55:43–50, 1986.
55. Letvin NL, King NW: Immunologic and pathologic manifestations of the infection of

rhesus monkeys with simian—immunodeficiency virus of macaques. *J Acquir Immune Defic Syndr* 3:1023–1040, 1990.
56. Rubinstein A. Pediatric AIDS. *Curr Probl Pediatr* 16:361–409, 1986.
57. Joshi VV, Gadol C, Connor E, et al: Dilated cardiomyopathy in children with acquired immunodeficiency syndrome: A pathologic study of five cases. *Hum Pathol* 19:69–73, 1988.
58. Woodruff JF: Viral myocarditis. A review. *Am J Pathol* 101:425–484, 1980.
59. Herskowitz A, Amari SS, Neumann DA: Cardiomyopathy in AIDS. Evidence for autoimmunity. *Circulation* 89:322a, 1989 (abstract).
60. Beschorner WE, Baughman K, Turnicky KP, et al: HIV-Associated myocarditis. *Am J Pathol* 137:1365–1371, 1990.
61. Calabrese LH, Proffitt MR, Yen-Lieberman B, et al: Congestive cardiomyopathy and illness related to AIDS associated with isolation of retrovirus from the myocardium. *Ann Intern Med* 107:691–692, 1987.
62. Dworkin BM, Antonecchia PP, Smith F, et al: Reduced cardiac selenium content in AIDS. *J Parenter Enteral Nutr* 13:644–647, 1989.
63. Bharati S, Joshi VV, Connor EM, et al: Conduction system in children with acquired immunodeficiency syndrome. *Chest* 96:406–413, 1989.
64. Joshi VV, Pawel B, Connor E, et al: Arteriopathy in children with acquired immune deficiency syndrome. *Pediatr Pathol* 7:261–275, 1987.
65. Kure K, Kim TS, Park YD, et al: Immunocytochemical localization of an HIV epitope in cerebral aneurysmal arteriopathy in pediatric AIDS. *Pediatr Pathol* 9:655–667, 1989.
66. Connor E, Gupta S, Joshi V, et al: Acquired immunodeficiency syndrome-associated renal disease in children. *J Pediatr* 113:39–44, 1988.
67. Strauss J, Abitbol C, Zilleruelo G, et al: Renal disease in children with the acquired immunodeficiency syndrome. *N Engl J Med* 321:625–630, 1989.
68. Calvelli TA, Rubinstein A: Intravenous gamma-globulin in infant acquired immunodeficiency syndrome. *Pediatr Infect Dis J* 5:S207–210, 1986.
69. Cohen AH, Sun NC, Shapshak P, et al: Demonstration of human immunodeficiency virus in renal epithelium in HIV-associated nephropathy. *Mod Pathol* 2:125–128, 1989.
70. Joshi VV, Connor EM, Dicarlo F: Neoplastic diseases in children with AIDS (Abstr TBP 259). In *Proceedings of Vth International Conference on AIDS* (Montreal, Canada, 1989) (abstract), p 330.
71. Chadwick EG, Connor EM, Harrison CG, et al: Tumors of smooth muscle origin in HIV infected children. *JAMA* 263:3182–3184, 1990.
72. Dicarlo FJ, Oleske JM, Connor EM: Personal communication, 1992.
73. Mueller BV, Butler KM, Hingham MC, et al: Smooth muscle tumors in children with HIV infection. *Pediatrics* 90:460–462, 1992.
74. Arico M, Caselli D, Argenio D, et al: Malignancies in children with HIV type 1 infection. *Cancer* 68:2473–2477, 1991.
75. Young JL Jr, Miller RW: Incidence of malignant tumors in U.S. children. *J Pediatr* 86:254–258, 1975.
76. Miller RW: Frequency and environmental epidemiology of childhood cancer. In *Principles and practice of pediatric oncology* (Pizzo PA, Poplack DG, Eds). Lippincott, Philadelphia, 1989, Chap 1, pp 3–18.
77. Joshi VV: Pathology of AIDS in children: Overview, update and future direction. *Ann NY Acad Sci* (in press).
78. Lyall EGH, Langdale-Brown B, Eden OB, et al: Ewing's sarcoma in a child with HIV (type 1) infection. *Med Pediatr Oncol* 21:127–131, 1993.
79. Larague D: Severe anogenital warts in a child with HIV infection. *N Engl J Med* 320:1220–1221, 1988.

80. Henry MJ, Stanley MW, Cruihshank S, et al: Association of HIV-induced immunosuppression with human papilloma virus infection and cervical intraepithelial neoplasia. *Am J Obstet Gynecol* 160:352–353, 1988.
81. Forman AB, Prendiville JS: Association of HIV seropositivity and extensive perineal condylomata in a child. *Arch Dermatol* 124:1010–1011, 1988.
82. Shafer MAB, Moscick AB: Sexually transmitted diseases: In *Rudolph's pediatrics* (Rudolph AM, Ed), 19th ed. Appleton & Lange, Norwalk, CT, 1987, Chap 4, pp 71–81.
83. Gutman LT, St. Claire KK, Weedy C, et al: HIV transmission by child sexual abuse. *Am J Dis Child* 145:137–141, 1991.
84. Zucker-Franklin D, Termin CS, Cooper MC: Structural changes in the megakaryocytes of patients infected with the human immune deficiency virus (HIV-1). *Am J Pathol* 134:1295–1303, 1989.
85. McLoughlin LC, Nord KS, Joshi VV, et al: Severe gastrointestinal involvement in children with the acquired immunodeficiency syndrome. *J Pediatr Gastroenterol Nutr* 6:517–524, 1987.
86. Jonas MM, Roldan EO, Lyons HJ, et al: Histopathologic features of the liver in pediatric acquired immune deficiency syndrome. *J Pediatr Gastroenterol Nutr* 9:73–81, 1989.
87. Witzleben CL, Marshall GS, Wenner W, et al: HIV as a cause of giant cell hepatitis. *Hum Pathol* 19:603–605, 1988.
88. Kahn E, Greco MA, Daum F, et al: Hepatic pathology in pediatric AIDS. *Hum Pathol* 22:1111–1119, 1991.
89. Dalakas MC, Pezeshkapour GH: Neuromuscular diseases associated with HIV infection. *Ann Neurol* 235:38–48, 1988.
90. Walter EB, Drucker RP, McKinney RE, et al: Myopathy in HIV-infected children receiving long-term zidovudine therapy. *J Pediatr* 119:152–155, 1991.
91. Polos PG, Wolfe D, Harley RA, et al: Pulmonary hypertension and HIV infection: Two reports and a review of the literature. *Chest* 101:474–478, 1992.
92. Bartlett JG, Belitsos PC, Sears CL: AIDS enteropathy. *Clin Infect Dis* 15:726–735, 1992.
93. Pomerantz RJ, de-la-Monte SM, Donegan SP, et al: Human immunodeficiency virus (HIV) infection of the uterine cervix. *Ann Intern Med* 108:321–327, 1988.
94. Wofsy CB, Cohen JB, Hauer LB: Isolation of AIDS-associated retrovirus from genital secretions of women with antibodies to the virus. *Lancet* 1:527–529, 1986.
95. Jauniaux E, Nessmann C, Imbert MC, et al: Morphological aspects of the placenta in HIV pregnancies. *Placenta* 9:633–642, 1988.
96. Chandwani S, Greco MA, Mittal K, et al: Pathology and human immunodeficiency virus expression in placentas of seropositive women. *J Inf Dis* 163:1134–1138, 1991.
97. Martin AW, Brady K, Smith SI, et al: Immunohistochemical localization of human immunodeficiency virus p24 antigen in placental tissue. *Hum Pathol* 23:411–414, 1992.
98. Maury W, Potts BJ, Robson AB: HIV-1 infection of first trimester and term human placental tissue: A possible mode of maternal-fetal transmission. *J Inf Dis* 160:583–588, 1989.
99. Peuchmaur M, Delfraissy JF, Pons JC, et al: HIV proteins absent from placentas of 75 HIV-1 positive women studied by immunohistochemistry. *AIDS* 5:741–745, 1991.
100. Hill WC, Bolton V, Carlson JR: Isolation of AIDS virus from the placenta. *Am J Obstet Gynecol* 157:10–11, 1987.
101. Mundy DC, Schinazi RF, Gerber AR, et al: HIV isolated from amniotic fluid. *Lancet* 2:459–460, 1987.
102. Sprecher S, Soumenkoff S, Puissant F, et al: Vertical transmission of HIV in 15 week fetus. *Lancet* 2:288, 1986.

103. Lyman WD, Kress Y, Kure K, et al: Detection of HIV in fetal central nervous system tissue. *AIDS* 4:917–920, 1990.
104. Papiernik M, Brossard Y, Mulliez N, et al: Thymic abnormalities in fetuses aborted from HIV type 1 seropositive women. *Pediatrics* 89:297–301, 1992.
105. Gourgnaud V, Laure F, Brossard A: Frequent and early in utero HIV-1 infection. *AIDS Res Hum Retroviruses* 7:337–341, 1991.
106. Daffos F, Forestier F, Mandelbrot A, et al: Prenatal diagnosis of HIV infection: Two attempts using fetal blood sampling. *J Acquir Immune Defic Syndr* 2:205–207, 1989.
107. Kamps WA, Cooper MD: Development of lymphocyte subpopulations identified by monoclonal antibodies in human fetuses. *J Clin Immunol* 4:36–39, 1984.
108. Ehrnst A, Lindgren S, Dictor M, et al: HIV in pregnant women and their offspring—evidence for late transmission. *Lancet* 338:203–207, 1991.
109. Borkowsky W, Krasinski K: Perinatal human immunodeficiency virus infection: Ruminations on mechanisms of transmission and methods of intervention. *Pediatrics* 90:133–136, 1992.
110. Eichberg JW, Lee DR, Allan JS, et al: In utero infection of an infant chimpanzee with HIV. *N Engl J Med* 319:722–723, 1988.
111. Gaudecker BV, Muller-Hermelink HK (Ed): The development of human thymus microinvolvement. In *The human thymus. Histophysiology and pathology*. Springer-Verlag, Berlin, 1986, pp 1–41.
112. Marion RW, Wiznia AA, Hutcheon RG, et al: Fetal AIDS syndrome score: Correlation between severity of dysmorphism and age at diagnosis of immunodeficiency. *Am J Dis Child* 141:429–431, 1987.
113. Qazi QH, Sheikh TM, Fikrig S, et al: Lack of evidence for cranifacial dysmorphism in perinatal HIV infection. *J Pediatr* 112:7–11, 1988.
114. Vogel RL, Alboliras ET, McSherry GD, et al: Congenital heart defects in children with HIV positive mothers. *Circulation* 78:II–17, 1988 (abstract).
115. Toltzis P, Marx CM, Kleinman N, et al: Zidovudine-associated embryonic toxicity in mice. *J Inf Dis* 163:1212–1218, 1991.
116. Jason JM, Stehr-Green J, Hohman RC: Human immunodeficiency virus in hemophiliac children. *Pediatrics* 82:565–570, 1988.
117. Joshi VV: Pathologic surveillance of pediatric HIV infection: Importance of biopsies and autopsies. *Pediatr AIDS HIV Infect Fetus Adolesc* 1:9–10, 1990.
118. Oleske J, Minnefor A, Cooper R, et al: Immune deficiency in children. *JAMA* 249:2345–2349, 1983.
119. Rubinstein A, Sicklick M, Gupta A, et al: Acquired immunodeficiency with reversed T4/T8 ratios in infants born to promiscuous and drug-addicted mothers. *JAMA* 249:2350–2356, 1983.
120. Horowitz ME, Pizzo PA: Cancer in the child infected with human immunodeficiency virus. *J Pediatr* 116:730–731, 1990.
121. Itescu S, Brancato LJ, Buxbaum J, et al: A diffuse infiltrative CDS lymphocytosis syndrome in human immunodeficiency virus (HIV) infection: A host immune response associated with HLA-DR5. *Ann Intern Med* 112:3–10, 1990.
122. Kline MW, Bohannon B, Kozinetz CA, et al: Characteristics of human immunodeficiency virus-associated mortality in pediatric patients with vertically transmitted infection. *Pediatr Infect Dis J* 11:676–677, 1992.

3 NEONATAL RESPIRATORY DISTRESS SYNDROME

INTRODUCTION

Neonatal respiratory distress syndrome (NRDS) is also known as "neonatal hyaline membrane disease." The former term is preferred since hyaline membranes are not present in the very early stages and do not play a primary role in the pathogenesis of the syndrome. Therapy with mechanical ventilation and oxygen has modified the natural history of NRDS as described below and shown in Figure 3-1. Therapeutic application of the pulmonary surfactant which took 30 years to develop[1] since the demonstration of surfactant deficiency in NRDS by Avery and Mead in 1959[2] may make a further impact on the natural history. NRDS at its various stages continues to be a significant lesion in the neonatal autopsies. Therefore, knowledge of the natural history, advances in therapy and of the impact of therapy on the natural history is essential for intelligent interpretation of pathologic findings in autopsies on infants who die at various times after the onset of the syndrome and in some instances even *before* its clinically recognizable onset.

INCIDENCE AND CLINICAL FEATURES

NRDS is a disease of prematurity. The incidence of prematurity is about 8%. About 14% of all premature infants and 1% of all liveborn infants develop NRDS. Maternal diabetes and elective cesarean sections are additional risk factors. Exceptional cases are seen at 37 weeks of gestation or beyond. The syndrome occurs throughout the world. Approximately 40,000 cases occur in the United States every year. Despite the reduction in mortality from about 30% in 1977 to less than 15% in 1985, about 6,000 infants die of NRDS every year in the United States.

Many of the infants who develop NRDS have had intrapartum depression with resuscitation being necessary at birth. Characteristically the syndrome has its onset a few hours after birth. However, the initially healthy appearing infant may exhibit tachypnea from the first minutes after birth. As described below pathologic changes precede the full-fledged clinical manifestations of the acute stage. Full-blown NRDS is characterized by chest retraction, grunting, cyanosis and characteristic chest x-ray findings (granular pattern and increase in the pulmonary density with airbronchograms).

NATURAL HISTORY OF NRDS AND ITS PATHOLOGIC IMPLICATIONS

The clinical picture reaches the peak within 3 days, following which there is gradual recovery in those infants who survive. In most fatal cases, the death occurs within the first 3 days. However, with the introduction of mechanical ventilation and oxygen therapy some of these infants who would have otherwise died survive for longer periods of time.[3] This prolongation and modification of natural history of NRDS is represented diagrammatically in Figure 3-1.

Recovery may be slower due to prolongation of healing stage and superimposed oxygen toxicity. Many of these infants ultimately recover but others die in the healing stage or go on to develop a chronic pulmonary disease labelled bronchopulmonary dysplasia (BPD) usually after one month of age although it can be seen earlier. BPD is seen in infants who require mechanical ventilation at high pressures (>35 cm of water) and high oxygen concentration (>40%) for relatively prolonged periods of time. Following the healing stage and before the development of BPD a transition stage is recognized between 10 and 20 days after the onset of the syndrome. Radiologic stages characterized by granular pattern (stage I), white-out of the lungs (stage II), bubbly pattern with multiple cystic areas (stage III), and hyperinflation alternating with dense sharply outlined strands (stage IV) generally correlate well with the four pathologic stages shown in Figure 3-1, but disagreement by one or rarely more stages may occur. Pathologic stage is generally greater than the radiologic stage in these cases. In recent years natural history as seen radiographically and pathologically has been modified further. Specifically: (1) a larger number of infants have started surviving the acute stage; (2) radiologic stage II is less frequent, stage III is less clearly marked, and there is more insidious progression to stage IV; and (3) in the autopsy cases, frequency of acute stage of NRDS is reduced, the healing stage is less clearly marked and the florid pathologic changes of BPD are less frequently seen. This has happened largely because of the increasing experience of the neonatologists in the management of NRDS so that lower pressures and lower concentrations of oxygen are now generally used for shorter duration with earlier weaning off the respirator.

Pathologic changes occurring in each of these stages will be described separately for the purpose of convenience and better understanding. It is to be emphasized that these stages represent a systematized version of the probable

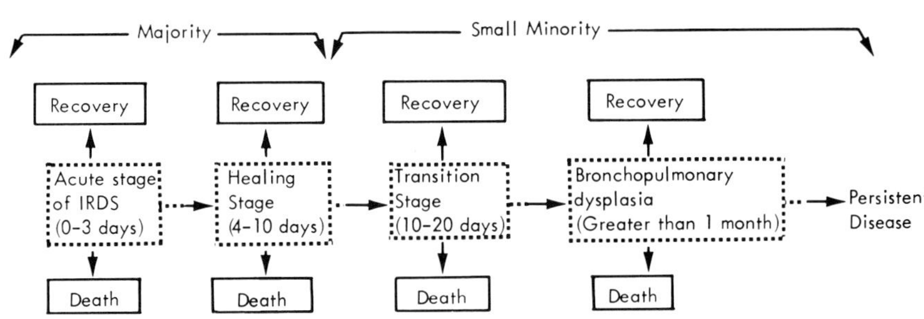

FIGURE 3-1. Diagrammatic representation of natural history NRDS modified by therapy.

sequence of events and not distinctive clinicopathologic entities. Some overlap between the time periods and between the pathologic changes in the different stages is to be expected and does occur in individual autopsy specimens. The description of the pathologic changes is based on the report by Northway et al[3] and personal experience of over 300 autopsy cases of NRDS[4] (Joshi VV: Unpublished data, 1991).

PROCESSING OF AUTOPSY SPECIMENS OF LUNGS IN NRDS

Since pattern of alveolar atelectasis and overdistension of terminal air passages (TAP) are diagnostic features of acute-stage NRDS (see below), fixation of lungs by perfusion through the blood vessels or respiratory tract is to be avoided. Such procedures will distort or destroy the characteristic pattern. The trachea and bronchi are left attached to the lungs. The lungs should be inspected and very lightly palpated. Deep transverse incisions are then made in the lung parenchyma by holding the lung by the main stem bronchus at the hilus and by using a new sharp scalpel blade. The lungs are then emersed in formalin for overnight fixation. Fixation in Kelly's fluid and Zenker's fixative may be used for demonstration of edema in the acute stage of NRDS. The lungs in all other stages of NRDS, including BPD, are processed similarly. The larynx is processed as described in the chapter on iatrogenic lesions. One section is made from each lobe of each lung (five sections).

PATHOLOGY OF DIFFERENT STAGES OF NRDS

Acute Stage (0–3 Days)

The knowledge of pulmonary pathologic changes in the acute-stage NRDS is almost exclusively derived from the autopsy study of patients dying during the first 3 days of life. It is generally presumed that similar but perhaps less severe pulmonary changes occur in those infants who ultimately recover fully. Grossly the lungs are usually uniformly red-purple and rubbery firm in consistency. There is diffuse loss of lobular markings. Focal loss of such markings and focal red-purple areas are seen in the very early stages (Figures 3-2A,B). In some cases the lungs may be tan in color. The rubbery firm consistency is however a consistent feature. The weight of the lungs is not significantly increased. The following are the main components of the pathologic lesion of acute-stage NRDS seen by light microscopy: atelectasis with dilatation of the terminal air passages (TAP), pulmonary edema, necrosis of epithelium of TAP and hyaline membranes lining exclusively or predominantly the TAP.

Atelectasis with Dilatation of TAP

There is diffuse alveolar atelectasis involving both the lungs uniformly. In contrast the TAP are dilated. The TAP include terminal bronchioles, respiratory bronchioles and alveolar ducts. This combination of atelectasis and dilatation produces a characteristic "Swiss cheese" pattern, which is best seen on a

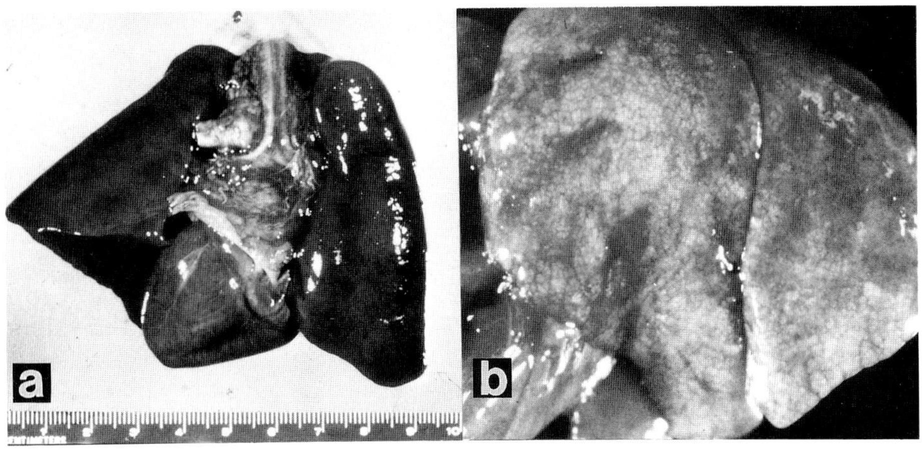

FIGURE 3-2. Gross appearance of lungs in acute stage of NRDS: (A) note the dark appearance of the lungs (due to red-purple color) and diffuse loss of lobular markings; (B) these features are focally present in the early phase of the acute stage.

low-power view of the section and is in marked contrast to the normal pattern of expansion in premature infants who do not have NRDS (Figures 3-3A,B). In the very early stages of NRDS the pattern of atelectasis with or without dilatation of TAP may be seen only focally. This pattern correlates with the gross findings (Figure 3-2B). Focal partial expansion related to mechanical ventilation of the alveoli may be seen in some sections but the predominant pattern is that of atelectasis.

Pulmonary Edema

Pulmonary edema of the TAP and interstitium is a consistent finding, particularly in the early phase of acute-stage NRDS.[5–7] However, it is difficult to

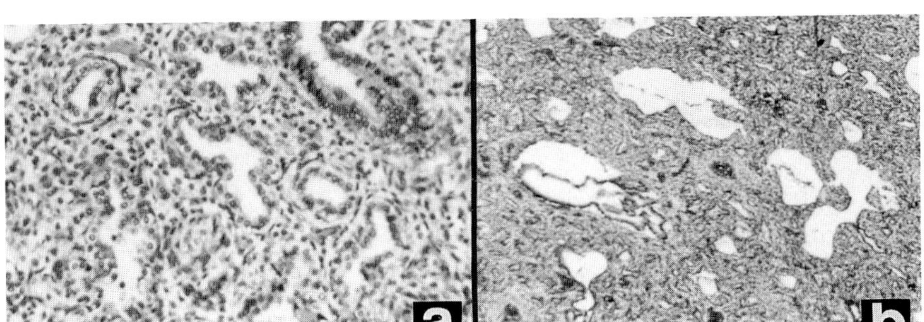

FIGURE 3-3. (A) Normal premature lung showing normal terminal bronchiole with intact epithelium and immature distended alveoli (H&E, ×100); (B) dilated terminal air passages (TAP) lined by hyaline membranes and atelectatic alveoli are seen in the acute stage (H&E, ×40).

demonstrate unless special fixatives such as Zenker's or Kelly's are used.[6,7] (Figure 3-4). It is possible that edema also involves the alveoli in the very early phase. But when atelectasis is fully developed, alveolar edema is not discernible.

Necrosis of Epithelium of TAP

The pyknotic nuclei of the necrotic epithelium, which may be focally piled up in several layers in some areas, may form plugs in the lumen or are incorporated in the hyaline membranes lining the TAP (Figure 3-5). These findings are best seen in the first 6–8 hours after onset of the disease. However, de la Monte et al[8] have shown that focal necrosis of TAP epithelium seldom accompanied by atelectasis can be demonstrated in infants surviving for 10 seconds to 4 hours. In my experience these foci of necrotic epithelium consist of a few pyknotic nuclei accompanied by variable degree of atelectasis (Figure 3-6). In such instances a pathologic diagnosis of early phase of the acute stage or preclinical incipient stage of NRDS is made, although characteristic clinical and radiologic features are not present.

Hyaline Membranes

The hyaline membranes are eosinophilic (Figure 3-7), although fine or clumped basophilic nuclear debris of necrotic epithelial lining of TAP is frequently present in the early stages (Figure 3-5). They are usually less than 50 μm in thickness. In occasional areas there may be thick clumps rather than membranes partially or even completely occluding the lumen of TAP (Figure

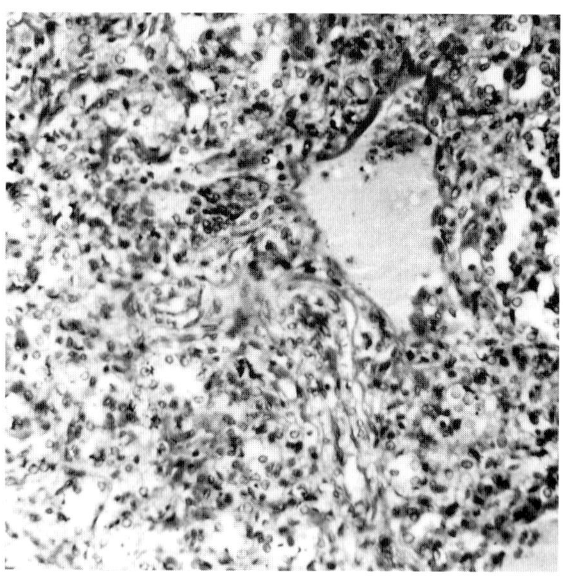

FIGURE 3-4. Pulmonary edema in the acute stage. Note the atelectatic alveoli. The edema involves a TAP. A hyaline membrane lining portion of the TAP is present (H&E, ×100).

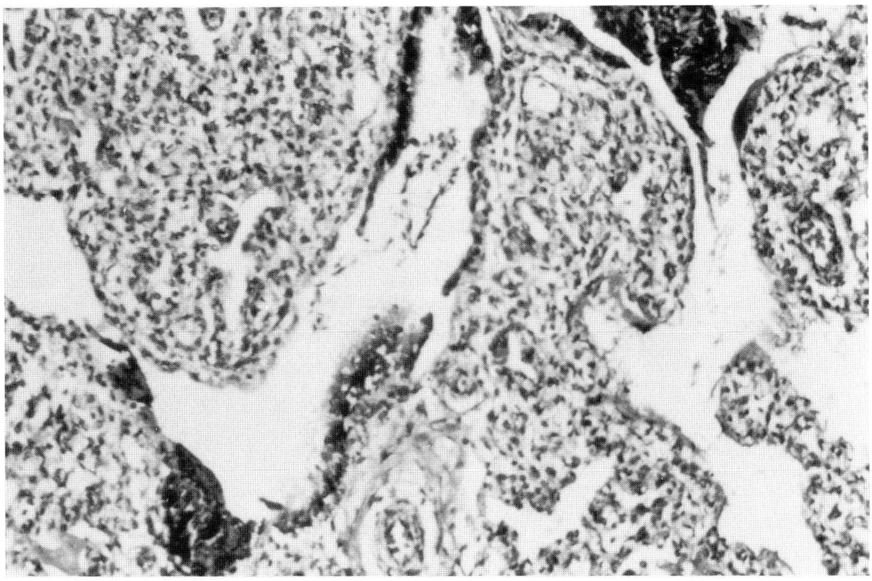

FIGURE 3-5. Dilated TAP showing necrotic epithelial lining with piled up pyknotic nuclei. Not focal presence of hyaline membranes and focal basophilic appearance of the hyaline membranes due to inclusion of nuclear debris (H&E, ×250).

3-8). It is important to note that the hyaline membranes are found predominantly or exclusively along the walls of TAP the epithelial lining of which is necrotic (Figure 3-7). In typical cases they are absent or rare along the alveolar septa. Various constituents including fibrin, hemoglobin-like compounds, amniotic debris, lipid, and mucoid material are present in the hyaline membranes. Hyaline membranes are generally not found in infants dying within a few hours (usually 2–4 hours) of onset of NRDS. Rarely the hyaline membranes may be yellow due to binding of unconjugated bilirubin.[9]

Other Components

These include pulmonary capillary and venous congestion, focal hemorrhage, and dilatation of the pulmonary lymphatics.[5] Pulmonary hemorrhage of varying degrees of severity is not infrequent in the acute stages of NRDS. Early features of healing stage of NRDS may be seen in the infants dying in the acute stage. For example, early evidence of regeneration of epithelium of TAP is not infrequently seen in the lungs of infants dying of NRDS 2–3 days after onset of the disease.

Electron Microscopic Changes

Besides the lesions seen by light microscopy as described above, the following ultrastructural changes have been reported.[5] The pulmonary capillaries show endothelial swelling and increased number of pinocytotic vesicles. The

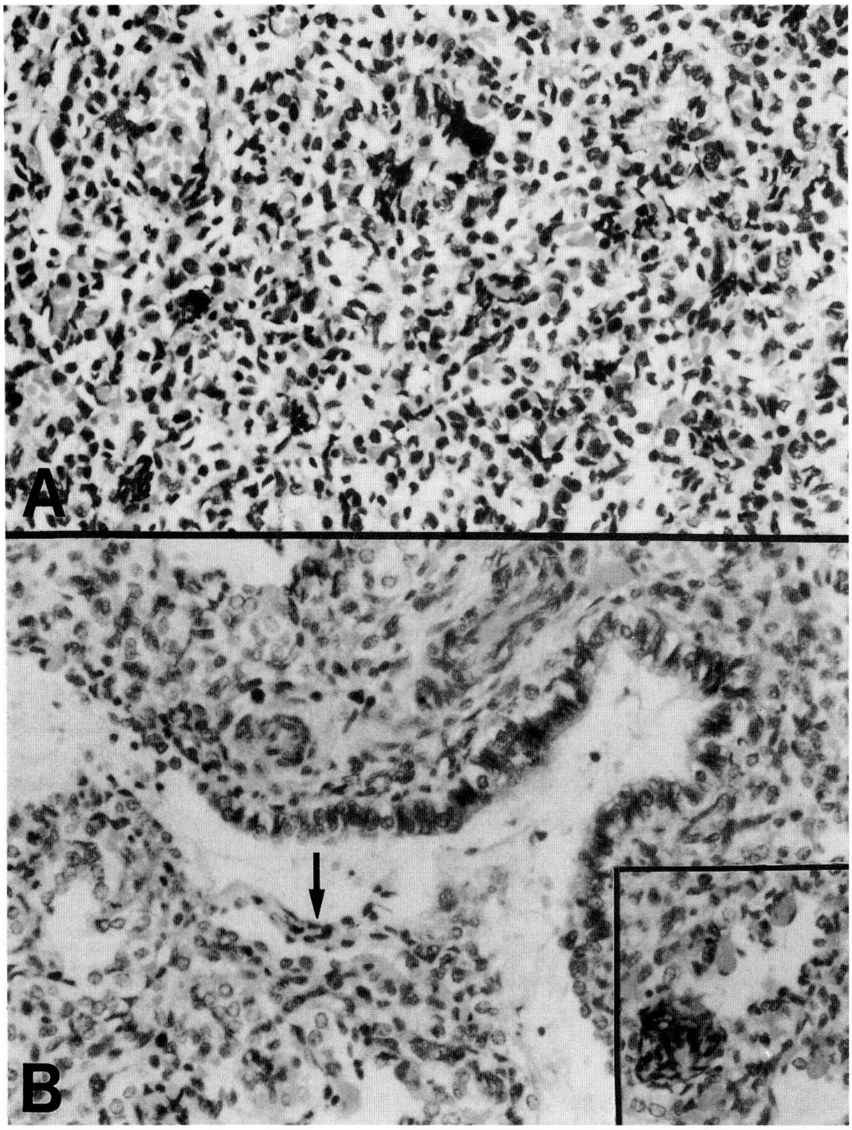

FIGURE 3-6. Necrosis of epithelium in "preclinical" stage. (A) Atelectasis of alveoli without dilatation of TAP—the pyknotic nuclei of the epithelium of TAP form darkly staining clusters (H&E, ×100); (B) slightly dilated TAP showing necrosis of the lining epithelium (arrow). The epithelium is sloughed off in some areas, while intact normal epithelium is seen in other areas. There is normally expanded alveolus. Note the cluster of pyknotic nuclei of TAP in the inset (H&E, ×250).

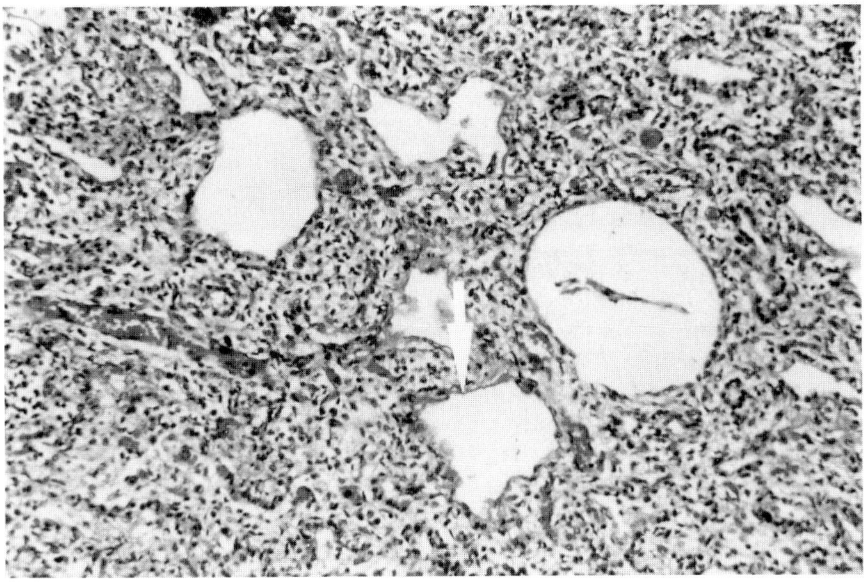

FIGURE 3-7. Note the dilated TAP lined by thin hyaline membranes (arrow). The alveoli are atelectatic (H&E, ×250).

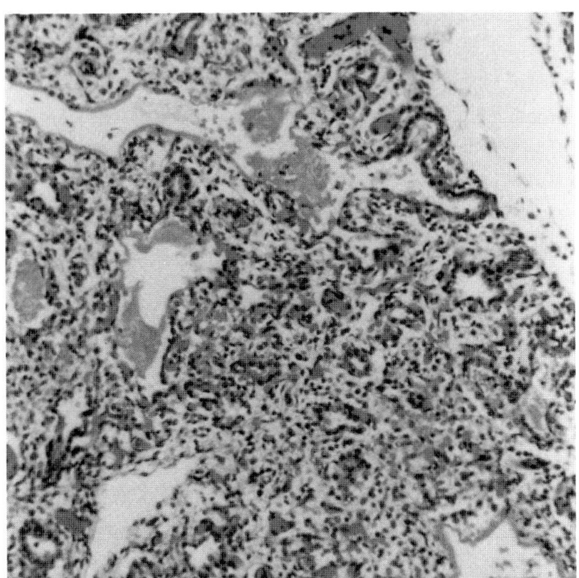

FIGURE 3-8. Note hyaline membranes and hyaline clumps partially occluding the TAP (H&E, ×100).

hyaline membranes are composed mainly of unidentifiable amorphous ground substance with granular or fibrillar matrix. Degenerating cell organelles, osmiophilic lamellar bodies, fibrin, and keratinized cells probably derived from amniotic fluid are frequently seen in the hyaline membranes. Lauweryns[5] also described the presence of variable but often impressive numbers of surfactant (surface-active agent) containing lamellar bodies in the type II alveolar cells.

Pathogenesis of Lesions of Acute-Stage NRDS

Pulmonary surfactant maintains the alveolar stability at low volumes. It consists mainly of phospholipids but also contains specific proteins. Dipalmitoylphosphatidylcholine, which is the major phospholipid component, is largely responsible for the surface activity. Surface-active material not only must be present in sufficient amounts at birth but also must be synthesized and released in sufficient amounts after birth. There is overwhelming evidence that the pulmonary atelectasis seen in the acute stage is related to deficiency of pulmonary surfactant in the lungs of infants with NRDS.[2,10] The deficiency is due primarily to immaturity of the pulmonary surfactant system, but inactivation of surfactant also plays a role. Gruenwald[11] had shown that when artificially inflated NRDS lungs removed at autopsy are deflated, they deflate at higher pressures and more thoroughly than the normal lungs. Therefore, he concluded that the atelectasis seen in NRDS is not resorption atelectasis. The type II alveolar cells synthesize the pulmonary sufactant, which is believed to be stored in the lamellar inclusions.[12] However, as decribed above, Lauweryns[5] reported that variable numbers of lamellar inclusions are seen ultrastructurally in the type II alveolar cells. It is possible that in the acute stage of NRDS the precursor of pulmonary surfactant may be present in alveolar epithelial cells but it may either be inactivated or not secreted from the cells. Lamellar bodies are converted to tubular myelin after secretion from the type II pneumocytes. Tubular myelin bodies then give rise to the functional surfactant at the air–fluid interphase in the alveolus. It should be noted that the tubular myelin is absent in NRDS lungs. De Mello et al[13] have shown that there is a deficiency of surfactant protein in NRDS lungs. The protein may be involved in the conversion of lamellar bodies to tubular myelin. This explains the finding of abundant lamellar bodies in the type II pneumocytes by Laweryns.[5] The overdistenstion of TAP appears to be due to stretching by the atelectatic alveoli and the mechanical ventilation.

The pathogenesis of pulmonary edema, which also is an important primary component of the pathologic lesion of NRDS, is related to continued secretion and delay in clearing of the pulmonary fluid that is present in premature infants. It is also related to increased permeability of the pulmonary epithelium and to surfactant deficiency. Increased surface tension leads to increased microvascular transmural pressure.[14] Edema further accentuates the surfactant deficiency by binding the surfactant.

The pathogenesis of necrosis of epithelium of the TAP and the hyaline membranes will be considered together because it appears that the two lesions are interrelated. Oxygen toxicity is probably the major factor in the pathogenesis of necrosis of the epithelium of TAP. Stretching due to interstitial edema may also play a role. In an experimental study McAdams et al[15] showed the presence of gastric pepsin in the hyaline membranes in the lungs of premature rhesus monkeys. They suggested that gastric contents may be aspirated in the lungs and pepsin may itself produce necrosis of the epithelium of TAP or may sensitize it to another necrotizing agent such as oxygen. De la Monte et al[8] suggested that asphyxia, ischemia and reflow injury may be causally related to the necrosis of TAP epithelium and the process may be initiated in the intrapartum period. They also raised the possibility of necrosis occurring in the type II pneumocytes leading to surfactant deficiency.

Because of necrosis of the epithelium of the TAP, the underlying capillaries are exposed. These capillaries also have increased permeability related to hypoxic damage to the endothelium in the first few hours after onset of NRDS. From these exposed damaged capillaries transudation of plasma occurs, which appears as hyaline membrane lining the walls of the TAP. The hyaline membranes thus consist predominantly of endogenous materials, i.e., plasma constituents and cell debris from necrotic TAP epithelium; the exogenous material such as amniotic fluid and its cellular contents may contribute slightly to the formation of hyaline membranes. A factor related to persistence but probably not to formation of hyaline membranes per se is the deficiency of plasminogen activity in the lungs of infants with NRDS.[16]

The precise pathogenesis of pulmonary congestion with focal hemorrhage in acute-stage NRDS is not known. There is evidence to suggest that the infants with NRDS may have left ventricular failure.[17] The pulmonary congestion seen frequently in NRDS and that imparts the characteristic red-purple color to the lungs may be related to left ventricular failure. Interstitial edema and focal pulmonary hemorrhage may be due to increased capillary pressure and capillary endothelial damage from congestive failure and hypoxia.

Lauweryns et al,[18] who used morphometric studies to demonstrate the presence of statistically significant dilatation of pulmonary lymphatics as compared with controls, suggested that the dilatation may be related to one or more of the following factors: increased transudation of fluid from the alveolar wall, delayed removal of fetal lung fluid, or stretching of thin-walled lymphatics by the surrounding collapsed alveoli.

Significance of Different Components of the Pathologic Lesion of Acute Stage of NRDS

In terms of morbidity, mortality, and devising proper management for NRDS, atelectasis is by far the most significant component of the lesion. The significance of hyaline membranes has been overemphasized. There is no evidence of any role of membranes in morbidity and mortality of NRDS.[19] First, the hyaline membranes are located predominantly or almost exclusively in the TAP, which are not important in the gas exchange. Second, they usually measure $< 50\ \mu m$ in thickness and oxygen can easily pass through them. Third, the hyaline membranes usually line the walls of the TAP without obstructing their lumina. Therefore, the atelectasis seen in acute stage of NRDS is not related to obstruction by the hyaline membranes. Hyaline membranes can be considered as scabs on a wound resulting from necrosis of the epithelium of TAP. Gruenwald[20] called the hyaline membranes the "eosinophilic herring" of NRDS. The only significance of hyaline membranes is that they are a convenient diagnostic tool for the pathologist when they are seen in the typical location in association with

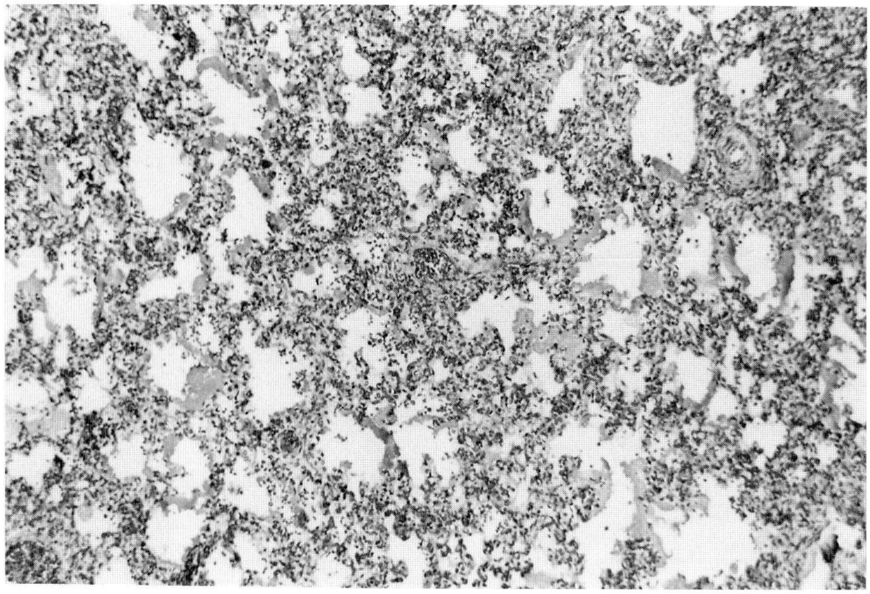

FIGURE 3-9. Note hyaline membrane lining the alveoli that are not atelectatic. The infant had severe asphyxia that required oxygen therapy (H&E, ×100).

pulmonary atelectasis. However, their absence in infants with NRDS dying within a few hours of onset of the disease does not rule out the diagnosis of NRDS.[20] Also the mere presence of hyaline membranes in the neonatal lung does not necessarily make a diagnosis of NRDS because hyaline membranes can be seen in other conditions such as pneumonia, asphyxia, and congenital heart disease (Figure 3-9) as a result of oxygen toxicity. It should be emphasized that pulmonary atelectasis and increased fluid content are the most significant component of the pathologic lesion in relation to pathophysiology and management.

Recovery from Acute-Stage NRDS

When recovery from NRDS occurs, the prognosis with respect to lung function is generally good in uncomplicated cases or in cases not requiring prolonged mechanical ventilation or oxygen therapy. Chest x-ray also returns to normal appearance. From clinical and radiologic data and on the basis of the findings in infants who die later than 3 days (to be described below) it is assumed that there is complete return of lung parenchyma to normal structure, pattern, and function, i.e., normal expansion of alveoli, regeneration of the epithelium of the TAP and gradual resorption and lysis of hyaline membranes. I have observed these changes in the lungs of a premature infant who had recovered from the acute stage of clinically and radiologically diagnosed NRDS but died of pneumonia at the age of 10 days (Figures 3-10 and 3-11).

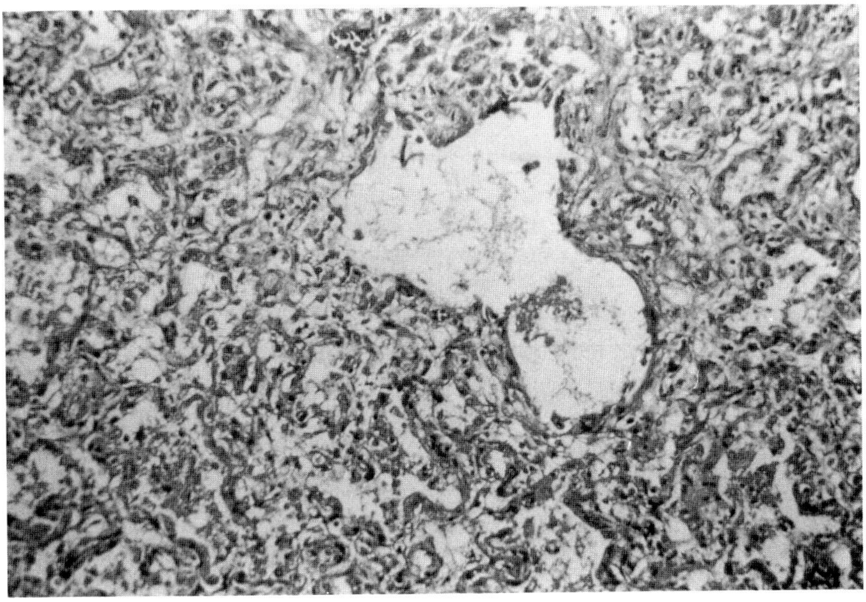

FIGURE 3-10. Note absence of hyaline membrane or lining epithelium in a TAP. The alveoli are partially expanded (H&E, ×100).

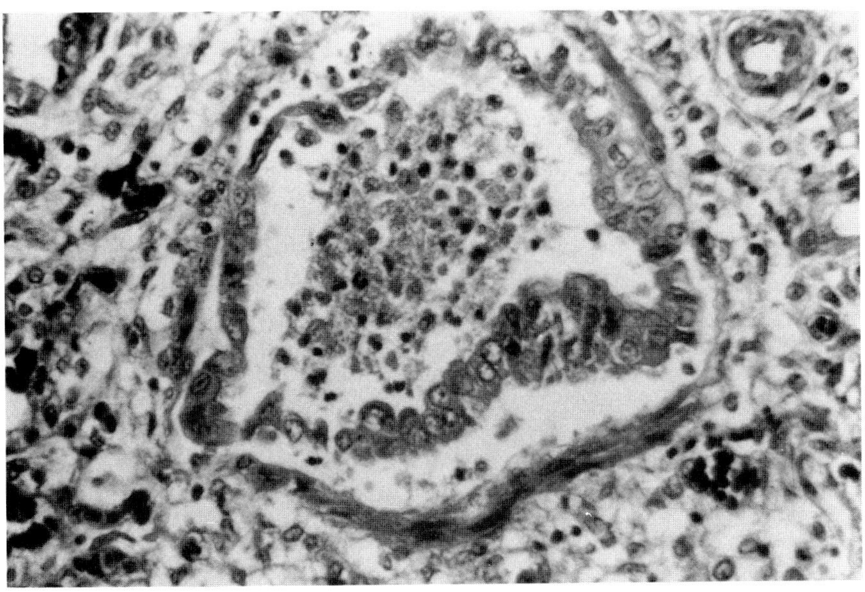

FIGURE 3-11. Note the regenerated epithelium lining of TAP. There is acute inflammatory infiltrate in the lumen (H&E, ×400).

Healing Stage of NRDS

This stage is seen in infants between about 4 and 10 days after the onset of NRDS. In the fatal cases gross changes in the lungs consist of yellow-tan color and a variable (crepitant to slightly firm) consistency. Microscopically, some of the TAP show focally persistent hyaline membrane while others are lined by regenerating epithelium (Figure 3-12). Focal mixed inflammatory infiltrate is present in the walls of some of the bronchioles. There is a mixed pattern of alveolar expansion. Some alveoli are normally expanded or emphysematous, while others still are atelectatic or incompletely expanded. In some areas alveolar lumina contain histiocytes and the alveolar epithelium shows cuboidal metaplasia (Figure 3-13). Slight focal fibroblastic proliferation in the alveolar septa and underneath the remaining membranes is evident in the later part of the healing stage (Figure 3-14). The remaining hyaline membranes are fragmented and eventually phagocytosed by histiocytes;[21] the cells in relation to the hyaline membranes may be histiocytic in nature or be regenerating epithelial cells.[22]

Transition Stage

This stage is seen usually between 10 and 20 days after the onset of NRDS. In fatal cases the pathologic changes in the lungs are intermediate between those seen in the healing stage as described above and those seen in BPD (see below).

Stage of Chronic Lung Disease—Bronchopulmonary Dysplasia (BPD)

BPD is defined as a disease associated with intensive therapy for respiratory difficulty in the newborn infant and leading to chronic lung disease character-

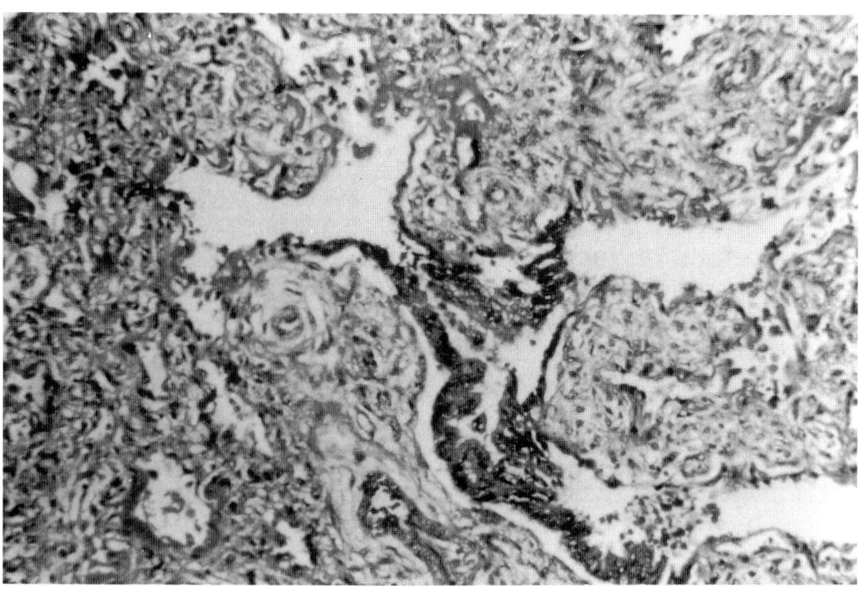

FIGURE 3-12. Regenerating epithelium lining a dilated TAP. Note the persistent patches of hyaline membrane (H&E, ×250).

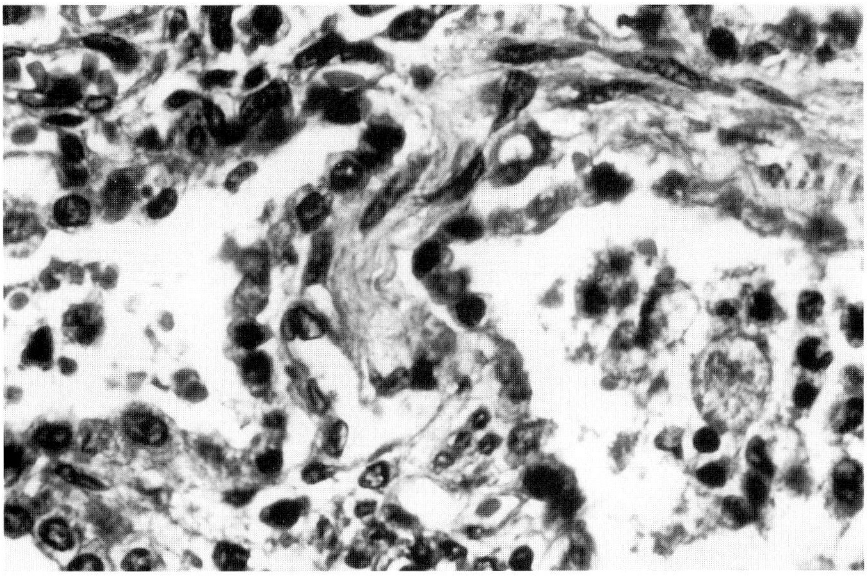

FIGURE 3-13. Note the cuboidal metaplasia of normally expanded alveoli; there is septal fibroblastic proliferation. A few macrophages are present in the lumen (H&E, ×400).

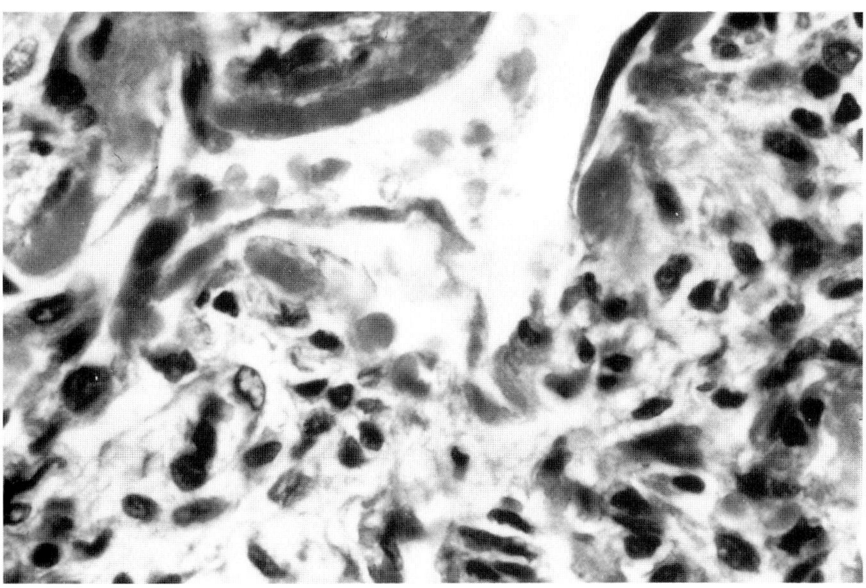

FIGURE 3-14. Note the hyaline membrane, which is discontinuous; there are cells with round or fusiform nuclei under the hyaline membrane (H&E, ×400).

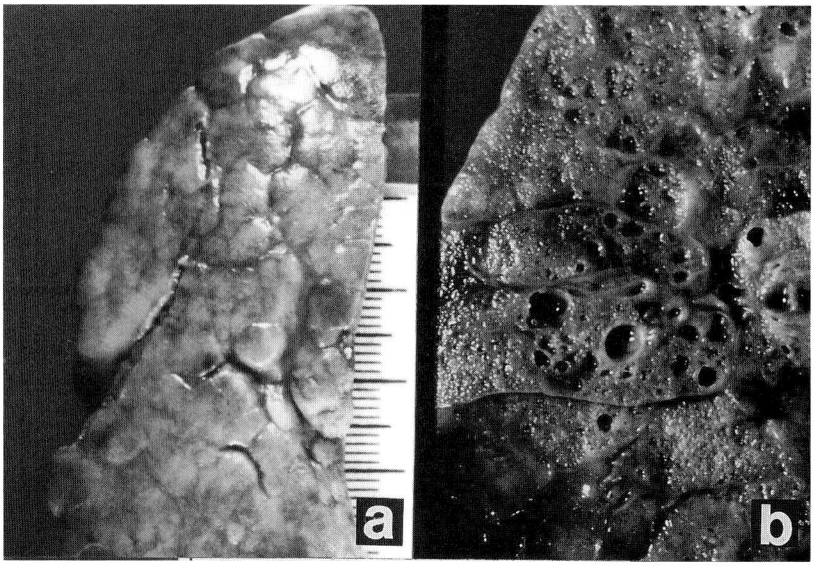

FIGURE 3-15. Gross photographs of lungs showing bronchopulmonary dysplasia. Note the prominent hyperinflated lobules on the external surface (A) and the honeycomb appearance on the cut surface (B).

ized by hypoxia, hypercarbia, and an oxygen dependence with an associated chest radiograph showing hyperexpansion and focal hyperdeficiency alternating with strands of opacification.[23] The term dysplasia implies abnormal growth and development of the lung (of acquired origin). This stage is seen in infants who continue to have respiratory problems and require hospitalization beyond one month after the onset of NRDS, although occasionally it may be seen earlier. In fatal cases the gross changes in the lungs consist of areas of hyperinflation and collapse and firm consistency. A honeycomb appearance is evident on the cut surface (Figures 3-15A,B). Microscopically some alveoli show emphysematous dilatation while others are atelectatic or only partially inflated (Figure 3-16). There are striking proliferative and hypertrophic changes in some of the lobules of the lungs.[3,24] The alveoli in these lobules show thickening of their walls due to marked fibroblastic proliferation with deposition of collagen (Figure 3-17). Focal smooth muscle proliferation and increase in elastic tissue are also seen in the alveolar walls (Figure 3-18). The alveolar lining cells are cuboidal (Figures 3-17, 3-19). The alveoli contain variable number of histiocytes (Figure 3-19). The bronchial and bronchiolar epithelium shows persistent necrosis with inflammatory infiltrate and fibroblastic proliferation in the wall (necrotizing bronchiolitis) or widespread squamous metaplasia (Figure 3-19). The walls of some of the bronchioles and bronchi show hypertrophic smooth muscle (Figure 3-20) or fibroblastic proliferation and fibrosis with bronchiolectasia (Figure 3-21). There may be collapse of some of the bronchioles with obliterated lumen and fibrosis of the wall (obliterative necrotizing bronchiolitis) (Figure 3-22). The pulmonary arteries may show mild to moderate medial hypertrophy. There is also recruit-

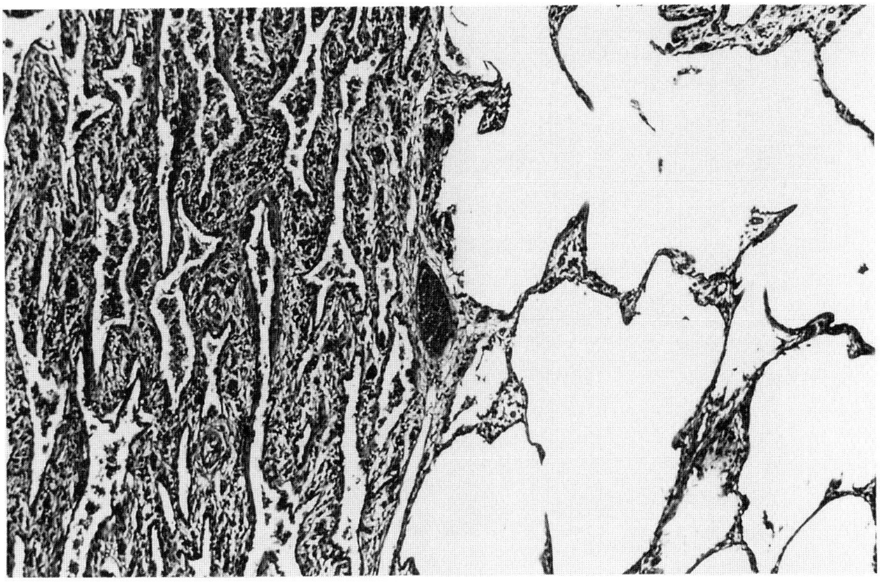

FIGURE 3-16. Note the areas of hyperinflation and atelectasis in BPD; the septa in the atelectatic area are thickened due to fibroblastic proliferation, and there is also cuboidal metaplasia of the alveolar epithelium (H&E, ×100).

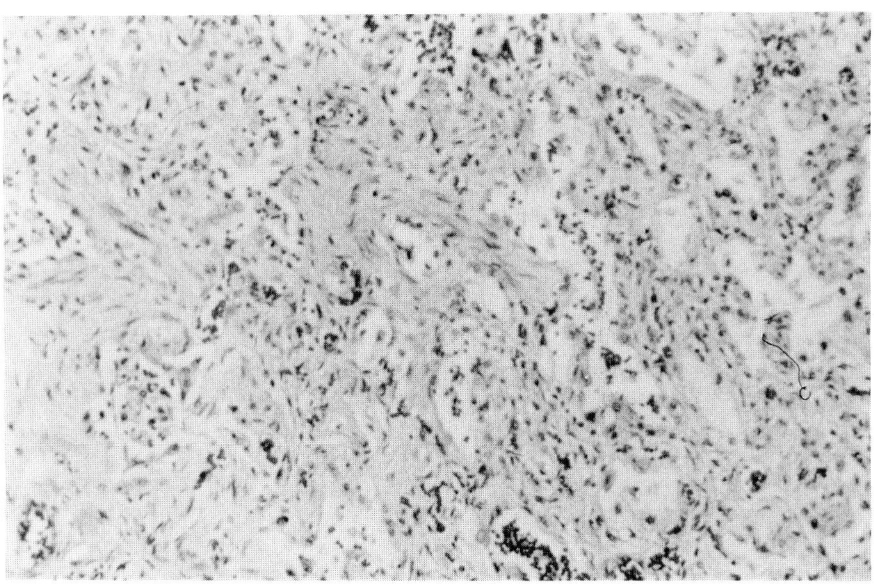

FIGURE 3-17. Severe BPD with marked thickening of alveolar septa due to fibrosis and fibroblastic proliferation (H&E, ×100).

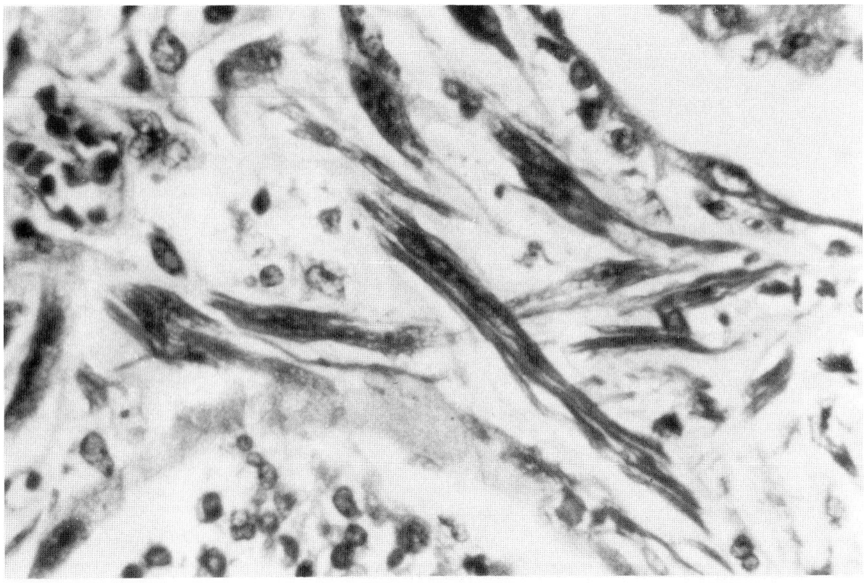

FIGURE 3-18. Smooth muscle proliferation in the alveolar septa in BPD (trichrome, ×400).

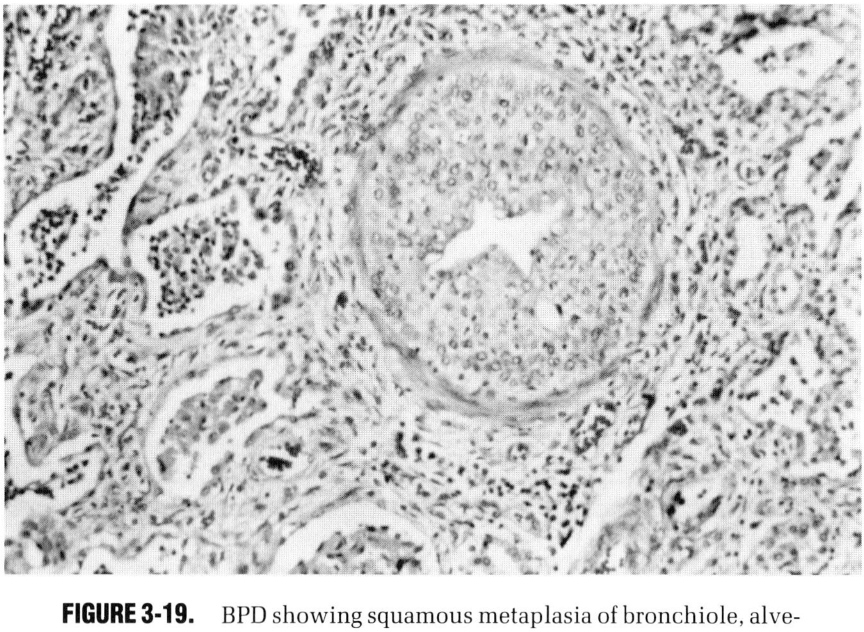

FIGURE 3-19. BPD showing squamous metaplasia of bronchiole, alveolar septal fibrosis, cuboidal metaplasia of alveolar epithelium, and histiocytes and neutrophils in the alveoli (H&E, ×250).

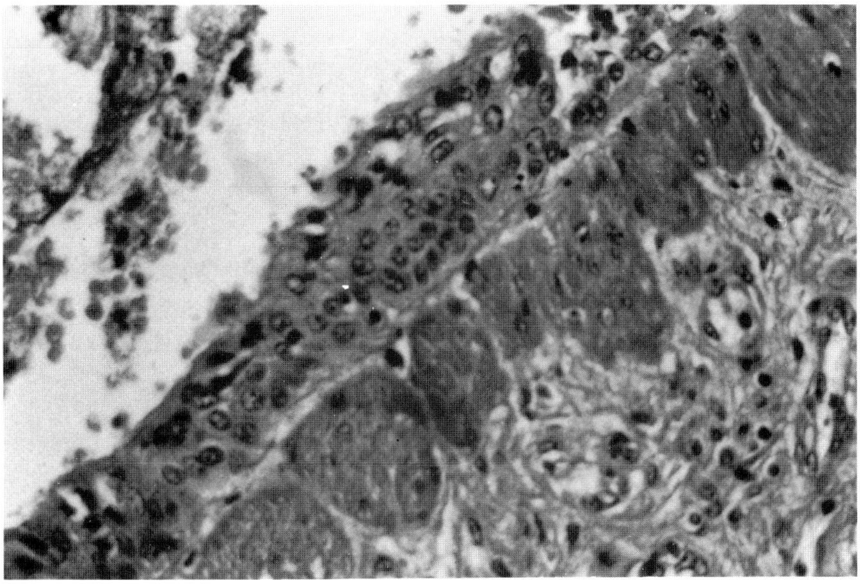

FIGURE 3-20. Squamous metaplasia and hypertrophy of smooth muscle in the wall of a small bronchus in BPD (H&E, ×400).

ment of systemic arteries into the lungs damaged by BPD. These systemic arteries have systemic blood pressure, which may make them more prone to rupture, resulting in pulmonary hemorrhage. These changes including the interstitial fibrosis show some variation in severity from lobule to lobule. Thus some lobules have mild septal fibrosis, while others show severe fibrotic changes. A few areas of the lungs may show nearly normal appearance. Electron microscopy reveals proliferation of type II cells lining the alveoli.[25]

Besides this varying severity within the lung there is variation in the severity of pathologic changes in BPD also in different cases. The major bronchiolar and the alveolar changes listed in Table 3-1 can be arbitrarily graded into mild, moderate, and severe on the basis of degree of severity and extent (i.e., proportion of lung parenchyma and bronchioles showing pathologic changes) of involvement.[26] In the early to mid-1970s, florid pathologic changes of the type described above and listed in Table 3-1 were seen frequently in autopsy cases of BPD. In recent years, the changes vary from mild to moderately severe with occasional cases showing florid changes (Figures 3-23, 3-24). The bronchiolar changes may be minimal or absent[27] (Figure 3-24).

Two phases can be recognized in fatal cases of BPD:

1. *Active BPD.* This phase of BPD is seen up to a few weeks of life but may be seen even later if there is continuing need for relatively high concentration of oxygen and mechanical ventilation. In this phase more fibroblastic proliferation than laying down of collagen and necrotizing and obliterative bronchiolitis rather than bronchiolectasia are present. The cuboidal metaplasia of alveolar epithelium and alveolar macrophages are more marked or more

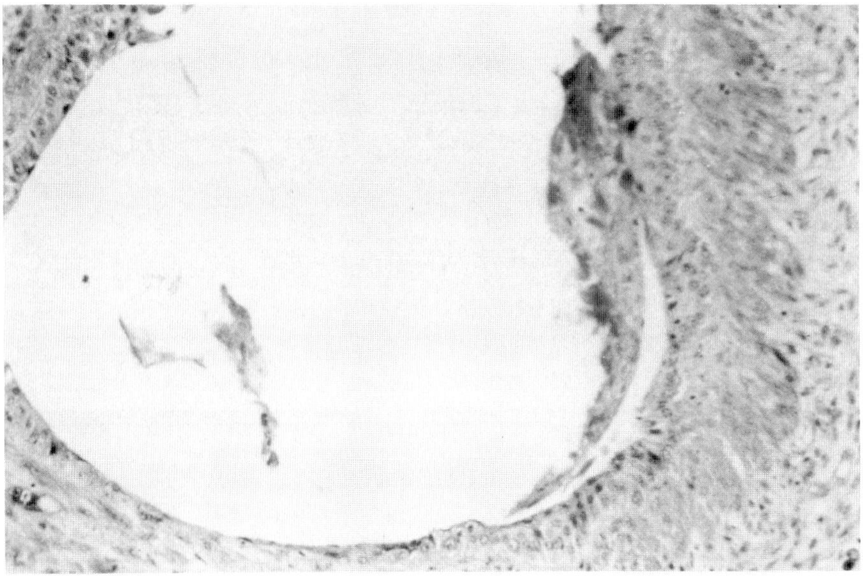

FIGURE 3-21. Bronchiolectasia in BPD; note the absence of epithelial lining, necrotic debris, hypertrophy of the muscle and fibrosis of the wall of the bronchiole (H&E, ×250).

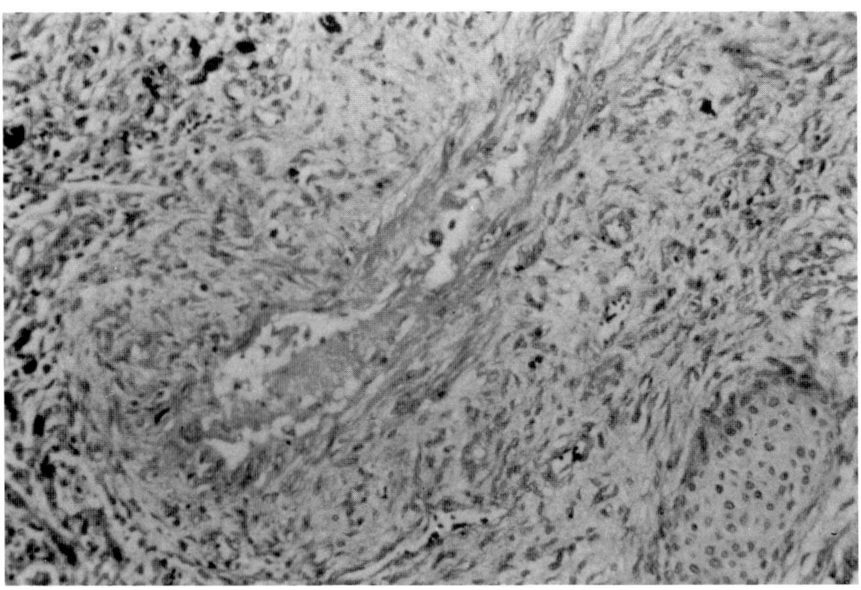

FIGURE 3-22. Obliterative bronchiolitis characterized by marked narrowing of the lumen and fibrosis of the wall (H&E, ×250).

TABLE 3-1 Pathologic Findings Considered in the Grading of Bronchopulmonary Dysplasia

Bronchi and bronchioles
Necrosis of lining epithelium
Necrotizing bronchiolitis
Squamous metaplasia
Hypertrophy of muscle
Fibroblastic proliferation in the wall
Fibrosis of the wall
Obliterative bronchiolitis
Bronchiolectasia
Alveoli
Atelectasis
Emphysema
Cuboidal metaplasia of lining epithelium
Alveolar macrophages
Septal thickening due to edema
Septal fibroblastic proliferation
Septal fibrosis
Smooth muscle hyperplasia in septa
Pulmonary artery branches
Thickening of muscle coat
Reduced vascularity

numerous than in the healed stage. Focal squamous metaplasia of the bronchial and bronchiolar epithelium and fibrosis of varying degrees are also present.

2. *Healed BPD.* This phase is seen usually beyond 3 months of age when the infant with BPD has been weaned off the respirator or is getting low concentration of oxygen. In this phase there is fibrosis of alveolar septa and bronchiolar walls. Emphysema of some of the lobules is also more marked than in active BPD. Squamous metaplasia and bronchioloectasia are more marked than in the active stage.

Other lesions frequently found in bronchopulmonary dysplasia include multifocal bronchopneumonia, patent ductus arteriosus, cardiomegaly with right ventricular hypertrophy and dilatation, retrolental fibroplasia, gliosis of the cerebral cortex and subependymal intraventricular hemorrhage.[3,4]

Northway et al[3] emphasized that in spite of the diffuse involvement of the lungs as seen on chest x-rays, some of these infants with BPD survived and became asymptomatic at age ranging from 16 to 19 months. It is likely that the pathologic changes in the lungs of infants with BPD who survive and subsequently become asymptomatic are less advanced and less extensive and do not lead to clinically significant functional impairment. However, in a long-term follow-up study of adolescents and young adults who had bronchopulmonary dysplasia in infancy, Northway et al[28] have shown persistence of some degree of pulmonary dysfunction (hyperinflation, airway hyperreactivity).

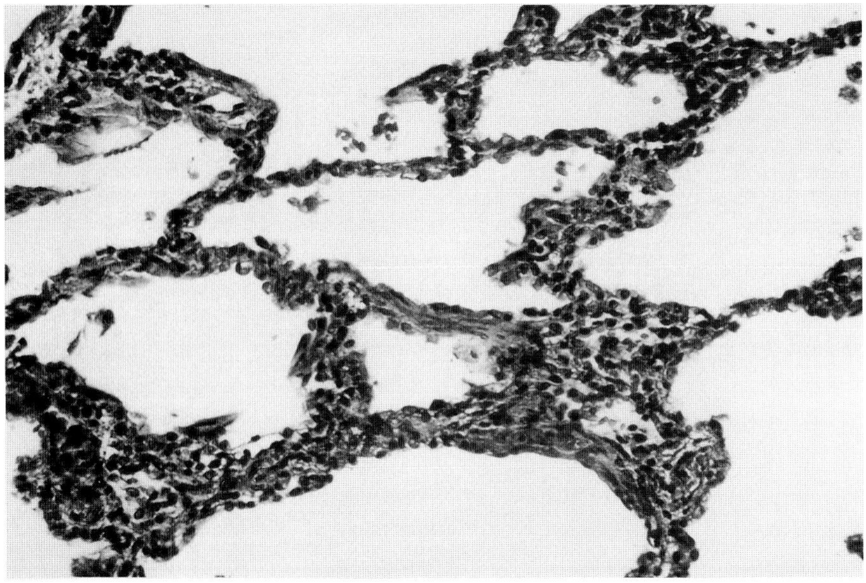

FIGURE 3-23. Minimal focal alveolar septal fibrosis and overdistention of alveoli in mild BPD (H&E, ×250).

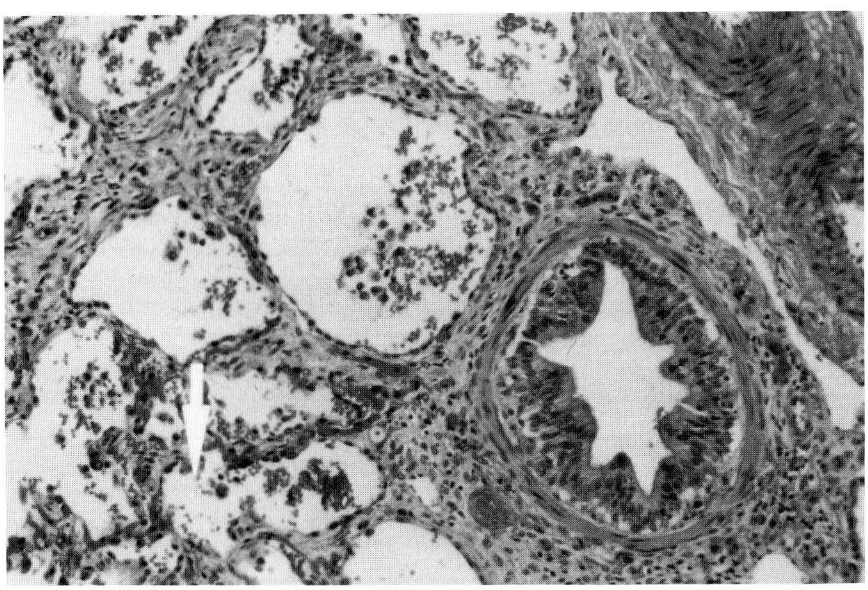

FIGURE 3-24. Mild to moderately severe BPD showing overdistension of alveoli and septal thickening; note absence of squamous metaplasia of the bronchiole.

Pathogenesis of Pulmonary Lesions of Bronchopulmonary Dysplasia

The pathogenesis of the pulmonary lesions of BPD is probably related to oxygen toxicity. Northway et al[3] and Banerjee et al[24] reported that the infants who developed BPD were treated with 60–80% oxygen for 105–156 hours. The necrotizing bronchiolitis and its sequelae (obliterative bronchiolitis and bronchiolectasia) are due to the destruction of the muscle by the inflammatory changes secondary to mucosal necrosis and ulceration and infections associated with stagnation of mucous secretions. Pulmonary changes similar to those seen in BPD are seen in lungs exposed to high concentration of oxygen for prolonged periods of time in experimental animals.[29] Oxygen concentration appears to be the more important determinant of BPD. Oxygen concentration of >40% and ventilatory pressure of >35 cm of water for relatively long periods of time are generally associated with development of BPD. There is an inverse relationship between concentration of oxygen and duration of therapy. Conditions other than NRDS such as congenital heart disease, meconium aspiration syndrome, congenital myopathy, and neonatal tetanus may require mechanical ventilation at relatively high pressures and oxygen in their management. BPD can be seen as a sequela of such therapy in these conditions.

As noted above, the pathologic changes are variable in different parts of the lungs. Stocker [30] suggested that the alveoli distal to the respiratory bronchiole, which shows epithelial necrosis, hyaline membrane, and fibroblastic proliferation in the wall, are protected from oxygen toxicity and barotrauma because of the narrowing or occlusion of the bronchiole. In the later stage the lumen of the bronchiole opens up and the alveoli distal to these bronchioles are expanded and resume their function (Figure 3-25). These alveoli show overdistension. The alveoli distal to the bronchiole, which shows less severe changes with patent lumen, suffer the full brunt of ventilatory pressure and oxygen concentration. Septal fibrosis will be more severe in these alveoli. The varying severity of pathologic changes in different cases of BPD can be explained on the basis of variations in the oxygen concentrations, ventilatory pressures, duration of therapy, individual susceptibility to barotrauma, and oxygen toxicity and the severity of acute-stage NRDS.

It has been shown by morphometric studies in BPD that there is marked reduction in the total number of alveoli. The total number of alveoli in a 10 month old infant was equivalent to that in a newborn infant.[31] The postnatal alveolar multiplication begins normally at two months of age. The premature injured lungs of BPD lag significantly in this growth phase. The emphysematous changes in BPD represent compensatory phenomenon secondary to atelectasis of some of the alveoli and reduced total number of alveoli. Acquired bronchomalacia resulting in bronchial collapse during expiration has been suggested as a cause of multilobar emphysema.[32] It is also partly a destructive emphysema related to infections associated with BPD.[33]

Differential Diagnosis of NRDS in Its Various Stages

The conditions in which hyaline membranes are seen in the lungs are to be considered in the acute stage of NRDS. Group B streptococcal (GBS) pneumonia is the most important consideration. GBS penumonia can resemble NRDS

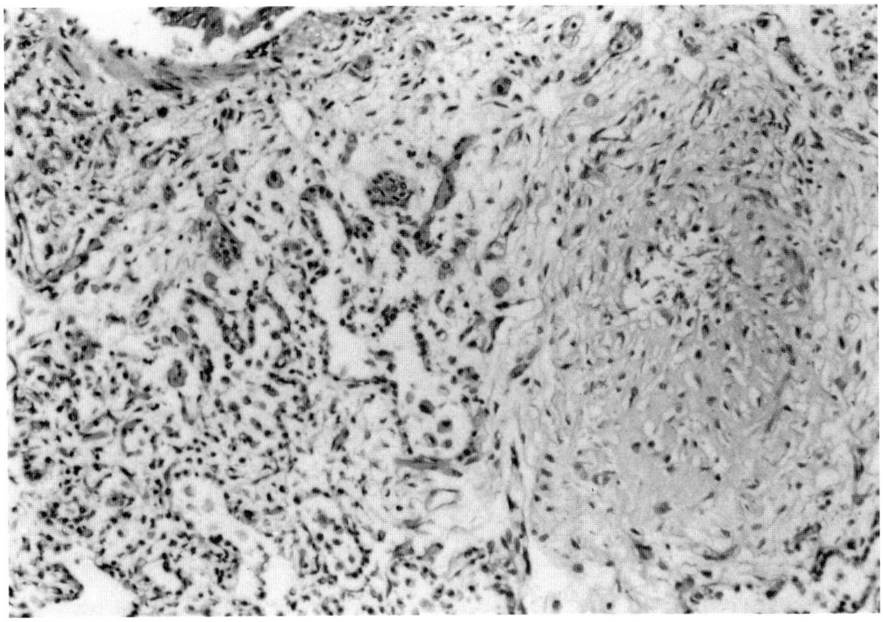

FIGURE 3-25. Note the severely damaged respiratory bronchiole with a small lumen and the relatively less affected alveoli in a case of bronchopulmonary dysplasia; the epithelial lining of the respiratory bronchioles is artifactually sloughed off (H&E, ×250).

clinically, radiologically, and pathologically.[34,35] Three features are helpful in the diagnosis of GBS pneumonia: (1) atelectasis is absent or only focally present, (2) the hyaline membranes are seen along the alveolar septa, and (3) Gram-positive cocci can be frequently demonstrated in the hyaline membranes and cultured from the lungs. If the number of organisms is very large, the membranes appear blue in the hematoxylin and eosin-stained sections.

Hyaline membranes can be seen in the neonates who are given oxygen for a variety of conditions other than NRDS such as asphyxia neonatorum, congenital heart disease, meconium aspiration syndrome, and pneumonia (Figure 3-9). Hyaline membranes are also seen in viral pneumonia. The hyaline membranes are along the alveolar septa in these conditions and there is no atelectatic pattern as seen in NRDS. The infants suffering from these conditions also require mechanical ventilation. Dilatation of TAP and epithelial necrosis without the atelectasis is frequently present in these conditions (Figure 3-26).

The main diagnostic considerations in BPD are Wilson–Mikity syndrome,[36] idiopathic pulmonary fibrosis, and cystic fibrosis.[37] A lung biopsy may be rarely done in some infants for diagnosis. In Wilson–Mikity syndrome there is atelectasis and overdistension but the epithelial and fibroblastic proliferation seen in BPD is characteristically absent (Figure 3-27). Atelectasis, emphysema and squamous metaplasia of bronchioles are absent in idiopathic pulmonary fibrosis. In cystic fibrosis the prominence of mucous glands of bronchi, prominent mucous secretions in the bronchial lumen, and presence of pneumonia are

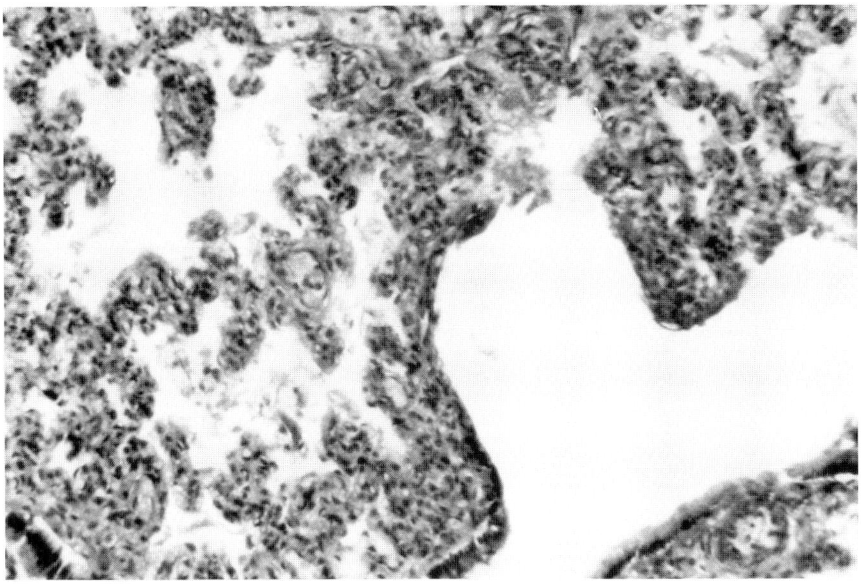

FIGURE 3-26. Dilatation of TAP and denudation of TAP epithelium without alveolar atelectasis in a newborn infant with severe congenital heart disease (H&E, ×250).

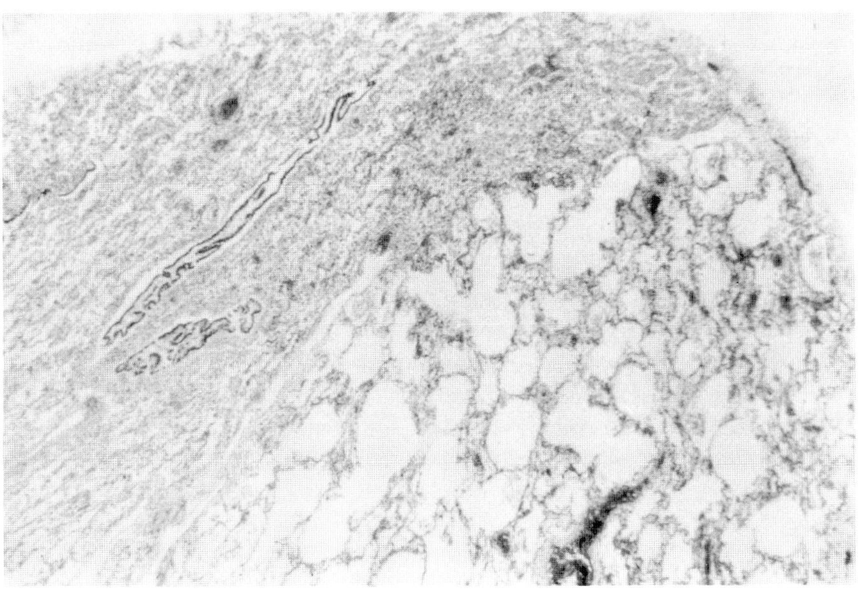

FIGURE 3-27. Wilson–Mikity syndrome showing hyperinflation and atelectasis without alveolar septal fibrosis or bronchiolar squamous metaplasia (H&E, ×100).

characteristically present. In these conditions, clinical history and/or laboratory data will be helpful in arriving at the correct diagnosis.

It should be noted that adult respiratory distress syndrome (ARDS) also occurs in full term neonates in association with severe perinatal asphyxia and GBS infection.[38] The pattern of atelectasis in ARDS is not the same as in NRDS. The atelectasis in the acute stage of ARDS is patchy, dilatation of TAP is focal and minimal to mild, pulmonary edema is more marked, and the hyaline membranes are formed along the alveolar septa. The pathologic changes of chronic stage of ARDS are difficult to distinguish from those of BPD. BPD associated with meconium aspiration syndrome, in fact represents the chronic stage of ARDS.

Complications of Bronchopulmonary Dysplasia

The following complications may be superimposed on the pathologic process of BPD: (1) bacterial pneumonia is related to squamous metaplasia of respiratory tract leading to defective clearing mechanism of the lung and also perhaps to immunologic deficiency due to severe thymic atrophy which is consistently present in the autopsy cases of BPD—a variable degree of bacterial pneumonia is almost always present in all autopsy cases of BPD; (2) viral pneumonia, particularly due to respiratory syncytial virus, may prove fatal; (3) cor pulmonale with or without failure is related to pulmonary fibrosis and pulmonary vascular thickening, which is seen in late and severe cases of BPD; (4) left ventricular hypertrophy with or without failure is related to persistent patent ductus arteriosus and hypoxia leading to high output; (5) wheezing noted clinically is related to the hypertrophy of the bronchial and bronchiolar muscle; and (6) sudden infant death syndrome (SIDS) is seven times more common in BPD than in control population.[39] Some pathologists may not consider such a case as that of SIDS. However, it appears that the infants with BPD who die suddenly, unexpectedly and without antecedent superimposed illness are usually stable and have adequate pulmonary function prior to death.

PATHOLOGY OF COMPLICATIONS OF MANAGEMENT OF NRDS

Endotracheal intubation, mechanical ventilation, high concentration of oxygen, and umbilical catheterization are frequently used in the management of NRDS. Various iatrogenic lesions related to these procedures are seen at autopsy on fatal cases of NRDS. Necrotizing and inflammatory lesions of the upper respiratory tract can result from endotracheal intubation. Endotracheal intubation, if associated with bacterial contamination, can lead to serious complications such as acute necrotizing tracheobronchitis and pneumonia.[40] Pulmonary interstitial emphysema, pneumomediastinum, and pneumothorax secondary to mechanical ventilation are not infrequently seen during the clinical course and at autopsy in fatal cases of NRDS. Rarely, pneumopericardium and air embolism may be seen. Thrombosis, embolism, infection, and hemorrhage are the major complications of umbilical catheterization, which can be seen in autopsy cases of NRDS. All these lesions are described and illustrated in detail in the chapter on iatrogenic lesions. The prolongation of healing stage of NRDS and occurrence of BPD could also be regarded as iatrogenic lesions related to oxygen toxicity.

In recent years, surfactant therapy has been used increasingly as a prophylactic or therapeutic measure and has shown significant reduction in neonatal morbidity and mortality from NRDS.[41] However, in a retrospective analysis of a multicenter study in which 1411 premature infants weighing $\geqslant$ 700 g were treated with the synthetic surfactant, Exosurf Neonatal (Burroughs Wellcome Co., Research Triangle Park, NC). In this study 1.9% of the infants were found to have developed clinical pulmonary hemorrhage (PH) (appearance of blood-stained fluid from the endotracheal tube suctioning). In contrast, only 1% of the 1420 air placebo-treated control infants developed the same complication ($p<.01$).[42] PH was rarely the major factor in death but it was associated with a high mortality in both groups. Review of clinical charts of infants with PH showed that the frequencies of bleeding in extrapulmonary sites (umbilicus, gastrointestinal tract, lateral ventricles of brain, etc.) were not significantly different in the two groups. Further, there were no significant differences with respect to platelet counts, hematocrit values, and the number of platelet or red blood cell transfusions. The authors concluded that clinical PH, which remains an important issue, was not caused by bleeding diathesis. They suggested that longer survival in surfactant treated group may be related to the increased frequency of PH. The same group of investigators reviewed autopsy reports of 159 infants of the 445 deaths occurring before the age of one year in the infants enrolled in the same study for presence or absence of pathologic evidence of PH.[43] The difference in frequency of PH in the study and control groups was not statistically significant (35 out of 69 vs. 54 out of 90). The severity of PH also was not significantly different. This review did not look for possible differences in the pattern and precise sites of intrapulmonary hemorrhage. Other investigators who have studied the pathology of PH with respect to these details have published preliminary reports of their findings.[44–46] Hagstrom and Waters[44] noted no differences in the frequency of PH in the surfactant treated versus the nontreated infants. Pappin et al[45] and Anderson[46] have described differences in the pattern of PH, intraalveolar hemorrhages (>5 mm in diameter), and hematomas being more frequent in surfactant treated infants. Anderson[46] has also reported presence of hyaline clumps or globoids surrounded by mononuclear cells or occasionally multinucleated foreign-body-type giant cells in the surfactant-treated infants. The observations reported by these authors have been made on a small number of cases and need to be confirmed on a larger series with appropriate control group for comparison. Pulmonary pathologic features of infants receiving surfactant for prophylactic and therapeutic purposes and of infants receiving different types of surfactant must also be compared.

MAJOR PATHOLOGIC LESIONS CONTRIBUTING TO DEATH IN FATAL CASES OF NRDS

In a retrospective analysis of 130 fatal cases of acute and healing stages NRDS (Joshi VV, Wigglesworth FW: Unpublished data, 1972) it was found that intraventricular hemorrhage was the commonest major contributing lesion

TABLE 3-2 Summary of Pathologic Findings in Various Stages of NRDS

Stage	Alveoli	Terminal air passages	Comments
Preclinical incipient stage	Focal atelectasis	Necrosis of epithelium	
Acute stage	Edema (alveolar and interstitial), diffuse atelectasis	Edema, necrosis of epithelium, dilatation, hyaline membranes	Focal alveolar hemorrhage, focal early evidence regeneration may be present; hyaline membranes may be absent until 6–8 hours after clinical onset
Healing stage	Focal normal expansion	Regeneration of epithelium, lysis and resorption of hyaline membranes, return to normal dimension	Focal persistence of findings of acute stage may be present
Transition stage	Focal overdistention, focal atelectasis, focal normal expansion, increased number of macrophages, cuboidal metaplasia of epithelium	Same as above but more marked	
Chronic stage of BPD	See Table 3-1	See Table 3-1	

(49%). The other major lesions in descending order of frequency found at autopsy which contribute to death in NRDS were pneumothorax (19%), other CNS lesions such as paraventricular leukomalasia, anoxic neuronal degeneration (15%), massive pulmonary hemorrhage (4%), and superimposed bacterial pneumonia (3%).

In a series of 35 autopsy cases of BPD (Joshi VV: Unpublished data, 1991), bacterial pneumonia, pulmonary hemorrhage, posthemorrhagic hydrocephalus, and respiratory syncytial virus pneumonia were the major contributing or terminal causes of death. In two cases, I considered the death as a manifestation of SIDS.

INTERPRETATION OF PATHOLOGIC FINDINGS

In general, the clinical and radiologic features, therapy given, and age of the infant at death are taken into consideration for the pathologic staging of NRDS as shown in Figure 3-1 because there is overlap of different findings in the different stages of NRDS. The typical clinical and pathologic findings of each stage as described above may not be present or fully developed in every case. Thus the atelectasis may be partial in some foci or may be focally developed. The necrosis of TAP epithelium may be minimal to mild. In such instances a diagnosis of early phase of acute stage of NRDS is justified even though such a stage has not been clinically or radiologically defined and the typical clinical features of NRDS may be absent. Although atelectasis is characteristically diffuse in the acute stage, a few alveoli may be partially or fully expanded because of the mechanical ventilation. The only discernible changes in the transition stage may be increased number of alveolar macrophages, alveolar septal widening due to edema and minimal fibroblastic proliferation, and a few hyaline clumps in the bronchioles. The alveolar septal fibroblastic proliferation and fibrosis may be minimal to mild in the transition stage and even in the stage of BPD. Pathologic findings seen in NRDS may be individually present in various other conditions listed in the section on differential diagnosis. The diagnosis of NRDS and its stages is based on the overall features described above. The pathologic findings in various stages are summarized in Table 3-2.

In cases of BPD, the pathologic changes should be characterized as active or healed and graded into mild, moderate, and severe. Mild or even moderately severe BPD may be associated with stable respiratory formation and BPD may not be immediate cause of death (see above).

REFERENCES

1. Horbar JD, Soll RF, Sutherland JM, et al: A multicenter randomized, placebo-controlled trial of surfactant therapy for respiratory distress syndrome. *N Engl J Med* 320:959–965, 1989.
2. Avery ME, Mead J: Surface properties in relation to atelectasis and hyaline membrane disease. *Am J Dis Child* 97:517–523, 1959.
3. Northway WH Jr, Rosan RC, Porter DY: Pulmonary disease following respiratory therapy of hyaline membrane disease. Bronchopulmonary dysplasia. *N Engl J Med* 276:357–368, 1967.
4. Joshi VV: Pathology of idiopathic respiratory distress syndrome of newborn infants. *Bull PGI* 9:178–187, 1975.
5. Lauweryns JM: Hyaline membrane disease in newborn infants. Macroscopic, radiographic, and light and electron microscopic studies. *Hum Pathol* 1:175–204, 1970.
6. deSa DJ: Pulmonary fluid content in infants with respiratory distress. *J Pathol* 97:469–479, 1969.
7. Shanklin DR: The influence of fixation in the histologic features of hyaline membrane disease. *Am J Pathol* 44:823–833, 1964.
8. de la Monte SM, Hutchins GM, Moore GW: Respiratory epithelial cell necrosis is the earliest lesion of hyaline membrane disease of the newborn. *Am J Pathol* 123:155–160, 1986.
9. Morgenstern B, Klionsky B, Doshi N: Yellow hyaline membrane disease. Identification of the pigment and bilirubin binding. *Lab Invest* 44:514–518, 1981.

10. Farrell PM, Avery ME: Hyaline membrane disease. *Am Rev Respir Dis* 111:657–688, 1975.
11. Gruenwald P: Pathology of the respiratory distress syndrome studied by artificial inflation of the lungs. *Arch Pathol* 80:30–37, 1965.
12. Askin FB, Kuhn C: The cellular origin of pulmonary surfactant. *Lab Invest* 25:260–268, 1971.
13. de Mello DE, Phelps DS, Patel G, et al: Expression of the 35kD and low molecular weight surfactant-associated proteins in the lungs of infants dying with respiratory distress syndrome. *Am J Pathol* 134:1285–1293, 1989.
14. Jefferies AL, Coates G, OBrodovich H: Pulmonary epithelial permeability in hyaline-membrane disease. *N Engl J Med* 311:1075–1180, 1984.
15. McAdams AJ, Coen R, Kleinman LI, et al: The experimental production of hyaline membranes in premature rhesus monkeys. *Am J Pathol* 70:277–290, 1973.
16. Lieberman J: The nature of fibrinolytic enzyme defect in hyaline membrane disease. *N Engl J Med* 265:363–369, 1961.
17. Stahlman M, Blankenship WJ, Shepard FM, et al: Circulatory studies in clinical hyaline membrane disease. *Biol Neonate* 20:300–320, 1972.
18. Lauweryns JM, Deleersnyder M, Boussauw L: The body lymphatics in neonatal hyaline membrane disease. *Pediatrics* 44:126–128, 1969.
19. Fujikura T: Pulmonary hyaline membranes: Killer or protector. *Pediatrics* 49:639–640, 1972.
20. Gruenwald P: Pulmonary hyaline membrane: Killer or protector. *Pediatrics* 49:640, 1972.
21. Larroche JC, Nessmann C: Hyaline membrane disease: Evolution, cicatrization, sequelae. Histological study. *Arch Fr Pediatr* 28:113–131, 1971.
22. Nakamura Y, Saitoh Y, Yamamoto I, et al: Regenerative process of hyaline membrane disease. Electron microscopic, immunohistochemical, and biochemical study. *Arch Pathol Lab Med* 112:821–824, 1988.
23. Anonymous: Recommendations of the workshop on bronchopulmonary dysplasia. Sponsored by Division of Lung Diseases, National Heart, Lung and Blood Institute, National Institutes of Health. *J Pediatr* 95:920, 1979.
24. Banerjee CK, Girling DJ, Wigglesworth JS: Pulmonary fibroplasia in newborn babies treated with oxygen and artificial ventilation. *Arch Dis Child* 47:509–518, 1972.
25. Anderson WR, Strickland MB, Tsai SH, et al: Light microscopic and ultrastructural study of the adverse effects of oxygen therapy on neonate lung. *Am J Pathol* 73:327–348, 1973.
26. Bonikos DS, Bensch KG, Northway WH jr, et al: Bronchopulmonary dysplasia: The pulmonary pathologic sequel of necrotizing bronchiolitis and pulmonary fibrosis. *Hum Pathol* 7:643–666, 1976.
27. McKay CA jr, Faulkner CS 2nd, Edwards WH: Unusual pulmonary reaction to respiratory therapy in a premature newborn. *Hum Pathol* 16:629–631, 1985.
28. Northway WH, Moss RB, Carlisle KB, et al: Late pulmonary sequelae of bronchopulmonary dysplasia. *N Engl J Med* 323:1793–1799, 1990.
29. Coalson JJ, Kuehl TJ, Escobedo MB, et al: A baboon model of bronchopulmonary dysplasia. *Exp Mol Pathol* 37:335–350, 1982.
30. Stocker JT: Pathologic features of long standing "healed" bronchopulmonary dysplasia: A study of 28 3 to 40 month old infants. *Hum Pathol* 17:943–961, 1986.
31. Sobonya RE, Logvinoff MM, Taussig LM, et al: Morphometric analysis of the lung in prolonged bronchopulmonary dysplasia. *Pediatr Res* 16:969–972, 1982.
32. Azizkhan RG, Grimmer DL, Askin FB, et al: Acquired lobar emphysema (overinflation): Clinical and pathological evaluation of infants requiring lobectomy. *J Pediatr Surg* 27:1145–1152, 1992.

33. Reid L: Bronchopulmonary dysplasia—pathology. *J Pediatr* 95:836–841, 1979.
34. Craig JM: Group B beta hemolytic streptococcal sepsis in the newborn. *Persp Pediatr Pathol* 6:139–151, 1981.
35. Katzenstein AL, Davis C, Braude A: Pulmonary changes in neonatal sepsis to group B beta hemolytic streptococcus: Relation of hyaline membrane disease. *J Inf Dis* 133:430–435, 1976.
36. Wilson MG, Mikity VG: A new form of respiratory disease in premature infants. *Am J Dis Child* 99:489–499, 1960.
37. Edwards DK: Bronchopulmonary dysplasia today. *Adv Perinat Med* 3:117–163, 1983.
38. Pfenninger J, Tschaeppeler H, Wagner BP, et al: The paradox of adult respiratory distress syndrome in neonates. *Pediatr Pulmonol* 10:18–24, 1991.
39. Werthammer J, Brown ER, Neff RK, et al: Sudden infant death syndrome in infants with bronchopulmonary dysplasia. *Pediatrics* 69:301–304, 1982.
40. Joshi VV, Mandavia SG, Stern L, et al: Acute lesions induced by endotracheal intubation. Occurrence in the upper respiratory tract of newborn infants with respiratory distress syndrome. *Am J Dis Child* 124:646–649, 1972.
41. Long W, Corbet A, Cotton R, et al: The American Exosurf Neonatal Study Group I, and the Canadian Exosurf Neonatal Study Group. A controlled trial of synthetic surfactant in infants weighing 1250 g or more with respiratory distress syndrome. *N Engl J Med* 325:1696–1703, 1991.
42. Long W, Corbet A, Allen A, et al: Retrospective search for bleeding diathesis among premature newborn infants with pulmonary hemorrhage after synthetic surfactant treatment. *J Pediatr* 120:S45–S48, 1992.
43. Houten JV, Long W, Mullet M, et al: Pulmonary hemorrhage in premature infants after treatment with synthetic surfactant: An autopsy evaluation. *J Pediatr* 120:S40–S44, 1992.
44. Hagstrom N, Waters BL: Morphometric analysis of exogenous surfactant's effect on neonatal lung: A retrospective, case-controlled postmortem study. Abstract presented at the Interim Meeting of Society for Pediatric Pathology, October 1–4, 1992, Louisville, KY.
45. Pappin AL, Shenker N, Hack M, et al: Differing patterns of pulmonary hemorrhage in the presurfactant and surfactant eras. Abstract presented at the Interim Meeting of Society for Pediatric Pathology, October 1–4, 1992, Louisville, KY. *Pediatr Pathol* 13:105, 1993.
46. Anderson V, Gibson J, Cobham A, et al: Hyaline membrane disease following rescue surfactant therapy. *Pediatr Res* 31:299A, 1992.

4 NEONATAL NECROTIZING ENTEROCOLITIS

INTRODUCTION

Neonatal necrotizing enterocolitis (NEC) is the commonest acquired abdominal emergency in neonates. There are about 2000–4000 cases of NEC every year in the United States.[1] Uncomplicated NEC can be managed by medical treatment. Complications such as perforation and lack of response to medical management are considered as indications for surgery. The mortality due to NEC has been considerably reduced in recent years, and pathologists tend to see it particularly as a surgical pathology specimen.

There is a tendency to consider NEC as a single entity. After reviewing the clinicopathologic features of NEC as seen in personal experience and as described in the literature,[2–9] four distinct clinicopathologic types and a miscellaneous group belonging to the spectrum of NEC emerged. Although there are similarities in some of the clinical features of the different types of NEC, other clinical features, known or proposed pathogenesis, pathologic changes, site of involvement, and mortality are different. The clinicopathologic features of these different types will be presented in this chapter. Kliegman and Fanaroff[9] have suggested an elaborate classification. I have used the following classification: (1) idiopathic NEC, (2) NEC following exchange transfusion (ET), (3) NEC following occlusive arterial thrombosis (OAT) due to umbilical arterial catheterization (UAC), (4) NEC following diarrhea, and (5) a miscellaneous group. Because of the differences mentioned above it is of practical importance to recognize these different types.[4]

PROCESSING OF THE NEC SPECIMEN

Because of the presence of necrosis, the possibility of an impending or actual perforation and paper thin segments, the specimen should be sent immediately after resection to the attention of the pathologist in the fresh state immersed in saline in a sterile container. The immediate transportation of the specimen and prompt fixation prevent autolytic changes and distortion of the specimen. On rare occasions, the surgeon may ask for a frozen section to confirm the presence of viable tissue at the margin of resection.

Before prompt fixation, cultures should be taken from the margins of perforation, if one is present. The intestine is opened by using sterile instruments and a swab is taken from areas of mucosal necrosis. The specimen should

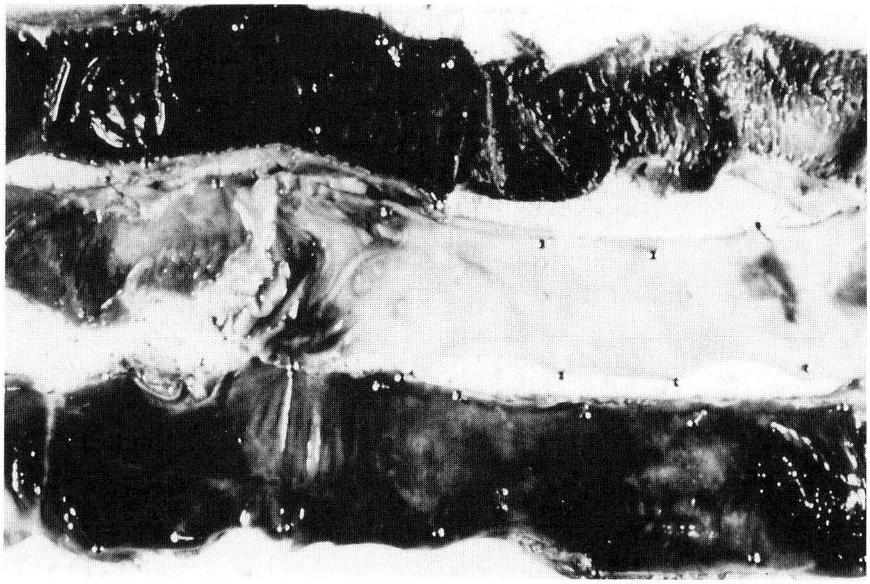

FIGURE 4-1. The resected segment is stretched and pinned for fixation in formalin; note the hemorrhagic appearance of the mucosa.

then be pinned down and fixed in formalin for several hours (or overnight) before sections are taken in the form of windows (Figure 4-1). The advantage is that the specimen remains intact. The following sections are recommended: margins of resection, area of mucosal necrosis, and perforation and thinning of the wall. In some cases there may be only an isolated area of mucosal necrosis with perforation. Multiple sections from such a specimen should be taken. Adequate fixation with firming up of the specimen is essential for proper orientation of the sections. Another method of fixation that I have used is the preparation of a roll from the entire specimen as one does for the placental membranes. After fixation of the roll in adequate amount of formalin for several hours, cross sections are taken (Figure 4-2).

IDIOPATHIC NEC (INEC)

This is easily the commonest of all types and serves as the prototype in the NEC spectrum. It has been labeled as "Idiopathic" because a single recognizable etiologic or associated factor is not consistently found although a set of "risk" factors that have the common denominator of hypoxia or hypotension can be recognized. The common associated perinatal conditions, which can produce hypoxia or hypotension, include apneic spells, respiratory distress syndrome, and hypothermia.[2,6,7] The disease is more frequent in infants who are given hypertonic formula feedings, but it also occurs in infants given exclusively human milk.[9] Besides the sporadic cases, INEC also occurs in epidemic form. INEC most commonly affects the premature low birth weight infants but cases have been reported in term infants.[8]

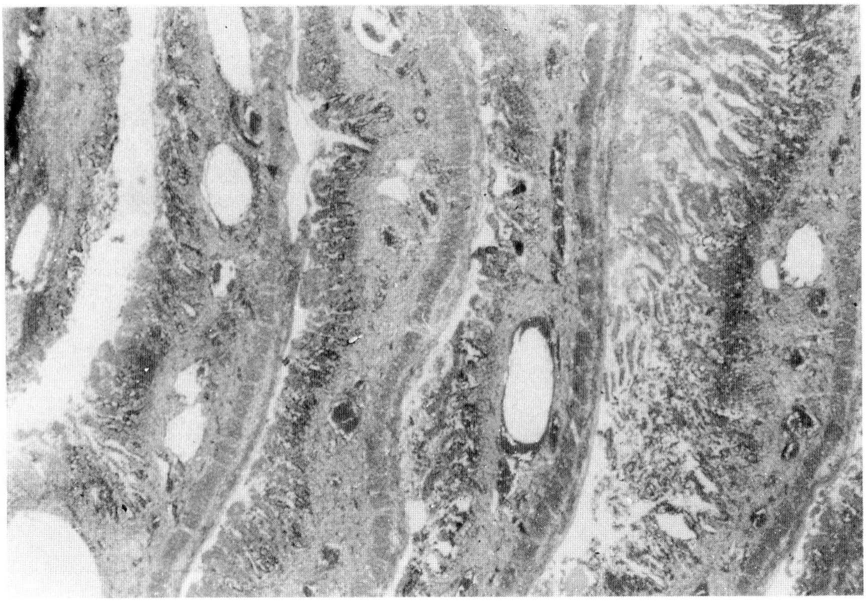

FIGURE 4-2. Photomicrograph of a Swiss roll-type preparation made from the entire resected segment; note mucosal necrosis, hemorrhage and pneumatosis intestinalis (H&E, ×20).

Clinical Features

The commonest clinical features are abdominal distension, lethargy, retention of gastric contents, vomiting, regurgitation, and Guaiac-positive or frankly bloody stools. Diarrhea is not observed in this type of NEC. The onset of the disease is between 1 and 90 days after birth but is most commonly seen between 3 and 10 days. The clinical diagnosis is confirmed by characteristic radiologic findings consisting of pneumatosis intestinalis (Figure 4-3). However, there may only be gaseous distension of intestinal loops without pneumatosis in a small proportion of cases.[10] Terminal ileum and proximal colon are most commonly involved, although any part of gastrointestinal tract from esophagus to rectum (excepting duodenum) can be involved.[6,7]

Pathologic Features

On gross examination the involved segment presents a red-purple dull external appearance, which is often described, particularly by the surgeons as "gangrenous" change (Figure 4-4). On opening the resected segment the mucosa shows a hemorrhagic dull appearance (Figure 4-1). Pneumatosis of the mucosa and submucosa may be present (Figure 4-5). Focal areas of extreme paper-like thinning and actual or impending perforation (Figure 4-4) are frequently present in the surgically resected specimen.

Acute, Healing, and Cicatricial Stages

Histologically three stages can be recognized.[2,11]

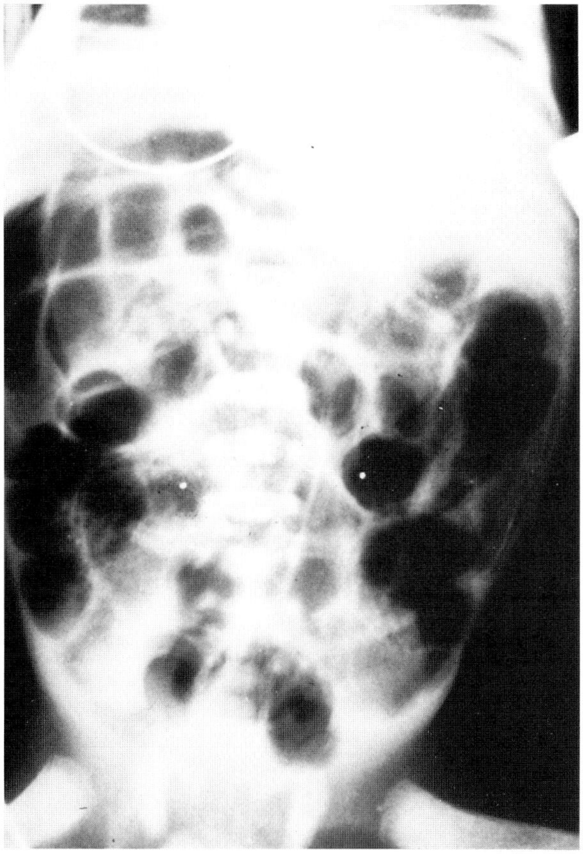

FIGURE 4-3. Radiograph of abdomen showing dilated bowel loops and pneumatosis intestinalis.

Acute Stage

In this the most prominent features are mucosal coagulative necrosis, hemorrhage with marked engorgement of blood vessels of all the coats of the segment (which gives the segment the red-purple color seen on gross examination) and pneumatosis intestinalis due to accumulation of hydrogen which is probably of bacterial origin (Figures 4-2, 4-6, 4-7).[12] In some areas only tips of the villi are necrotic. Thrombosis may be seen in the small submucosal arteries (Figure 4-8). In most of the involved segment the muscle coat is viable and intact (Figures 4-6, 4-9). Wavy muscle fibers, which are a manifestation of ischemia, may be present focally (Figure 4-10).[13] In the areas of perforation there is transmural necrosis. In some areas there may be disruption of muscle coat due to hemorrhage (Figure 4-11), or the necrotic mucosa, submucosa, and muscle coat may be completely sloughed off leaving behind only serosa. These areas correspond to the paper thin areas seen on gross examination (Figure 4-12). Besides these areas, occasional smaller foci of necrosis of portion of muscle coat may also be seen in some of the sections (Figure 4-13). In my experience and the

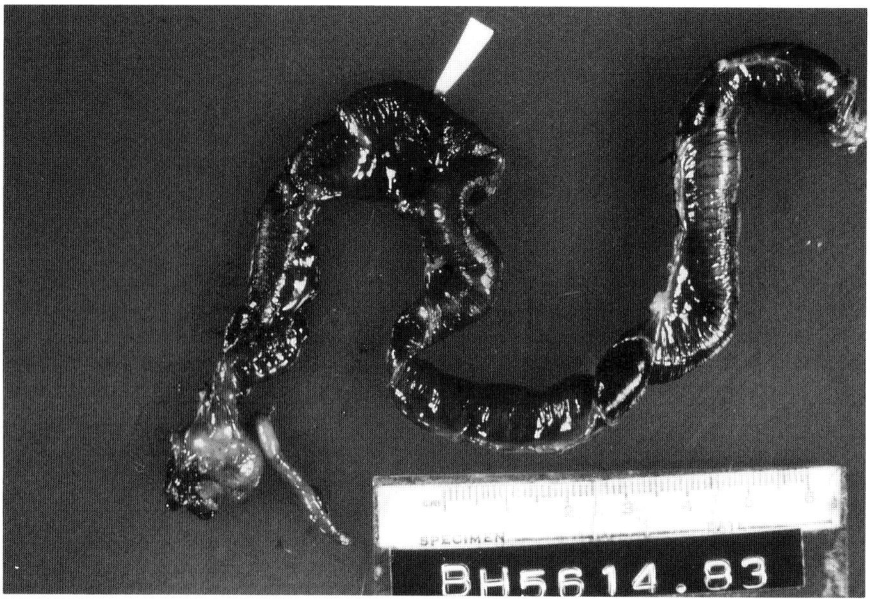

FIGURE 4-4. Resected specimen of NEC showing hemorrhagic appearance of serosal surface. There was an impending perforation in one area (white arrow).

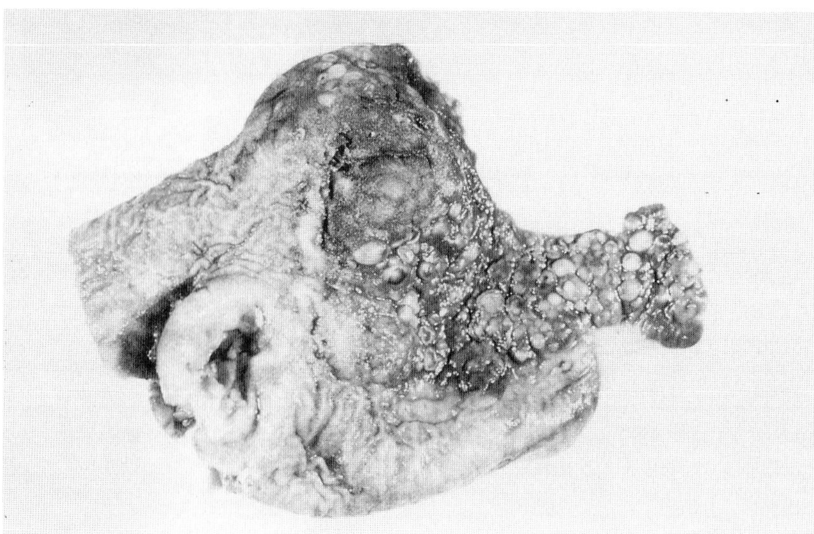

FIGURE 4-5. Specimen of stomach involved in NEC showing pneumatosis of the mucosa.

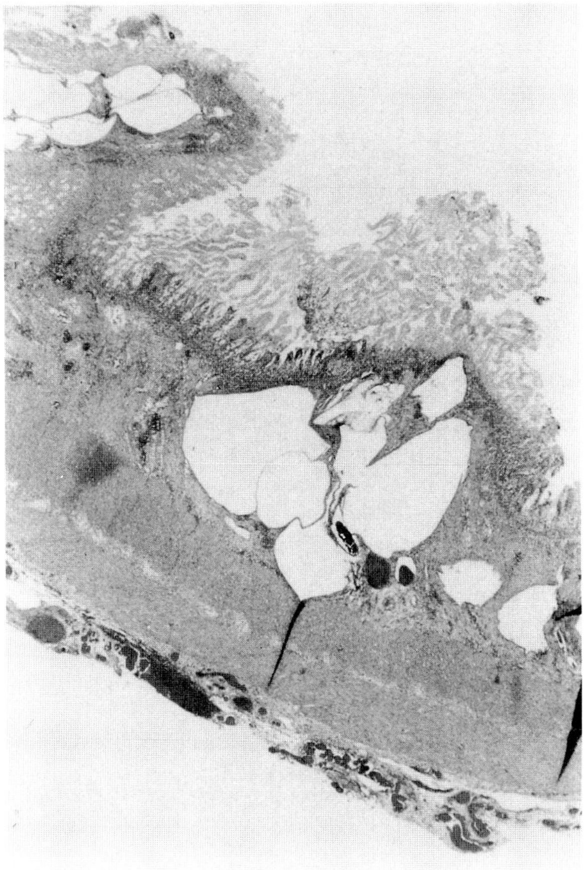

FIGURE 4-6. Mucosal necrosis and pneumatosis in the involved intestinal segment; there is no inflammatory reaction, and the muscle coat is intact (H&E, ×40).

experience of others,[14] the inflammatory reaction in the involved segment except at the site of perforation is characteristically minimal or absent (Figures 4-2, 4-6, 4-7). However, in some cases the inflammatory reaction is more marked (Figure 4-14) even in the nonperforated areas of the affected segment. Pseudomembrane formation may be seen in some cases (Figure 4-15). The changes described above involving a segment of intestine are the most characteristic. However, in some cases there may only be an isolated perforation in a segment of intestine without extensive mucosal necrosis.

Healing Stage

In this stage epithelization, granulation tissue formation and submucosal fibroblastic proliferation in the involved segment of intestine are noted.[2] Epithelialization is present as early as 3 days after the onset of the disease (Figure 4-16). The formation of granulation tissue and fibroblastic proliferation are seen around 9 days after the onset (Figure 4-17)[2]. The areas of partially necrotic

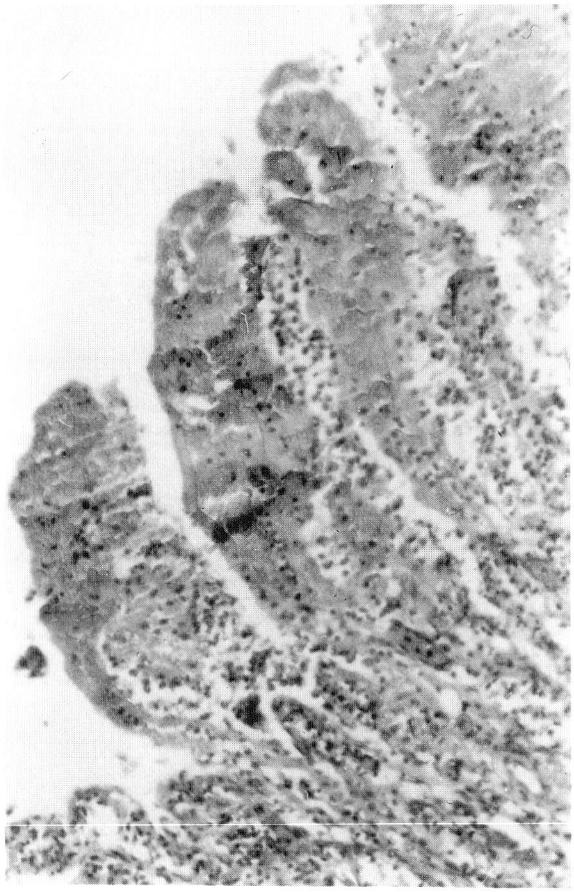

FIGURE 4-7. Hemorrhagic necrosis of mucosa with slight inflammatory reaction (H&E, ×250).

mucosa are reconstituted to a variable degree (Figure 4-18). In some areas the reconstituted mucosa is flat (Figure 4-18).

Cicatricial Stage

Excessive submucosal fibrosis and scarring of the muscle coat leads to stricture formation in occasional cases.

Pathogenesis

Ischemia Due to Segmental Hypoperfusion

Mucosal damage or actual necrosis resulting from hypoperfusion of a segment of the gastrointestinal tract appears to play an important role in the pathogenesis. The hypoperfusion is due to shunting of the blood from mesenteric bed to the vital organs in a 'stressed' infant and not to any irreversible structural obstructive lesions such as thrombosis of the arteries or veins.[2,15] No thrombosis of the regional arteries or veins is detected in the fatal cases at

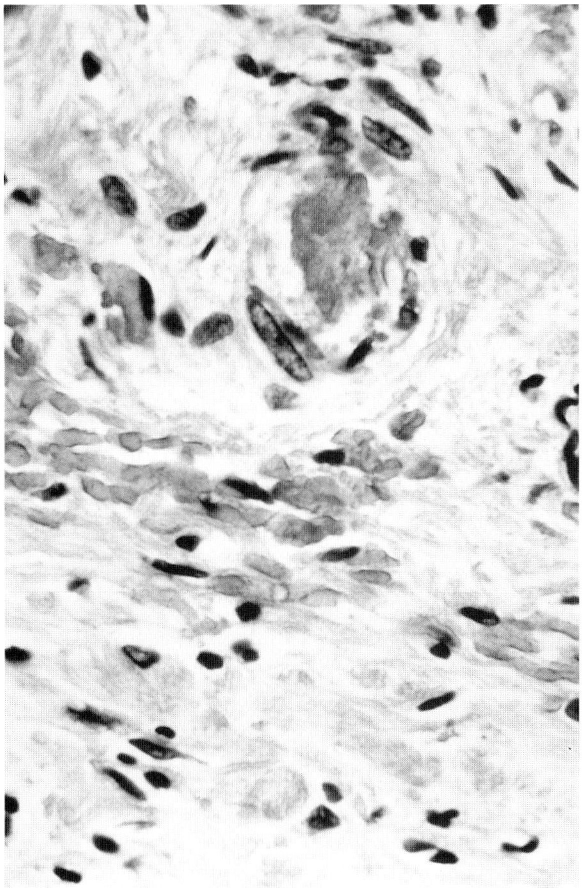

FIGURE 4-8. Thrombus in a submucosal blood vessel (H&E, ×200).

autopsy. Touloukian et al[15] have demonstrated that in newborn piglets asphyxia results in hypoperfusion of gut as demonstrated by radioindium distribution and radiorubidium fractionation technique. Intestinal hypoperfusion is due to shunting of blood flow from less vital organs to more vital organs (i.e., brain and heart). Following resuscitation there was rebound above normal in the gut perfusion, and the pathologic features of the affected segment resembled those of INEC. The pathologic findings (segmental distribution, mucosal necrosis, hemorrhage) in the affected segment in the neonate support the pathogenetic role of hypoperfusion. The hemorrhages probably result from the rebound of gut perfusion through the capillaries damaged previously during the episode of ischemia. The small thrombi seen in the submucosal blood vessels are probably the result and not the cause of mucosal necrosis.

Susceptibility of Mucosa to Hypoxia

Of the different layers of the intestine, the mucosa is the most susceptible layer to hypoxic and ischemic insult. The necrosis following hypoxic insult first occurs at the tips of the villi. In hypovolemic shock in experimental animals, the

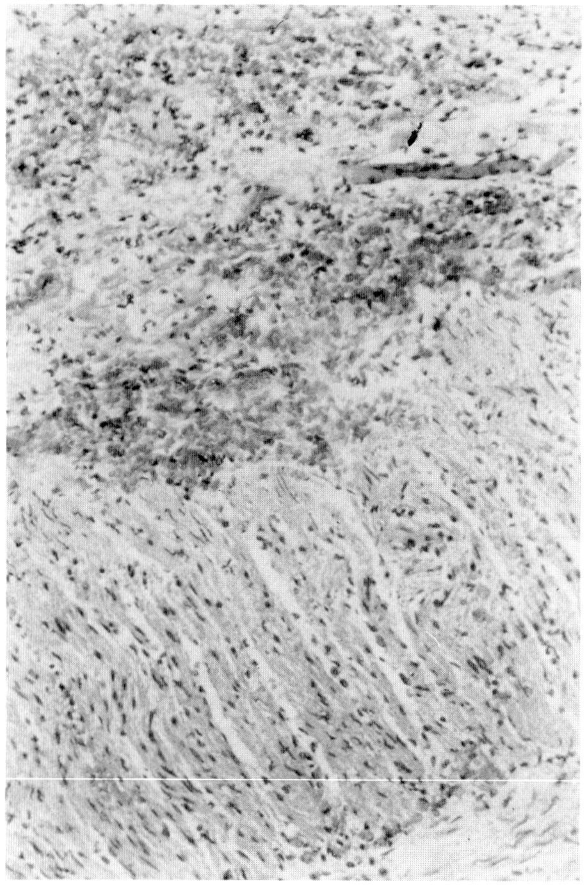

FIGURE 4-9. Submucosal hemorrhage; the muscle coat is intact (H&E, ×200).

mucosal blood flow is reduced to 16%, whereas the blood flow to the muscle layer is reduced to 33% of the normal level.[16] This profound reduction of the mucosal blood flow explains why damage to the mucosal layer rather than other layers is the predominant feature of NEC.

Temporal Disparity between Ischemia and Clinical Onset of NEC

The main criticism of the intestinal ischemia theory is the temporal disparity between the occurrence of ischemic insult and relatively late clinical onset of NEC.[17] Experimental evidence indicates that the sympathetic stimulation leading to vasoconstriction of intestinal resistance vessels and closure of precapillary sphincters occurs immediately after the insult.[18] It is postulated that the asphyxial or hypoxemic insult in infants with NEC occurs during delivery, whereas NEC has its onset usually in the second week of life. However, it is possible that during postnatal life these sick premature infants develop clinically unrecognized episode(s) of hypoxemia or hypotension, which set the stage for ischemic mucosal damage.

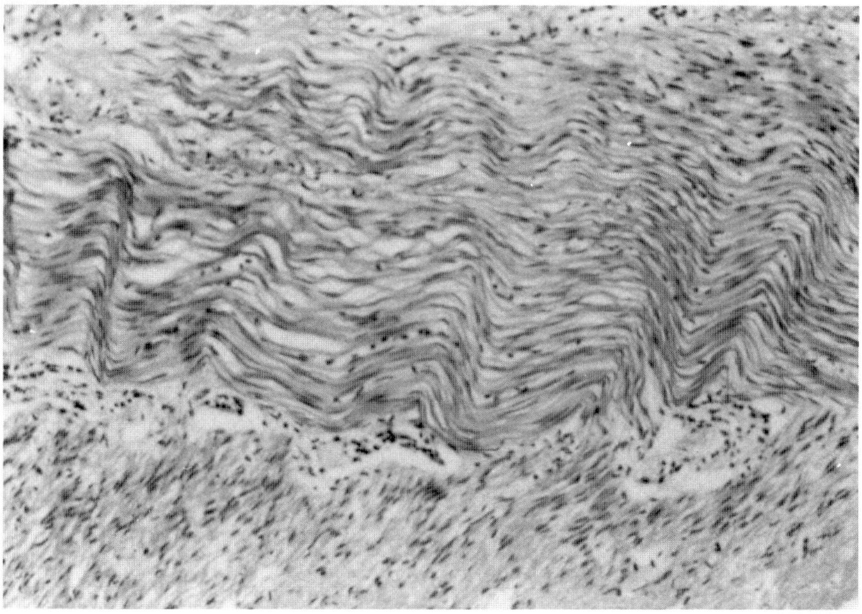

FIGURE 4-10. Wavy fibers of the muscle coat of the segment of small intestine affected by necrotizing enterocolitis (H&E, ×200).

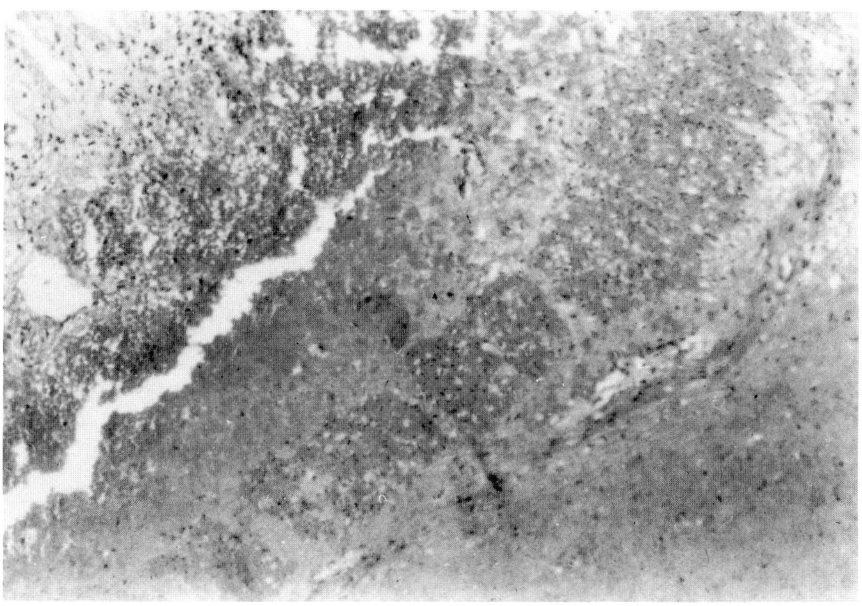

FIGURE 4-11. Submucosal hemorrhage extending into the muscle coat (H&E, ×200).

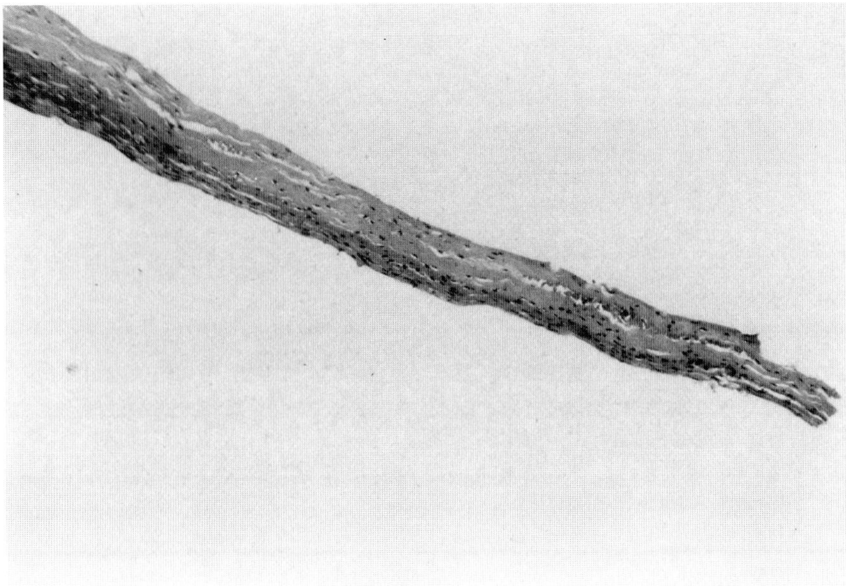

FIGURE 4-12. Section for paper-thin portion of the involved segment showing sloughed-off necrotic mucosa, submucosa, and muscle coat; only viable serosa is present in the paper thin area (H&E, ×200).

Chemical Mediators of Mucosal Necrosis in NEC

Role of the platelet activating factor (PAF) and endotoxin in the mucosal necrosis of the intestine has been studied by Gonzalez-Crussi and Hsueh.[19,20] By injecting PAF or a combination of PAF and Salmonella typhi derived lipopolysaccharide into the aorta of rats, they produced lesions similar to NEC. The mucosal necrosis was ischemic in nature and was related to release of vasoconstricting agents such as leukotriene C4 and not to thrombosis.[21] Leukotrienes are derived from the metabolic pathway of arachidonic acid, and some of these compounds are effective stimulators of smooth muscle, resulting in vasoconstriction.[22] The vasoconstriction may also be related to release of norepinephrine from the damaged intestinal tissue.[23]

Release of oxygen-derived free radicals (ODFR) following PAF injection in the rats has also been implicated in the pathogenesis of mucosal necrosis in NEC.[24] The available evidence suggests that ODFR, which are present in large amounts in ischemic tissues, account at least partly for the damage. It appears that these radicals are produced during the reperfusion following ischemic episode. Cueva and Hsueh[24] have shown that pretreatment with superoxide dismutase which metabolizes superoxide anions attenuated the mucosal necrosis following injection of PAF. It may be noted that PAF, which is an endogenous phospholipid produced by a wide variety of cells, acts as a mediator of numerous physiological responses.

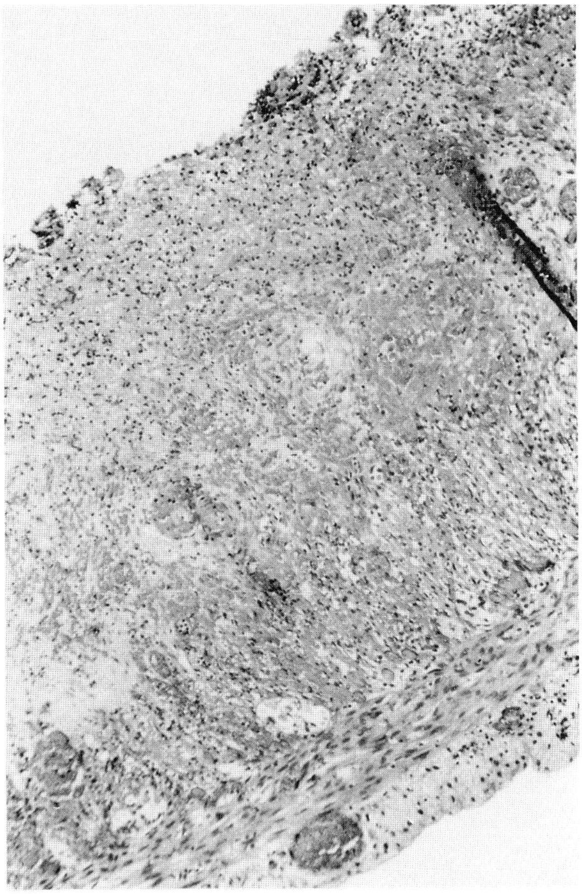

FIGURE 4-13. The necrotic mucosa is sloughed off. There is focal necrosis of the submucosa and inner layer of the muscle (note the pyknotic nuclei of the muscle fibers) (H&E, ×200).

Formula Feeding

Other factors such as oral feeding with formula have been implicated as the causes of mucosal markedecrosis.[25–27] In a prospective multicenter study on 926 premature infants randomly assigned to pasteurized banked breast milk or to an enriched preterm formula, NEC was ≤10 times more common in exclusively formula-fed babies than in those given breast milk alone.[28] Hyperosmolarity of the formula can produce mucosal damage.[25]

Infection

The infectious etiology is implicated because of the occurrence of INEC in the epidemic form in some instances and the possibly increased susceptibility of infants given formula feeds to infection apparently due to the absence of immunologic factors such as SIgA, IgG, lymphocytes, macrophages, specific antibodies, and complement components.[27,29,30] The GI tract of the formula-fed

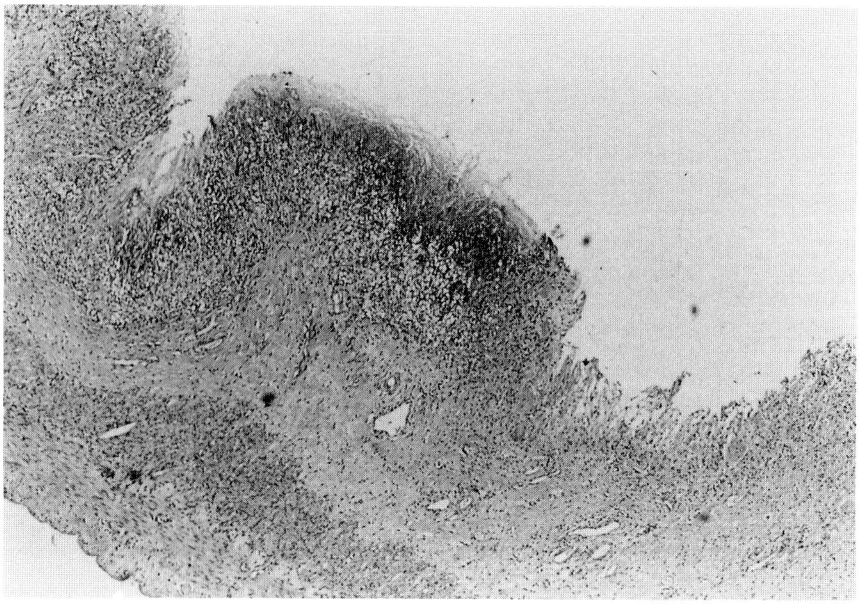

FIGURE 4-14. Mucosal necrosis with marked inflammatory reaction (H&E, ×40).

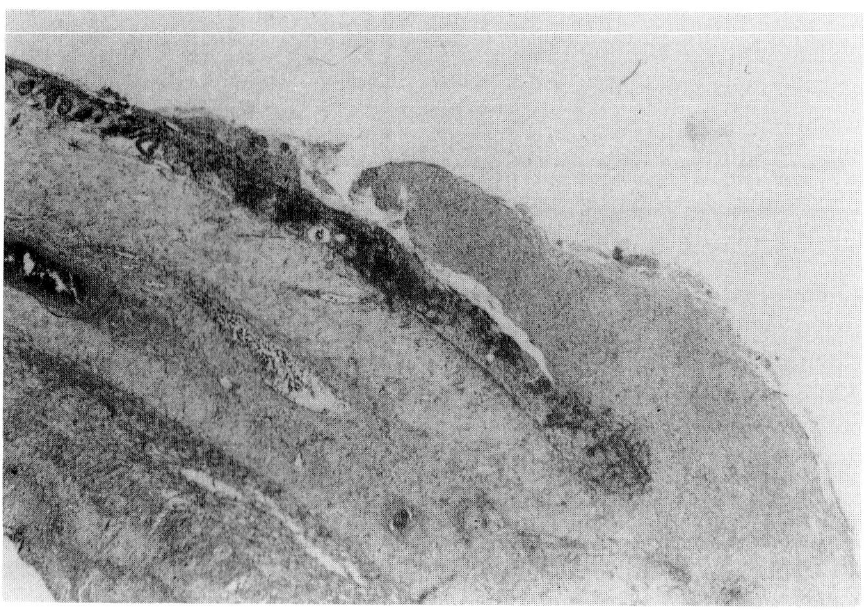

FIGURE 4-15. Mucosal necrosis with inflammatory reaction resulting in formation of a pseudomembrane (H&E, ×40).

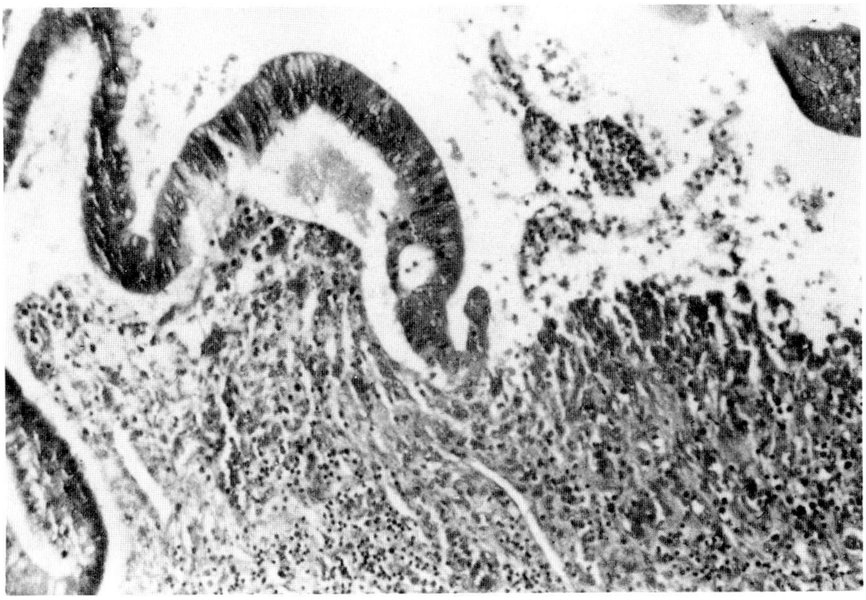

FIGURE 4-16. Epithelialization and granulation tissue formation in the early healing stage (H&E, ×400).

infant is colonized predominantly by enteric organisms such as *E. coli*, *Clostridium welchii*, bacteroides, proteus, and klebsiella.[30] (The GI tract of breast fed infants is colonized mainly by *Lactobacillus bifidus*.) Epidemics of INEC have been associated with these bacteria and also viruses such as coronavirus, enterovirus, and rotavirus.[31] But the responsible pathogen has not been demonstrated in the majority of the epidemics of INEC. Primary infectious etiology does not explain the segmental and hemorrhagic features of the lesion of INEC.

Secondary Role of Bacteria

In my opinion the role of bacteria is secondary as invaders of a previously damaged mucosa. The invading organisms accentuate the mucosal damage and may incite an inflammatory reaction. However, absence of inflammatory reaction in majority of the pathologic specimens of INEC suggests that microorganisms may not always be involved in its pathogenesis. From the evidence reviewed above it is reasonable to conclude that INEC is primarily an ischemic and not an infectious type of lesion. It is neither inflammatory nor of primary infectious etiology. "Ischemic gastroenteropathy" is the appropriate term for it. Microorganisms when present in the NICU (neonatal intensive care unit) environment and the gut play a secondary role as invaders of the mucosa compromised as a result of other factors.

Epidemics of INEC

There is no good explanation as to why INEC occurs in epidemics at certain times and in certain NICUs. I would like to offer the following hypothesis. Transient hypoperfusion of the gut is not an uncommon event in the sick

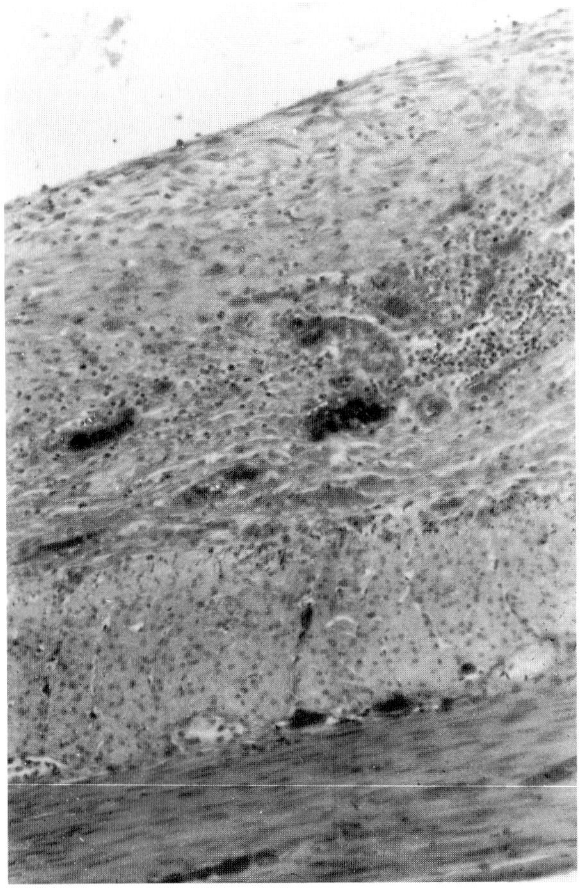

FIGURE 4-17. Fibroblastic proliferation (in the previously necrotic mucosa and submucosa) in the early healing stage (H&E, ×250).

newborn babies. In most instances the mucosal damage which is minimal to mild after such an event does not produce any clinical manifestations and is repaired readily. The microorganisms listed above when present in the environment and in the gut do not invade intact mucosa but can do so when even minimal to mild mucosal damage due to hypoperfusion is present. The result is an epidemic of INEC. Besides ischemia and infection, other factors such as tumor necrosis factor (TNF) and PAF can produce mucosal injury to the intestine. TNF synthesis is stimulated directly by endotoxin.[31]

Complications

Perforation and septicemia are the dreaded immediate complications of INEC.[6] Shock, leukopenia, thrombocytopenia, and renal failure also occur.[9] Late complications include short-gut syndrome, malabsorption syndrome, stricture, enterocyst, and aganglionosis[9,32,33] (Figures 4-18–4-21). Short-gut syndrome results when there is extensive involvement of the small and large intestine requiring resection of long segments. Malabsorption is likely to occur if there is

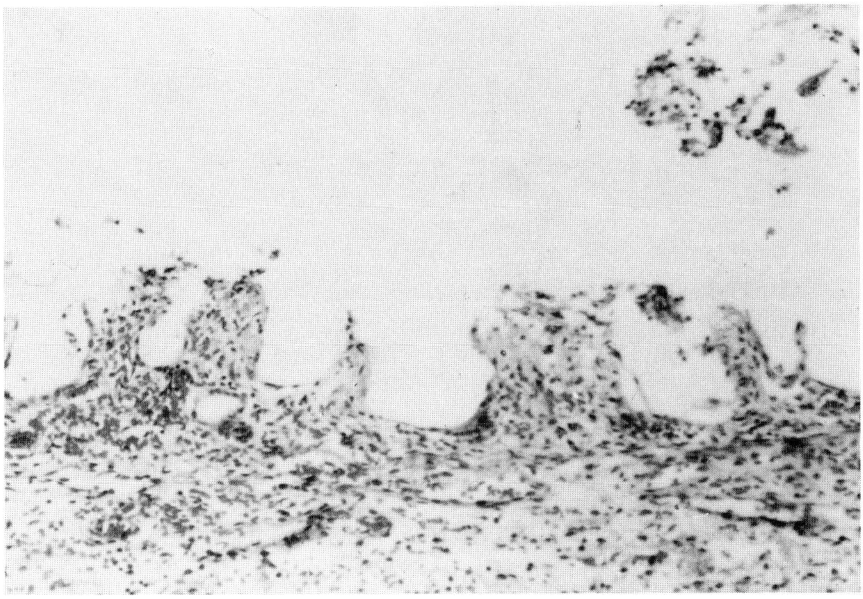

FIGURE 4-18. Partial reconstitution of the mucosa in the late healing stage (H&E, ×250).

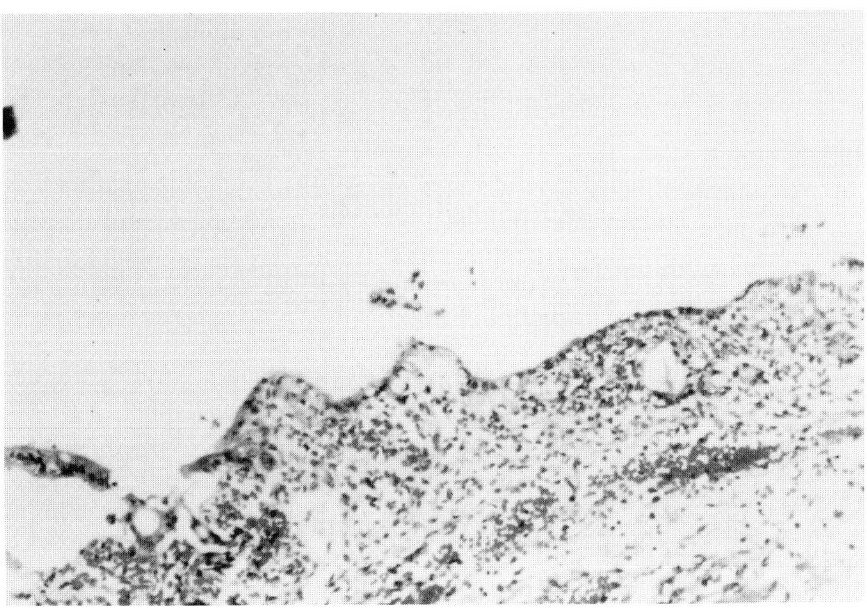

FIGURE 4-19. Flattened reconstituted mucosa in the late healing stage (H&E, ×250).

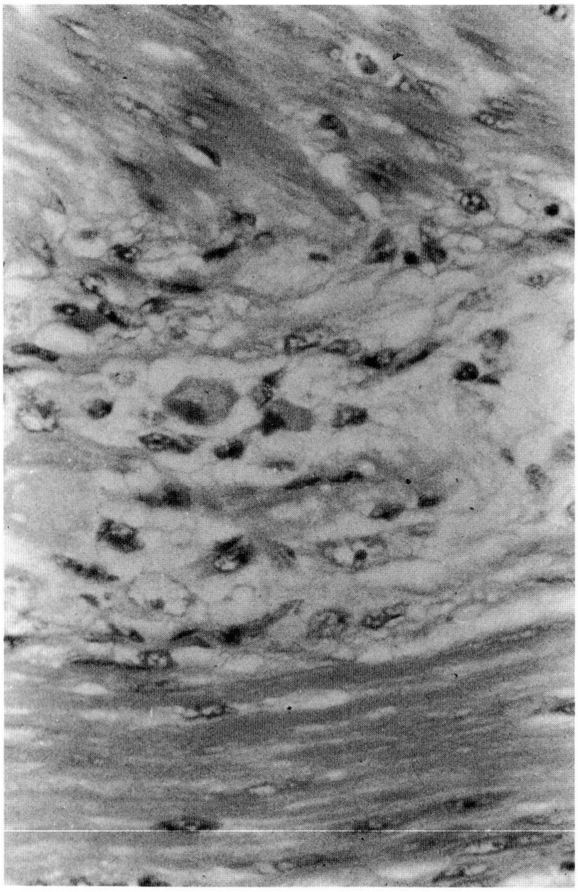

FIGURE 4-20. Degeneration and necrosis of ganglion cells in the myenteric plexus in the acute stage of NEC (H&E, ×400).

only a partial reconstitution of the affected mucosa (Figures 4-18, 4-19). Degeneration and necrosis of ganglion cells in the myenteric and submucosal plexuses is not infrequently seen in the surgically resected segment of INEC (Figure 4-20). In an infant with INEC who has responded to medical therapy, it is conceivable that the ganglion cells in the affected segment may have been damaged. The mucosa heals and gets reepithelialized as described above, but the ganglion cells do not regenerate. The segment would then be an adynamic segment. The result is what could be labelled as acquired Hirschsprung's disease. Formation of stricture is seen between 1 and 20 months after the acute stage of INEC (34) (Figure 4-21). Fibrosis of submucosa and muscle coat with flattening of the mucosa are noted histologically. These features represent the sequelae of the healing stage of INEC described above and illustrated in Figure 4-17.

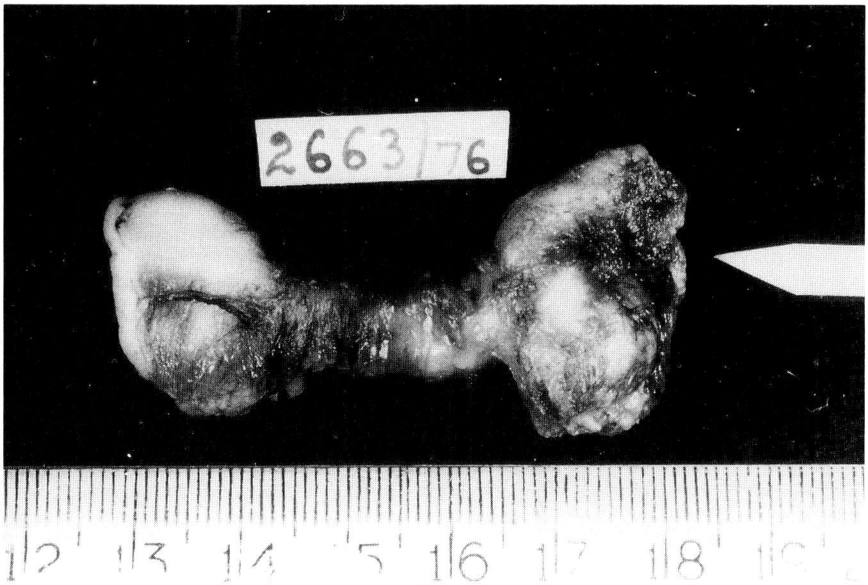

FIGURE 4-21. Stricture of colon in 6-month-old infant who had NEC in the neonatal period treated by medical regimen.

NEC FOLLOWING EXCHANGE TRANSFUSION (ET)

Clinical Features

This is a well-recognized complication of exchange transfusion. Abdominal distension, blood-streaked or bloody stools, and bilious vomiting are the most frequently observed clinical features.[35] The commonest condition that necessitates exchange transfusion is Rh incompatibility. The other perinatal complications such as asphyxia and respiratory distress seen in NEC are not commonly seen in infants with NEC following ET. The majority of infants (60%) of 29 cases reviewed by Hardy et al weighed >2500 g and in 13 of the 29 cases two or more exchange transfusions were given before the onset of the disease. The interval between ET and onset of the disease ranged from 4 to 96 hours.[36] Perforation is more common in this type of NEC than in INEC. The perforations may be multiple. It is possible that the impression of a high incidence of perforation is obtained because only the complicated cases tend to be reported in the literature. The colon is the most frequently involved part of the GI tract,[37] although stomach and small intestine also can be involved.[35]

Pathologic Features

The pathological changes are variable. There may be a single perforation in an otherwise normal-appearing colon or diffuse total thickness necrosis of the involved segment resembling venous infarction. Congestion, hemorrhage, and mild to moderate inflammation are also noted on microscopic examination. The mortality in promptly operated infants is low.[35]

Pathogenesis

The pathogenesis of the lesion is not completely understood, but it appears that it is related to impedance of venous outflow from the intestine due to portal hypertension produced by one or more of the following factors: (1) presence of tip of the catheter in the portal vein, (2) presence of narrow segment of ductus venosus, or (3) entrance of injected blood into the portal circulation in a restless crying infant with raised central venous pressure[35,36] (Figure 4-22). Other factors such as excessive speed of exchange, change in blood viscosity, manipulation of the catheter, injection of cool blood, and dislodgment of a small thrombus with retrograde embolization into portal venous circulation may also play a role. Touloukian et al[35] have shown that significant increase in portal venous pressure occurs during the injection phase of exchange transfusion carried out through the umbilical vein in newborn piglets. On the basis of these findings they recommend that a radiopaque catheter should be used for exchange transfusion and the tip of the catheter should be placed in the inferior vena cava.

NEC FOLLOWING OAT DUE TO UAC

Nine cases were reported until 1975.[3] Ballance et al[38] have recently described this type of NEC in five of their series of 84 cases of NEC. Most of the infants were critically ill due to a variety of conditions such as asphyxia, respiratory distress syndrome, hypoglycemia, or congenital heart disease. All five infants in whom data are given were of low birth weight. Details of clinical

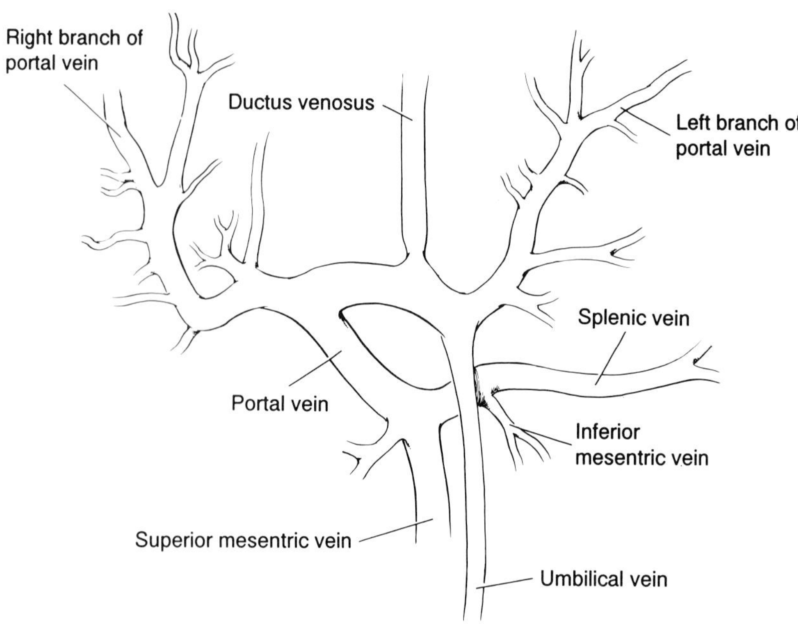

FIGURE 4-22. Diagrammatic representation of umbilical vein, ductus venous, and portal vein with its branches.

features which are given only in a few cases, were similar to those of INEC. Small intestine and/or colon are involved, depending on the site of thrombosis, which may be in the abdominal aorta or superior or inferior mesenteric artery. The mortality in this type of NEC has been 100%. The diagnosis of arterial thrombosis in all cases was made at autopsy. The involved segment of the intestine shows total-thickness necrosis, i.e., true arterial infarction (Figure 4-23).[3] The pathogenesis of this lesion is obviously related to occlusive thrombosis of the major arterial trunk supplying the involved segment of intestine (Figures 4-24, 4-25). All infants with this type of NEC are prone to develop thrombosis. The presence of the foreign body in the form of the catheter may precipitate thrombosis in such an infant. Another factor which may be related to thrombosis following UAC is giving of hypertonic solutions particularly dextrose through the arterial catheter. It has been suggested that the arterial catheter should be inserted to the level of diaphragm and hypertonic solutions should not be injected through the catheter.[39]

NEC FOLLOWING DIARRHEA

Clinical Features and Subtypes

This type of NEC differs clinically from other types of NEC in that diarrhea is an antecedent or initial feature of the disease.[8,40–42] There appear to be two

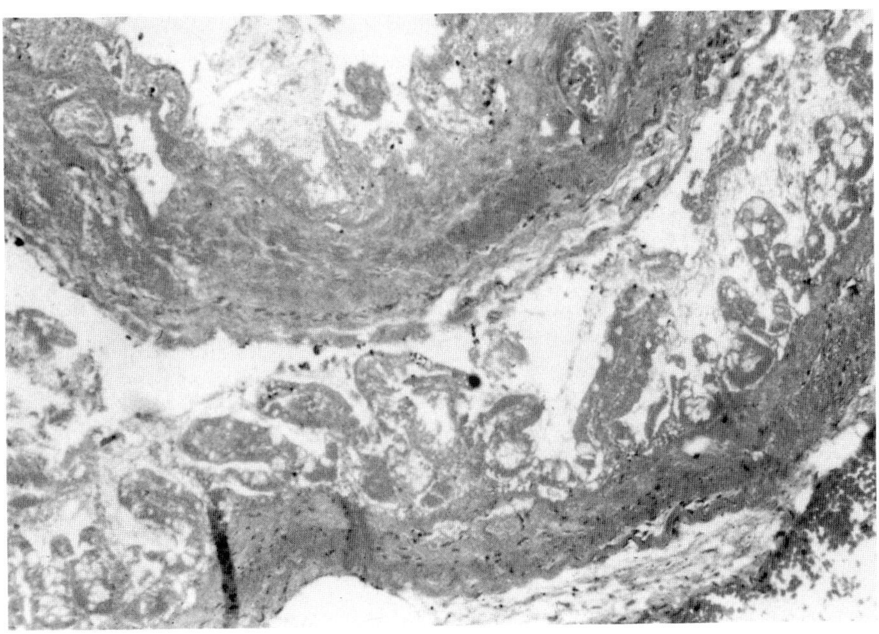

FIGURE 4-23. Total thickness necrosis of involved segment in a case of neonatal necrotizing enterocolitis following occlusive thrombosis of the ostium of the inferior mesenteric artery associated with umbilical arterial catheterization (H&E, ×100).

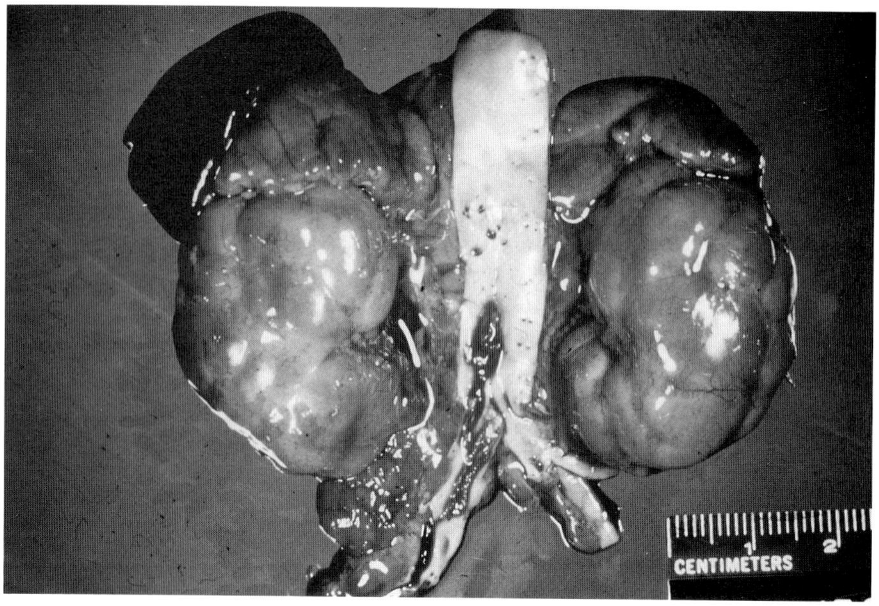

FIGURE 4-24. Thrombus occluding the ostium of inferior mesenteric artery in a newborn infant with NEC associated with umbilical arterial catheterization.

subtypes in this group. In one subtype the diarrhea was due to demonstrable infectious agents such as salmonella, *E. coli*,[40–42] or rotavirus[43] as shown by positive stool cultures. Other associated features such as low birth weight, asphyxia, respiratory distress, apneic spells, and hypothermia were the same as in INEC. Data on the type of oral feeding is not given in these reports. Almost all the affected infants were of low birth weight. In all patients reported by Stein et al[40] dehydration and peripheral circulatory failure were present. Small and/or large intestine can be involved. In contrast to other types of NEC prominent inflammatory reaction with or without pseudomembrane formation in the involved mucosa is seen on microscopic examination more frequently in this type of NEC than in other types (Figure 4-26). Other pathologic findings such as mucosal necrosis, hemorrhage, and pneumatosis intestinalis are similar to those seen in INEC. The mortality is about 100%. In the other subtype the diarrhea was of a chronic idiopathic nature and all infants were full-term. In most cases dehydration and acidosis were present. The pathologic picture in the involved intestine was identical with that in INEC.[8]

Pathogenesis

The pathogenesis is probably the same as INEC with an added element of pre-existing or coexisting infectious gastroenteritis in the first subtype. Thus in a dehydrated infant with peripheral circulatory failure or in an infant with various perinatal complications leading to hypoxia, hypoperfusion of the gut mucosa due to shunting of blood supply from mesenteric bed might occur. This will in

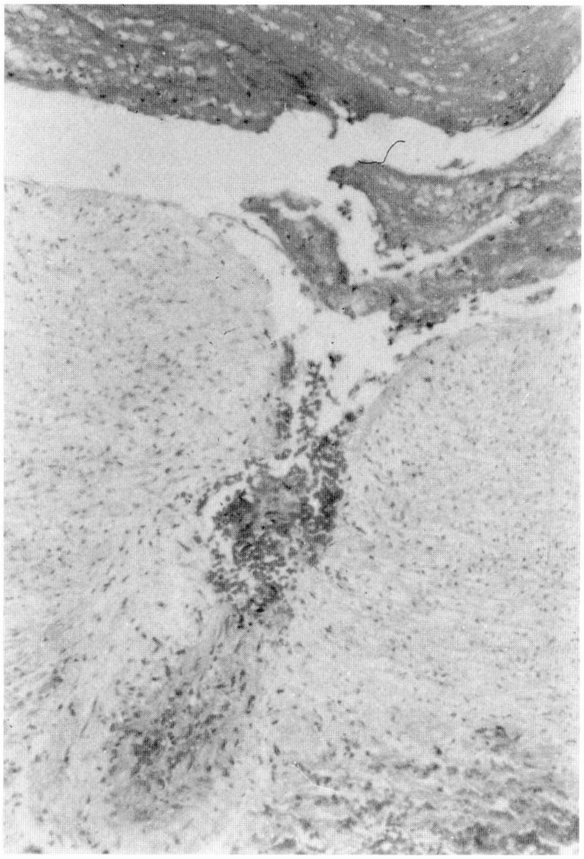

FIGURE 4-25. Thrombus occluding the ostium of inferior mesenteric artery (H&E, ×200).

turn lead to mucosal necrosis. In infants with infectious diarrhea the pathogenic organisms may further invade the devitalized mucosa. This explains the prominent inflammatory component of the lesion in the first subtype. Since they noted vascular thrombi in their cases, Stein et al[40] suggested that the Schwartzman reaction in their patients with Gram-negative infection may play a role in the pathogenesis of this type of NEC. In the other subtype the dehydration associated with chronic idiopathic diarrhea appears to be related to segmental hypoperfusion of the GI tract.

MISCELLANEOUS GROUP

NEC Associated with Hemodynamic Abnormalities

Besides the four types of NEC described above there is a miscellaneous group of patients with NEC in whom various predisposing factors are present. These include recent surgery,[44] congenital heart disease,[8,44] hyperviscosity syn-

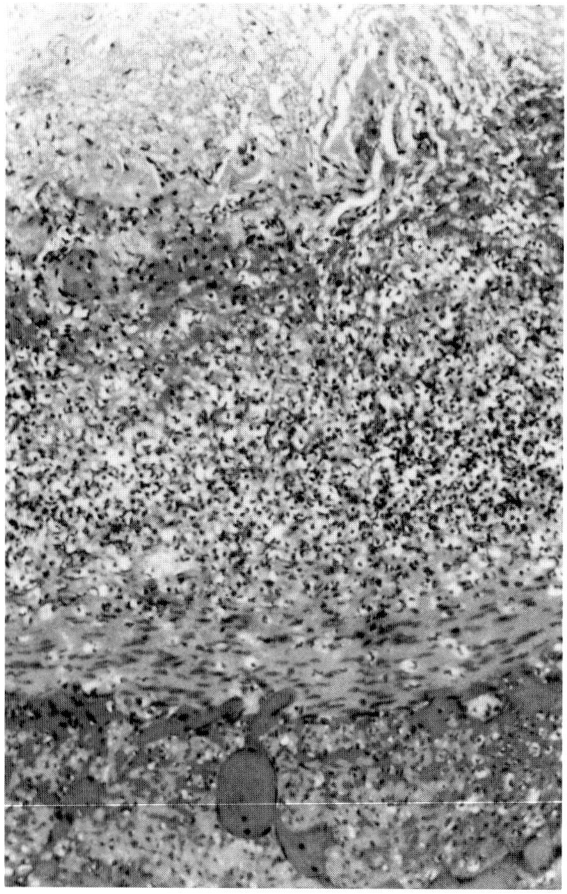

FIGURE 4-26. NEC following bacterial gastroenteritis; note the marked inflammatory reaction in the submucosa (H&E, ×200).

drome,[45,46] and perinatal cocaine exposure.[47] The final common pathogenetic pathway in these patients appears to be segmental hypoperfusion of the gut.

Idiopathic Gastrointestinal Perforation

The occurrence of idiopathic gastrointestinal perforation in the neonate also probably belongs to this miscellaneous group.[48] The perforation can occur in the stomach, small intestine, and colon. Small intestine appears to be the commonest site. Maternal obstetric complications, prematurity and perinatal stress were common in the series reported by Zamir et al.[48] Meyer et al[49] described a similar lesion in newborn infants weighing <1000 g. They considered these perforations as distinct from NEC. However the presence of extreme prematurity and respiratory distress requiring mechanical ventilation suggests that episodes of hypoxia and low hypertension might have occurred in these infants. Thus the final common pathway in the pathogenesis of perforation appears to be segmental hypoperfusion of the gut.

Necrotizing Enterocolitis Beyond Neonatal Period

Necrotizing enterocolitis can also occur beyond neonatal period.[50,51] Gastroenteritis with hypovolemia, acute lymphoblastic leukemia, congenital immune deficiency syndromes, aplastic anemia, congenital heart disease, etc. were the primary clinical diagnoses in these infants. NEC occurred as a complication or terminal event in these infants. The final common pathway in these infants also appears to be segmental hypoperfusion associated with shock, hypovolemia, hypoxia, and hypotension. NEC occurring in infants with Hirschsprung's disease also belongs to this group. Mucosal hypoperfusion due to increased intaluminal pressure appears to be the pathogenetic mechanism.

COMMENTS

Salient Pathologic Features

The following features of idiopathic NEC are not sufficiently stressed, and their implications in the treatment of INEC are not appreciated:

1. A common misconception is that the dark-red dull appearance of the affected intestinal segment of INEC is indicative of "infarction" of that segment, i.e., total thickness necrosis. But in fact the necrosis is almost exclusively confined to the mucosa and is transmural only in a focal area or areas in cases in which a perforation or perforations occur.[52]
2. Inflammatory reaction, although variable in severity, is frequently minimal or absent in the damaged mucosa. The presence of a relatively severe inflammatory reaction may be related to secondary bacterial invasion and/or extent of reperfusion injury (release of oxygen derived free radicals).
3. In INEC, there is no occlusion of the major arteries or the veins of the affected segment. This can be demonstrated in an autopsy case in which the affected segment was not resected. The thrombi seen in small submucosal blood vessels are probably secondary to the mucosal necrosis and not its cause. Mucosal necrosis related to PAF in the rat model is not due to thrombus formation but to vasoconstriction produced by a number of biochemical mediators. Thus hypoperfusion, thought to be the central mechanism in the pathogenesis of INEC, is due to reversible systemic and hemodynamic phenomenon and not due to irreversible luminal obstruction of the major blood vessels of the affected segment.
4. After the acute phase of the disease is over and presumably normal blood flow to the affected intestinal segment is reestablished, the areas of mucosal necrosis are capable of partial or near complete reconstitution.[2]

Clinical Implications of Pathologic Features

What are the implications of these findings in the treatment of NEC? Since there is no structural obstruction to the blood supply of the affected intestine and since the lesion is almost exclusively mucosal, medical management consisting of giving rest to the intestine and general systemic support can lead to healing of the lesions and reconstitution of the necrotic mucosa. If the complication of perforation occurs and surgical intervention is required, extensive resections of all the intestine that looks dark black and dull is not essential—only the portion that appears the worst grossly and/or shows perforation needs to be resected. Dark black but nonperforated intestine left behind and used for formation of stoma or mucous fistula has been observed to turn pink in 24–48 hours and remain viable (Hutcher NE: Personal communications, 1975). The pathologist by doing frozen sections of the margins of the resected portion can determine that there is no transmural necrosis at the margins of resection. If the surgeon will take such a conservative approach, immediate and remote postoperative morbidity and mortality of NEC can probably be much reduced. Avoidance of resection of excessive lengths of intestine would also reduce the long-term morbidity and mortality due to short-bowel syndrome.

Spectrum of NEC

From the description of various features of NEC it will be apparent that there are differences in some of the clinical features, associated conditions, pathologic changes, mortality, and known or proposed pathogenesis between the different types of NEC (Table 4-1). Thus increased frequency of stools, which is a prominent clinical feature of NEC following infectious gastroenteritis or idiopathic diarrhea, is not present in other types of NEC. Perinatal "stress" factors are commonly associated with NEC of all types except that following ET. All types of NEC except the one following ET are seen most commonly in premature and low-birth-weight infants, although INEC and NEC following diarrhea can occur in term infants. Only mucosal necrosis is seen in INEC and NEC following diarrhea, whereas total-thickness necrosis is present in the other two types of NEC. Inflammatory reaction is prominent in NEC following bacterial gastroenteritis. Incidence of perforation is higher in NEC following ET than in other types of NEC. In INEC the principal pathogenetic mechanism appears to be hypoperfusion of the intestine due to redistribution of blood supply in a "stressed" infant and not to irreversible structural obstruction of the arterial supply, which is the principal mechanism in infants with NEC following OAT due to UAC. In NEC following ET the pathogenesis is related to impedance of venous outflow and the lesion resembles a venous infarct. The mortality in NEC following ET, despite the high incidence of perforation, is low, that in INEC about 20–40% whereas the mortality in the remaining two types of NEC is almost 100%. The clinical features, pathogenesis and pathologic features of the cases in the miscellaneous NEC group are somewhat similar to those of INEC.

Because of the differences in the clinicopathologic features, pathogenesis and mortality of the different types of NEC as described above, it is recommended that these should be recognized as different clinicopathologic types belonging to the NEC spectrum.

TABLE 4-1 Differences in Clinicopathologic Features of Different Types of NEC[a]

Type of NEC	Antecedent features	Common site	Characteristic pathologic lesion	Pathogenesis	Comment
Idiopathic NEC	Prematurity, LBW perinatal stress	Terminal ileum, proximal colon	Bland mucosal necrosis	Hypoperfusion of intestine due to shunting off of blood to more vital organs, followed by reflow injury	Variable degree of inflammation may be present in the involved segment in occasional cases, mortality: 20–40%
NEC following ET	Majority >2500 g, hyperbilirubinemia requiring ET	Colon	Hemorrhagic venous infarction	Impedance of venous outflow due to portal hypertension secondary to ET	Isolated perforation may be the only lesion, mortality: low
NEC following OAT due to UAC	Prematurity, LBW, perinatal stress	Small and/or large intestine	Total thickness infarction	Thrombotic occlusion of ostium or lumen of mesenteric artery	Rare occurrence, 100% mortality
NEC following diarrhea	Prematurity, LBW, perinatal stress, diarrhea	Small and/or large intestine	Mucosal necrosis with prominent inflammatory reaction	Hypoperfusion of intestine in a dehydrated infant	Occurrence mainly in developing countries, virtually 100% mortality
Miscellaneous group	Newborn infants, older children with a variety of predisposing factors[b]	Small intestine	Mucosal necrosis with variable degree of inflammatory reaction	Hypoperfusion of intestine in an infant with shock or hypotension	High mortality

[a] Abbreviations: NEC—neonatal necrotizing enterocolitis; LBW—low birth weight; ET—exchange transfusion; OAT—occlusive arterial thrombosis; UAC—umbilical arterial catheterization.

[b] These include recent surgery, congenital heart disease, gastroenteritis, and hemorrhagic disorders.

REFERENCES

1. Brown EG, Sweet AY: Neonatal necrotizing enterocolitis. *Pediatr Clin North Am* 29:1149–1170, 1982.
2. Joshi VV, Winston YE, Kay S: Neonatal necrotizing enterocolitis: Histologic evidence of healing. *Am J Dis Child* 126:113–116, 1973.
3. Joshi VV, Draper DA, Bates KD: Neonatal necrotizing enterocolitis: Occurrence secondary to thrombosis of abdominal aorta following umbilical arterial catheterization. *Arch Pathol* 99:540–543, 1975.
4. Joshi VV: Clinicopathologic spectrum of neonatal necrotizing enterocolitis. *Indian Pediatr* 15:447–450, 1978.
5. Stevenson DK, Graham CB, Oliver TK, et al: Neonatal necrotizing enterocolitis. A report of 21 cases with 14 survivors. *Am J Surg* 118:260–272, 1969.
6. Santulli TV, Schullinger JN, Heird WC, et al: Acute necrotizing enterocolitis in infancy: A review of 64 cases. *Pediatrics* 55:376–387, 1975.
7. Frantz ID, Lheureux P, Engel RR, et al: Necrotizing enterocolitis. *J Pediatr* 86:259–263, 1975.
8. Polin RA, Pollack PF, Barlow B, et al: Necrotizing enterocolitis in term infants. *J Pediatr* 89:460–462, 1976.
9. Kliegman RM, Fanaroff AA: Necrotizing enterocolitis. *N Engl J Med* 310:1093–1103, 1984.
10. Kliegman RM, Fanaroff AA: Neonatal necrotizing enterocolitis in the absence of pneumatosis intestinalis. *Am J Dis Child* 136:618–620, 1982.
11. Hopkins GB, Gould VE, Stevenson JK, et al: Necrotizing enterocolitis in premature infants. A clinical and pathologic evaluation of autopsy material. *Am J Dis Child* 120:229–232, 1970.
12. Engel RR, Virning VL, Hunt CE, et al: Origin of mural gas in necrotizing enterocolitis. *Pediatr Res* 7:292, 1973.
13. Salinas-Madrigal L, Bruk A, DeMello DE: Myofibrillar degeneration and necrosis of the visceral smooth musculature: An ischemic visceral myopathy. *Hum Pathol* 18:815–823, 1987.
14. Ballance WA: Personal communication, 1992.
15. Touloukian RJ, Posch JN, Spencer R: The pathogenesis of ischemic gastroenterocolitis of the neonate: Selective gut mucosal ischemia in asphyxiated neonatal piglets. *J Pediatr Surg* 7:194–205, 1972.
16. Norris HT: Re-examination of the spectrum of ischemic bowel disease. In *Pathology of colon, small intestine and anus* (Norris HT, Ed). Churchill Livingstone, New York, 1991, Chap 5, pp 121–136.
17. Norwicki P: Intestinal ischemia and necrotizing enterocolitis. *J Pediatr* 117:S14–S19, 1990.
18. Shepherd AP, Mailman D, Burks TF, et al: Effects of norepinephrine and systematic stimulation on extraction of oxygen and ^{86}Rb in perfused canine small bowel. *Circ Res* 33:166–174, 1973.
19. Gonzales-Crusi F, Hsueh W: Experimental model of ischemic bowel necrosis: The role of platelet-activating factor and endotoxin. *Am J Pathol* 112:127–135, 1983.
20. Hsueh W, Gonzales-Crussi F, Arroyave JL: Platelet activating factor is an endogenous mediator in endotoxin induced bowel necrosis. *FASEB J* 1:403–405, 1987.
21. Hsueh W, Gonzales-Crussi F, Arroyave JL: Platelet activating factor induced ischemic bowel necrosis. An investigation of secondary mediators in its pathogenesis. *Am J Pathol* 122:231–239, 1986.
22. Lefer AM: Leukotrienes as mediators of ischemia and shock. *Bioch Pharmacol* 35:123–127, 1986.

23. Hsueh W, Gonzales-Crussi F, Arroyave JL: Sequential release of leukotrienes and norepinephrine in rat bowel after platelet activating factor. A mechanistic study of platelet-activating factor-induced bowel necrosis. *Gastroenterology* 94:1412–1418, 1988.
24. Cueva JP, Hsueh W: Role of oxygen derived free radicals in platelet activating factor induced bowel necrosis. *Gut* 29:1207–1212, 1988.
25. Book LS, Herbst JJ, Jung AL: Necrotizing enterocolitis in infants fed an elemental formula. *Pediatr Res* 8(379):105, 1974.
26. deLemos RA, Rogers JH, McLaughlin GW: Experimental production of necrotizing enterocolitis in newborn goats. *Pediatr Res* 8(380):106, 1974.
27. Kliegman RM: Neonatal necrotizing enterocolitis: Implications for an infectious disease. *Pediatr Clin N Am* 95:327–344, 1979.
28. Lucas A, Cole T: Breast milk and neonatal necrotizing enterocolitis. *Lancet* 336:1519–1523, 1990.
29. Pitt J, Barlow B, Heird WC, et al: Macrophages and the protective action of breast milk in necrotizing enterocolitis. *Pediatr Res* 8(384):110, 1974.
30. Barlow B, Santulli TV, Heird WC, et al: An experimental study of acute neonatal enterocolitis—the importance of breast milk. *J Pediatr Surg* 9:587–595, 1974.
31. Kliegman RM: Models of the pathogenesis of necrotizing enterocolitis. *J Pediatr* 117:S2–S5, 1990.
32. deSa DJ, Mucklow ES, Gough MH: Neonatal gut infarction. *J Pediatr Surg* 5:454–459, 1970.
33. Lloyd DA, Cywes S: Intestinal stenosis and enterocyst formation as late complications of neonatal necrotizing enterocolitis. *J Pediatr Surg* 8:479–486, 1973.
34. Janik JS, Ein SH, Mancer K: Intestinal stricture after necrotizing enterocolitis. *J Pediatr Surg* 16:438–443, 1981.
35. Touloukian RJ, Kadar A, Spencer RP: The gastrointestinal complications of neonatal umbilical venous exchange transfusion: A clinical and experimental study. *Pediatrics* 51:36–43, 1973.
36. Corkery JJ, Dubowitz V, Lister J, et al: Colonic perforation after exchange transfusion. *Br Med J* 4:345–349, 1968.
37. Hardy JD, Savage TR, Shirodaria C: Intestinal perforation following exchange transfusion. *Am J Dis Child* 124:136–141, 1972.
38. Ballance WA, Dahms BB, Shenker N, et al: Pathology of neonatal necrotizing enterocolitis: A ten year experience. *J Pediatr* 117:S6–S13, 1990.
39. Gupta JM, Robertson NRC, Wigglesworth JS: Umbilical artery catheterization in the newborn. *Arch Dis Child* 43:382–387, 1968.
40. Stein H, Beck J, Solomon A, et al: Gastroenteritis with necrotizing enterocolitis in premature babies. *Br Med J* 2:616–619, 1972.
41. Karan S, Pathak A: Necrotizing enterocolitis in the newborn. *Indian Pediatr* 10:279–286, 1973.
42. Bhargava SK, Mittal SK, Saxena HM, et al: An outbreak of necrotizing enterocolitis in a special care newborn nursery. *Indian Pediatr* 10:551–553, 1973.
43. Rotbart HA, Levin MJ, Yolken RH, et al: An outbreak of rotavirus associated neonatal necrotizing enterocolitis. *J Pediatr* 103:454–459, 1983.
44. Amoury RA, Goodwin CD, McGill CW, et al: Necrotizing enterocolitis following operation in the neonatal period. *J Pediatr Surg* 15:1–8, 1980.
45. Kliegman RM, Walsh MC: Neonatal necrotizing enterocolitis. Pathogenesis, classification, and spectrum of illness. *Curr Prob Pediatr* 17:213–288, 1987.
46. Dunn SP, Gross KR, Scherer LR, et al: The effect of polycythemia and hyperviscosity on bowel ischemia. *J Pediatr Surg* 20:324–327, 1985.
47. Telsey AM, Merrit TA, Dixon SD: Cocaine exposure in a term neonate: Necrotizing enterocolitis as a complication. *Clin Pediatr* 27:547–550, 1988.

47. Telsey AM, Merrit TA, Dixon SD: Cocaine exposure in a term neonate: Necrotizing enterocolitis as a complication. *Clin Pediatr* 27:547–550, 1988.
48. Zamir O, Goldberg M, Udassin R, et al: Idiopathic gastrointestinal perforation in the neonate. *J Pediatr Surg* 23:335–337, 1988.
49. Meyer CL, Payne NR, Roback SA: Spontaneous isolated intestinal perforations in neonates with birth weight <1000 g not associated with necrotizing enterocolitis. *J Pediatr Surg* 26:714–717, 1991.
50. Takayanagi K, Kapila L: Necrotizing enterocolitis in older infants. *Arch Dis Child* 56:468–471, 1981.
51. Moss TJ, Adler R: Necrotizing enterocolitis in older infants, children and adolescents. *J Pediatr* 100:764–766, 1982.
52. Joshi VV: Implications of pathologic findings in NEC in its treatment. *Pediatrics* 59:954, 1977.

5 PERINATAL LESIONS OF THE HEAD AND BRAIN

INTRODUCTION

Perinatal lesions of the head and brain include hemorrhagic and nonhemorrhagic lesions. Hemorrhages may be extracranial (in relation to the scalp, aponeurosis, and periosteum) or intracranial (in relation to the dura and arachnoid matter and the brain). Birth trauma is the main pathogenetic factor in the extracranial hemorrhages. Asphyxia may act as a contributory factor. Birth trauma or asphyxia is the main factor in the pathogenesis of different types of intracranial hemorrhage. These hemorrhagic lesions are represented diagrammatically in Figure 5-1. Nonhemorrhagic lesions of the brain related to ischemia also are commonly seen in neonatal autopsies.

HEMORRHAGIC LESIONS

Extracranial Hemorrhage

Caput succedaneum, subaponeurotic hemorrhage, and cephalhematoma constitute the different types of extracranial hemorrhages.

Caput succedaneum. There is a hemorrhagic edema of the scalp and superficial fascia. Caput succedaneum, which is commonly observed (Figure 5-1), is of no specific clinical significance.

Subaponeurotic hemorrhage. This is also called subgaleal hemorrhage (Figure 5-2). The hemorrhage is located under the epicranial aponeurosis. The aponeurosis represents the tendon of the occipitofrontal muscle. This type of hemorrhage may involve large portions of scalp and may extend into the subcutaneous tissue of the lateral and posterior parts of the neck. Extensive hemorrhage of this type may be a major factor in death of the infant.[1]

Cephalhematoma. This term is generally confined to the subperiosteal hemorrhage most commonly in the parietal bones (Figure 5-3). Periosteal attachments at the margins of the parietal bones tend to limit the extent of cephalhematoma. Therefore, it is rarely of clinical significance.

Pathogenesis of Extracranial Hemorrhage

Prolonged or obstructed labor, cephalopelvic disproportion, and instrumental intervention (vacuum extraction; forceps) are predisposing factors. Caput succedaneum occurs as a result of venous compression of the presenting part against uterine and pelvic wall. Some of these infants have intrauterine asphyxia, which renders them more vulnerable to bleeding.

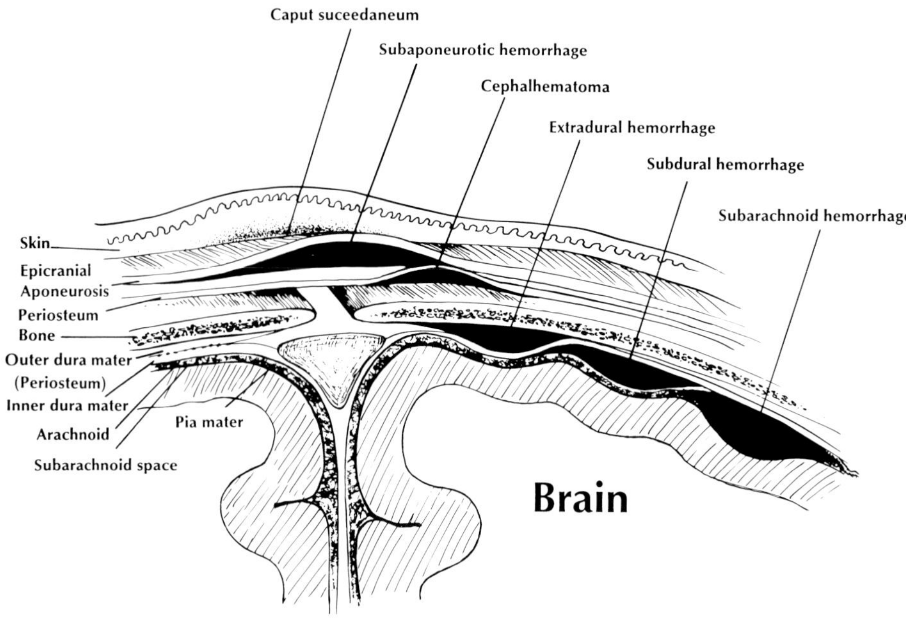

FIGURE 5-1. Diagrammatic representation of various sites of extracranial and intracranial hemorrhages.

Intracranial Hemorrhage

These include extradural, subdural, subarachnoid, and germinal matrix hemorrhages with or without intraventricular and/or parenchymal extension.

Extradural Hemorrhage

In this type, the hemorrhage occurs between the periosteum and the inner surface of the skull bone (Figure 5-1). Extradural hemorrhage is usually associated with fracture of the skull bones.

Subdural Hemorrhage

This type of hemorrhage[2–6] is seen at the following intracranial locations:

1. *Blood clot over the cerebral convexity.* Hemorrhage at this site occurs as a result of rupture of the superficial cerebral veins which drain into the superior sagittal sinus. In severe cases subarachnoid hemorrhage with or without cerebral contusion is present. The hematoma is located more towards the lateral aspect of the temporal lobe.
2. *Blood clot in the longitudinal cerebral fissure covering the corpus callosum.* Hemorrhage at this site occurs as a result of tear of falx cerebri near its junction with the tentorium cerebelli. The inferior sagittal sinus is ruptured at this site.
3. *Blood clot in the posterior fossa.*
   a. Hemorrhage at this site occurs as a result of tear of tentorium cerebelli. The tear, which may be partial- or full-thickness, involves the free margin of the tentorium near its junction with the falx. The straight sinus, vein of Galen, or lateral sinus is ruptured. The blood clot may be both supra and

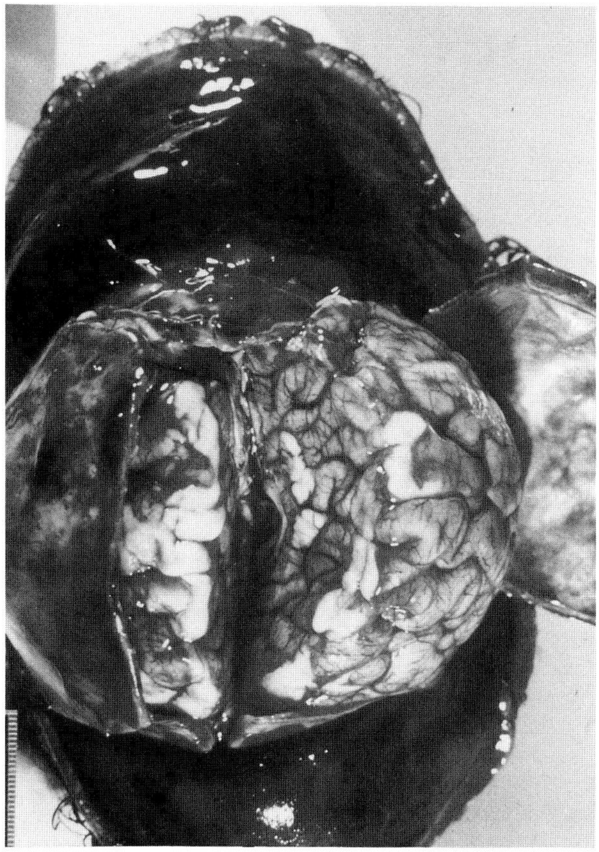

FIGURE 5-2. Diffuse subaponeurotic (subgaleal) hemorrhage of the scalp.

infratentorial. The infratentorial bleeding is often more severe than the supratentorial bleeding (Figure 17 in chapter 1). The bleeding produces severe compression of brain stem with fatal outcome. Rupture of vein of Galen with massive infratentorial hemorrhage may occur without demonstrable tentorial tear.

b. Posterior fossa hemorrhage can also occur particularly in breech delivery with application of forceps,[5,7] as a result of upward and inward bending of the squamous portion of the occipital bone into the posterior fossa (occipital osteodiastasis). The projecting bony edge tears the dura matter and ruptures the occipital sinuses. Laceration of cerebellum with intracerebellar hematoma may be present in these cases.

Pathogenesis of Subdural Hemorrhage. Subdural hemorrhage is related to birth trauma and occurs almost exclusively in a full-term newborn infant. Cephalopelvic disproportion, rigid pelvis of a primipara, and prolonged—or, in contrast, unusually short—duration of labor are the predisposing factors. In the past, delivery in abnormal presentations (such as breech, foot, face, brow) was

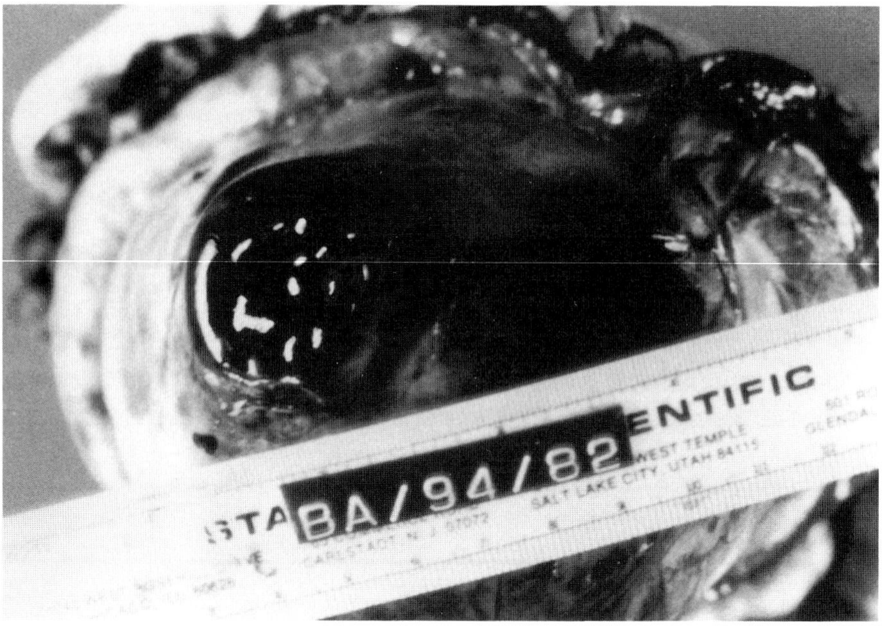

FIGURE 5-3. Subperiosteal hemorrhage (cephalhematoma) of the cranium.

facilitated by forceps extraction or rotational maneuvers. Under these circumstances the head is subjected to unusual deforming stresses and undergoes excessive vertical molding and anteroposterior elongation. Excessive stretching of falx and tentorium can occur resulting in tearing of these structures. The veins or sinuses are also "stretched" and are liable to rupture.[2,4] The dural compartments, the various intracranial sinuses and veins are represented diagrammatically in Figure 5-4. In recent years the incidence of these complications is virtually eliminated because of the progress in obstetric practice and increasing use of cesarean section. However, these lesions are seen in rare instances, and the pathologist should verify the intactness of the various dural compartments and intracranial sinuses at autopsy.

Subarachnoid Hemorrhage

Subarachnoid hemorrhage may be primary or secondary to subdural, intraventricular, or intracerebellar hemorrhage. Focal primary subarachnoid hemorrhage is a common finding in perinatal autopsies (Figure 5-5). These hemorrhages are of no clinical significance. More severe primary hemorrhages may be manifested by seizures or recurrent apnea. The hemorrhage is of venous origin and is related to hypoxia. Birth trauma also plays a role in the pathogenesis, particularly in full-term newborn infants. Hydrocephalus may occur as a late sequela of severe primary basal arachnoid hemorrhage due to adhesions around the foramina of Magendie and Luschka (see discussion of posthemorrhagic hydrocephalus following intraventricular hemorrhage below).

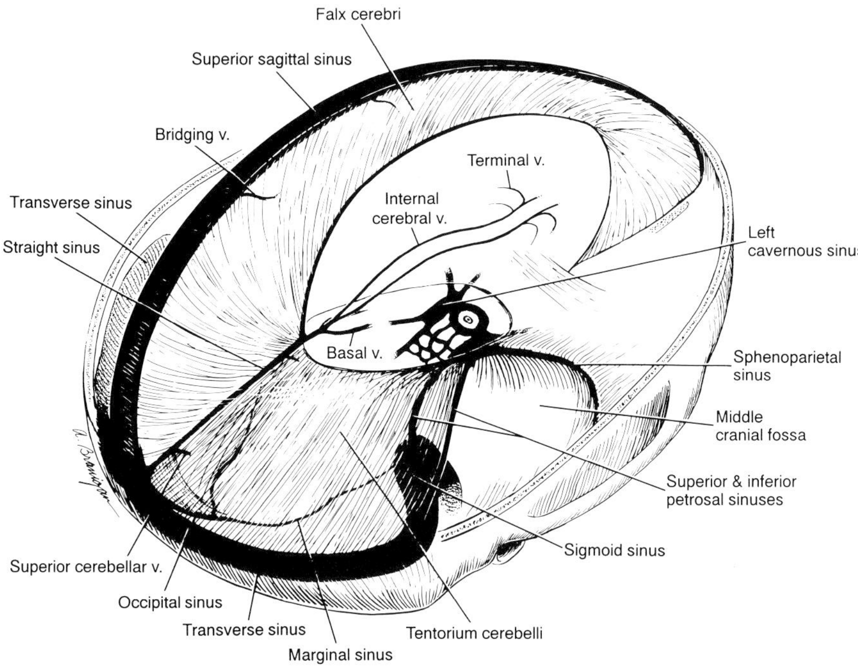

FIGURE 5-4. Diagrammatic representation of various intracranial sinuses and veins and dural compartments.

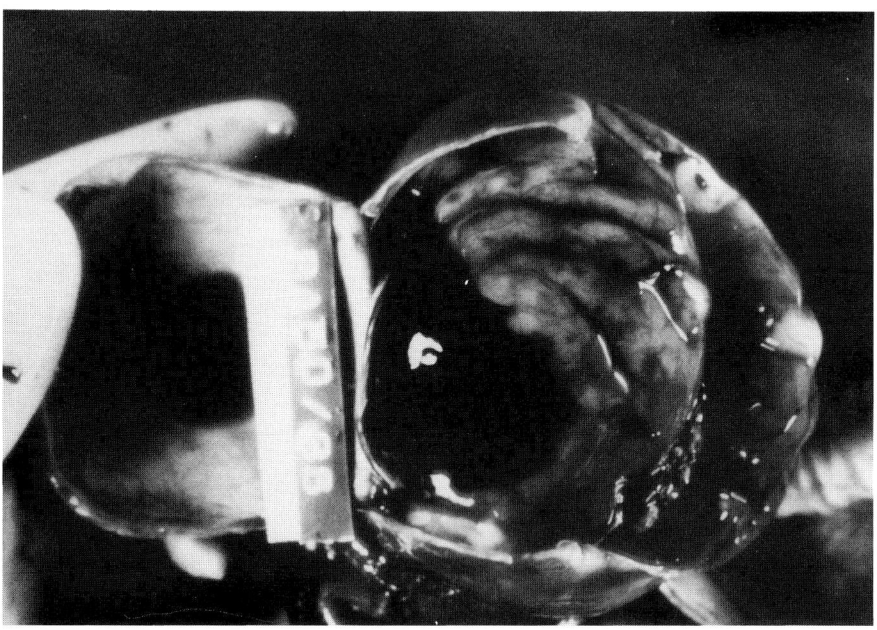

FIGURE 5-5. Localized subarachnoid hemorrhage.

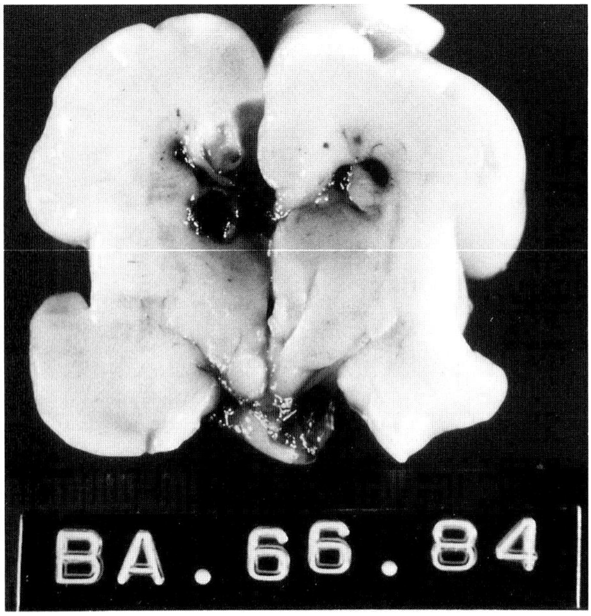

FIGURE 5-6. Bilateral subependymal hemorrhage with extension to the ventricles.

Subependymal Germinal Matrix Hemorrhage with Periventricular and Intraventricular Extension

This type of hemorrhage, abbreviated as PV/IVH, is essentially a lesion seen in premature infants, particularly at <30 weeks' gestation.[8] These lesions have aroused great interest in recent years because a larger number of infants who develop PV/IVH are surviving as a result of improvements in the management of neonatal disorders and also because of the advent of ultrasound and computerized tomography, which enables the neonatologist to document the lesion in its early stages and follow its evolution or resolution.[9]

The hemorrhage originates in the subependymal germinal matrix zone (GMZ) located between the caudate nucleus and thalamus (Figures 5-6, 5-7). The hemorrhage may extend into the ventricles and subsequently into the basal subarachnoid space (Figure 5-6) and even the subarachnoid space of the spinal cord and/or into the surrounding parenchyma. The severity of the hemorrhage is graded on the basis of extent of ventricular filling, dilatation of ventricles, and extension to the surrounding parenchyma. The blood clot may form casts of the lateral ventricles (Figure 5-8). A number of grading systems of PV/IVH have been described. The following system, described by Papile et al[10] is used commonly: *grade I*—subependymal hemorrhage only; *grade II*—IVH without dilatation; *grade III*—IVH with ventricular dilatation; *grade IV*—IVH with involvement of surrounding brain tissue (Figures 5-9, 5-10). It is important that the neonatologists (who monitor the PV/IVH by ultrasound) and the pathologist should use the same grading system so that valid comparisons can be made between the

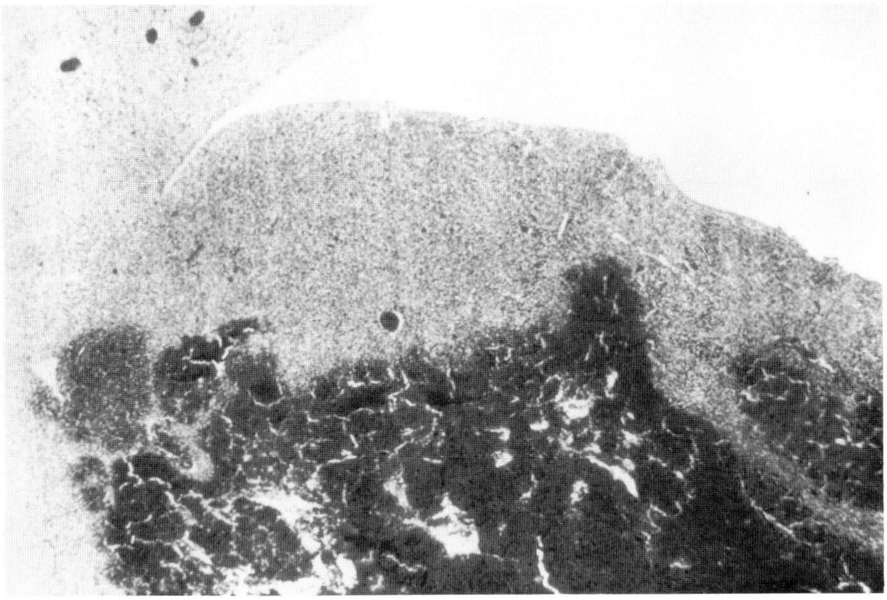

FIGURE 5-7. Subependymal hemorrhage on microscopic examination.

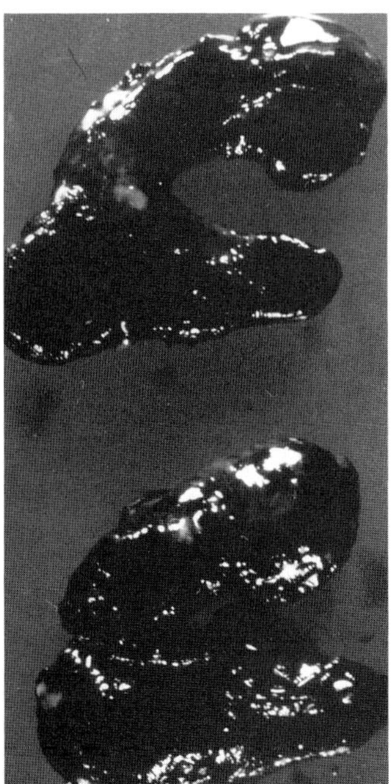

FIGURE 5-8. Casts of the lateral ventricle on subependymal hemorrhage with massive intraventricular extension.

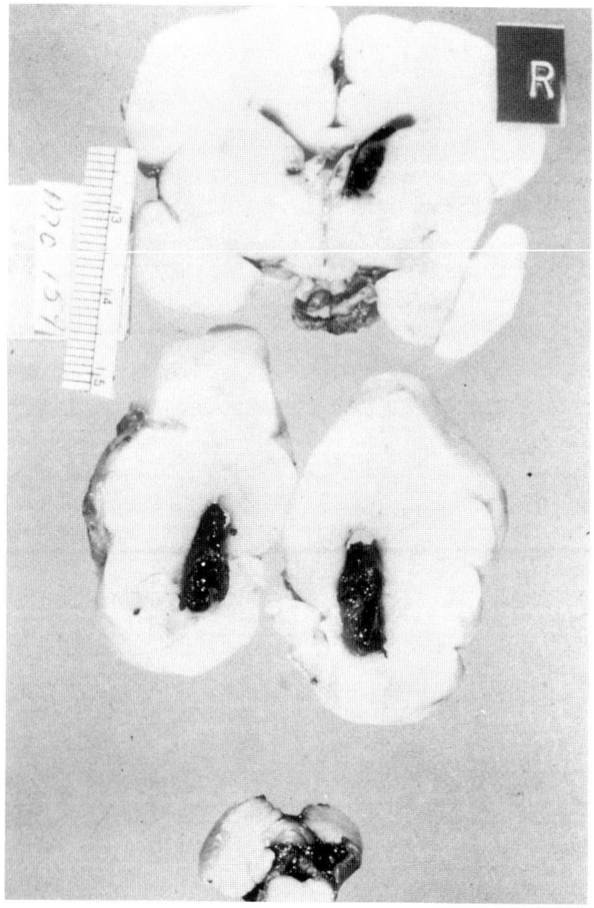

FIGURE 5-9. Intraventricular extension of subependymal hemorrhage without dilatation of the ventricles (grade II).

sonographic and pathologic findings. It has been shown that small subependymal hemorrhages documented by ultrasound examination may resolve over a period of several days. In such fatal cases the hemorrhage will not be seen at autopsy.

On histologic examination marked disruption of the GMZ may be seen in severe lesions. The ependymal lining is destroyed, and the blood fills the ventricular cavity and may extend into the surrounding brain parenchyma. The overlying white matter may show necrosis. It is difficult to demonstrate ruptured blood vessels.

Timing, Source, and Pathogenesis of PV/IVH

A number of factors related to gross and microanatomy, vascularity, hemodynamics, oxygenation, and acid–base balance are involved in the timing, source, and pathogenesis of PV/IVH.[2,8,9] Sonographic studies indicate that the hemorrhage occurs by the eighth day in majority of the cases.[11] It appears that the hemorrhage can occur either rapidly or over a period of time.[12]

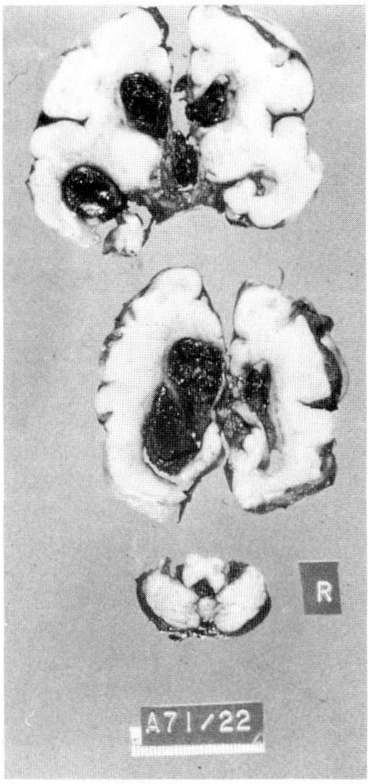

FIGURE 5-10. Intraventricular extension of subependymal hemorrhage with dilatation of the ventricles (grade III). There is also extension to the basal subarachnoid space.

GMZ is of a relatively large size up to 34 weeks' gestation[9] (Figure 5-11). It consists mostly of immature neuroblasts with virtually no supporting glial tissue. In contrast, the GMZ in the term newborn infant contains recognizable glial tissue, although a few immature neuroblasts still persist (Figure 5-12). The blood flow through the GMZ is higher than in the surrounding brain tissue.[13] The blood vessels of the GMZ which have been studied in newborn infants and puppies show the following notable features. The blood vessels are of relatively large size, have thinner walls and are poorly supported because of the paucity of glial tissue in the GMZ.[13–16] The frequent sites of hemorrhage within the GMZ correspond to the zones of convergence of veins of the GMZ.[14] These peculiar gross and microscopic anatomic features of the GMZ and its vascularity explain the occurrence of hemorrhage in the GMZ rather than in other parts of the brain. Arteries, veins, and capillaries have been implicated as the source of PV/IVH by various authors.[17–19] A study involving injection of arteries and veins has shown that the hemorrhage is of venous origin.[19] It appears that veins or the capillary vein junctions are the most likely source of PV/IVH.[8,18]

The disturbances of oxygenation (hypoxia) and acid–base balance (acidosis) associated with the common disorders in premature infants play an important role in the pathogenesis of PV/IVH. Endothelial injury, venous stasis with raised venous pressure, and impaired autoregulation of the cerebral blood flow resulting from hypoxia and acidosis can lead to PV/IVH. Normally autoregulation involving constriction and dilatation of arterioles in appropriate conditions maintains a constant cerebral blood flow. Impairment of this mechanism can lead to bursts of high flow and high pressure through a damaged vasculature,

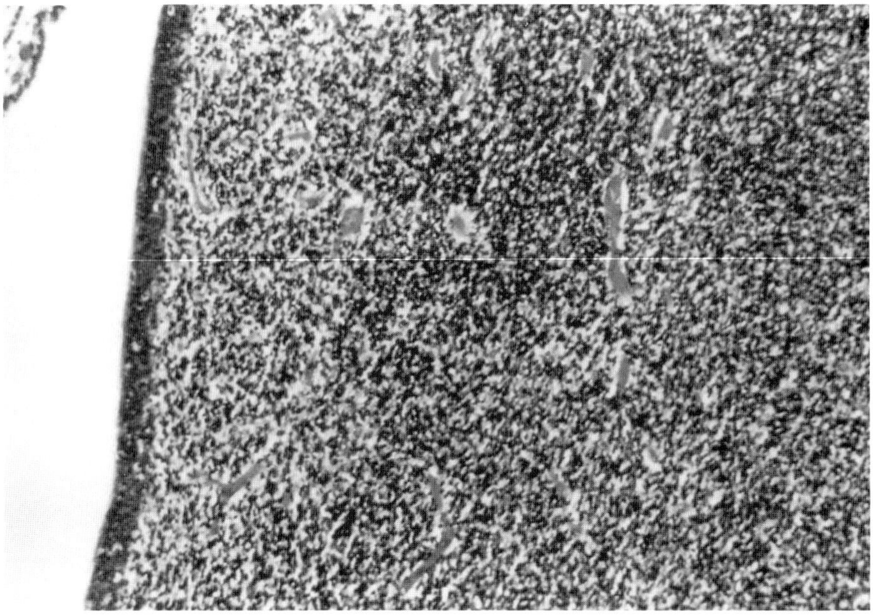

FIGURE 5-11. Subependymal germinal matrix zone in the premature infant. Note the undifferentiated neuroblasts without any glial (or neuronal) differentiation. The blood vessels are prominent. (H&E, ×100.)

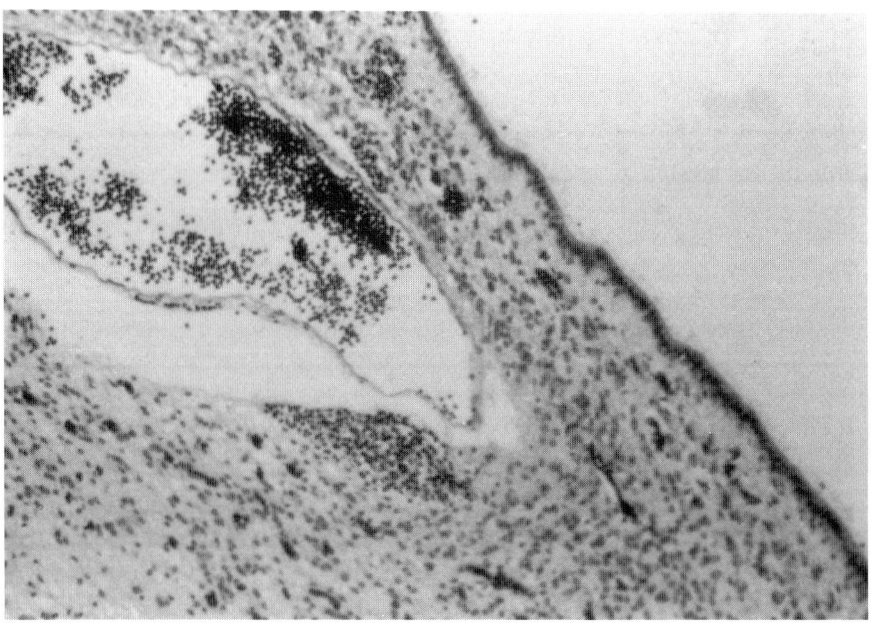

FIGURE 5-12. Subependymal germinal matrix zone in a full-term newborn infant; note the differentiation into glial tissue and persistent small foci of undifferentiated neuroblasts (H&E, ×100).

resulting in their rupture.[13] Other factors such as coagulation defects, high fibrinolytic activity of the GMZ, hypothermia, and hyperosmolarity produced by administration of excess sodium bicarbonate are also of importance in prolonging and increasing the severity of PV/IVH.[21–23] The various pathogenetic factors in PV/IVH are summarized in Table 5-1.

Sequelae of PV/IVH

Milder degrees of subependymal and even intraventricular hemorrhage can become absorbed and do not result in any significant neurologic deficit. However, more severe degrees of PV/IVH may be associated with neurologic deficit in about one-third to one-half of the cases. The morphologic sequelae include posthemorrhagic hydrocephalus. The dilated ventricle may show a persistent old blood clot (Figure 5-13). The generally accepted mechanism relates to the basal obliterative arachnoiditis associated with basal subarachnoid extension of PV/IVH, resulting in the blockage of the pathways of cerebrospinal fluid circulation in the posterior fossa (foramina of Luschka and Magendie).[24] The blood in the subarachnoid space is lysed and absorbed within about a week. But the associated inflammatory reaction with accumulation of the hemosiderin laden macrophages and fibrosis produces brownish discoloration and thickening of the leptomeninges and obstruction of CSF (cerebrospinal fluid) pathways (Figures 5-14–5-16). In some cases the site of obstruction to the CSF circulation is the aqueduct.[24]

It takes several days for this sequela to develop fully. However, sonographic studies have shown that hydrocephalus starts developing within a few days of PV/IVH. Small fragments of blood clot and fibrin visualized as particulate matter

TABLE 5-1 Factors in Pathogensis of Periventricular and Intraventricular Hemorrhage

Factor	Mechanisms	Effect
Prematurity	Presence of germinal matrix zone	Characteristic location of hemorrhage
Hypoxia/acidosis	Endothelial injury, myocardial failure, impaired autoregulation of cerebral circulation	Edema and/or hemorrhage Venous stasis, raised venous pressure, rupture of blood vessels Bursts of high flow and high pressure
Germinal matrix zone	Absence of glial elements, Normally high blood flow as compared with other areas of the brain, large number of thin-walled blood vessels, high fibrinolytic activity	Lack of support to the blood vessels→rupture Hemorrhage through previously damaged blood vessels Tendency to rupture Prolongs the hemorrhage
Hypothermia, hyperosmolarity, and coagulation defects	Endothelial injury, blood pressure fluctuation, and increased tendency to bleed	Rupture of blood vessels and prolongation of bleeding

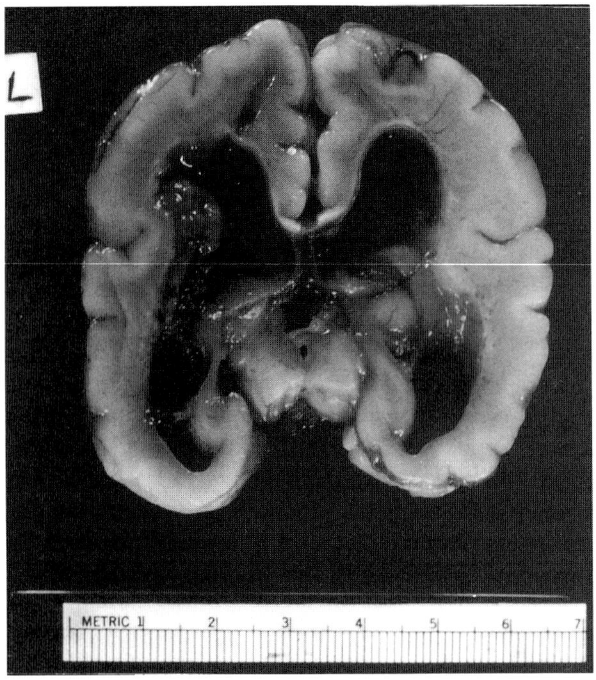

FIGURE 5-13. Posthemorrhagic hydrocephalus in a premature infant. Note the persistent blood clot in the left lateral ventricle.

on the sonograms may block the arachnoid villi, resulting in decreased CSF reabsorption and early development of hydrocephalus.[25]

Intraventricular Hemorrhage in the Term Infant

Intraventricular hemorrhage (IVH) in the full-term infant, is usually confined to the ventricular cavity since choroid plexus rather than the GMZ is the source of bleeding.[26,27] Hemorrhage into the GMZ with intraventricular extension also occurs in the full-term neonate.[27] In rare instances hemorrhage can occur at both the sites.[27] On gross and histologic examination there is marked

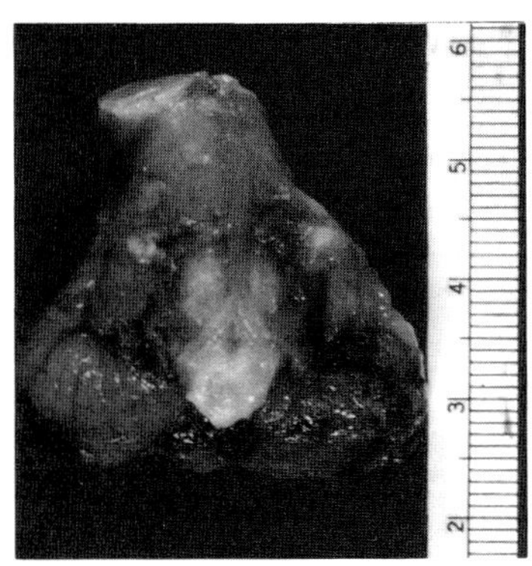

FIGURE 5-14. Note brownish staining of the basal leptomeninges due to old hemorrhage (in a case of posthemorrhagic hydrocephalus).

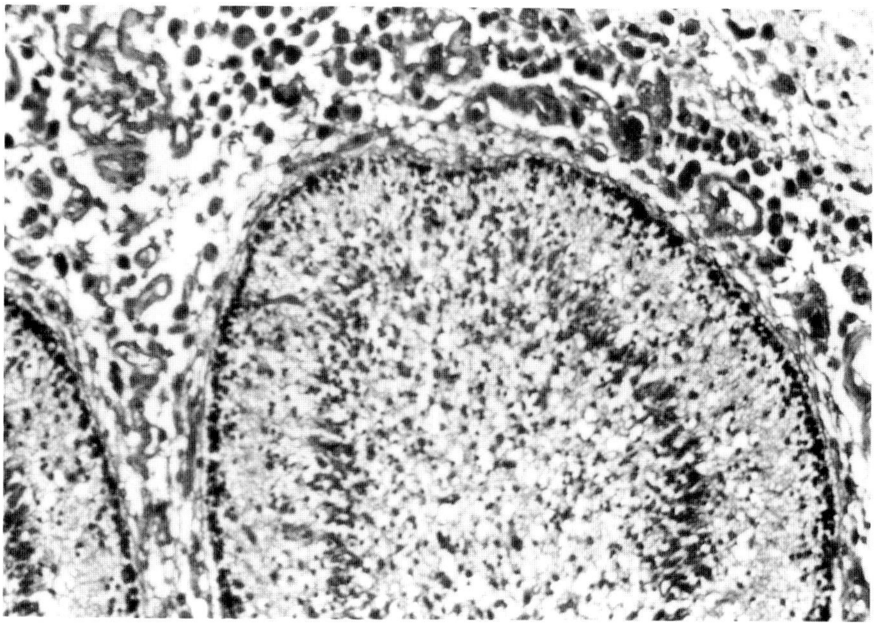

FIGURE 5-15. Note the numerous hemosiderin-laden macrophages in the leptomeninges of the cerebellum in a case of posthemorrhagic hydrocephalus (H&E, ×250).

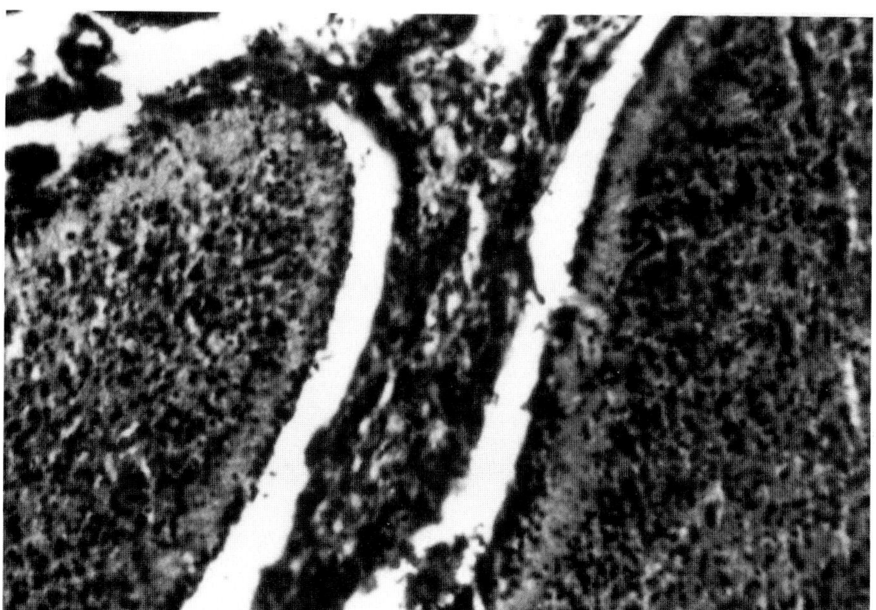

FIGURE 5-16. Fibroblastic proliferation in the leptomeninges of the cerebellum in a case of posthemorrhagic hydrocephalus (H&E, ×250).

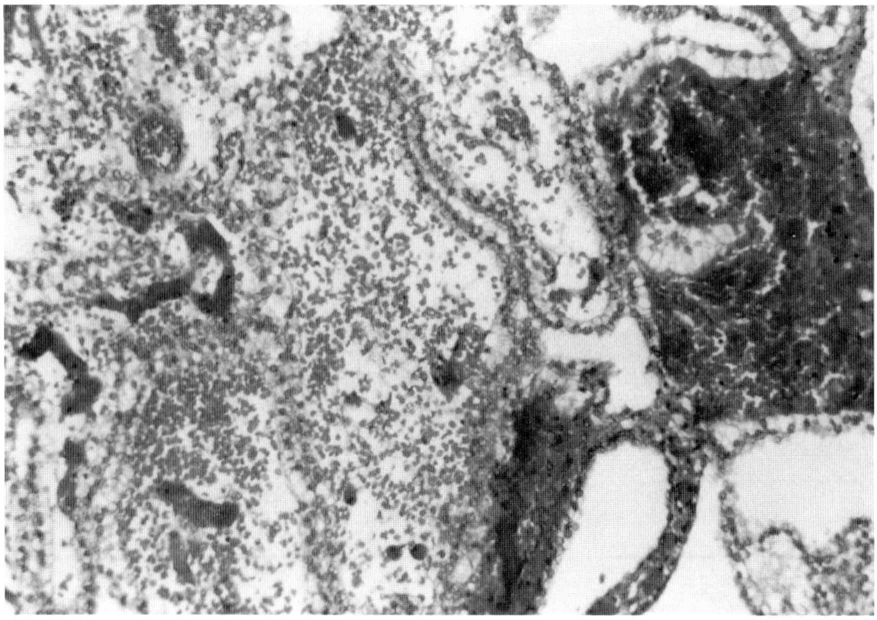

FIGURE 5-17. Hemorrhage in the choroid plexus of a full term newborn infant (H&E, ×250).

engorgement of the choroid plexus and hemorrhage into the matrix of the plexus is present (Figure 5-17).

Pathogenesis of IVH in the Term Infant

In the series of 32 cases reported by Lacey et al[27] mean Apgar scores at 1 and 5 minutes were 3.5 and 5 respectively. Hypotonia, hyporeflexia, and seizures were the characteristic neurologic features. Other findings consisted of visceral congestion, IRDS (idiopathic respiratory distress syndrome), and meconium aspiration, and interestingly in 13 cases severe forms of congenital heart disease (transposition of great vessels, large ventricular septal defect, hypoplastic chambers and blood vessels, etc.) were present. All these findings indicated that these full term infants with IVH had asphyxia. Therefore, all the factors described above in the pathogenesis of PV/IVH in the preterm neonate may also be implicated in the IVH in the term infant.

Although GMZ is not completely mature in the term infant, it is significantly reduced in size (Figure 5-12). The difference in the source of hemorrhage can be explained by this marked diminution of the GMZ at term. The regional blood flow also changes from predominant orientation to basal ganglia to the cortical pattern by 34 weeks' gestation.[28] This change of blood flow away from the GMZ explains the relative infrequency of hemorrhage at that site in the term infant. Thinness of venous walls and poor support of the vascular structures of the choroid plexus have been implicated in predilection for that site in the term infant.[27] The presence of congenital heart disease in the series reported by Lacey et al[27] suggested the possible role of venous stasis of the choroid plexus as a contributory factor. A vascular malformation or blood dyscrasia (hemophilia, isoimmune neonatal thrombocytopenia) may be the primary factors in the pathogenesis in some cases.[29,30]

Intracerebral Hemorrhage

Intracerebral hemorrhage is generally not considered as a separate entity. There is an intracerebral component in PV/IVH. There may also be a hemorrhagic component in the hypoxic ischemic lesions (to be described below). Thalamic hemorrhage may occur in association with PV/IVH, particularly in the full-term newborn infants.[31]

Intracerebellar Hemorrhage

Intracerebellar hemorrhage is more common than is generally appreciated (Figure 5-18). It is reported to have the incidence of 15–25% in premature infants of <32 weeks' gestation.[32,33] The hemorrhage may vary from slight to massive. The mechanism is not known. Occipital compression caused by the band of the face mask has been implicated[34] but not confirmed by others.[32,33] It has been suggested that the pathogenesis may be the same as PV/IVH.[2] The external granular layer of the cerebellar foliae composed of immature neuroblasts with poorly supported blood vessels may play a role in the localization of the hemorrhage to the cerebellum.

NONHEMORRHAGIC LESIONS

Hypoxic-Ischemic Encephalopathy (HIE)

Although hemorrhage may occur in HIE, the lesions represent primarily neuronal or white-matter necrosis. These lesions are distinctive from PV/IVH. We owe the initial recognition of HIE used in this restricted sense to ultrasonographic scanning used in the neonatal intensive nursery.[35] These observations, which indicated that besides PV/IVH, there was parenchymal necrosis in the

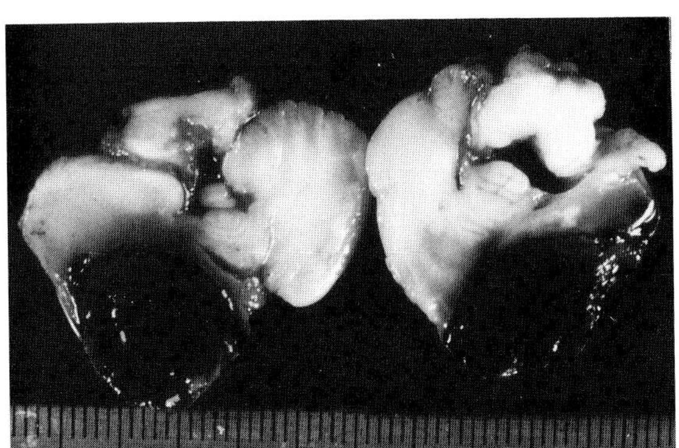

FIGURE 5-18. Intracerebellar hemorrhage.

cerebral hemisphere, were substantiated by clinical and pathologic studies.[36] The following clinical features are seen characteristically in newborn infants with HIE: (1) history of significant perinatal distress (Apgar scores <3); (2) sustained blood gas and pH abnormalities; (3) neurologic features such as hypotonia, seizures, stupor, and even coma; (4) increased CSF protein lactate and pyruvate; (5) diffuse CNS injury evidenced by imaging and electroencephalographic studies; and (6) absence of other CNS, metabolic, infectious, or structural abnormalities.

There are two distinctive types of pathologic lesions in HIE: selective neuronal necrosis (SNN) and periventricular leukomalasia (PVL).[8]

Selective Neuronal Necrosis

On gross examination the brain is edematous and diffusely softened with flattening of gyri and narrowing of sulci. Uncal or cerebellar tonsillar herniation may be present. On cut section the brain is edematous and pale and may disintegrate even with minimal handling.

The following patterns of SNN have been described:[8,37,38] (1) descending pattern involving the cerebral cortex and the thalamus; (2) ascending pattern involving the spinal cord, brain stem, midbrain, and thalamus; and (3) pontosubicular pattern, in which the pons and subicular segment of the Ammon's horn are affected. Overlapping patterns and involvement of neurons in other areas of the brain (e.g., dentate nucleus of the cerebellum) are not uncommon. The neuronal necrosis is characterized by nuclear pyknosis, eosinophilia or vacuolation of the cytoplasm (Figures 5-19, 5-20). Fragmentation of nucleus

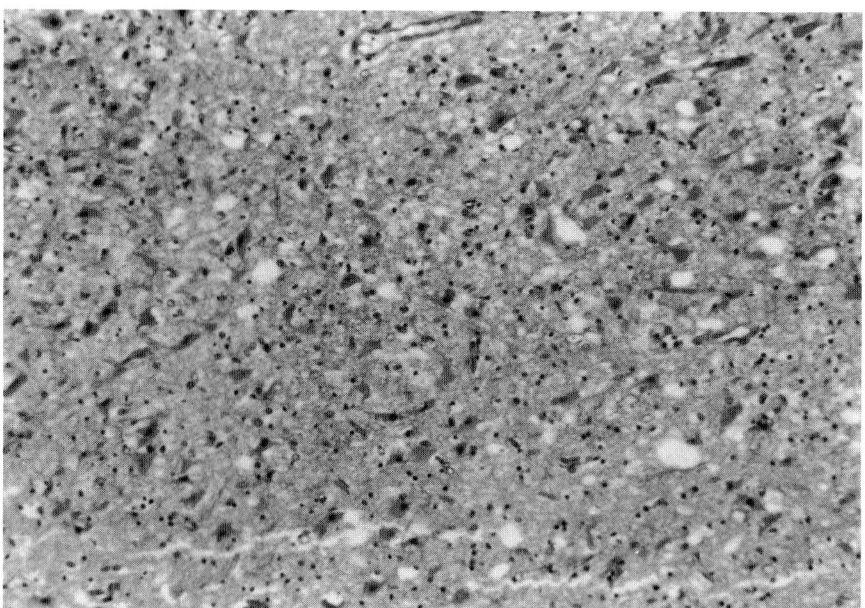

FIGURE 5-19. Hypoxic ischemic encephalopathy characterized by necrosis of cortical neurons (H&E, ×100).

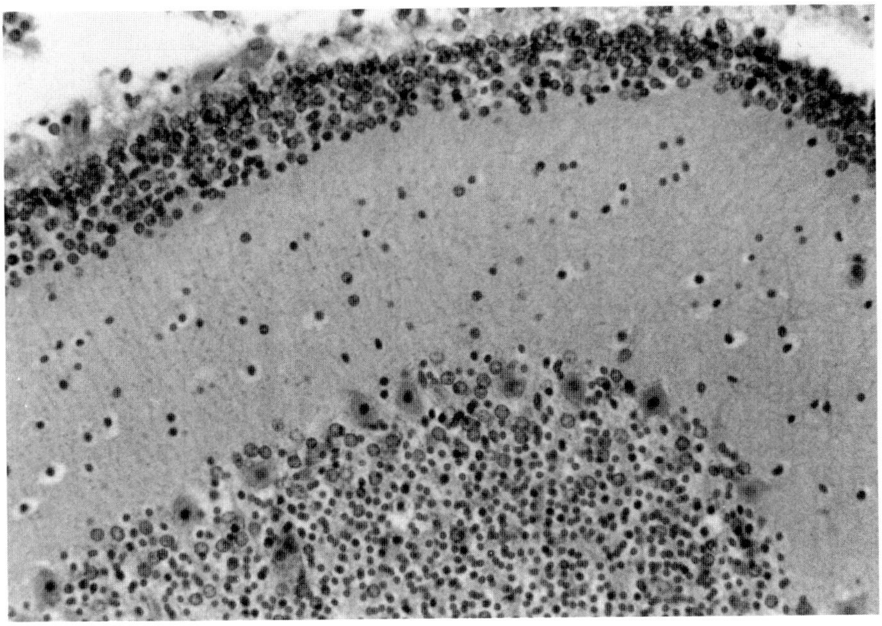

FIGURE 5-20. Hypoxic ischemic encephalopathy characterized by necrosis of Purkinje cells of the cerebellum (H&E, ×250).

(karyorrhexis) may also be seen. In later stages neuronal loss, encrustation (calcium and/or iron deposition) of neurons, glial reaction and prominent vascularity are seen in the areas of SNN.

Sequelae of SNN include cerebral atrophy with dilated ventricles, shrinkage of convolutions with widening of the sulci (ulegyria), and extensive liquefaction with multicystic encephalomalacia (porencephaly).

Periventricular Leukomalacia (PVL)

PVL is characterized by presence of poorly defined white spots measuring a few millimeters in diameter in the periventricular white matter of optic radiation at the trigone of the lateral ventricle and at the junction of corpus callosum with internal and external capsules (Figure 5-21). In the early stages coagulative necrosis is seen on microscopic examination (Figure 5-22). The areas of necrosis are infiltrated by lipophages. These lipophages give the spotty white appearance to the lesion. PVL may have a hemorrhagic component. These lesions have been considered as periventricular infarcts or periventricular hemorrhage. Such terminology invites confusion. These lesions are better described as hemorrhagic PVL[35] since the basic pathologic lesion is related to ischemia with the hemorrhagic component superimposed due to vascular damage or venous stasis (see below).

Sequelae of PVL include gliosis with or without calcification of the small lesions and liquefaction with cystic change of the larger lesions which usually appears by 2–3 months of age (Figures 5-23, 5-24).

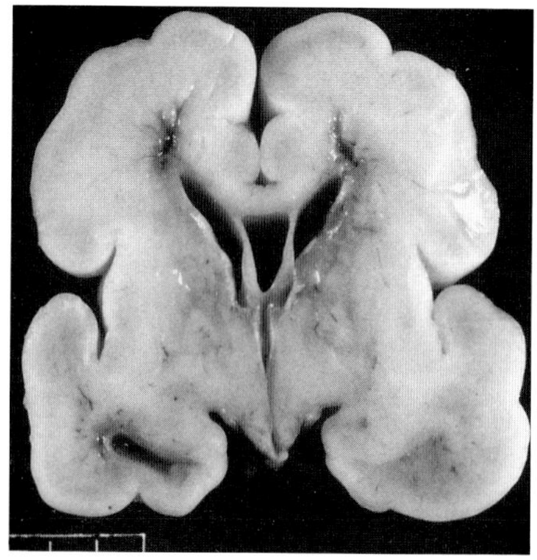

FIGURE 5-21. Hypoxic ischemic encephalopathy characterized by periventricular leukomalacia; note discoloration and breakdown in the white matter around the angles of the lateral ventricles (courtesy of Dr. L. S. Harris).

Pathogenesis of HIE

The pathogenesis of HIE is closely linked to the disorders in the newborn infant, which result in asphyxia. The brain is subjected to ischemia, hypercarbia, and hypoxia in prolonged asphyxia. Changes in the blood flow due to asphyxia play an important role in the pathogenesis of HIE. In the initial stages of asphyxia, redistribution of blood flow occurs. The blood flow is shunted from less vital organs to the more vital organs. There may also be a transient rise in

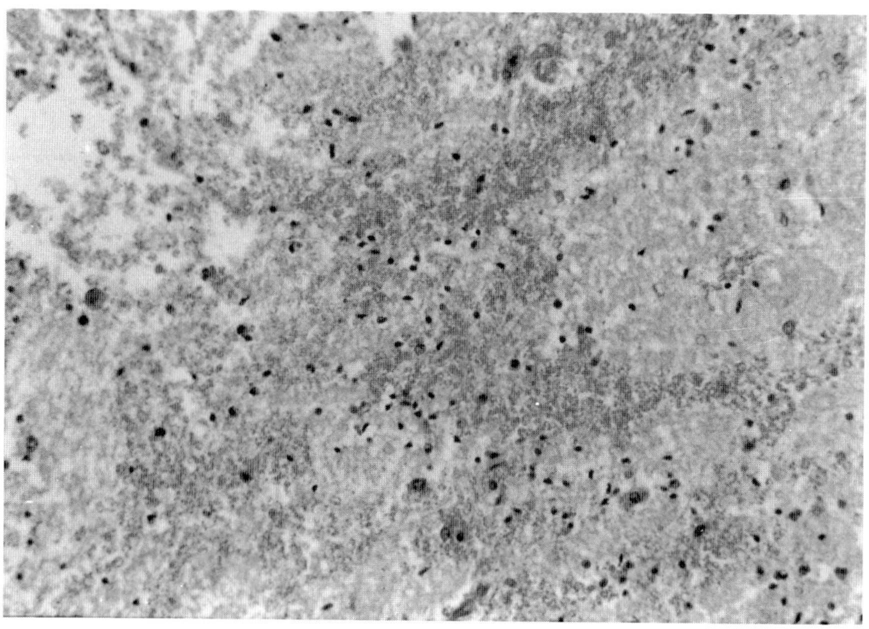

FIGURE 5-22. Hypoxic ischemic encephalopathy characterized by periventricular leukomalacia; note the necrosis of white matter (H&E, ×100).

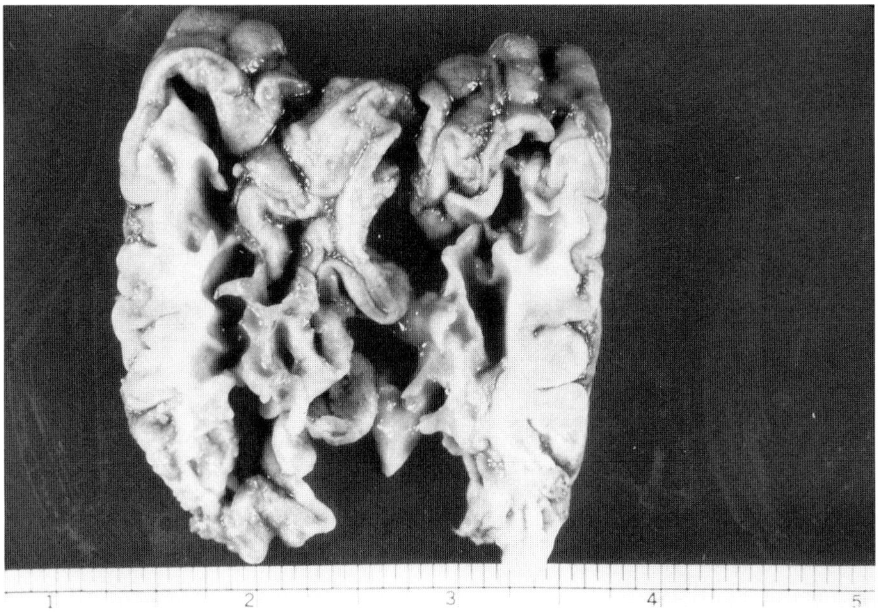

FIGURE 5-23. Gross photograph of cystic encephalomalacia representing a late sequela of periventricular leukomalacia.

blood pressure.[41] Loss of cerebral vascular autoregulation also occurs at the same time.[20] The cerebral arteries do not respond to these changes in the perfusion pressure. This results in an increase in the cerebral blood flow and sets the stage for PV/IVH.

With persistent asphyxia, cardiac output drops resulting in hypotension. Normally, the cerebral blood flow is independent of variations in the arterial blood pressure, and cerebral circulation is not significantly decreased when hypotension occurs.[39] In asphyxia, maximal vasodilatation has already developed since hypercapnia and hypoxia are potent vasodilator stimuli. Further vasodilatation cannot therefore occur in response to hypotension. With this loss of cerebral autoregulation, the cerebral blood flow decreases significantly. There is also associated edema, which further compromises the perfusion. The result is severe ischemic necrosis of the neurons in various locations and/or periventricular white matter in HIE.[8,40,41] Venous stasis and vascular damage, when present, add a hemorrhagic element to these necrotic lesions.

This sequence of events led Wigglesworth and Pape to develop an integrated model for hemorrhagic and ischemic lesions in the newborn brain[28] (Figure 5-25). The model explains how two different types of cerebral lesions occur in asphyxiated infants. Each lesion is an entity in itself but may also occur in association with the other lesion. Both types of event noted in Figure 5-25 may occur sequentially in an asphyxiated infant with occurrence of both types of lesion.

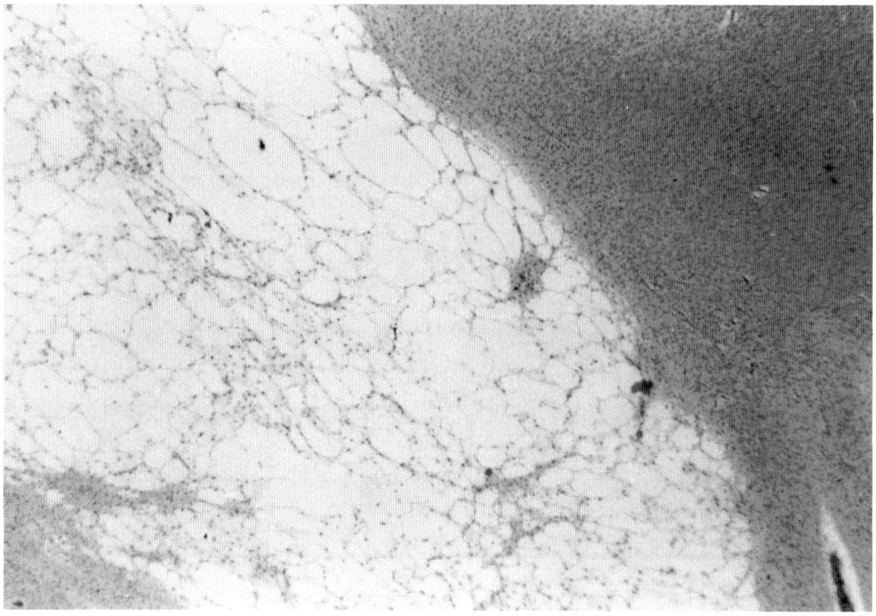

FIGURE 5-24. Photomicrograph of cystic encephalomalacia representing a late sequela of periventricular leukomalacia (H&E, ×100).

Infarcts of the Brain

Barmada and Moossy have described cerebral infarcts resulting from arterial occlusion.[42] Catheters, disseminated intravascular coagulation, infection, and exchange transfusion can be the source of thromboemboli. The infarcted cortex is fairly well demarcated from the normal tissue. The white-matter lesions may be hemorrhagic. Histologic examination reveals necrotic neurons, lipophages, and gliosis.

Kernicterus (KCT)

KCT is also called "billirubin encephalopathy." It was originally described in full-term infants with hemolytic disease. Depressed Moro reflex, opisthotonus, vomiting, high-pitched cry, and seizures are typical clinical features. With improvements in controlling hyperbilirubinemia by phototherapy and exchange transfusions, in recent years, KCT is rarely observed as a clinical entity. However, it continues to be seen occasionally at autopsy, as a pathologic entity. Yellow coloration is noted in the spinal fluid, meninges, cerebellum (dentate nucleus), hippocampus, basal ganglia, thalamus, and cranial nerve nuclei. On histologic examination, necrosis of the neurons in the affected areas is seen. Bilirubin pigment is demonstrable in severe KCT.

Pathogenesis of KCT

Free bilirubin is lipophilic; therefore, it is presumed to have relatively free access to the brain. A free bilirubin level of <20 mg/100 ml is considered safe in

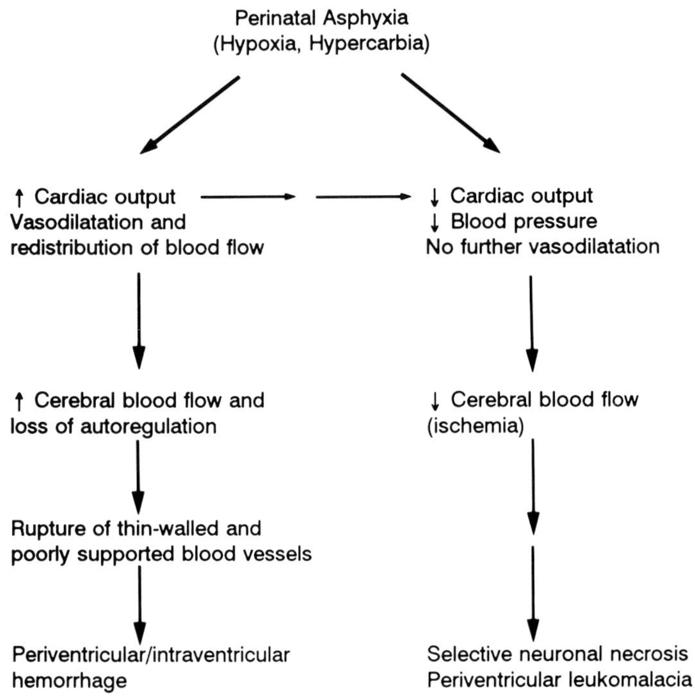

FIGURE 5-25. The initial events on the left-hand side may not always lead to hemorrhage. In such a case persistent asphyxia may lead to the end point on the right side of the diagram with occurrence of leukomalacia and neuronal necrosis. In some infants only hemorrhage may occur, in others hemorrhage and leukomalacia or neuronal necrosis may occur. (Adapted from references 28 and 41.)

the full-term newborn infant. However, in premature infants with asphyxia KCT can occur with levels of less than 12 mg.[43] The albumin-bound bilirubin is confined to the intravacular compartment by the blood–brain barrier. Increased permeability of the blood–brain barrier may lead to entry of even albumin-bound bilirubin into the brain.[44] Neuronal injury may result from intracellular bilirubin, which interferes with cell respiration, glucose metabolism, and protein synthesis.

COMMENT

Lesions of the head and brain are not uncommon in the neonatal autopsies. As indicated above, asphyxia plays an important primary or contributory role in the pathogenesis of these lesions. Lesions related to trauma have become vanishingly rare in recent years. However, the pathologist should look for these lesions during the various stages for removal of the brain. The diener is commonly called on to remove the brain while the pathologist or trainee is busy examining and dissecting the thoracic and abdominal organs. The pathologist should carefully inspect the structures of the head *before* each structure is reflected and/or cut. The blood clots associated with subdural hemorrhage may get misplaced if one is not on the lookout for them before the falx or tentorium is cut. Documentation of the various sites of SNN requires adequate sampling of the brain for histologic examination.

Intracranial hemorrhage at various sites and cerebral infarcts may also be associated with extracorporeal membrane oxygenation. The pathogenesis of these lesions relates to an increased tendency to bleed due to heparinization and increased venous pressure and to fibrin or aluminum-containing thromboemboli.[45–47]

REFERENCES

1. Plauche WC: Subgaleal hematoma. A complication of instrumental delivery. *JAMA* 244:1597–1598, 1980.
2. Volpe JJ: Neonatal intracranial hemorrhage. Pathophysiology, neuropathology, and clinical features. *Clin Perinatol* 4:77–102, 1977.
3. Chase WH: An anatomical study of subdural haemorrhage associated with tentorial splitting of the newborn. *Surg Gynecol Obstet* 51:31–41, 1930.
4. Haller ES, Newbitt REL Jr, Anderson GW: Clinical and pathologic concepts of gross intracranial hemorrhage in perinatal mortality. *OB Gynecol Surv* 11:179–204, 1956.
5. Menezes AH, Smith DE, Bell WE: Posterior fossa hemorrhage in the term neonate. *Neurosurgery* 13:452–456, 1983.
6. Hanigan WC, Morgan AM, Stahlberg LK, et al: Tentorial hemorrhage associated with vacuum extraction. *Pediatrics* 85:534–539, 1990.
7. Hemsath FA: Birth injury of occipital bone with a report of 32 cases. *Am J Obstet Gynecol* 27:194–203, 1934.
8. Wigglesworth JS: Problems in brain pathology in the perinatal period. In *Perinatal brain lesions* (Pape KE, Wigglesworth JS, Eds). Blackwell Scientific Publications, Boston, 1989, pp 1–24.
9. Rorke LB: Hemorrhages. In *Pathology of perinatal brain injury*. Raven Press, New York, 1982, pp 13–44.
10. Papile LA, Bernstein J, Burstein R, et al: Incidence and evolution of subependymal and intraventricular hemorrhage. A study of infants with birth weight less than 1500 g. *J Pediatr* 92:529–534, 1978.
11. Martin DJ: Cranial sonography in perinatology. In *Perinatal brain lesions* (Pape KE, Wigglesworth JS, Eds). Blackwell Scientific Publications, Boston, 1989, pp 55–98.
12. Emerson P, Fujimura M, Howat P, et al: Timing of intraventricular haemorrhage. *Arch Dis Child* 52:183–197, 1977.
13. Volpe JJ: Evaluation of neonatal periventricular-intraventricular hemorrhage. A major advance. *Am J Dis Child* 134:1023–1025, 1980.
14. Nakamura Y, Okudera T, Hashimoto T: Microvasculature in germinal matrix layer. Its relationship to germinal matrix hemorrhage. *Mod Pathol* 4:475–480, 1991.
15. Trommer BL, Groothuis DR, Pasteynak JF: Quantitative analysis of cerebral vessels in newborn puppy. The structure of germinal matrix vessels may predispose to hemorrhage. *Pediatr Res* 22:23–28, 1987.
16. Gruenwald P: Subependymal cerebral hemorrhage in premature infants and its relation to various injurious influences at birth. *Am J Obstet Gynecol* 61:1285–1292, 1951.
17. Coen RW, Sutherland JM, Bove K, et al: Anatomic and epidemiologic features of stroke lesions of newborn infants. *Trans Am Neurol Assoc* 95:36–40, 1970.

18. Hambleton G, Wigglesworth JS: Origin of intraventricular hemorrhage in the preterm infant. *Arch Dis Child* 51:651–659, 1976.
19. Nakamura Y, Okudera T, Fukuda S, et al: Germinal matrix hemorrhage of venous origin in preterm neonates. *Hum Pathol* 21:1059–1062, 1990.
20. Lou HC, Lassen NA, Friis-Hansen B: Impaired autoregulation of cerebral blood flow in the distressed newborn infant. *J Pediatr* 94:118–124, 1979.
21. Gilles FH, Price RA, Kevy SV, et al: Fibrinolytic activity in the ganglionic evidence of the premature human brain. *Biol Neonate* 18:426–431, 1971.
22. Beverley DW, Chance GW, Inwood MJ, et al: Intraventricular hemorrhage and hemostasis defects. *Arch Dis Child* 59:444–448, 1984.
23. Huseby JS, Gumprecht DG: Hemodynamic effects of rapid bolus hypertonic sodium bicarbonate. *Chest* 79:552–554, 1981.
24. Larroche JC: Posthemorrhagic hydrocephalus in infancy. *Biol Neonate* 20:287–299, 1972.
25. Hill A, Shackleford GD, Volpe JJ: A potential mechanism of pathogenesis of early posthemorrhagic hydrocephalus in the premature newborn. *Pediatrics* 73:19–21, 1984.
26. Donal JF, Okazaki H, Kleinberg F, et al: Intraventricular hemorrhage in the full term and preterm infants. *Mayo Clin Proc* 53:437–441, 1979.
27. Lacey DJ, Terplan K: Intraventricular hemorrhage in full-term neonates. *Dev Med Child Neurol* 24:332–337, 1982.
28. Wigglesworth JS, Pape KE: An integrated model for haemorrhagic and ischaemic lesions in the newborn brain. *Early Hum Dev* 2:179–199, 1978.
29. Yoffe G, Buchanan GR: Intracranial hemorrhage in newborn and young infants with hemophilia. *J Pediatr* 113:333–336, 1988.
30. Herman JH, Jumbelic MI, Ancona RJ, et al: In utero cerebral hemorrhage in alloimmune thrombocytopenia. *Am J Pediatr Hematol Oncol* 8:312–317, 1986.
31. Roland EH, Flodmark O, Hill A: Thalamic hemorrhage with intraventricular hemorrhage in the full term newborn. *Pediatrics* 85:737–742, 1990.
32. Grunnet ML, Shields WD: Cerebellar hemorrhage in the premature infant. *J Pediatr* 88:605–688, 1976.
33. Martin R, Roessmann V, Fanaroff A: Massive intracerebellar hemorrhage in low birth weight infants. *J Pediatr* 89:290–293, 1976.
34. Pape KE, Armstrong DL, Fitzhardinge PM: Central nervous system pathology associated with mask ventilation: A new etiology for the intracerebellar hemorrhage. *Pediatrics* 58:473–483, 1976.
35. Hill A, Melson GL, Clark HB, et al: Hemorrhagic periventricular leukomalacia: Diagnosis by real time ultrasound and correlation with autopsy findings. *Pediatrics* 69:282–284, 1982.
36. Skullerud K, Westre B: Frequency and prognostic significance of germinal matrix hemorrhage, periventricular leukomalacia and pontosubicular necrosis in preterm neonates. *Acta Neuropathol* 70:257–261, 1986.
37. Friede RL: Pontosubicular lesions in perinatal atoxia. *Arch Pathol Lab Med* 94:343–354, 1972.
38. Larroche JC, Encha-Razavi F: Fetal and neonatal brain damage: Central nervous system. In *Textbook of fetal and perinatal pathology*. (Wigglesworth JS, Singer DB, Eds). Blackwell Scientific Publications, Boston, 1991, pp 775–842.
39. Olesen J, Paulson OB, Lassen NA: Regional cerebral blood flow in man determined by the initial slope of the clearance of intra-arterially injected 133Xe. *Stroke* 2:519–540, 1971.
40. Kopelman AE: Blood pressure and cerebral ischemia in very low birth weight infants. *J Pediatr* 116:1000–1002, 1990.

41. Volpe JJ: Hypoxic-ischemic encephalopathy: Neuropathology and pathogenesis. In *Neurology of the newborn*. (Volpe JJ, Ed). Philadelphia, Saunders, 1987, pp 209–235.
42. Barmada MA, Moossy J: Cerebral infarcts with arterial occlusion in neonates. *Ann Neurol* 6:495–502, 1979.
43. Gartner LM, Snyder RN, Chalson RS, et al: Kernicterus: High incidence in premature infants with low serum bilirubin concentration. *Pediatrics* 45:906–917, 1970.
44. Levine RL: Neonatal jaundice. *Acta Pediatr Scand* 77:177–182, 1988.
45. Taylor GA, Fitz CR, Miller MK, et al: Intracranial abnormalities in infants treated with extracorporeal membrane oxygenization: Imaging with US and CT. *Radiology* 165:675–678, 1987.
46. Vogler C, Sotela C, Fulling K: Extracorporeal membrane oxygenization (ECMO) therapy: An analysis of 23 autopsies. *Pediatr Pathol* 7:496, 1987.
47. Vogler Sotelo-Avila C, Lagunoff D, et al: Aluminum-containing emboli in infants treated with extracorporeal membrane oxygenation. *N Engl J Med* 319:75–79, 1988.

6 PERINATAL IATROGENIC LESIONS

INTRODUCTION

Numerous diagnostic and therapeutic invasive procedures are done in sick premature and term newborn infants and also in the fetus. The diagnostic procedures are of benefit to the patient by providing guidelines to the neonatologist for continuation or modification of the therapeutic measures. The various therapeutic measures are of direct benefit to the patient by correcting the imbalances and deficiencies, by providing nutritional and other types of support and ultimately recovery from the disease process. However, there is a certain price in terms of iatrogenic complications to be paid by the patient. Andrews[1] considered these complications as the sixth finger representing pediatrica iatrogenica in a six-finger exercise of areas of concern in neonatology. The main fingers represent the following five areas: cardiorespiratory, hematologic, nutrition and metabolism, infection, and congenital anomalies.

These iatrogenic complications or lesions have varying frequency and degree of severity. Certain complications, such as interstitial pulmonary emphysema associateed with mechanical ventilation, are not uncommon. The exact incidence of these complications cannot be determined on the basis of autopsy studies alone since only the severe cases of different neonatal conditions with a fatal outcome will come to the attention of the pathologist. Therefore, the denominator in the autopsy studies is small and suffers from a selection bias. The severe complications of diagnostic and therapeutic measures may be associated with severe morbidity and in rare instances even mortality.

Despite the complications, it should be noted that the cost/benefit ratio of these procedures is greatly in favor of benefit, and therefore these procedures continue to be used in the neonatal intensive care units. In earlier years when neonatology had just begun to develop as a subspecialty, the severity and incidence of complications were higher than seen currently. With greater experience of using various techniques and sophistication in the biochemical and physiological monitoring, the complications are less severe and less common than in the past.

But the iatrogenic lesions continue to occur and documenting the previously recognized lesions, and looking out for new ones, especially when new diagnostic and therapeutic procedures are introduced are among the main objectives of neonatal autopsy. The reason is not to point fingers at the clinicians but to enable them to learn from the autopsy findings and take appropriate steps to prevent such lesions or if these are unavoidable, reduce their severity, and detect them early so that appropriate management decisions can be taken. Banagale[2] recommended that a regular and frquent internal review of individual cases showing iatrogenic lesions should be undertaken. These lesions, as he suggested, should be looked upon as constructive learning experiences. Besides their occurrence at autopsy, some of the iatrogenic lesions may be detected in biopsy specimens or surgically resected tissues. In the following description of iatrogenic lesions seen mainly at autopsy, those lesions for which incisional biopsy or surgical resection may be done will be specifically mentioned. Only lesions related to or associated with invasive procedures will be described. Drug toxicity and drug reactions are excluded except when a morphologic lesion related to the toxicity of drugs or infusions (e.g., diuretics, amino acid solution, and Intralipid given for nutritional support) is present.

Diagnostic and therapeutic procedures used in the fetus include intrauterine transfusion, fetal monitoring by a scalp electrode, and obstetric maneuvers during delivery. Other procedures, such as endotracheal intubation; umbilical, arterial, or venous catheterization; and total parenteral nutrition, are done in the neonate. The documentation and study of the lesions associated with these procedures can be done in a better manner if the catheters, tubes, etc. are left in place when the body is sent to the morgue. However, in my experience, it is difficult to have this practice followed consistently and regularly.

LESIONS ASSOCIATED WITH DIAGNOSTIC AND THERAPEUTIC PROCEDURES

Fetal Monitoring by Scalp Electrodes

Direct electronic evaluation of fetal heart rate by inserting a small electrode in the fetal scalp, which appears to be helpful in improving the obstetric management and perinatal outcome may be used in complicated labor. The following iatrogenic complications have been reported:[3] (1) scalp abscess, (2) septic dermatitis, (3) cellulitis, (4) necrotizing fasciitis, (5) osteomyelitis, and (6) meningitis. These complications are detected by the clinicians and are successfully treated, but late sequela such as hydrocephalus may occur. In rare cases of neonatal deaths due to other causes, one of the aforementioned lesions related to the fetal heart monitoring may be present. The scalp should be carefully examined at autopsy for evidence of these complications and appropriate cultures and sections for histology should be taken from the scalp lesion, if present.

Amniocentesis and Intrauterine Transfusions

Although with ultrasonic guidance and rigorous aseptic precautions, the incidence of complications associated with these procedures is markedly reduced, lesions listed below may be seen in rare instances. These lesions may lead to fetal death on rare occasions. The lesions associated with amniocentesis include (1) trauma to the fetus, placenta, or (rarely) umbilical cord; (2) infection; and (3) abortion or preterm labor associated with stimulation of uterine contractions or placental abruption.[4]

Intrauterine transfusion for treatment of erythroblastosis fetalis may be given via the intraperitoneal route or the umbilical cord (intravascular route).[5]

Fetal death associated with exsanguination due to laceration of fetoplacental blood vessel has been reported. Laceration of abdominal and thoracic organs may occur.[6,7] Compression of the umbilical vein due to inadvertent injection of the blood into Wharton's jelly can lead to fetal demise. Examination of the placenta is essential in the cases in which these procedures have been performed.[5]

Obstetrical Maneuvers, Including Application of Forceps during Delivery

At present these maneuvers are used in difficult vaginal deliveries much less frequently than in the past. The severity of birth trauma associated with the maneuvers is variable. Asphyxia plays a contributory role in the hemorrhagic lesions associated with birth trauma. Excessive traction or pressure applied to fetal parts in normal or abnormal presentations during delivery may result in a variety of injuries to the bones, extracranial and intracranial structures, soft tissues, viscera, and nerves.[8] Fractures of bones, including those of the skull and spine, are associated with hemorrhage and injury to underlying structures such as brain and spinal cord. Injury to extracranial and intracranial structures such as bone or dural and arachnoid membranes is associated with hemorrhages. These are described in the chapter on perinatal lesions of the head and brain. Hemorrhage in soft tissues involves most frequently skeletal muscle. Liver and adrenals are the most frequent sites of visceral injury. Subcapsular hematoma of liver with or without rupture into peritoneal cavity is associated with birth trauma. Massive bilateral adrenal hemorrhages (Figure 19 in chapter 1) are seen in traumatic breech deliveries. The adrenal hematomas may become infected and present as bilateral abdominal abscesses in the late neonatal period in rare instances.[9] Brachial plexus is probably the most common site of nerve injury. Injuries to other nerves such as cervical, phrenic and facial nerves can also occur.

Endotrachial Intubation

Endotrachial intubation (EI) is used for positive-pressure mechanical ventilation, which is frequently needed in the management of sick newborn infants. In recent years as a result of improvement in the choice of correct size, in the material from which the tubes are made, in the pulmonary toilet, heating and humidification of the inspired gas, and reduced pressure for mechanical ventilation the frequency and severity of the lesions seen in the upper respiratory tract related to EI are reduced as compared with those in the early 1970s.[10]

However, more recently necrotizing inflammatory lesions of the upper respiratory tract (URT) have been reported in newborn infants in whom high-frequency mechanical ventilation was used.[11–13] It should be noted that such lesions occur also in infants who are given conventional positive-pressure mechanical ventilation.[10] Following types of acute lesions associated with EI are seen in the upper respiratory tract: (1) mucosal necrosis (Figure 6-1), (2) mucosal and submucosal necrosis, (3) mucosal and submucosal necrosis with mild to moderate acute inflammatory reaction, and (4) mucosal and submucosal necrosis with severe acute inflammation (Figures 6-2, 6-3). In rare instances the cartilage of the trachea may show damage.[13] The extreme form of these lesions is

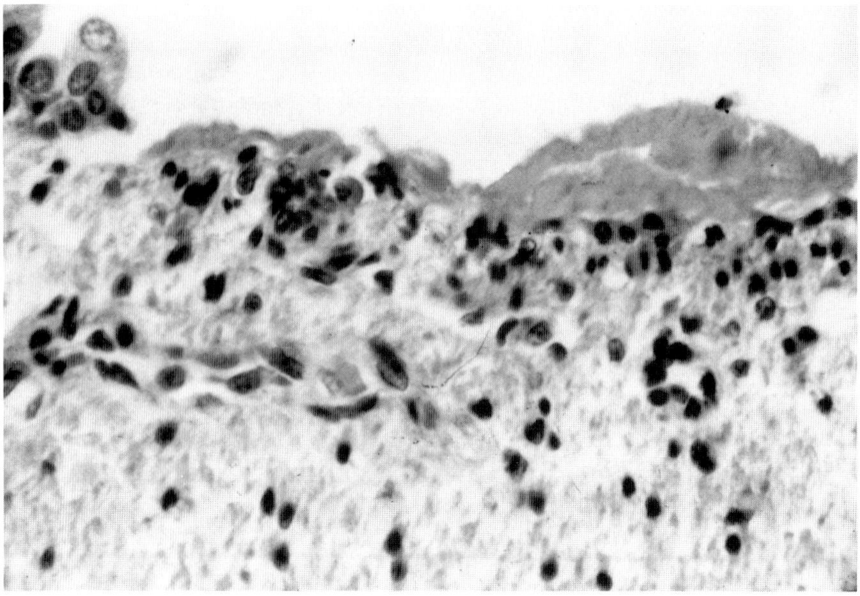

FIGURE 6-1. Mucosal necrosis of the vocal cord associated with endotracheal intubation; note a few intact epithelial cells on the left (H&E, ×400).

the acute diffuse necrotizing tracheobronchitis with extensive sloughing of the mucosa (Figure 6-4). These lesions, seen mainly in the true vocal cords and subglottic region of the trachea, are best demonstrated in the longitudinal sections taken from a specimen of larynx and trachea fixed in formalin in a stretched position (Figures 6-2, 6-5). If the endotracheal tube slips into one or the other main stem bronchus, similar lesions are also seen in the bronchus. However, the bronchial lesions are most likely related to excessive or improper use of suction catheters[14] (see below).

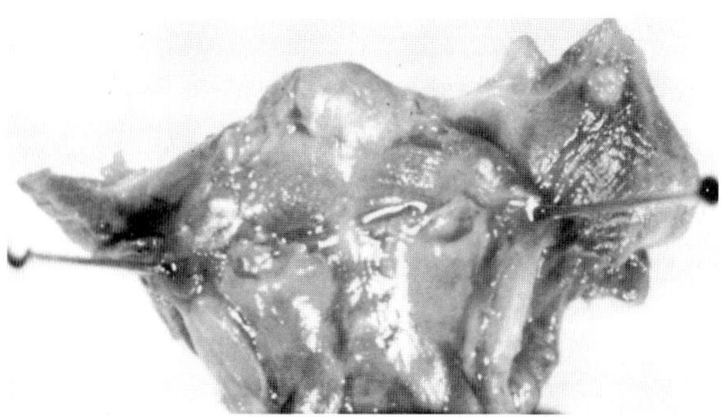

FIGURE 6-2. Gross specimen of larynx and subglottic portion of trachea fixed in a stretched position showing diffuse purulent exudate.

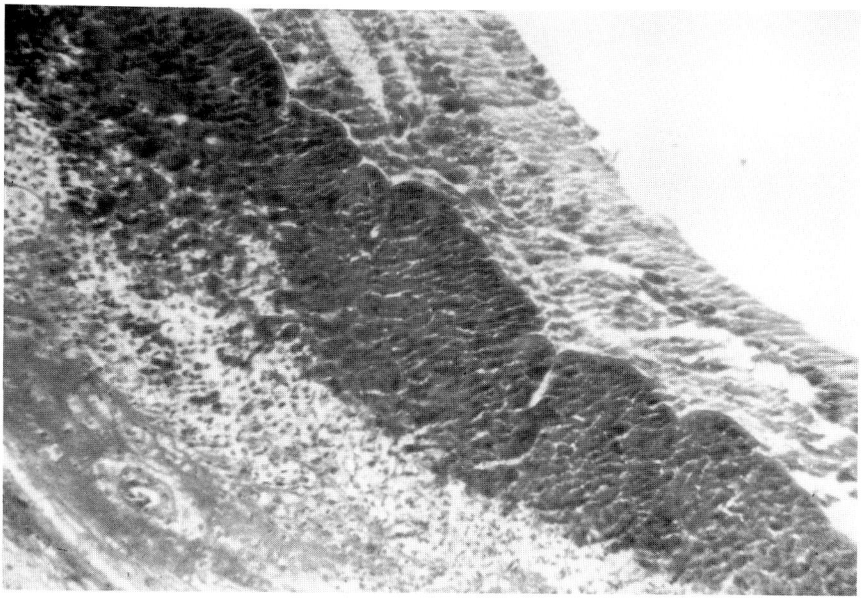

FIGURE 6-3. Severe acute necrotizing tracheitis. There was similar involvement of the larynx and main stem bronchi. (H&E, ×250.)

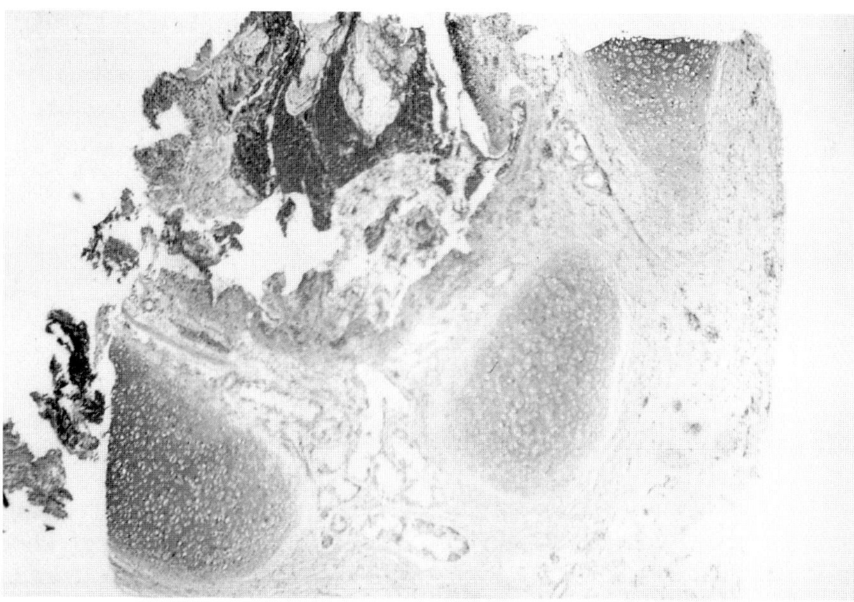

FIGURE 6-4. Sloughed-off necrotic mucosa forming a plug in the lumen in a case of necrotizing laryngotracheobronchitis (H&E, ×100).

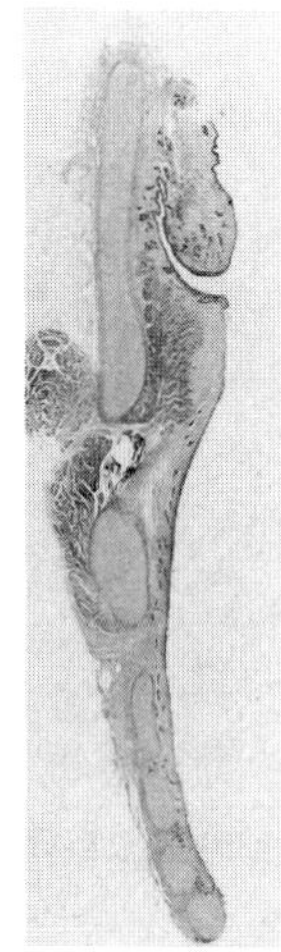

FIGURE 6-5. Whole mount of longitudinal section of false and true vocal cords and subglottic portion of trachea.

These acute lesions were seen with relatively high frequency in the early 1970s.[10] Thus URT lesions were present in 95.77% infants with IRDS in whom EI was done. The relationship between duration of intubation and severity of lesions was also noted. With longer duration of EI, more severe lesions were seen.

Perforation of trachea, main stem bronchus or esophagus may rarely occur due to EI (Figures 6-6, 6-7).[15] I have seen placement of endotracheal tube in the esophagus instead of the trachea in one case (Figure 6-8). All the aforementioned

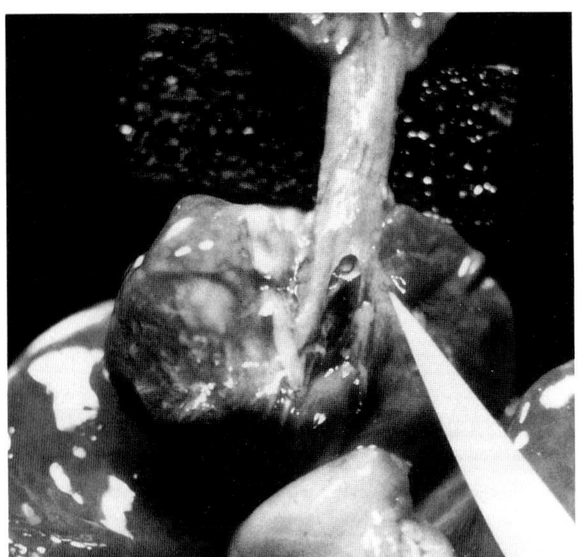

FIGURE 6-6. Perforation of trachea at the carina by the endotracheal tube.

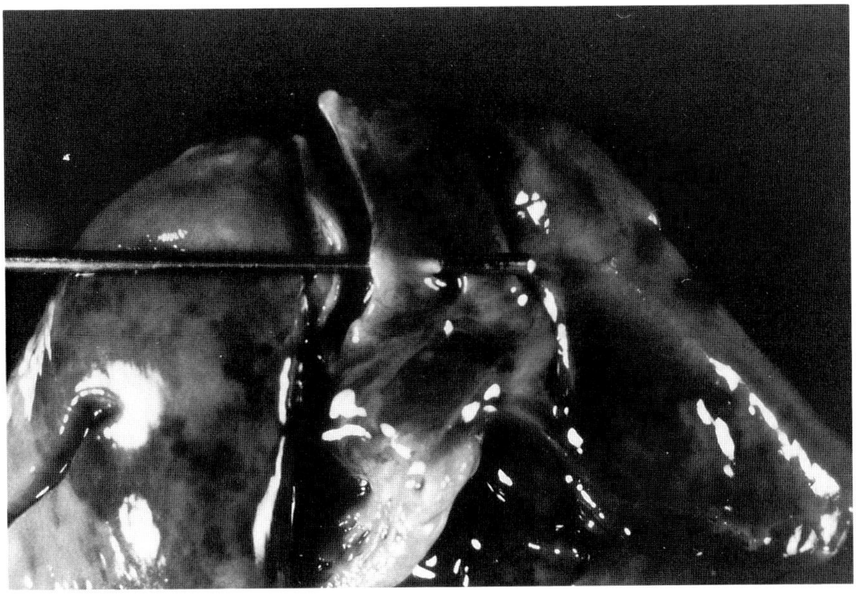

FIGURE 6-7. Perforation of right main stem bronchus due to suction catheter.

complications are related to the internal portion of the endotracheal tube. One rare preventable complication related to the external portion of the tube tapered to the nose is the gangrene of the tip and lateral aspects of the nose (Figure 6-9).

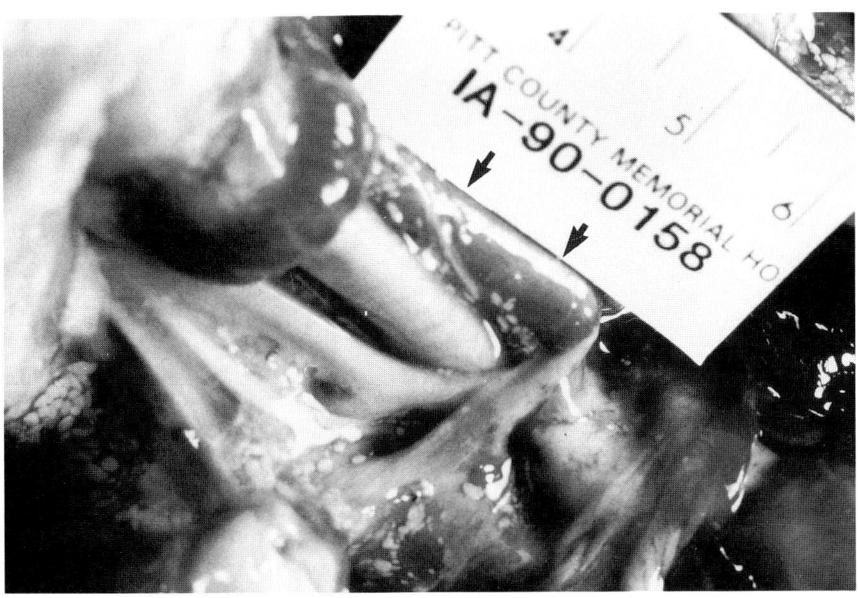

FIGURE 6-8. Endotracheal tube located in the esophagus (arrows).

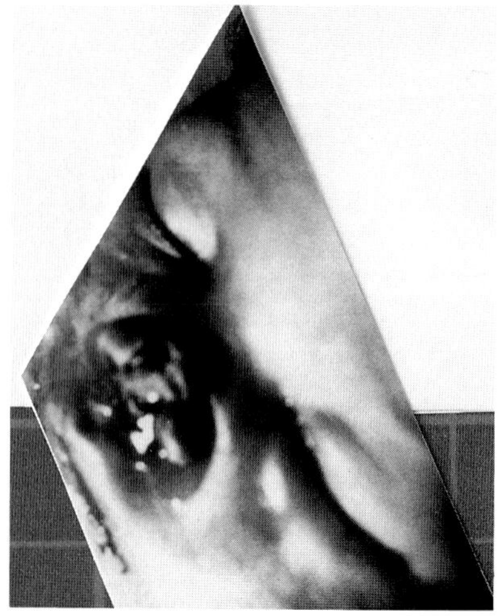

FIGURE 6-9. Gangrene of the nose due to compression by the taped external portion of the endotracheal tube.

Pathogenesis and Clinical Significance of Acute URT Lesions Associated with EI

Various pathogenetic mechanisms such as direct pressure, abrasive effect, transmitted piston effect of mechanical ventilation, chemical toxic factors of the tube, the number of times intubation and extubation is performed, injury due to suction catheter (in the lower portion of trachea and main-stem bronchi), bacterial contamination, inadequate humidification, excessive airway temperature, and ischemic injury have been implicated.[10,13,16] Bacterial contamination due to pseudomonas resulting in pseudomonas pneumonia or septicemia was observed in our series published in 1972.[10] I have also seen two cases of candida infection of the URT lesions in infants with prolonged EI (Figure 6-10). However, with improvement in pulmonary toilet and shorter duration of EI, bacterial or fungal contamination is a rare factor. It is possible that pathogenesis of the URT lesions associated with EI is multifactorial. One of the most significant factors is probably ischemia.[13,17] Weymuller has demonstrated the presence of hypoperfusion in the intubated dogs by fluorescein perfusion.[17] Ischemic injury occurs when the airway pressure exceeds the capillary perfusion pressure. The arterial and capillary perfusion pressures may be low in the sick newborns. This ischemic theory explains the presence of lesions that are distal to the endotracheal tube or to the suction catheters and the greater severity of lesions in location (trachea) where the endotracheal tube is not tightly positioned.[13]

The clinical significance of these lesions relates to the immediate direct effects and long term sequelae. The mild or moderately severe lesions do not probably produce significant morbidity and heal completely when the infant is extubated. The extremely severe lesion of necrotizing tracheobronchitis in a neonate with high-frequency mechanical ventilation may be associated with extensive sloughing of the necrotic mucosa. Severe obstruction due to luminal plug consisting of the sloughed off necrotic mucosa, inflammatory exudate, and mucous secretions may occur with serious consequences (Figure 6-4).[18,19] These can be avoided if the luminal plug is suctioned immediately. The suctioned

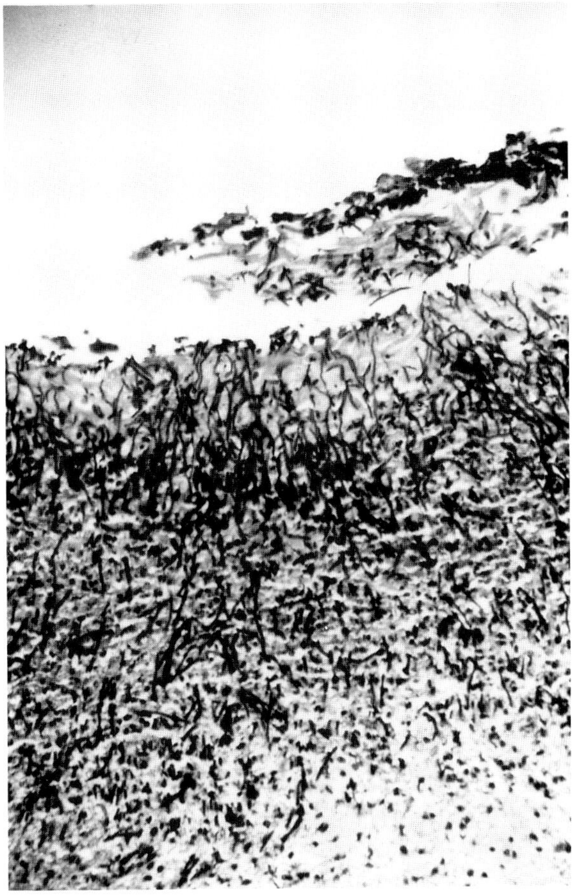

FIGURE 6-10. Candida infection of the ulcerated lesion of the vocal cord due to prolonged endotracheal intubation (PAS, ×400).

luminal plug should be sent to the surgical pathology laboratory for histologic examination. The long-term sequelae consist of formation of obstructing granulation tissue, polypoid lesions consisting of fibrous tissue covered with metaplastic squamous epithelium, submucosal fibrosis with stenosis, and even acquired atresia particularly of one of the bronchi (Figures 6-11–6-14) .[20] These obstructive lesions in the lobar bronchi may lead to acquired lobar emphysema due to a ball-valve effect when the bronchial lumen narrows during expiration.[21] The granulation tissue formation may recur after excision. Surgical pathologist will encounter these different types of specimens (polyps, lobectomy specimens, etc.).

Suction Catheters

At birth and during the subsequent clinical course as indicated, secretions are suctioned out from the pharynx, esophagus, stomach, and upper respiratory tract. Suction catheters may cause mucosal and submucosal necrosis of the

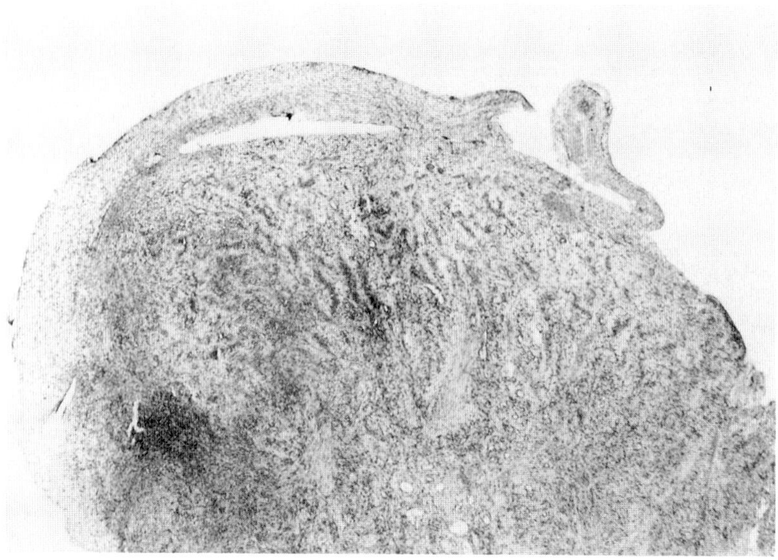

FIGURE 6-11. Granulation tissue removed surgically from trachea in an older infant with history of endotracheal intubation during the neonatal period (H&E, ×100).

bronchi followed by granulation tissue formation and polypoid fibroepithelial lesions obstructing the lumen (Figure 6-12).[14] A transient severe esophagitis with ulceration has been described in the neonates by Deneyer et al.[22] These authors attributed these lesions which are more severe in the upper esophagus and occur shortly after birth to the "trauma" associated with suction catheters.

Mechanical Ventilation

Many changes have occurred in the techniques of mechanical ventilation in recent years. Air-leak phenomena are the main lesions related to mechanical ventilation. Thus pneumomediastinum, pulmonary interstitial emphysema, pneumothorax, and subcutaneous emphysema may occur as acute phenomena (Figures 6-15, 6-16). In rare instances pneumopericardium, pneumoretroperitoneum and even pulmonary vascular air embolism may occur[23] (Figure 6-17A,B). Rupture of alveolar septa, airflow along the alveolar and lobular septa and perivascular sheaths, followed by rupture of pleura account for these phenomena.[24] Further dissection into the retroperitoneum, pericardium, or pulmonary vascular system explains the remaining lesions. Although air-leak phenomena can occur as a result of vigorous respiratory effort by the newborn infant, in most instances these lesions are iatrogenic, i.e., resulting from barotrauma due to mechanical ventilation. In newborn infants given prolonged mechanical ventilation (10–13 days) persistent interstitial pulmonary emphysema (PIPE) may develop.[25] PIPE is characterized by formation of single or multiple cysts of ≤ 3 cm in diameter localized to the interlobular septa (Figure 6-18). The cyst wall

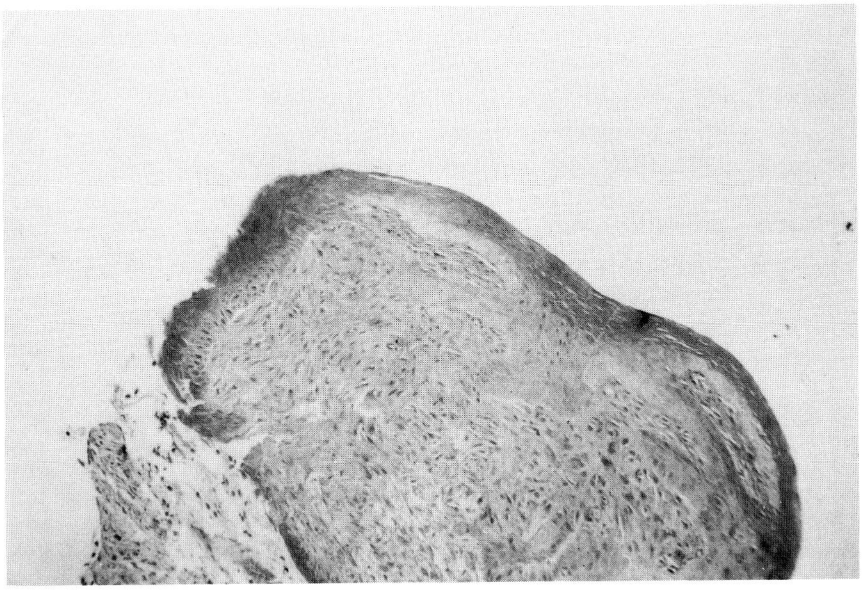

FIGURE 6-12. Bronchial fibroepithelial polypoid lesion obstructing the main stem bronchus in an infant with history of endotracheal intubation during the neonatal period; note the fibrous core and squamous epithelial lining (H&E, ×100).

consists of membranous fibrous tissue and is surrounded by compressed pulmonary parenchyma. The cysts are lined focally by multinucleated reactive giant cells (Figure 6-18). Increasing respiratory distress can occur in infants with PIPE. PIPE is seen in localized (confined to a segment of the lung) and diffuse (panlobar bilateral) forms. The localized form of PIPE is amenable to surgical resection, which is followed by clinical improvement. The surgical pathologist will encounter such a specimen, which should be distinguished from congenital localized cystic lesions of the lung (see chapter 8 on bronchopulmonary vascular malformations).

An interesting sequela of prolonged uninterrupted mechanical ventilation for ≥12 days immediately before death has been described by Knisely et al.[26] The diaphragmatic muscle mass appeared to be reduced in size on gross examination. Histologic examination revealed significantly small size of the diaphragmatic muscle fibers as compared with the control specimens. They suggested that the small size of the muscle fibers, which may be due to disuse atrophy or to failure of normal growth, may make weaning from ventilatory support more difficult.

Oxygen Therapy

Two major complications occur in relation to the oxygen therapy.

1. *Lung injury.* Lung injury is seen in the form of necrosis of epithelium of terminal air passages and hyaline membrane formation in the acute stage of

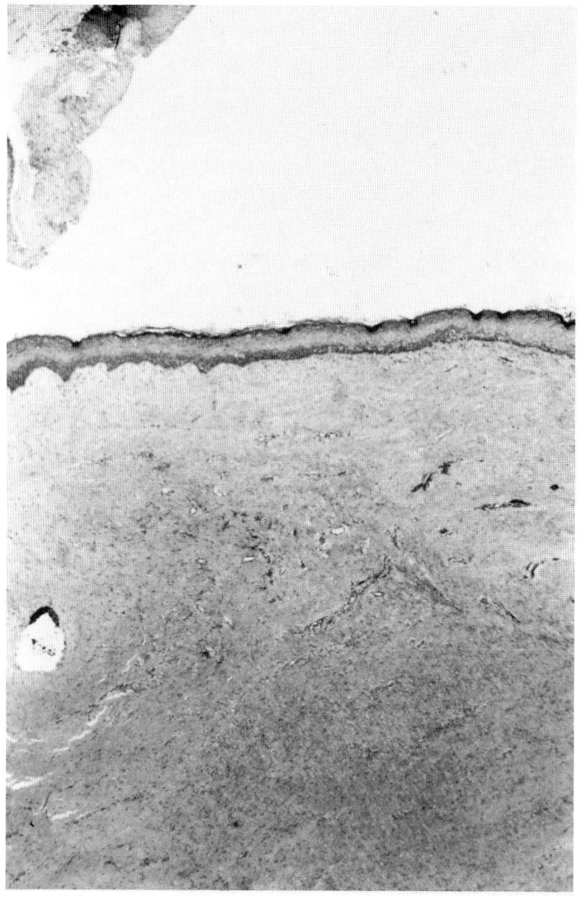

FIGURE 6-13. Squamous metaplasia and submucosal fibrosis of trachea in an infant with history of endotracheal intubation during the neonatal period (H&E, ×100).

idiopathic respiratory distress syndrome (IRDS). Bronchopulmonary dysplasia (BPD) can be regarded as the chronic proliferative stage of lung injury due to oxygen therapy (barotrauma due to positive-pressure mechanical ventilation also plays a role in the pathogenesis of BPD) (see chapter 3 NRDS).

2. *Retinopathy of prematurity* (ROP).[27–29] The conventional term "retrolental fibroplasia" reflects solely the subsequent scarring of the eye of the most severely affected infants. The term "ROP" is preferred because it describes all phases of retinal changes. Hyperoxia appears to be the major factor in the pathogenesis of ROP. However, other factors such as hypercarbia, metabolic acidosis, sepsis, vitamin E deficiency, bright-light exposure, and even hypoxia have also been implicated.[27] Since eyes are not routinely examined in neonatal autopsies, I have no personal experience of this lesion.

The following features have been described by Kushner et al.[28] Three clinicopathologic stages of ROP are recognized: vasoobliterative, proliferative,

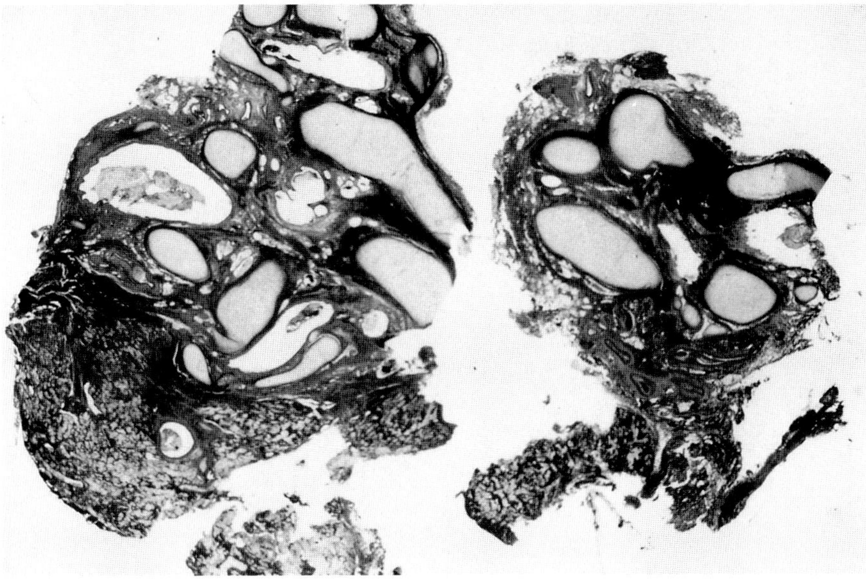

FIGURE 6-14. Acquired bronchial atresia related to endotracheal intubation; note the fibrous obliteration of the lumen in the main stem bronchus (H&E, ×25).

and cicatricial. In the vasoobliterative stage the walls of retinal vessels show degenerative changes and become adherent to each other. Small endothelial nodules in the inner portion of the retina represent the earliest manifestation of the proliferative stage. The neovascularization extends up to the retinal surface and in more severe cases into the vitreous. The cicatricial stage is characterized by fibrosis, which can lead to traction and retinal detachment. The proliferative changes may not progress to the cicatricial stage if oxygen therapy is discontinued. The mild proliferative changes are reversible in majority of the cases. In

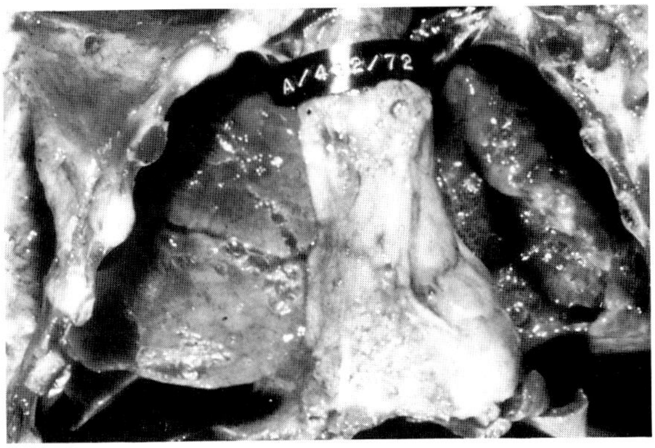

FIGURE 6-15. Acute interstitial pulmonary emphysema and pneumomediastinum. Pneumothorax was also present.

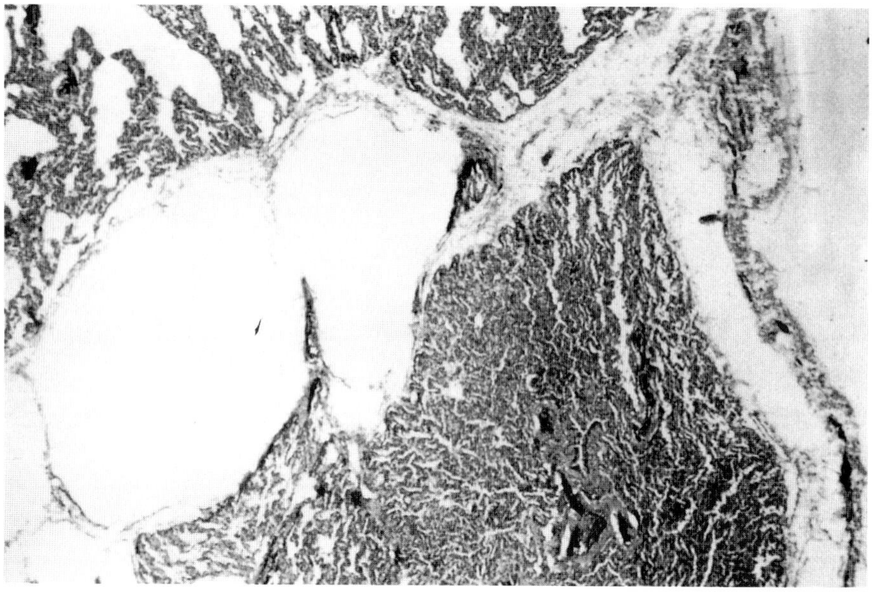

FIGURE 6-16. Acute interstitial pulmonary emphysema on histologic examination. Note the compression atelectasis of the surrounding alveoli (H&E, ×100).

severe cases a retrolental mass consisting of detached retina and organized vitreous is present.

Chest Tubes

Chest tubes are inserted as a therapeutic measure for pneumothorax. Penetration of lung tissue with or without hemorrhage may occur (Figure 6-19). The

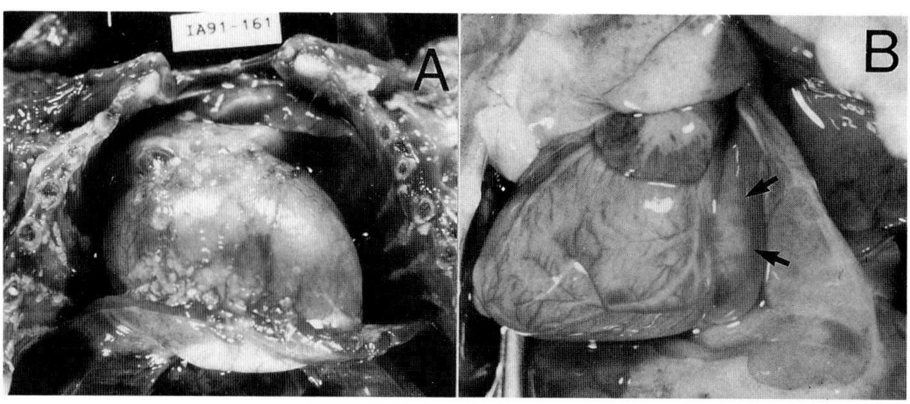

FIGURE 6-17. (A) Note the ballooning of the pericardial sac due to pneumopericardium; (B) note the air bubbles in the left atrium (arrows).

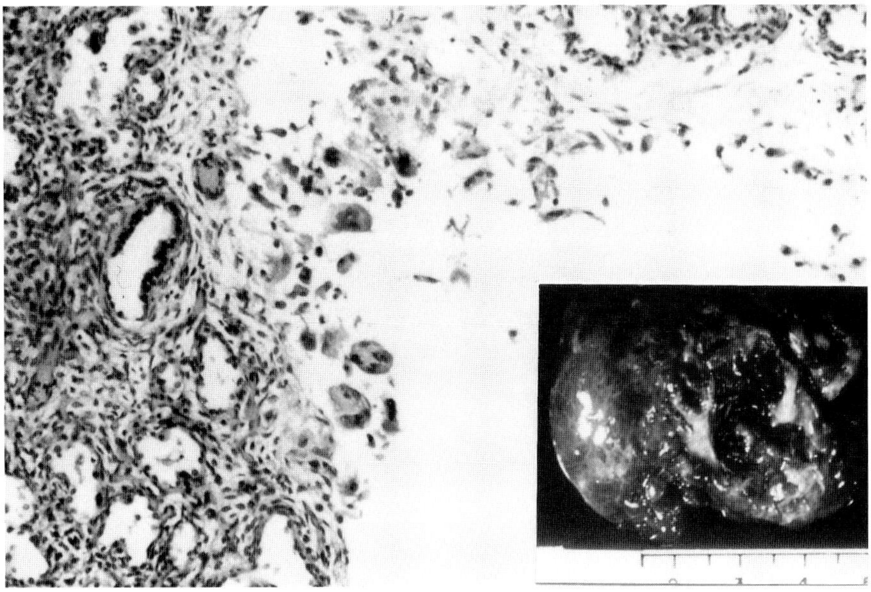

FIGURE 6-18. Localized persistent interstitial pulmonary emphysema on gross (inset) and histologic examination of a surgically resected specimen; note the multinucleated giant cells lining the emphysematous cyst (H&E, ×250).

hemorrhage is usually mild and localized. I have seen two cases in which the pericardium was penetrated by chest tube(s). In one of these cases there was hemopericardium leading to cardiac tamponade (Figure 6-20).

Extracorporal Membrane Oxygenation (ECMO)

ECMO involves placement of catheters in the jugular vein and in the common carotid artery. The blood flow is then diverted through a bypass circuit. The purpose of ECMO is to provide surrogate heart–lung functions in very sick newborn infants.[30,31]

Hemorrhage is the main complication since heparinized blood is required for ECMO. Various sites of hemorrhage have been reported.[8] These include intracranial, retroperitoneal, GI, URT, and pleural. Bleeding may occur at the site of surgical incision. Intracranial hemorrhage may prove to be fatal. In the series reported by Taylor et al[30] the intracranial sites included subependymal, intraventricular, parenchymal, and subarachnoid hemorrhage.

Multiple fibrin or aluminum-containing thromboemboli in arteries, arterioles, and capillaries with or without infarcts in various organs, including brain in infants who were treated with ECMO for more than a week, have been described by Vogler et al.[32] The aluminum-containing emboli which were granular, lamellar, and basophilic (in contrast to eosinophilic fibrin emboli) and could be demonstrated by aluminon stain[33] were found only in the extrapulmonary sites in all cases except one.

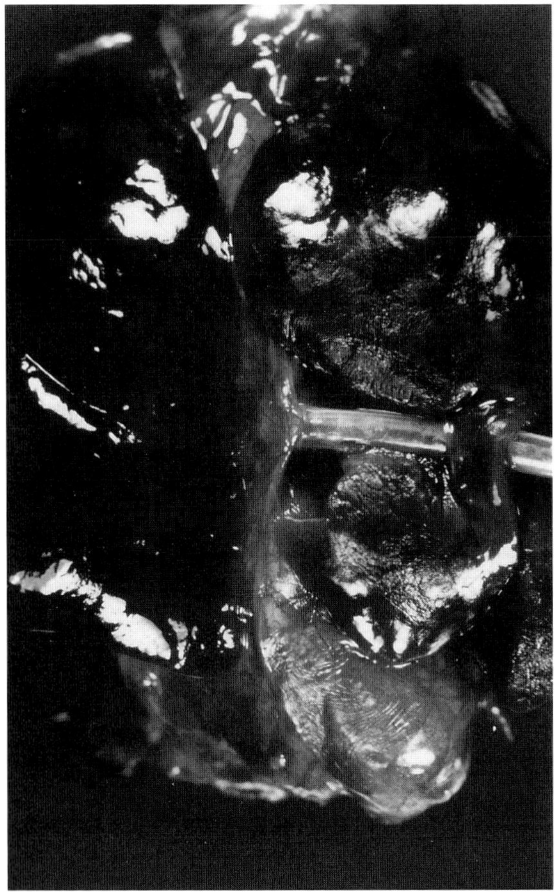

FIGURE 6-19. Chest tube penetrating the lung tissue. There was no significant hemorrhage associated with it.

Lesions demonstrated by CT (computed tomographic) scan of the central nervous system in the infants who were treated by ECMO include cerebral edema; atrophy; cystic encephalomalacia; infarcts involving cerebrum, cerebellum, and brain stem; and sagittal sinus thrombosis.[30,31]

Although the purpose of ECMO is to provide "rest" to the lungs, pulmonary changes such as bronchopulmonary dysplasia, interstitial and intraalveolar hemorrhage, hyaline membrane formation, squamous metaplasia, smooth muscle hyperplasia, and interstitial fibrosis have been noted by different observers.[34,35] Focal alveolar and bronchiolar calcification and mucinous metaplasia of bronchiolar and alveolar epithelium have also been described.[34] Pulmonary cystic lesions can also occur in patient with ECMO therapy.[36] It is not clear whether the pulmonary changes mentioned above are the result of ECMO alone. It should be noted that the infants who are given ECMO therapy have preexisting primary or secondary lung disease related to meconium aspiration syndrome, persistent pulmonary hypertension, neonatal respiratory distress syndrome,

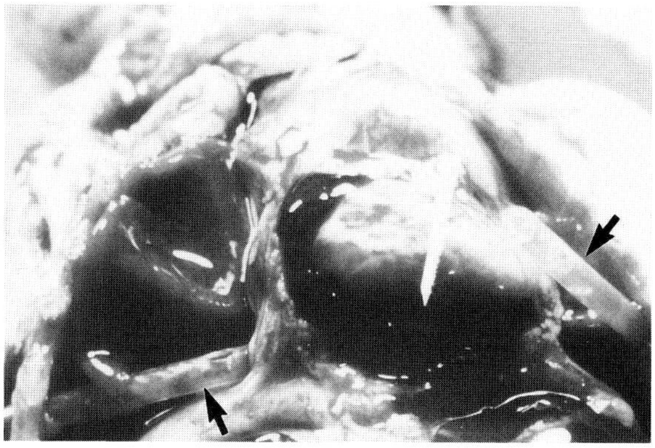

FIGURE 6-20. Two chest tubes (one on either side) (small arrows) penetrating the pericardium resulting in hemopericardium (large white arrows).

sepsis, congenital heart disease, etc. Therefore it is likely that a combination of factors such as the original disease process requiring ECMO therapy, respiratory failure, and ECMO itself may be associated with the pathogenesis of the pulmonary changes.[35,37] These changes may be related to the long-term pulmonary sequelae in ECMO survivors.[38,39]

Pathogenesis and Clinical Significance of Lesions Related to ECMO

Heparinization of blood, platelet destruction, and increased venous pressure due to ligation of internal jugular vein and arterial hypertension due to elevation of chemical mediators are implicated in the pathogenesis of hemorrhagic lesions. Nonhemorrhagic CNS lesions are probably related to persistent hypoxia and hypoperfusion. For locating the source of aluminum emboli, Vogler et al[31] investigated the mixing rods of heat exchangers, which were used for warming the blood in the ECMO circuit. Friable aluminum-containing concretions were found to be adhering loosely to these rods. It was suggested that these concretions formed the emboli. The aluminum-containing concretions were thought to be formed by exposure of aluminum after wearing away of the silicone coating.[32]

The clinical significance relates to immediate and remote effects on CNS function of the survivors. While many of the patients may survive with normal neurologic function, microcephaly, seizures, and neurologic impairment have been observed in a few long-term survivors.[30,40]

Umbilical Arterial Catheterization (UAC)

UAC is used extensively for monitoring of therapy of premature infants with IRDS, extrinsic perinatal asphyxia, etc. Complications include thrombosis with occlusion of aorta or ostia of its major branches, peritoneal perforation, hemorrhage due to vascular perforation, and infection.[41] Atheromatous lesions and aneurysm formation are the late complications.[42,43]

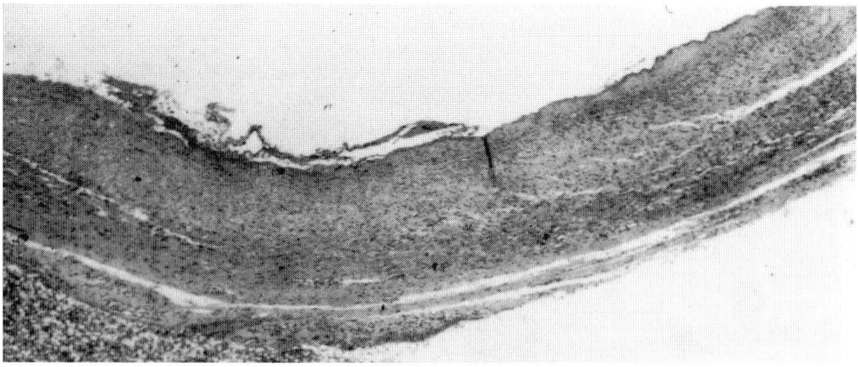

FIGURE 6-21. Endothelial ulceration of aorta associated with umbilical arterial catheterization (H&E, ×200).

Endothelial Injury and Thrombus Formation in the Aorta

The umbilical catheter causes endothelial injury and formation of minute thrombi that can be demonstrated only by microscopic examination of the aorta (Figures 6-21, 6-22). Although the catheter tip appears smooth and shiny to the naked eye, scanning electron-microscopic (SEM) study of tips of umbilical artery catheters reveals relatively rough thrombogenic surface.[44] Thrombi associated with UAC are of three different types: pericatheteric, mural, and both pericatheteric and mural.[45] Pericatheteric thrombi may be entirely pulled out with the catheter when it is withdrawn (Figures 6-23, 6-24). However, small emboli may get dislodged from the pericatheteric and mural thrombi.[41,45] Blanching or small infarcts of the toes may occur in these infants.[41] The mural thrombi may be small. Significant aortic luminal narrowing is not seen in such cases. On the other hand, mural thrombi may occlude the lumen of common iliac artery or the ostia of major branches of the aorta (see Figures 4-24 and 4-25 in chapter 4 neonatal necrotizing enterocolitis). Occlusion of the renal artery can result in renal hypertension due to infarction of that kidney (Figure 6-25). Infarction of small or large intestine mistaken clinically for neonatal necrotizing enterocolitis occurs when there is occlusion of ostium of superior or inferior mesenteric artery[46] (Figure 4-23 of chapter 4 neonatal necrotizing enterocolitis).

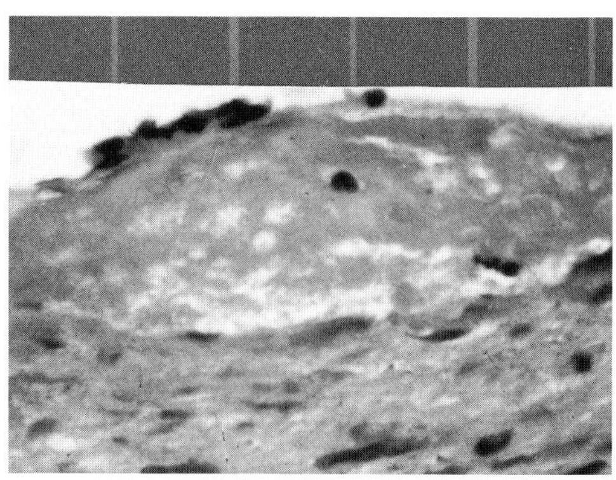

FIGURE 6-22. Microscopic thrombus in an aorta secondary to umbilical arterial catheterization (H&E, ×400).

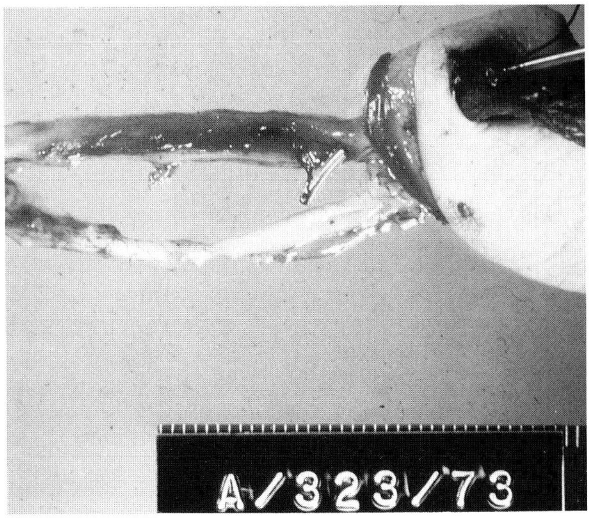

FIGURE 6-23. Pericatheteric thrombus of the umbilical artery.

Peritoneal Perforation and Rupture of Bladder

Peritoneal perforation and rupture of urinary bladder due to the umbilical arterial catheter have also been reported.[47,48] Perforation of the umbilical or hypogastric artery with severe hemorrhage can occur.[46] Clinically suspected arterial perforation can be demonstrated by radiologic studies and ligated

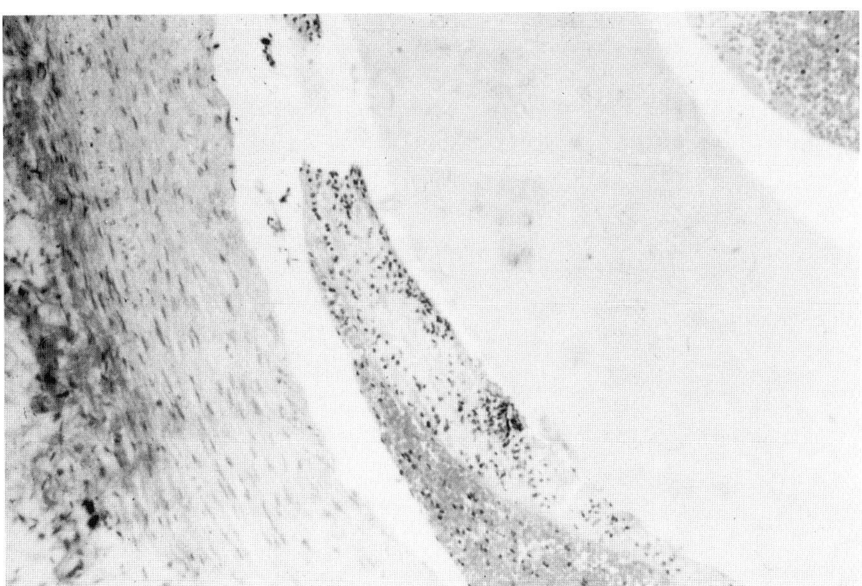

FIGURE 6-24. Pericatheteric thrombus on histologic examination (H&E, ×250).

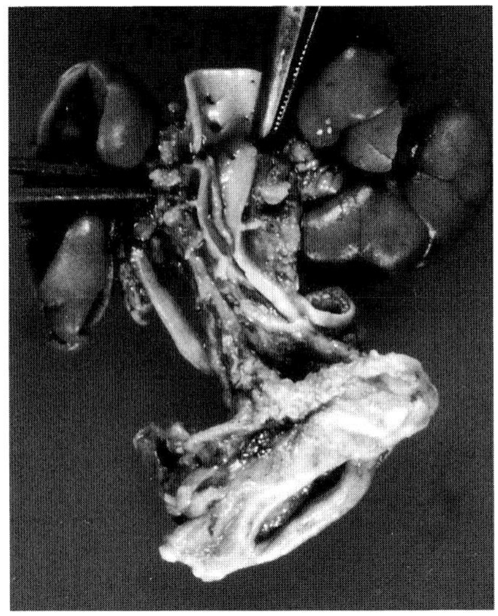

FIGURE 6-25. Occlusion of the ostium of left renal artery due to (an old calcified) thrombus associated with umbilical arterial catheterization. Note the smaller infarcted left kidney.

surgically.[49] Hemorrhage along the abdominal wall and perivesical, intraperitoneal, or retroperitoneal hemorrhage is noted at autopsy in fatal cases (Figures 6-26, 6-27). The site of perforation can be demonstrated at autopsy by injecting milk or any colored fluid through the aorta (Figure 6-28).

Sequelae of Thrombosis and Infection

Late sequelae of thrombosis and infection associated with UAC include atheromatous lesions and mycotic aneurysm of the aorta respectively.[42,43]

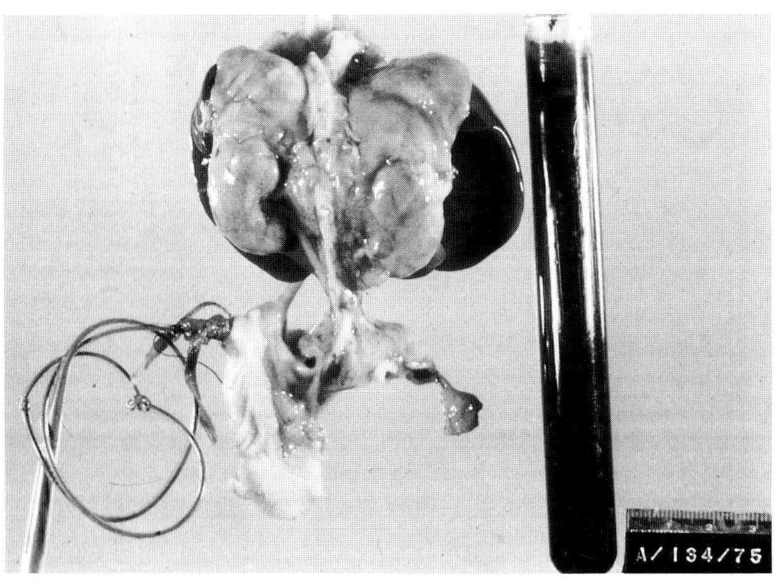

FIGURE 6-26. Intraperitoneal hemorrhage (blood in the test tube) in newborn infant with umbilical arterial catheterization.

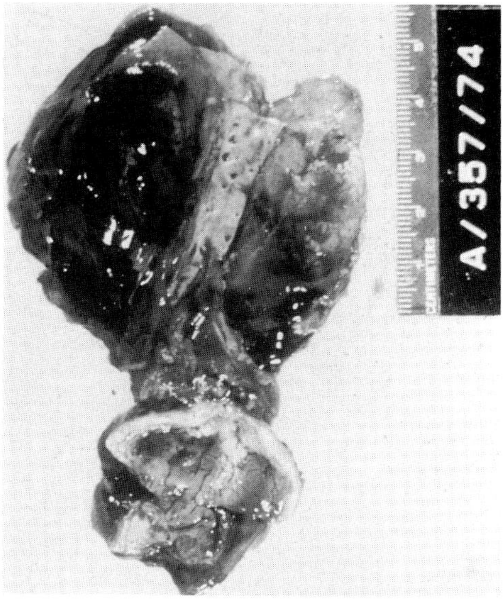

FIGURE 6-27. Retroperitoneal hemorrhage associated with perforation of umbilical artery due to umbilical arterial catheter.

Atheromatous lesions, which were seen in infants surviving for long periods of time (≤184 days) after UAC, consisted of fatty deposits within the thrombus, intima, and media. Smooth muscle cell hyperplasia and accumulation of mucopolysaccharide were noted in the media of the aorta. Organization of the thrombus leading to the formation of fibrous plaque with lipid and calcification was seen in infants who survived longer.[42] The microthrombus demonstrated in Figure 6-22 may represent an early stage leading to subsequent atheromatous changes. Tyson et al[42] also describe minute scars of aortic media with focal destruction of internal elastic lamina in a 7-year-old girl who had UAC done at birth. Colclough and Barson[43] have reported a case of true aneurysm of thoracic aorta in a premature infant who died of pseudomonas septicemia at 14½ weeks of age. The authors suggested that elastases produced by pseudomonas organisms were responsible for destruction of elastic tissue in the aortic wall. Lobe et al have recently reviewed 16 cases of mycotic aneurysm following umbilical arterial catheterization in preterm infants.[50] The infection was due to *Staphylococcus aureus*, *Klebsiella pneumoniae*, or *Candida albicans*.

Umbilical Venous Catheterization (UVC)

UVC is done for exchange transfusion in newborn infants. Thrombosis, necrotizing enterocolitis (NEC) (related to impedance of portal venous flow), and infection are the main iatrogenic lesions associated with UVC.[51] The thrombus may involve the umbilical vein, the ductus venosus (Figure 6-29), and even the portal vein branches. NEC associated with UVC is described in the chapter on NEC. Impedance of portal venous blood flow due to misplaced catheter tip, rate of exchange transfusion, or thrombosis is the main pathogenetic factor related to this type of NEC. Infection with phlebitis and septicemia is rarely seen. A late sequelae of UVC is portal hypertension due to portal vein thrombosis.[52]

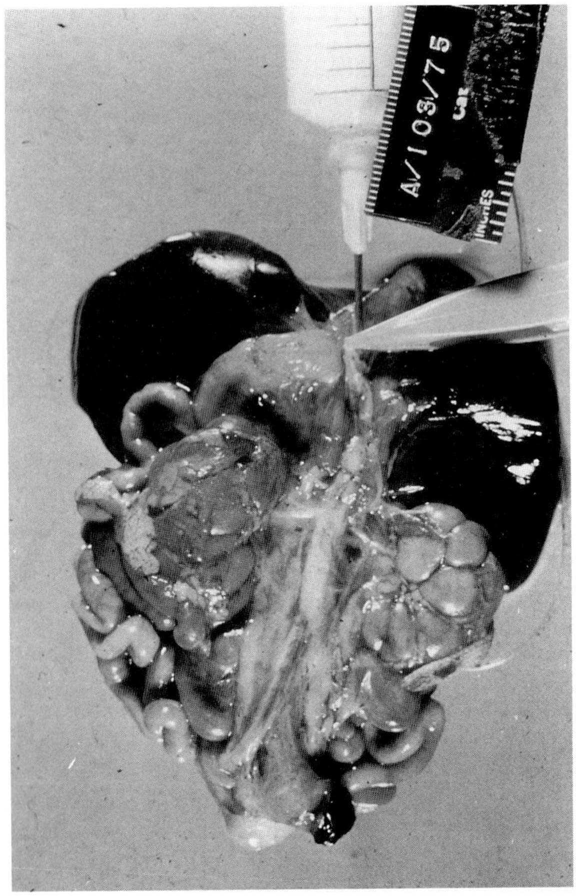

FIGURE 6-28. Method of demonstrating site of perforation of umbilical artery by injection of milk.

Total Parenteral Nutrition (TPN)

TPN is used in premature infants since those with IRDS are incapable of adequate oral feeds and have inadequate reserve of nutrient, rapid growth rate, and possible propensity to suffer an irreversible neurologic damage due to nutritional deficiency. Numerous good-quality nutrient preparations, including those containing amino acids, fat, and multivitamin additions, are available for TPN. The complications associated with TPN are those related to (1) the central catheter, (2) possible "toxic" action of the constituents, and (3) overload of nutrients—particularly fat.

Complications Related to Central Venous Catheter

A recent review of 587 instances of central venous catheter (CVC) placements[53] for TPN (and other procedures) revealed an overall complication rate of 28%. Dislodgement (11%), perforation (5%), obstruction (5%), sepsis (4%), and caval thrombosis (1%) were seen in these infants. There were two deaths related to cardiac tamponade due to perforation with leakage of TPN fluid into the

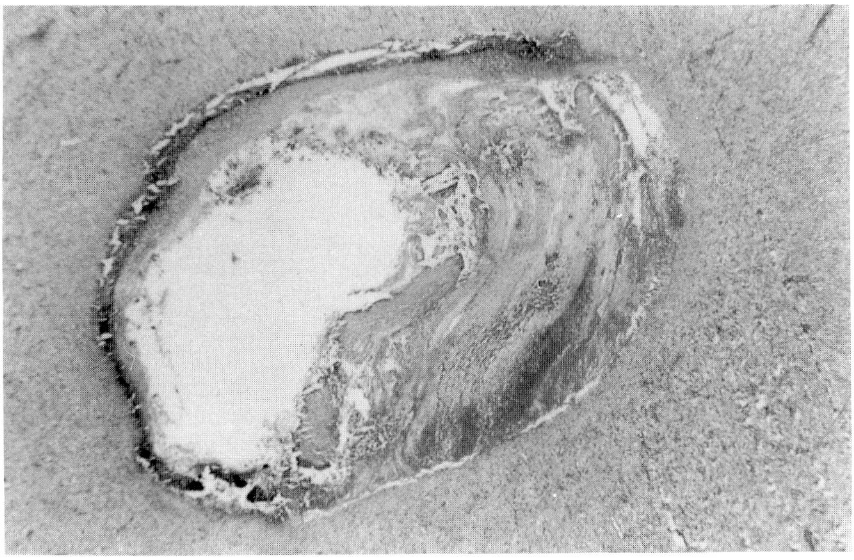

FIGURE 6-29. Thrombosis of ductus venosus associated with umbilical venous catheterization (H&E, ×100).

pericardial cavity. Pleural effusions also occur as a complication of CVC placement. Three cases of sudden death due to wedging of the CVC against the myocardium followed by myocardial necrosis and pericardial effusion have been reported.[54] Sepsis, particularly that due to Candida, was one of the first infectious complications of parenteral nutrition (hyperalimentation) to be reported.[55] Fungal sepsis may be followed by delayed right-sided endocarditis (Figure 6-30).[56]

Another fungus that has been reported to cause systemic infections, particularly in patients who receive intralipid therapy, is *Malassezia furfur* (MF).[57,58] MF causes tinea versicolor and seborrheic dermatitis. It requires high concentration of fatty acids for growth. Patients receiving intralipid therapy are therefore susceptible to infection by MF. The diagnosis of MF infection is made by blood culture, demonstration of the organisms in the lung tissue by culture or morphology, or by culture of catheter tip. The characteristic lesion seen in the lung biopsy or autopsy specimen is vasculitis. Small branches of pulmonary arteries show a mixed inflammatory infiltrate (lymphocytes, mononuclear cells, and neutrophils) extending through the wall. MF has hyphal and yeast forms. The budding is characteristically unipolar. Gomori's methenamine silver stains the organisms which are barely visible in the routine H&E stain. Fat stain demonstrates deposition of fat in the affected vessel wall.

Complications Related to Possible "Toxic" Action of the Constituents of Preparations Used for TPN

The main lesion in this category is TPN-associated liver disease. The development and progression of liver disease is clearly related to TPN, but the precise etiopathogenesis is not known. Direct hepatotoxicity of amino acid

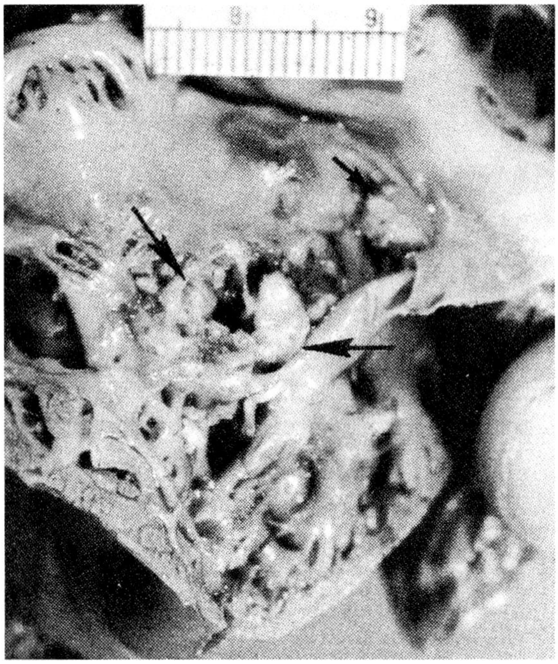

FIGURE 6-30. Candida endocarditis of tricuspid valve as a late sequela of catheter-related sepsis; note the large nodular vegetations on the cusps of tricuspid valve (arrows).

infusate, high glucose content of infusions, immaturity of the liver, and sepsis have been implicated.[59–62] Cholestatic jaundice in the absence of extrahepatic biliary obstruction is the most commonly observed early manifestation. The incidence of cholestasis in <1000 g infants after 2 weeks of TPN is about 50%.

Pathologic changes related to TPN liver disease include the following: (1) *parenchyma*—fatty change, giant cell transformation, and ballooning degeneration of hepatocytes, centrilobular cholestasis, scattered foci of hepatocyte necrosis, pericellular fibrosis, and persistent hematopoiesis; (2) *portal tracts*—mixed inflammatory infiltrate (lymphocytes, eosinophils, and neutrophils), fibrosis, bile duct proliferation, and rarely bile plugging; and (3) *Kupffer cells*—foamy cytoplasm containing lipofuscin (Figures 6-31, 6-32).[61,63] Ultrastructural study has revealed the presence of membrane bound inclusions and cytoplasmic degenerative changes.[61]

With persistent use of TPN over long periods of time (usually >2 months) progression to marked portal fibrosis and even to micronodular cirrhosis can occur (Figures 6-33, 6-34).[63] Liver biopsy may be done for the diagnosis of type of liver disease in an infant on prolonged TPN. Portal fibrosis, bile ductular proliferation, and bile plugging in ductules and hepatocytes seen at this stage of TPN liver disease simulate hepatic changes in biliary atresia.[64] Hepatocellular carcinoma has been reported as a late sequela in a 26-month-old prematurely born infant who had received TPN for a total of 395 days.[65]

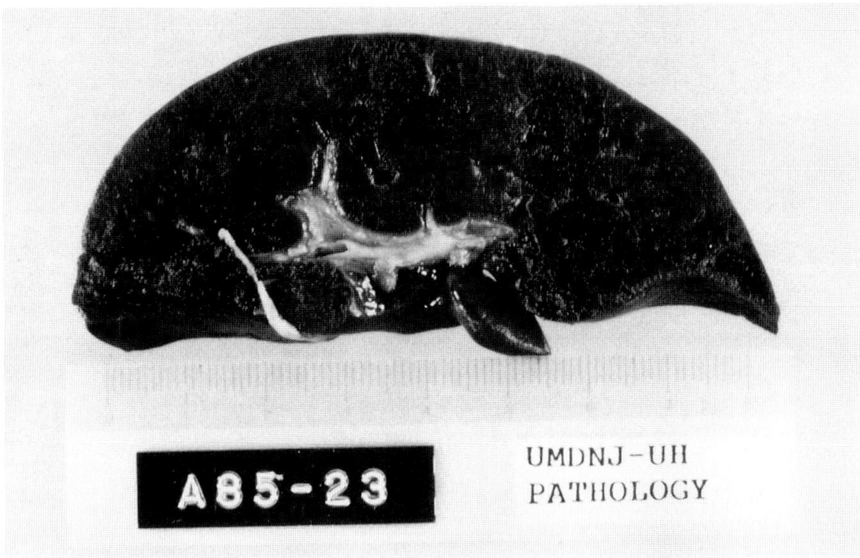

FIGURE 6-31. Dark (green) color of the liver due to cholestasis associated with total parenteral nutrition.

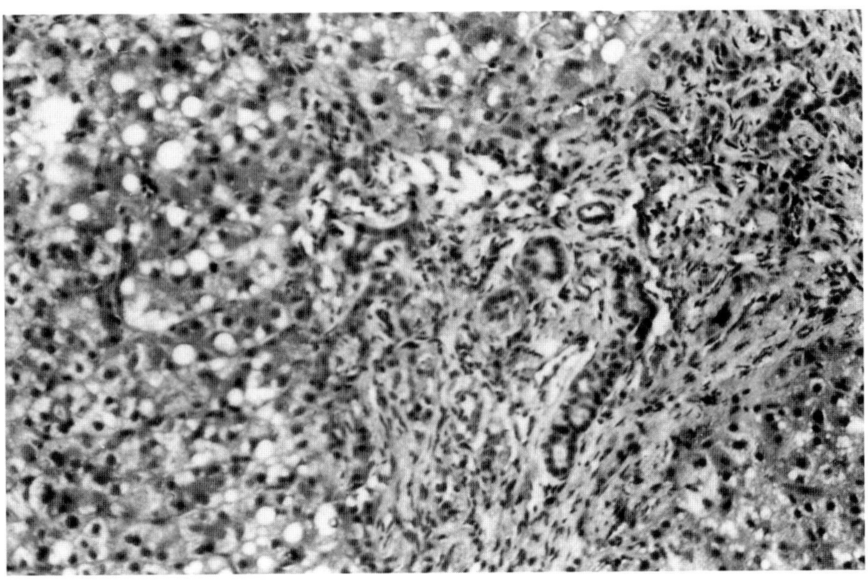

FIGURE 6-32. Note the fatty change, portal fibrosis, and bile ductular proliferation in liver disease associated with total parenteral nutrition; there was also hepatocellular and canalicular cholestasis (not shown) (H&E, ×250).

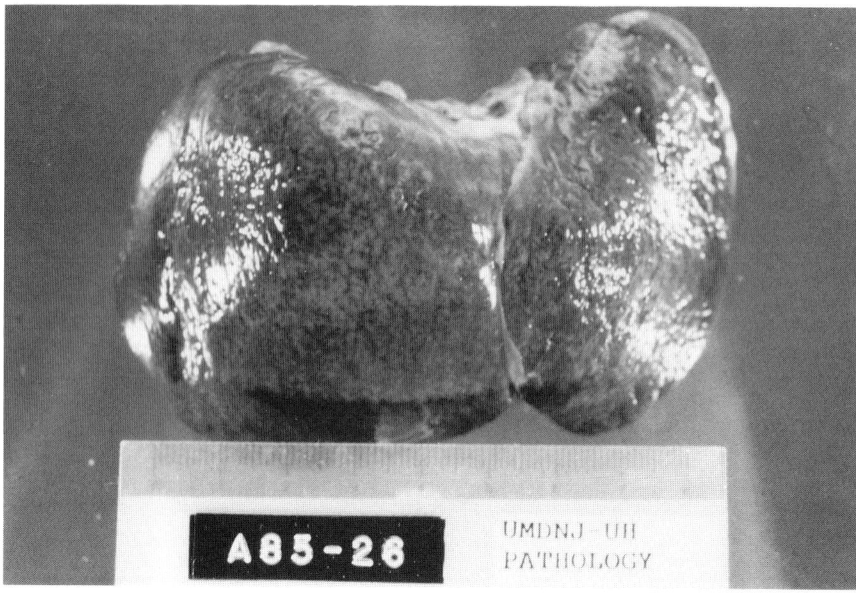

FIGURE 6-33. Liver cirrhosis associated with prolonged total parenteral nutrition; note the granular external appearance of the micronodular cirrhosis of the liver.

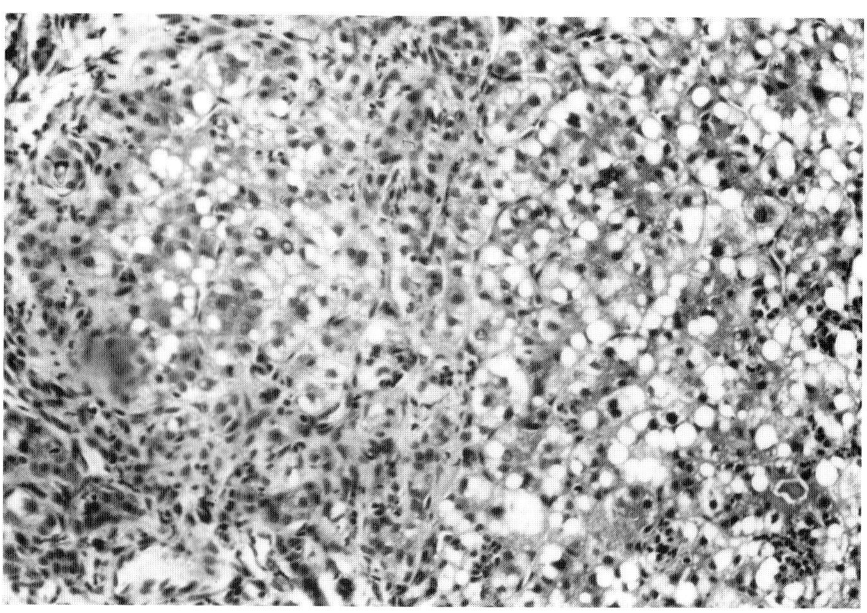

FIGURE 6-34. Note the micronodular cirrhosis with fatty change of liver cells on histologic examination (H&E, ×250).

Complications Related to Overload of Fats

The commercially available lipid infusion called "Intralipid" is widely used for TPN. The main pathologic changes are seen in the lungs. Fat emboli and fat accumulation in the macrophages in the alveoli and subintima of small muscular pulmonary arteries with narrowing of the lumen have been described.[66–68] The latter occurs in infants with pulmonary hypertension due to chronic lung disease or congenital heart disease.[67] Dahms et al[67] suggested that the increased luminal pressure in these infants resulted in the injury to the pulmonary vessel wall facilitating the passage and deposition of lipid. They also showed that subintimal lipid accumulation accentuates the pulmonary hypertension. A lung biopsy may be done in an infant with bronchopulmonary dysplasia who shows persistent respiratory insufficiency despite what appears to be adequate supportive therapy and absence of severe changes on radiologic examination of the chest. I have seen such a case in which the discontinuation of intralipid infusion following the detection of subintimal arterial lipid deposition in a lung biopsy led to marked improvement (Figure 6-35). A full-fledged fat overload[69] syndrome has not been described in newborn infants. Infection due to MF with intralipid infusion is described above.

Hepatic Lesion Related to Vitamin E Supplementation

A rare hepatic lesion in very low-birth-weight infants (<1500 g) related to vitamin E supplementation (E-Ferol) of TPN solution has been described in an autopsy study.[70] Kupffer cell exfoliation, centrilobular cell debris, and panlobular congestion, which was particularly more marked in the central portion of

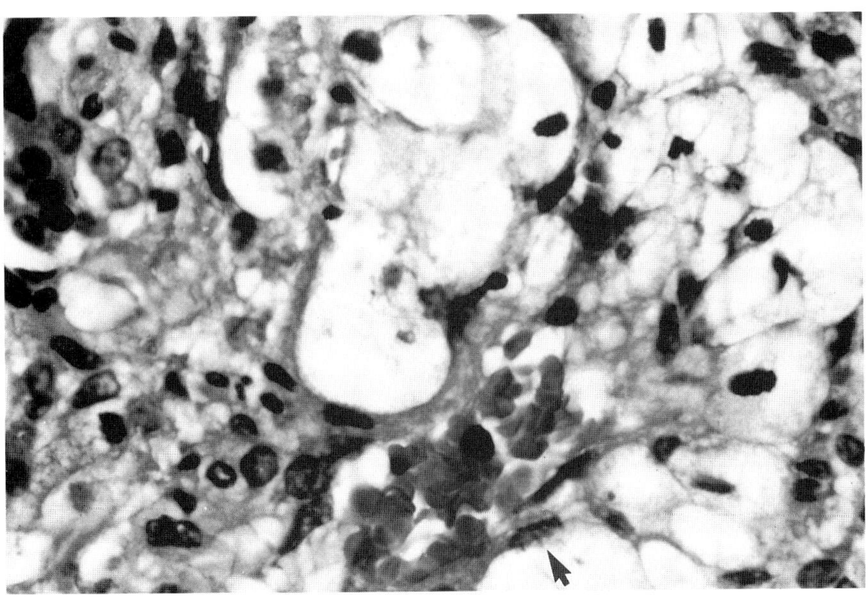

FIGURE 6-35. Pulmonary artery in an infant with bronchopulmonary dysplasia showing lipid macrophages in the subintima with marked narrowing of the lumen (arrow).

the lobule, were noted as initial evidence of hepatic injury. Prolonged use of vitamin E supplementation led to progressive cholestasis, inflammation of hepatic venules, and extensive sinusoidal occlusion by fibrosis. Clinically the infants showed hepatomegaly, jaundice, ascites, hypotension, thrombocytopenia, and renal dysfunction.

Morphologic Lesions Related Side Effects of Drugs

Gastric Outlet Obstruction Related to Prostaglandin E1

Prostaglandin E1 is used for maintaining patency of the ductus arteriosus in infants with congenital heart disease and persistent pulmonary hypertension. Peled et al[71] have described five infants who were given prostaglandin E1 for long periods of time and who developed gastric outlet obstruction. Pathologic examination of the gastric antrum in one of these infants revealed increased thickness of the antral mucosa (three times normal) with marked hyperplasia of cells of the gastric pit (foveolar cells) and increased secretion of mucin. The antral mucosal thickening was documented by ultrasonography in all the cases. In two cases reversal of the hyperplastic antral mucosa after discontinuation of the prostaglandin therapy was documented by ultrasonography. Prostaglandin E1 (and E2) has been shown to produce gastric antral hyperplasia in experimental animals and in adults. It is also possible that the clearance of prostaglandin may be slower in sick neonates.

Renal Calcification Associated with Diuretics and Corticosteroids

Renal calcification is a well-recognized complication of prolonged furosemide therapy.[72–74] It can be detected by sonographic examination. At autopsy, focal tubular calcification is seen on microscopic examination. In a recent brief report Kamitsuka and Peloquin have described renal calcification in a preterm infant on prolonged dexamethasone therapy.[74] Furosemide, a patent diuretic, is used commonly in the infants with bronchopulmonary dysplasia. It causes hypercalciuria which is an important factor in the pathogenesis of renal calcification. Other factors such as alkaline urine, oliguria, hypercalcemia, and hypophosphatemia may also play a role.[73] Follow-up studies have shown improvement or resolution in renal calcification with normal renal growth.[73] No pathologic studies of long-term sequelae are available.

Hypertrophic Cardiomyopathy Related to Dexamethasone Therapy

Werner et al[75] carried out echocardiographic monitoring of the cardiac changes in infants with bronchopulmonary dysplasia (BPD) who were given high-dose dexamethasone therapy. Significant thickening of the interventricular septum and diastolic left ventricular wall was noted. These changes were transient. The transient nature of the cardiac changes may explain the lack of pathologic description of the lesion. The pathogenesis of the cardiac changes, which are also seen in neonatal rats given dexamethasone, is not clear.

Pulmonary Lesions Possibly Related to Surfactant Therapy

These are described in the chapter on neonatal respiratory distress syndrome.

TABLE 6-1 Iatrogenic Lesions That May be Seen in the Surgical Pathology Specimen from Neonates and Young Infants

Tissue or Organ	Lesion
Placenta	Traumatic lesions related to amniocentesis and intrauterine transfusion
Tracheal, broncheal mucosa, and submucosa	Sloughed-off necrotic mucosa, granulation tissue, stenosis due to scarring, fibroepithelial polypoid lesion related to endotracheal intubation and suction catheters
Lung biopsy	Bronchopulmonary dysplasia, lipid deposition in the arterial wall accentuating pulmonary hypertension (intralipid therapy), persistent interstitial pulmonary emphysema related to mechanical ventilation, pulmonary vasculitis associated with *Malassezia furfur* infection (intralipid therapy)
Segment of intestine	Necrotizing enterocolitis associated with exchange transfusion or occlusive arterial thrombosis secondary to umbilical arterial catheterization
Liver biopsy	Liver disease associated with total parenteral nutrition
Stomach, antral biopsy	Mucosal hyperplasia related to prostaglandin E1 therapy

COMMENT

Many of the iatrogenic lesions detected at autopsy in newborn infants who have been subjected to various invasive diagnostic and therapeutic procedures are of direct or indirect clinical significance. They may be indicative of the early acute stage, which leads to long-term sequelae in the survivors. Thus acute lesions of the upper respiratory tract related to EI seen at autopsy are the precursors of the granulation tissue formation and stenosis of trachea seen in the surviving older infants. Thrombosis of aorta associated with UAC serves as an example of an iatrogenic lesion causing immediate or late morbidity and mortality. Certain lesions such as pulmonary arterial lipid accumulation may accentuate already existing clinical problems. The surgical pathologist should be alert to the possibility that some of these early and late lesions may be encountered in biopsy specimens (Table 6-1). *At autopsy, efforts should be made for proper demonstration of the iatrogenic lesions described in this chapter and summarized in Table 6-2.

*The lesions described in this chapter are summarized in Table 6-2. New lesions are being studied in a prospective manner by a multidisciplinary group (Study Group for Complications of Perinatal Care—SGCPC) established in 1984. Systematic retrospective reviews of previously known lesions are also conducted by SGCPC. Individual and institutional memberships of the SGCPC are offered. Those interested can write to the Office of SGCPC at the Department of Pathology, Magee Womens Hospital, Pittsburgh, PA 15213.

TABLE 6-2 Perinatal Iatrogenic Lesions

Procedure	Lesion	Pathogenesis	Comment
Amniocentesis	Injuries to fetus, placenta, umbilical cord; infection	Trauma	Examination of placenta is essential
	Abortion; preterm labor	Stimulation of uterine contraction, placental abruption	—
Intrauterine transfusion	External injury to fetus, traumatic fetal hemorrhage, visceral injury	Trauma	—
	Fetal demise	Compression of umbilical vein by inadvertent injection of blood in Wharton's jelly	Examination of placenta is essential
Obstetrical maneuvers	Injuries to bones, soft tissues, viscera, nerves	Trauma	—
	Hemorrhages in various sites	Trauma, asphyxia	In situ examination of tentorium cerebelli and falx is essential
Endotracheal intubation	Necrosis and inflammation of mucosa and wall of the upper respiratory tract of varying severity	Multifactorial (trauma, microbial contamination, ischemia, etc.)	Sloughing of necrotic mucosa may produce severe obstruction
	Perforation of trachea, bronchi	Trauma	In situ examination with the tube in place is essential
	Gangrene of tip of nose	Ischemia due to pressure	—
	Granulation tissue, submucosal fibrosis, fibroepithelial polypoid lesion	Healing of acute lesion	The lesions may recur after surgical excision
Mechanical ventilation	Acute air-leak phenomena including pulmonary vascular air embolism	Barotrauma with extension of air via connective tissue planes	—
	Persistent interstitial pulmonary emphysematous bulla(e) lined by multinucleated giant cells	Persistent barotrauma	It should be differentiated from congenital pulmonary cystic lesions
	Reduced size of diaphragm	Disuse atrophy and/or failure of growth	Sections for histology from the diaphragm should be taken routinely at autopsy

TABLE 6-2 Continued

Procedure	Lesion	Pathogenesis	Comment
Oxygen therapy	Acute and chronic lung injury (diffuse alveolar damage)	Oxygen toxicity	—
	Retinopathy of prematurity (vasoobliterative, proliferative, and cicatricial stages)	Multifactorial with hyperoxia as the major factor	Examination of the eyes at autopsy may require special permission
Chest tubes	Lung injury, pericardial injury with hemopericardium	Trauma	In situ examination is essential
Extracorporeal membrane oxygenation	Intracranial and extracranial hemorrhages	Heparinization of blood, platelet dysfunction, increased venous and arterial pressure	—
	Cerebral edema, cystic encephalomalacia	Persistent hypoxia and hypoperfusion	—
	Thromboemboli and infarct in viscera	Disseminated intravascular coagulation	—
	Aluminum emboli and infarcts in extrapulmonary sites	Fragmentation of aluminum of mixing rods of the heat exchangers	Aluminon stain for aluminum should be done
Umbilical arterial catheterization	Thrombosis	Thrombogenic surface of the catheter, endothelial injury	Thrombi may occlude ostia of major arteries with infarction of the respective organ (NEC, renal infarction); emboli may lodge in peripheral circulation
	Atheromatous lesions	Sequelae of acute lesions	—
	Aneurysm formation	Mycotic aneurysm	Staphylococci, klebsiella, and candida
	Peritoneal perforation, perforation of umbilical artery, rupture of urinary bladder	Trauma	Intraperitoneal or retroperitoneal hemorrhage due to arterial perforation
Umbilical venous catheterization	Thrombosis, infection	—	The ductus venosus and veins of the liver should be routinely examined at autopsy

(continued)

TABLE 6-2 Continued

Procedure	Lesion	Pathogenesis	Comment
	NEC	Impedance of portal venous flow	—
	Portal hypertension	Thrombosis of portal vein	Late sequela
Total parenteral nutrition	Dislodgement, perforation, (leakage of fluid), obstruction, sepsis, thrombosis, myocardial necrosis	Trauma, infection, faulty placement of catheter	Careful in situ examination of the catheter with appropriate cultures and histologic section from thrombus, when present, is essential
	Liver disease (cholestasis, fatty change, bile cut proliferation)	?"Toxic" action of aminoacid infusate, sepsis, immaturity of the liver	Liver biopsy may be done; neonatal hepatitis and extrahepatic biliary atresia are to be considered in the differential diagnosis
	Fat deposition in the alveoli and subintima of pulmonary artery branches	Increased intraluminal pressure in infants with pulmonary hypertension may injure the vessel wall facilitating the passage and deposition of lipid	Lung biopsy may be done; careful assessment of the pulmonary artery branches is essential
Diuretics and corticosteroids	Renal calcification	Hypercalcemia, alkalinity of urine, hypophosphatemia may play a role	Renal calcification may be detected by ultrasound
Prostaglandin E1	Mucosal hyperplasia of gastric antrum	Prostaglandin E1 induces hyperplasia	Produces gastric outlet obstruction
Corticosteroids	Hypertrophic cardiomyopathy	Not known	Transient change

REFERENCES

1. Andrews BF: Six finger exercise. *Am J Dis Child* 166:334, 1968.
2. Banagale RC: Iatrogenous complications in the fetus and newborn. The dilemma (editorial). *Am J Dis Child* 138:621–622, 1984.
3. Sola A, Bednarek FJ, Davidson R, et al: Meningitis, ventriculitis, and hydrocephalus: A complication of fetal monitoring. *Obstet Gynecol* 56:663–665, 1980.
4. Cunningham FG, MacDonald PC, Grant NF: *Williams Obstetrics*, 18th ed. Appleton and Lange, Norwalk, CT, 1989, p 278.
5. Bowman JM: Hemolytic disease (erythroblastosis fetalis). In *Maternal fetal medicine: Principles and practice*, 2nd ed. (Creasy RK, Resnick R, Eds). Saunders, Philadelphia, 1989, pp 613–655.
6. Wade ME, Ogden JA, Anderson GG, et al: Intrauterine fetal transfusions. Experience with 101 transfusions in 48 mothers. *Am J Obstet Gynecol* 105:962–971, 1969.

7. Valdes-Dapena M: Iatrogenic disease in perinatal period as seen by the pathologist. In *Perinatal diseases.* (Naeye RL, Kissane JM, Kaufman N, Eds). Williams & Wilkins, Baltimore, 1981, pp 382–418.
8. Valdes-Dapena M: Iatrogenic disease in the perinatal period. *Pediatr Clin N Am* 36:67–93, 1989.
9. Carty A, Stanley P: Bilateral adrenal abscesses in a neonate. *Pediatr Radiol* 1:63–64, 1973.
10. Joshi VV, Mandavia SG, Stern L, et al: Acute lesions induced by endotracheal intubation. Occurrence in the upper respiratory tract of newborn infants with respiratory distress syndrome. *Am J Dis Child* 124:646–649, 1972.
11. Metlay LA, MacPherson TA, Doshi N, et al: Necrotizing tracheobronchitis in intubated newborns: A complication of associated ventilation. *Pediatr Pathol* 7:575–584, 1987.
12. Boros S, Mammel MC, Lewallen PK, et al: Necroting tracheobronchitis: A complication of high-frequency mechanical ventilation. *J Pediatr* 109:95–100, 1986.
13. Hanson JB, Waldstein G, Hernandez JA, et al: Necrotizing tracheobronchitis. An ischemic lesion. *Am J Dis Child* 142:1094–1098, 1988.
14. Friedberg J, Forte V: Acquired bronchial injury in neonates. *Int J Pediatr Otorhinolaryngol* 14:223–228, 1987.
15. Clarke TA, Coen RW, Feldman B, et al: Esophageal perforations in premature infants and comments on the diagnosis. *Am J Dis Child* 134:367–368, 1980.
16. Stetson JB, Guess WL: Causes of damage to tissues by polymers and elastomers used in the fabrication of tracheal devices. *Anesthesiology* 33:635–652, 1970.
17. Weymuller EA Jr: Laryngeal injury from prolonged endotracheal intubation. *Laryngoscope* 98:1–15, 1988.
18. Carlton GC, Kahn RC, Howland WS, et al: Clinical experience with high frequency jet ventilation. *Crit Care Med* 9:1–6, 1981.
19. Pokora T, Bing D, Mammel M, et al: Neonatal high frequency jet ventilation. *Pediatrics* 72:27–32, 1983.
20. Ratner I, Whitfield J: Acquired subglottic stenosis in the very low birth weight infant. *Am J Dis Child* 137:40–43, 1983.
21. Azizkhan RG, Grimmer DL, Askin FB, et al: Acquired lobar emphysema (overinflation): Clinical and pathological evaluation of infants requiring lobectomy. *J Pediatr Surg* 27:1145–1152, 1991.
22. Deneyer M, Goossens A, Pipeleers-Marichal M, et al: Esophagitis of likely traumatic origin in newborns. *J Pediatr Gastroenterol Nutr* 15:81–84, 1992.
23. Lee SK, Tanswell AK: Pulmonary vascular air embolism in the newborn. *Arch Dis Child* 64:507–510, 1989.
24. Caldwell EJ, Powell RD, Mullooly JP: Interstitial emphysema: A study of physiologic factors involved in experimental induction of the lesion. *Am Rev Resp Dis* 102:516–525, 1970.
25. Stocker JT, Madewell JE: Persistent interstitial pulmonary emphysema: Another complication of the respiratory distress syndrome. *Pediatrics* 59:847–857, 1977.
26. Knisely AS, Leal SM, Singer DB: Abnormalities of diaphragmatic muscle in neonates with ventilated lungs. *J Pediatr* 113:1074–1077, 1988.
27. Avery GB, Glass P: Retinopathy of prematurity: Progress report. *Pediatr Annals* 17:528–533, 1988.
28. Kushner BJ, Essner D, Cohen IJ, et al: Retrolental fibroplasia. II. Pathologic correlation. *Arch Ophthalmol* 95:29–38, 1977.
29. Committee for the classification of retinopathy of prematurity: An International Classification of Retinopathy of Prematurity. *Pediatrics* 74:127–133, 1984.
30. Taylor GA, Fitz CR, Miller MK, et al: Intracranial abnormalities in infants treated with

extracorporeal membrane oxygenization: Imaging with US and CT. *Radiology* 165:675–678, 1987.
31. Vogler C, Sotela C, Fulling K: Extracorporeal membrane oxygenation (ECMO) therapy: An analysis of 23 autopsies. *Pediatr Pathol* 7:498, 1987.
32. Vogler C, Sotelo-Avila C, Lagunoff D, et al: Aluminum-containing emboli in infants treated with extracorporeal membrane oxygenation. *N Engl J Med* 319:75–79, 1988.
33. Maloney NA, Ott SM, Alfrey AC, et al: Histological quantitation of aluminum in iliac bone from patients with renal failure. *J Clin Lab Med* 99:206–216, 1982.
34. Taylor GA, Lotze A, Kapur S, et al: Diffuse pulmonary opacification in infants undergoing extracorporeal membrane oxygenation: Clinical and pathologic correlation. *Radiology* 161:347–350, 1986.
35. Chou P, Blei ED, Shen-Schwarz S, et al: Pulmonary changes following extracorporeal membrane oxygenation: An autopsy study of 23 cases. *Hum Pathol* 24:405–412, 1993.
36. Gross GW, Cullen J, Desai HJ: Progression of pulmonary cystic disease during ECMO. *Pediatr Radiol* 20:191, 1990.
37. Pratt PC, Vollmer RT, Shelburne JD, et al: Pulmonary morphology in a multihospital collaborative extracorporeal membrane oxygenation project. *Am J Pathol* 95:191–214, 1979.
38. Toomasian JM, Snedocor SM, Cornell RG, et al: National experience with extracorporeal membrane oxygenation for newborn respiratory failure: Data from 715 cases. *ASAIO Trans* 11:140–147, 1988.
39. Glass P, Miller M, Short B: Morbidity for survivors of extracorporeal membrane oxygenation. Neurodevelopmental outcome at one year of age. *Pediatrics* 83:72–78, 1989.
40. Andrews AF, Nixon CA, Cilley RE, et al: One-to-three-year outcome for 14 neonatal survivors of extracorporeal membrane oxygenation. *Pediatrics* 78:692–698, 1986.
41. Kitterman JA, Phibbs RH, Tooley WH: Catheterization of umbilical vessels in newborn infants. *Pediatr Clin N Am* 17:895–912, 1970.
42. Tyson JE, DeSa DJ, Moore S: Thromboatheromatous complications of umbilical arterial catheterization in the newborn period. Clinicopathological study. *Arch Dis Child* 51:744–754, 1976.
43. Colclough AB, Barson AJ: Infantile aortic aneurysm complicating umbilical arterial catheterization. *Arch Dis Child* 56:795–797, 1981.
44. Hecker JF: Thrombogenicity of tips of umbilical catheters. *Pediatrics* 67:467–471, 1981.
45. Neal WA, Reynolds JW, Jarvis CW, et al: Umbilical artery catheterization: Demonstration of arterial thrombosis by aortography. *Pediatrics* 50:6–13, 1972.
46. Joshi VV, Draper DA, Bates RD: Neonatal necrotizing enterocolitis. Occurrence secondary to thrombosis of abdominal aorta following umbilical arterial catheterization. *Arch Pathol* 99:540–543, 1975.
47. Van Leeuwen G, Patney M: Complications of umbilical vessel catheterization: Peritoneal perforation. *Pediatrics* 44:1028–1030, 1969.
48. Diamond DA, Ford C: Neonatal bladder rupture: A complication of umbilical artery catheterization. *J Urol* 142:1543–1544, 1989.
49. Miller D, Kirkpatrick BV, Kodroff M, et al: Pelvic exsanguination following umbilical artery catheterization in neonates. *J Pediatr Surg* 14:264–269, 1979.
50. Lobe TE, Richardson J, Boulden TF, et al: Mycotic thromboaneurysmal disease of the abdominal aorta in preterm infants: Its natural history and its management. *J Pediatr Surg* 27:1054–1060, 1992.
51. Scott JM: Iatrogenic lesions in babies following umbilical vein catheterization. *Arch Dis Child* 40:426–429, 1965.
52. Oski FA, Allen DM, Diamond LK: Portal hypertension—a complication of umbilical vein catheterization. *Pediatrics* 29:297–302, 1963.

53. Goutail-Flaud MF, Sfez M, Berg A, et al: Central venous catheter-related complications in newborns and infants: A 587 case survey. *J Pediatr Surg* 26:645–650, 1991.
54. Franciosi RA, Ellefson RD, Uden D, et al: Sudden unexpected death due to central hyperalimentation. *Pediatrics* 69:305–307, 1982.
55. Curry CR, Quie PG: Fungal septicemia in patients receiving parenteral hyperalimentation. *N Engl J Med* 285:1221–1225, 1971.
56. Joshi VV, Wang N-S: Repeated pulmonary embolism in an infant with subacute Candida endocarditis of the right side of the heart. *Am J Dis Child* 125:257–259, 1973.
57. Redline RW, Dahms BB: Malassezia pulmonary vasculitis in an infant on long-term intralipid therapy. *N Engl J Med* 305:1395–1398, 1981.
58. Redline RW, Redline SS, Boxerbaum B, et al: Systemic Malassezia furfur infections in patients receiving intralipid therapy. *Hum Pathol* 16:815–822, 1985.
59. Postuma R, Trevenen CL: Liver disease in infants receiving total parenteral nutrition. *Pediatrics* 63:110–115, 1979.
60. Manginello FP, Javitt NB: Parenteral nutrition and neonatal cholestasis. *J Pediatr* 92:296–298, 1979.
61. Dahms BB, Halpin TC Jr: Serial liver biopsies in parenteral nutrition-associated cholestasis of early infancy. *Gastroenterol* 69:136–144, 1981.
62. Moss RL, Das JB, Ansari G, et al: Hepatobiliary dysfunction during total parenteral nutrition is caused by infusate, not the route of administration. *J Pediatr Surg* 28:391–397, 1993.
63. Gutcher G, Cutz E: Complications of parenteral nutrition. *Sem Perinatol* 10:196–207, 1986.
64. Body JJ, Bleiberg H, Bron D, et al: Total parenteral nutrition-induced cholestasis mimicking large bile duct obstruction. *Histopathology* 6:787–792, 1982.
65. Vileisis RA, Sorensen K, Gonzalez-Crussi F, et al: Liver malignancy after parenteral nutrition. *J Pediatr* 100:88–90, 1982.
66. Barson AJ, Chistwick ML, Doig CM: Fat embolism in infancy after intravenous fat infusions. *Arch Dis Child* 53:218–223, 1978.
67. Dahms BB, Halpin TC Jr: Pulmonary arterial lipid deposit in newborn infants receiving intravenous lipid infusion. *J Pediatr* 97:800–805, 1980.
68. Levene MI, Wigglesworth JS, Desai R: Pulmonary fat accumulation after intralipid infusion in the preterm infant. *Lancet* 2:815–820, 1980.
69. Haber LM, Hawkins EP, Seilheimer DK, et al: Fat overload syndrome. An autopsy study with evaluation of the coagulopathy. *Am J Clin Pathol* 89:223–227, 1988.
70. Bove KE, Kosmetatos N, Wedig KE, et al: Vasculopathic hepatotoxicity associated with E-Fesol syndrome in low-birth-weight infants. *JAMA* 254:2422–2430, 1985.
71. Peled N, Dagan O, Belnjm P, et al: Gastric outlet obstruction induced by prostaglandin therapy in neonates. *N Engl J Med* 327:505–510, 1992.
72. Hufnagle KG, Khan SN, Penn D, et al: Renal calcifications. A complication of long term furosemide therapy in preterm infants. *Pediatrics* 70:360–363, 1982.
73. Ezzedeen F, Adelman RD, Ahlfors CE: Renal calcification in preterm infants: Pathophysiology and long-term sequelae. *J Pediatr* 113:532–539, 1988.
74. Kamitsuka MD, Peloquin D: Renal calcification after dexamethasone in infants with bronchopulmonary dysplasia. *Lancet* 337:626, 1991.
75. Werner JC, Sicard RE, Hansen TWR, et al: Hypertrophic cardiomyopathy associated with dexamethasone therapy for bronchopulmonary dysplasia. *J Pediatr* 120:286–291, 1992.

7 HIRSCHSPRUNG'S DISEASE

INTRODUCTION

Harald Hirschsprung (a Danish pediatrician) presented 20 cases of congenital megacolon at the Pediatric Congress in Berlin in 1886. Tittel described absence of ganglion cells in 1901. Robertson and Kernohan from Mayo Clinic correlated distal aganglionosis with intestinal obstruction in 1938. Swenson and Bill introduced corrective surgery in 1948. Swenson and his colleagues introduced rectal biopsy as a diagnostic procedure in 1959.[1]

The incidence is one in 5000 live births. About 700 infants with Hirschsprung's disease (HD) are born in the United States every year. It is more common in white children and in boys. Familial incidence has been observed in long-segment HD. HD usually occurs as a solitary anomaly. But other anomalies (Down's syndrome, anomalies of cardiovascular system, GI tract, CNS, etc.) are present in some patients.

CLINICAL FEATURES

In recent years the diagnosis is most frequently made in the newborn period. When a full-term otherwise healthy (male) infant does not pass meconium for more than 48 hours since birth, HD should be suspected. Older children with HD present with constipation, abdominal distension, and wasting. Characteristically evacuation occurs after a rectal examination. Acute appendicitis and cecal perforation may be the initial presenting features in the newborn period.

DIAGNOSTIC WORKUP

Barium enema is confirmatory when it demonstrates the length of aganglionic segment. Confirmatory results are usually obtained in older patients, but roentgen examination may not be helpful in the newborn period in some cases. Anorectal manometry is valuable in diagnosis (normally transient rectal distention causes relaxation of the internal anal sphincter, in HD contraction instead of relaxation occurs).[2] However, rectal biopsy is the only way of making definitive diagnosis and is mandatory before definitive surgery. In the past, HD, which was usually diagnosed in older children, was characterized by typical findings on barium enemas. Suction biopsy technique was not yet developed. This explains why in the past the primary diagnosis of HD by frozen section on a full-thickness biopsy was requested by the surgeon before doing a colostomy or a definitive surgery. Some surgeons did not do a biopsy in the past when barium enema was typical. However, with the disease now being diagnosed most frequently in the newborn period and with lack of development of demonstrable x-ray abnormalities in some of the neonatal cases of HD, the role of suction rectal biopsy and the need for its systematic processing for definitive preoperative diagnosis from permanent section have become crucial (see below).

ENTERIC PLEXUSES

Embryology of Enteric Neural Plexus

Okamoto and Ueda[3] examined human embryos by silver impregnation method and showed that there is migration of neuroblasts of cephalic neural crest between 6 and 8 weeks along the vagal nerve in the craniocaudal direction starting from the esophagus. The migration of neuroblasts to distal colon and rectum with formation of ganglion cells in the plexuses is present at 12 weeks of gestation. In the distal intestine fibers enter the bowel via the sacral plexus. There is still controversy as to whether there is any contribution to the rectal ganglion cells from the lumbosacral neural crest.[4] The submucosal plexuses form by migration of neuroblasts across the circular muscle layer into the submucosa. The cells of the enteric nerve plexuses are immature in the newborn infant. Maturity is gained subsequently.

Normal Enteric Plexus

Three plexuses are present; these plexuses are also called *ganglia*: (1) Auerbach's myenteric plexuses between circular and longitudinal muscle layers, (2) Henle's deep submucosal plexuses along the inner aspect of circular layer of muscle, and (3) Meissner's superficial submucosal plexuses beneath the muscularis mucosae.

The plexus consists of nerve cell processes supported by Schwann cells with round to oval nuclei. The Schwann cells are arranged randomly (Figure 7-1). Small groups of ganglion cells are seen at the junction of neural processes, which do not have well-defined perineurium or collagen fibers. An incomplete layer of collagen is present around the ganglion, but unlike other ganglia, no collagen is present within it. The nerve trunks of unmyelinated fibers surrounded by perineurium and containing appreciable amounts of collagen penetrate the longitudinal muscle layer of the intestine (Figure 7-2). They show branching, lose the perineurium and connective tissue, and blend with the myenteric plexuses. The nerve fibers in these trunks and plexuses are largely cholinergic. A few adrenergic fibers are also present in the myenteric and Henle's plexuses but not in the superficial submucosal plexuses. The ganglion cells are mostly cholinergic and represent peripheral parasympathetic ganglion. However, by demonstrating numerous other neurotransmitter substances (purine nucleotide, substance P, VIP, serotonin, etc.) besides acetyl choline and adrenaline, immunocytochemical and histochemical studies have shown that the neural constitution of the enteric nervous system is extremely complex.

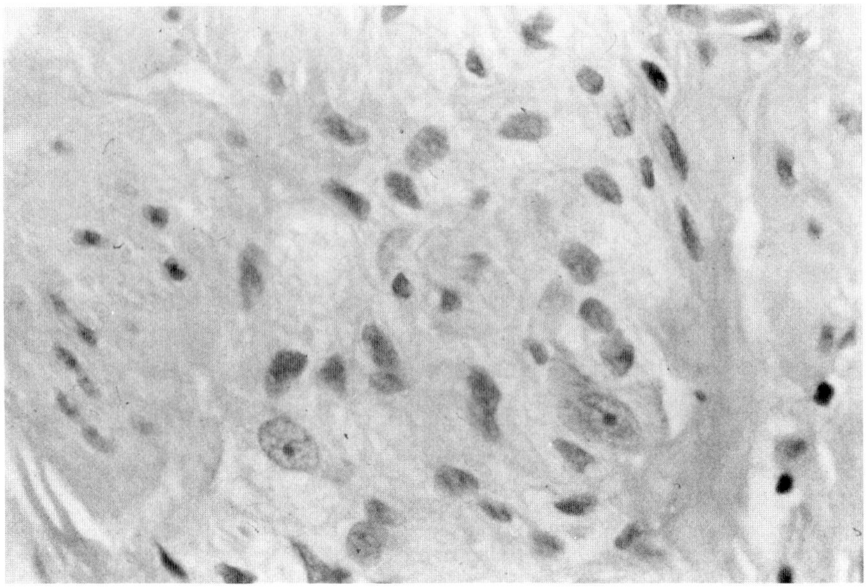

FIGURE 7-1. Myenteric plexus consisting of ganglion cells, Schwann cells with round to oval nuclei and neuritic processes; the Schwann cells are randomly arranged (H&E, ×400).

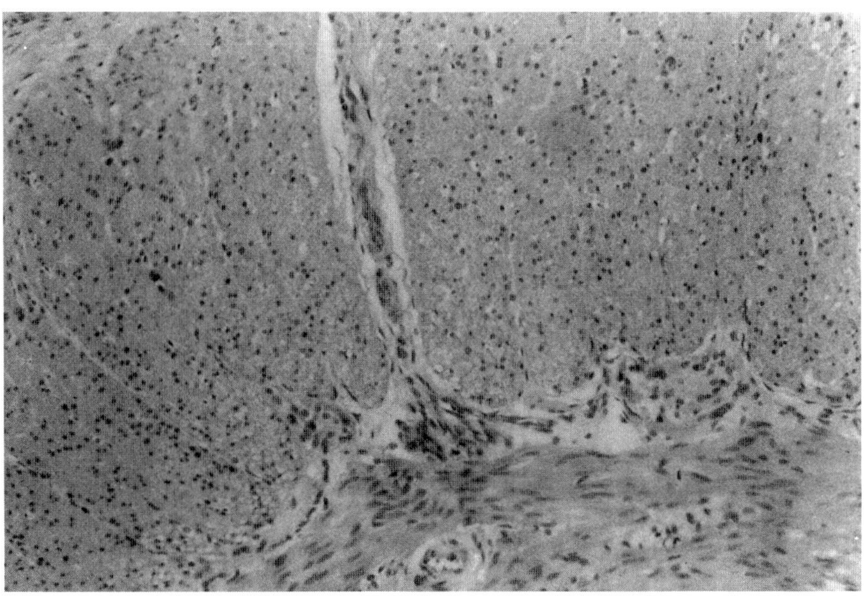

FIGURE 7-2. The penetrating nerve blends with the myenteric nerve plexus (H&E, ×100).

The normal ganglion cells measuring 15–40 μm have multipolar polygonal shape with amphophilic to eosinophilic vacuolated cytoplasm and oval to round 10–15-μm nucleus containing a prominent nucleolus (Figure 7-1). The myenteric ganglion or plexus contains 1–19 ganglion cells showing measurements of individual ganglion cells at the upper limit of normal. The submucosal ganglia contain 1–5 ganglion cells (mostly 1 or 2 ganglion cells) that are smaller in size.[5] But occasionally clusters of up to 10 ganglion cells may be seen in the submucosal ganglia. These characteristic morphologic features may be obscured to some extent because of inadequate fixation and processing or other artifacts (Figure 7-3).

Anal Enteric Plexus

There is a zone in the region of internal anal sphincter in which there is paucity or absence of ganglion cells. In children this zone extends to about 1.8 cm proximal to the pectinate (dentate) line (anal mucocutaneous junction) for the submucosal plexuses and to about 1.4 cm for the myenteric plexuses.[5,6] In addition to the paucity or absence of ganglion cells, there are prominent nerve trunks similar to those found in HD. Because of the presence of this normal hypoganglionic zone, it is generally recommended that a biopsy for diagnosis of HD should be obtained about 2 cm above the pentinate line in infants and 3 cm in children. However, Venugopal et al[7] have shown that in normal children suction biopsies taken at a distance of 1–1.5 cm from the pectinate line show ganglion cells and are therefore appropriate for diagnosis of HD.

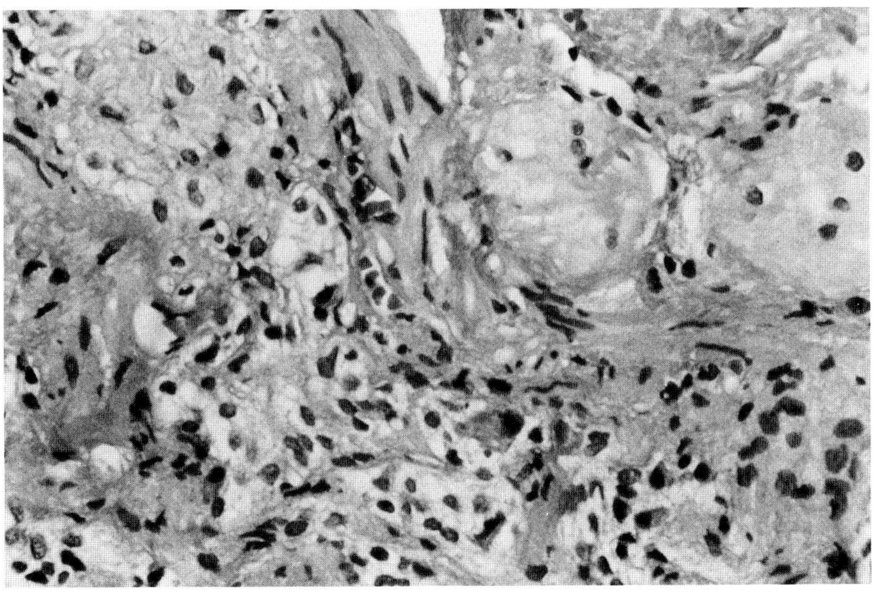

FIGURE 7-3. Artifactual changes resulting in more condensed appearance of the nucleus and shrinkage of the ganglion cells (H&E, ×250).

BASIC ABNORMALITY IN HIRSCHSPRUNG'S DISEASE

Histologic Findings

In a typical case of HD, the sigmoid colon and proximal rectum are involved. The involved segment of intestine is characteristically narrow. The colon proximal to the involved segment is dilated and hypertrophic. Between the narrow and dilated segments is the transition zone (Figure 7-4). The margins of the transition zone are poorly defined on macroscopic examination.

There is absence of ganglion cells in all the plexuses (myenteric and submucosal) of the involved segment of intestine. Large nerve trunks are found instead of the normal plexuses. The nerve trunks appear more compact than the normal plexuses. The elongated nuclei of Schwann cells of the nerve trunks are arranged in a longitudinal parallel pattern, in contrast to the round nuclei and random arrangement of Schwann cells as normally seen in the plexuses (Figures 7-1, 7-5). Presence of collagen and distinct perineurium is also seen in the nerve trunk in contrast to absence of these features in the normal plexuses.

The absence of ganglion cells probably results from failure of neural crest derived neuroblasts to migrate to the colon. However, in a murine model of HD [homozygous lethal spotted (*ls/ls*) mutants] it has been suggested that local mesenchymal defects result in an unfavorable environment for neural crest migration and colonization.[8,9] The mesenchymal defects consist of differences

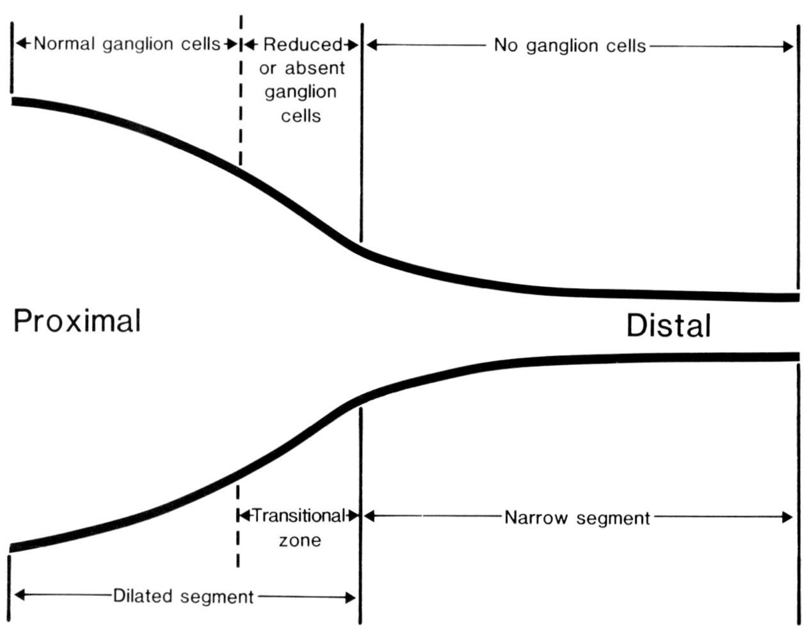

(Adapted from: Bodian, et al: Lancet 1949, 1, 6–11)

FIGURE 7-4. Diagrammatic representation of the involved distal segment of Hirschsprung's disease with the dilated transition zone and proximal segment.

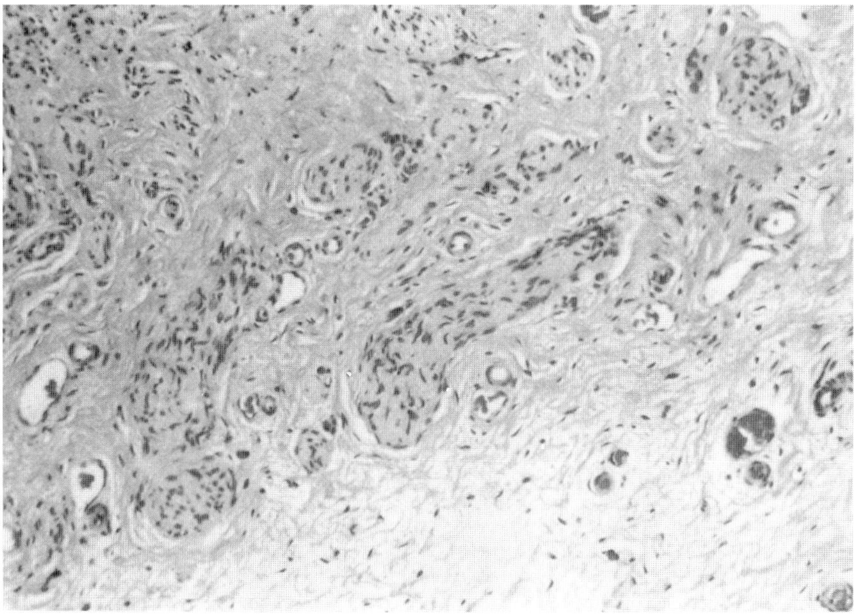

FIGURE 7-5. Hyperplastic nerve trunks between the two layers of the muscle in the affected segment of Hirschsprung's disease. Ganglion cells are absent. Note the more compact and parallel arrangement of the Schwann cells and neuritic processes and the elongated nuclei of the Schwann cells (compare with Figure 7-1). (H&E, ×100.)

in distribution and quantity of laminin, type IV collagen, and other extracellular matrix components. These types of mesenchymal abnormalities have also been demonstrated in the segment involved by HD in humans.[10]

Degenerative changes in ganglion cells have been described in HD. However, it should be noted that ganglion cells in the normal intestine show a wide variation in their morphology, partly related to degree of fixation and variations in the processing for histology (Figure 7-3). Therefore it is difficult to ascertain whether degenerative changes in the ganglion cells in the involved segment are indeed present. Such changes may also at times make definitive recognition of ganglion cells difficult for the uninitiated. Stain for neuron-specific enolase (NSE) may be helpful in such instances (see below). Tangentially cut smooth muscle in the walls of the submucosal arteries or the muscularis mucosae may be mistaken for hyperplastic nerve plexuses without ganglion cells of Hirschsprung's disease (Figures 7-6–7-8). As indicated in the section on complications below, special attention should also be paid to the changes in the crypts and lamina propria for predicting onset of necrotizing enterocolitis associated with HD.

The transition zone between the narrow segment and the dilated segment shows prominent nerve trunks and markedly reduced numbers of ganglion cells. A gradual transition from aganglionic to normoganglionic bowel is usually seen. The proximal margin of the transition zone may not always correlate with the gross appearance.

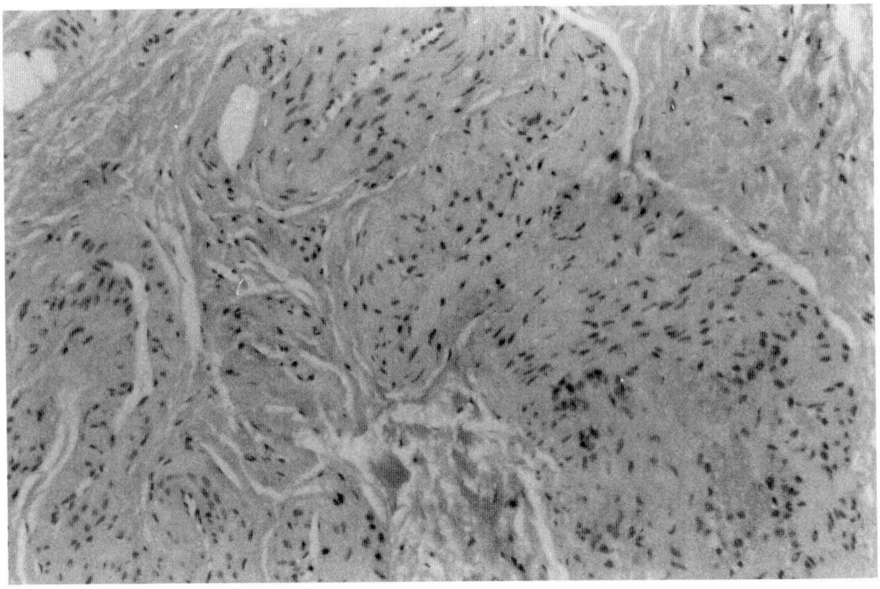

FIGURE 7-6. Tangentially cut smooth muscle in the walls of large submucosal arteries in a rectal biopsy. These smooth muscle bundles should not be mistaken for hyperplastic nerve trunks seen in Hirschsprung's disease. (H&E, ×100.)

Histochemical Findings

In addition to these histologic findings, the following findings have been demonstrated by histochemical methods: (1) intense acetyl cholinesterase (AChE) activity in the nerve trunks of the submucosa and muscle coat and (2) increase in cholinergic fibers in the mucosa, muscularis mucosae, submucosa, and muscle coat. (Increased numbers of adrenergic fibers in the muscle coat of the aganglionic bowel demonstrated by some investigators could not be confirmed by others.[4])

The increased numbers of coarse cholinergic nerve fibers in the muscularis mucosae and lamina propria are demonstrated by histochemical stain for AChE on frozen section of rectal suction biopsy containing mucosa and submucosa. In normal infants no appreciable fibers or only a few delicate fibers may be present (Figure 7-9).[11] Two patterns of positive acetylcholinesterase staining are described: *pattern A*—positivity in both lamina propria and muscularis mucosae (Figure 7-10); *pattern B*—positivity only in the muscularis mucosae and lower third of mucosa.[12] Pattern B, which is seen in patients of HD up to 6 months of age, is often described as the neonatal pattern (Figure 7-11).

The great merit of this procedure is that it enables the pathologist to make the diagnosis of HD on the basis of a positive finding. A technologist trained in histochemical procedures can readily perform the stain.[11] However, false-negative results may be obtained due to technical problems, inexperience, and misinterpretation (e.g., lack of awareness of the neonatal pattern). Most centers

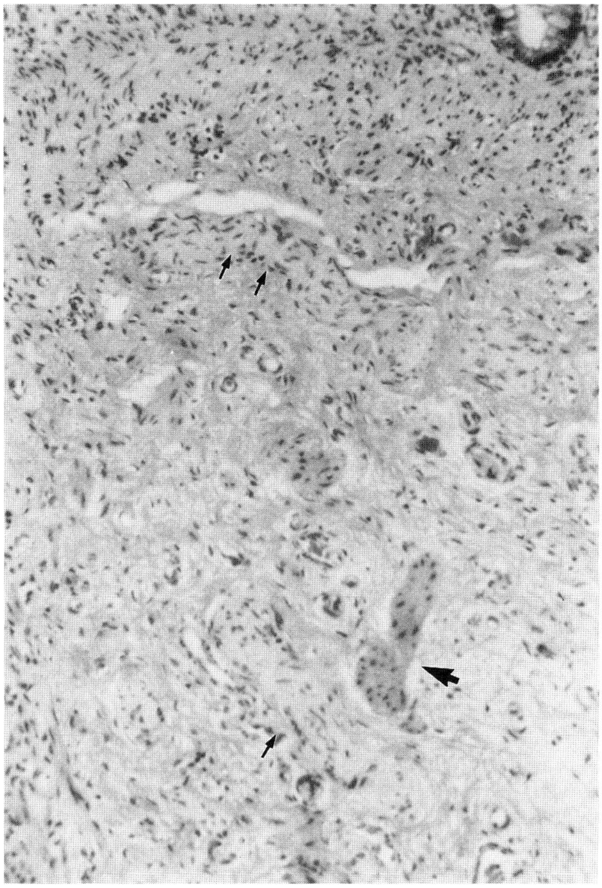

FIGURE 7-7. Rectal biopsy showing small bundles of smooth muscle (large arrow) which should be distinguished from the hyperplastic nerves (small arrows) (H&E, ×100).

that use the technique also routinely process portions of biopsy specimens for histologic study.[11] In many centers, full-thickness biopsies are used only if the original specimen of suction biopsy is inadequate or if there is uncertainty about the level of the suction biopsy specimens.

In a recent brief review of their experience of 324 cases of HD, Lake and associates at the Hospital for Sick Children, London, England[13] have pointed out the following aspects of histochemical staining for AChE in HD:

1. Detection of ganglion cells in the submucosa rules out the diagnosis of HD—even if only one is found and whatever else is seen in the AChE preparation.
2. The earliest change in HD is an increase in coarse nerve fibers in the muscularis mucosae and submucosa. There is increase in nerve fibers in the lamina propria over a period of time (≤6 months of age). Therefore in the neonate with HD special attention must be given to muscularis mucosae and submucosa since the AChE stain would show negative pattern in the lamina propria.

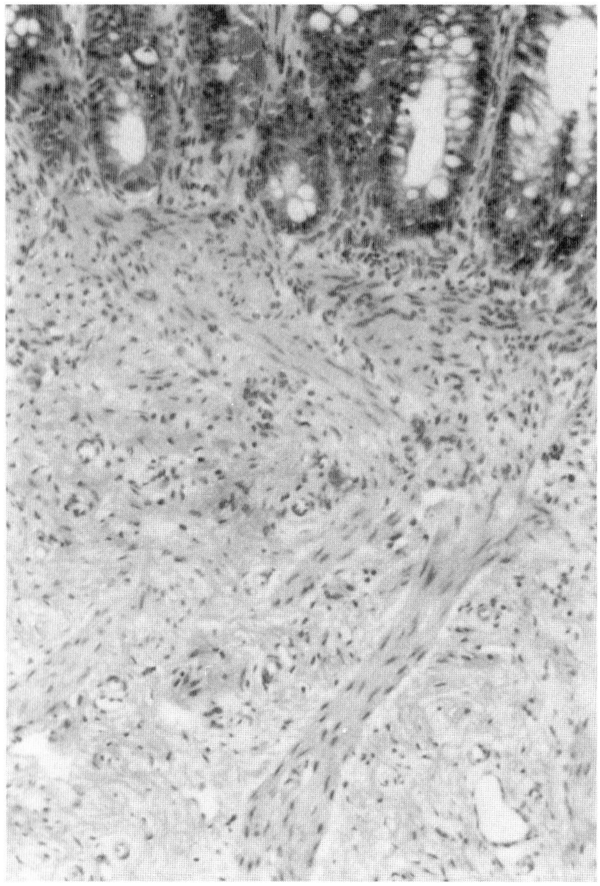

FIGURE 7-8. Rectal biopsy showing smooth muscle bundles of muscularis mucosae, which should be distinguished from the hyperplastic nerves (H&E, ×100).

3. False-negative staining occurs in some cases of total colonic HD, and under the following circumstances:
   a. Incorrect interpretation, i.e., lack of familiarity with the neonatal pattern described above.
   b. Incorrect biopsy site, i.e., proximal to involved segment.
   c. The density of AChE-positive nerve fibers drops to normal at the splenic flexure, therefore negative staining is seen in biopsies and pull-through specimens proximal to splenic flexure.
4. AChE staining can be suitably modified for rapid results (45 minutes vs. the usual 2 hours).

Immunohistologic Findings

Immunoperoxidase stain for neuron-specific enolase (NSE) and S-100 are helpful in demonstrating the basic abnormality of HD. The S-100 stain lights up

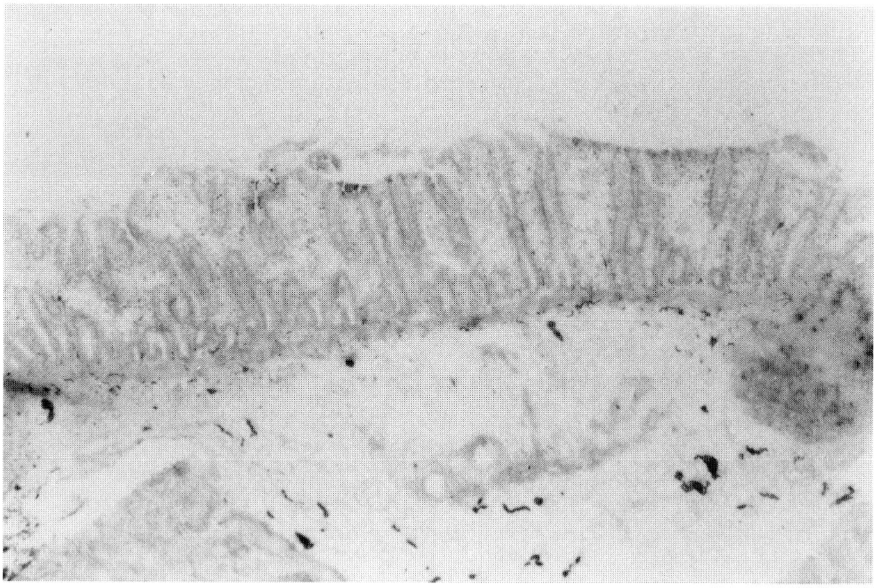

FIGURE 7-9. Rectal biopsy in whom Hirschsprung's disease was not present; note the positive staining in the normal submucosal nerve plexuses, rare delicate short nerve fibers in the muscularis mucosae, and absence of nerve fibers in the lamina propria (acetylcholinesterase stain, ×50).

(illuminates) the plexuses and the NSE stain demonstrates the ganglion cells. The ganglion cells are usually negative for S-100 stain. The NSE stains the immature ganglion cells in the newborn infant. Thus immunoperoxidase stains for NSE and S-100 may be used as adjuvant aids in the diagnosis. Unfortunately, the S-100 stain does not demonstrate the AChE-positive nerve fibers that are present in the muscularis mucosae and lamina propria in HD (Figure 7-12).[14] However, Tam and Owen[15] have shown recently that these AChE-positive fibers can be demonstrated by immunofluorescence when monoclonal antibodies against neuronal microtubule-associated proteins are employed. The prominent nerves in the submucosa and muscle coat in the involved segment can also be demonstrated effectively by immunoperoxidase stain for neurofilaments by using monoclonal antibodies.[16] But these techniques should not distract from the meticulous attention to the routine techniques of proper processing with multiple sections of the biopsy and the recognition of immature ganglion cells in routine H&E stained preparations as described below.

TYPES OF BIOPSY

Two types of biopsy may be done on infants suspected of having HD: full thickness rectal biopsy and suction biopsies, which include mucosa and submucosa.

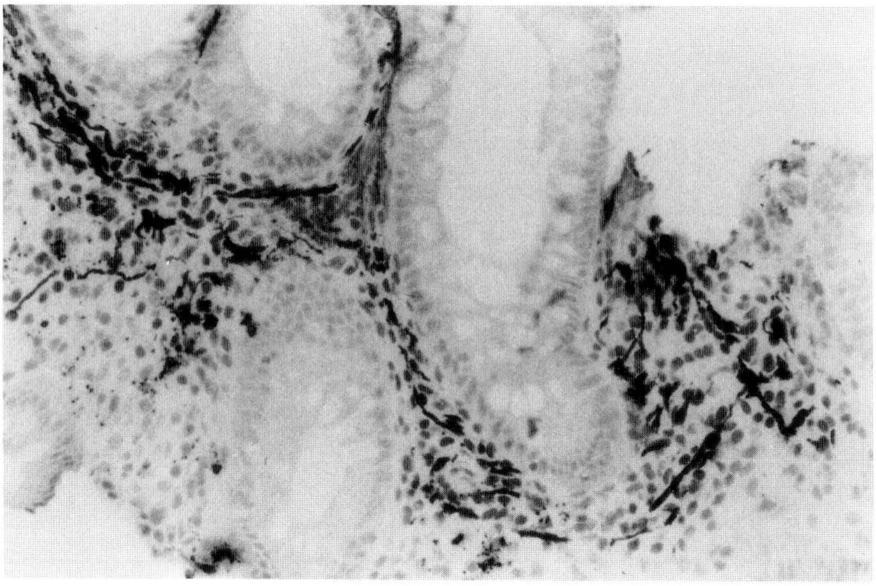

FIGURE 7-10. Rectal biopsy from a 9-month-old child with Hirschsprung's disease. Note the coarse nerve fibers in the lamina propria of the mucosa. Similar fibers were present in the muscularis mucosae (not shown). (Acetylcholinesterase stain, ×400.)

Full-Thickness Rectal Biopsy

This includes the mucosa, submucosa, and muscle coat. The full-thickness biopsy, in comparison with the section biopsy containing only mucosa and submucosa (see below), has the following advantages:

1. Relatively large size of the specimen (0.5–1-cm strip), which facilitates the orientation of the specimen for histologic sections and makes available a larger number of both myenteric and submucosal nerve plexuses to be evaluated.
2. The distance between the site of the biopsy and the pectinate line can be judged better since the infant is under general anesthesia, thus avoiding the normal hypoganglionic zone.
3. A large number of sections can be relatively readily studied if necessary.
4. Some surgical pathologists have grown up with and hence are more familiar and comfortable with this type of biopsy, which had been the standard practice until the 1970s.
5. The ganglion cells in the myenteric plexuses are larger, more mature, and more numerous than in submucosal plexuses.
6. The normal myenteric plexus extends a few millimeters beyond the normal submucosal plexus.[5] The disadvantages are that it requires general anesthesia; in some cases, due to inexperience of the surgeon, inadequate tissue may be removed for biopsy; and the procedure may be associated with postopera-

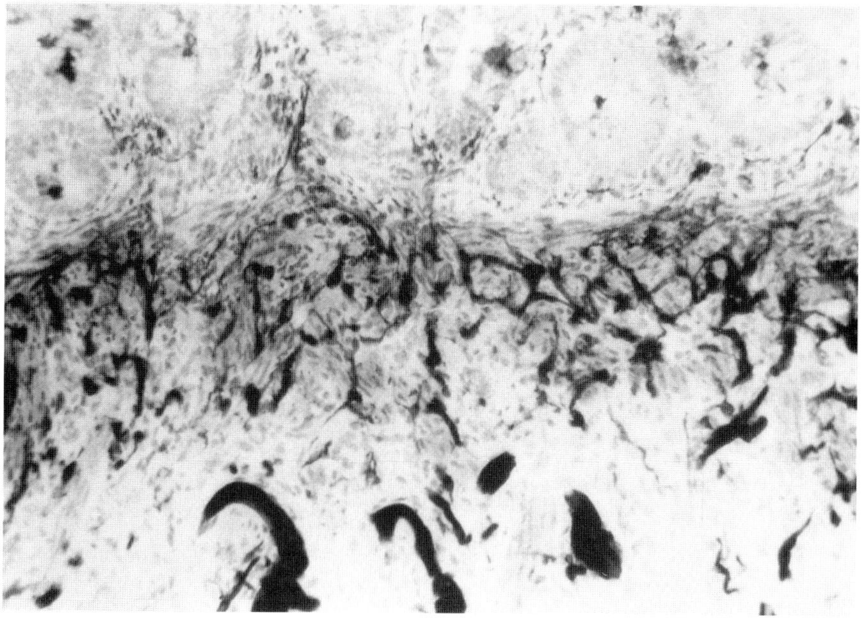

FIGURE 7-11. Rectal biopsy from a 3-month-old infant with Hirschsprung's disease. Note the numerous coarse nerve fibers in the muscularis mucosae and a few fibers in the lower portion of the lamina propria. There are large darkly staining submucosal nerve trunks. (Acetylcholinesterase stain, ×400.)

tive complications that can be serious. However, the incidence of these complications is extremely low.

Suction Biopsy

Suction biopsy has the following advantages and disadvantages: (1) it can be obtained without anesthesia; (2) the area biopsied is small (2–3 mm in length and 1 mm in width with a 2-mm breadth of submucosa); (3) it makes available only submucosal plexuses for evaluation since it consists of mucosa and submucosa only; (4) the ganglion cells in the submucosal plexuses are smaller, less numerous, and less mature than those in myenteric plexuses; (5) multiple samples (~3) can be taken; (6) it may be difficult to judge the distance from the pectinate line; (7) orientation of biopsy may be difficult because of the small size (occasionally a lymphoid nodule may occupy much of the submucosa, further reducing the effective size of the specimen); and (8) the rate of complication is extremely low. Ability to perform the biopsy without anesthesia and to obtain multiple samples are distinct advantages.

PROCESSING OF THE BIOPSY

If a full-thickness rectal biopsy is performed, it should be stretched out and properly pinned down or flattened out on a filter paper. The surgeon can take

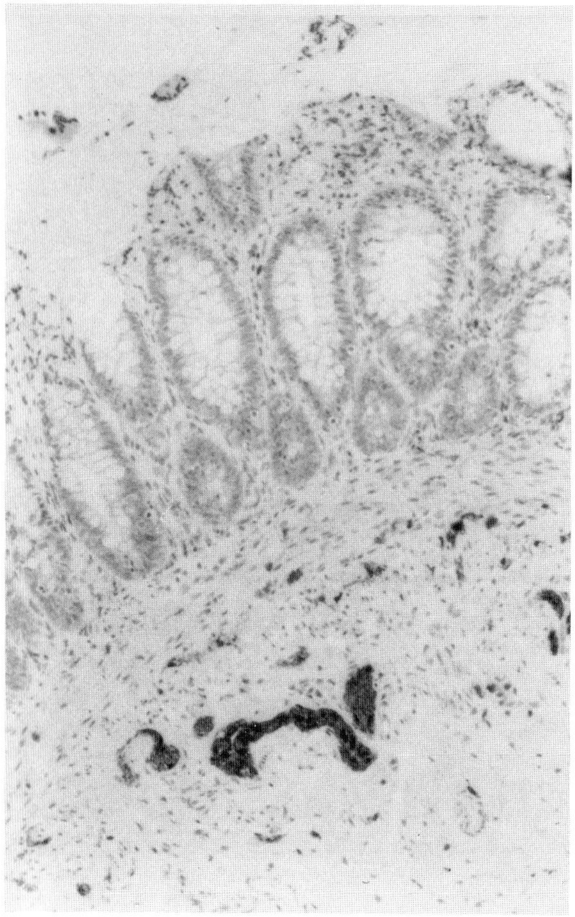

FIGURE 7-12. Immunoperoxidase stain for S-100 demonstrating prominent nerve trunks in the submucosa of rectal biopsy in a child with Hirschsprung's disease; note the absence of any staining in the muscularis mucosae or lamina propria (×100).

these steps in the operating room or should send the specimen immediately to the pathologist. The proximal and distal ends of the biopsy should be identified particularly in the specimen of anorectal myectomy done for treatment of ultrashort HD. A small portion of the biopsy should be processed for frozen sections to demonstrate AChE activity. The remaining biopsy should be adequately fixed in formalin and may be bisected before submitting for histology if of a sufficient size. If it is relatively small, the whole specimen should be embedded on edge as it is. A large number of sections are usually not necessary to recognize the abnormalities in the plexuses noted above. However, it is advisable to examine at least 15–20 sections to be certain about the absence of ganglion cells. Importance of proper orientation and rapid fixation of the specimen cannot be overemphasized in the assessment of the biopsy specimen.

If submucosal biopsies are obtained, these should be flattened out on a filter paper as soon as they are obtained. One of the biopsy specimens should be processed for a frozen section if the acetylcholinesterase histochemical stain is available in the laboratory and the remaining pieces should be immediately fixed in formalin. The biopsies should be properly oriented for frozen and permanent sections (Figures 7-13, 7-14). The biopsies processed for permanent sections should be placed in the smallest mold for embedding and the face of the block should be trimmed closely so that 15–20 sections can be mounted on a single slide (Figures 7-15, 7-16). Two pieces may be placed in a single block. A total of 60–80 serial sections should be obtained. In a patient without HD, ganglion cells are usually demonstrable within the first 15–20 sections (if a sufficient amount of submucosa is present). Before the diagnosis of HD is given on the basis of absence of ganglion cells, 60–80 sections should be carefully examined. The diagnosis of HD means a definitive major surgery for the infant or the child. A diagnosis based on absence of a particular structure should be made only after the plexuses are examined in the serial sections. Technical difficulties related to orientation, poor quality of serial sections, insufficient number of sections, and misjudgment regarding the site of biopsy may interfere with proper interpretation of the biopsy specimens.

EXTENT OF DISEASE

HD involves variable portions of large and small intestine. The disease process extends proximally from anal canal or rectum to variable points along the large and small intestine. The following categories are recognized: A—limited segment or short segment (involvement of anal canal, rectum, rectosigmoid or up to sigmoid colon) (60–75%); B—ultrashort segment (involvement of distal third of rectum/anal canal) (~20%); C—total colonic (1–2%); D—extension to small intestine (2%) (Figure 7-17) (in total colonic aganglionosis and disease extending into the small intestine, hyperplastic nerve plexuses without ganglion cells are present in the rectum but there is total absence of nerve elements in the rest of the involved bowel) (Figure 7-18); E—segmental HD with skip areas also called *zonal HD*. Normally there is involvement of distal rectum and anal canal with variable extension of aganglionosis in direct continuity proximally as in the categories C and D above. However, in rare instances there may be aganglionosis of a proximal segment with normal plexuses in the distal portion of colon, or

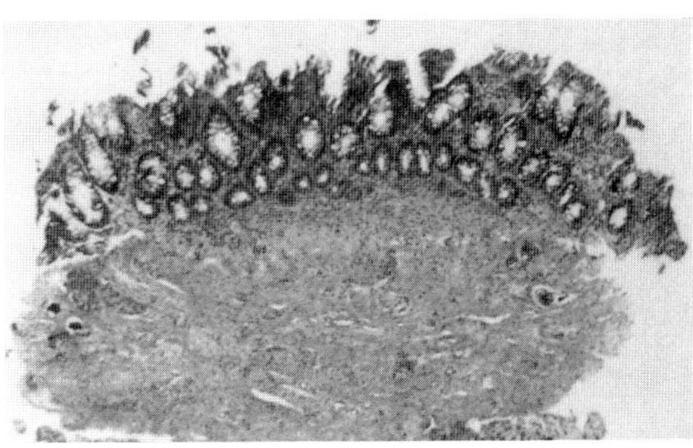

FIGURE 7-13. Fairly oriented rectal suction biopsy with adequate amount of submucosa; a few nerve plexuses are present (H&E, ×40).

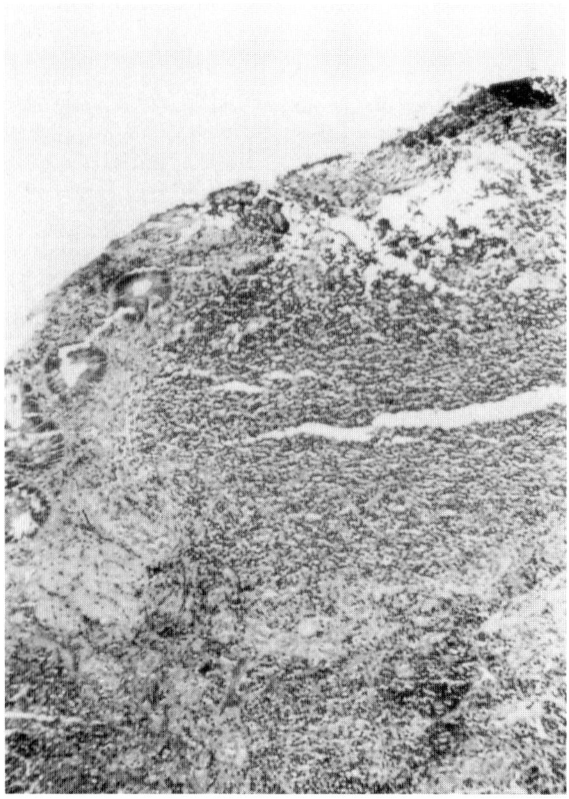

FIGURE 7-14. Poorly oriented rectal suction biopsy with a large lymphoid follicle in the mucosa and submucosa; there is inadequate amount of submucosa in this case (H&E, ×50).

there may be two segments of aganglionosis with normoganglionic segment in between. Detailed pathologic studies of this type of HD are not available.

PROBLEMS ENCOUNTERED IN DIAGNOSIS OF HD

There are three situations in which problems may be encountered in the diagnosis of HD: (1) HD in the newborn infant, (2) ultrashort HD, and (3) inadequate suction biopsies.

HD in the Newborn

HD has been diagnosed more frequently in the newborn period in recent years (>70% of the cases are diagnosed in newborn infants). The ganglion cells in the biopsy specimen tend to be immature in this age group. During the process

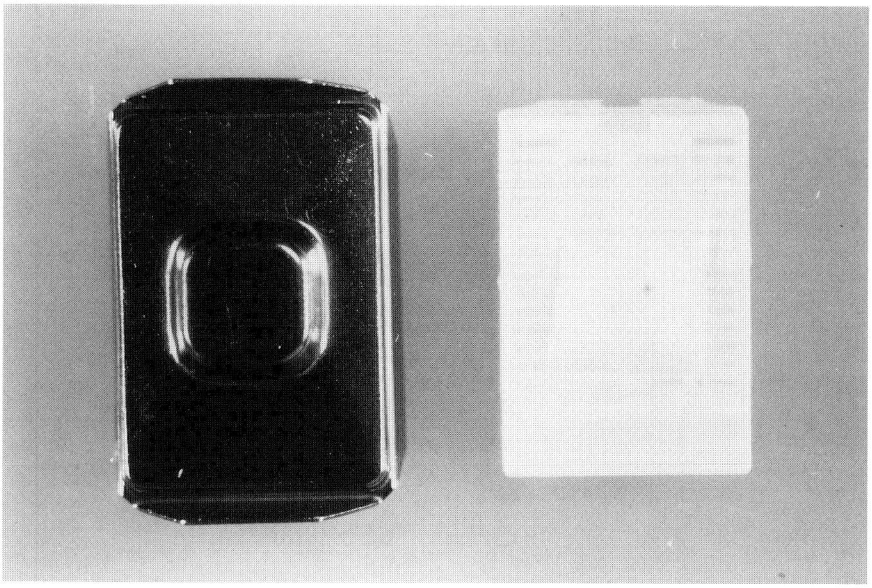

FIGURE 7-15. The smallest mold for preparing paraffin block should be used for embedding the rectal biopsies. The face of the block should be trimmed to make it as small as possible. This enables multiple sections to be mounted on a single slide (see Figure 7-14).

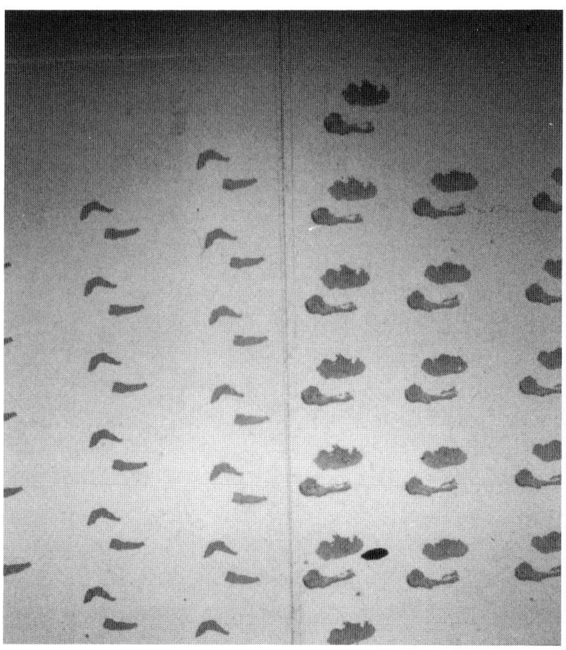

FIGURE 7-16. Up to three ribbons of sections, each ribbon with five to seven sections, can be mounted on a single slide.

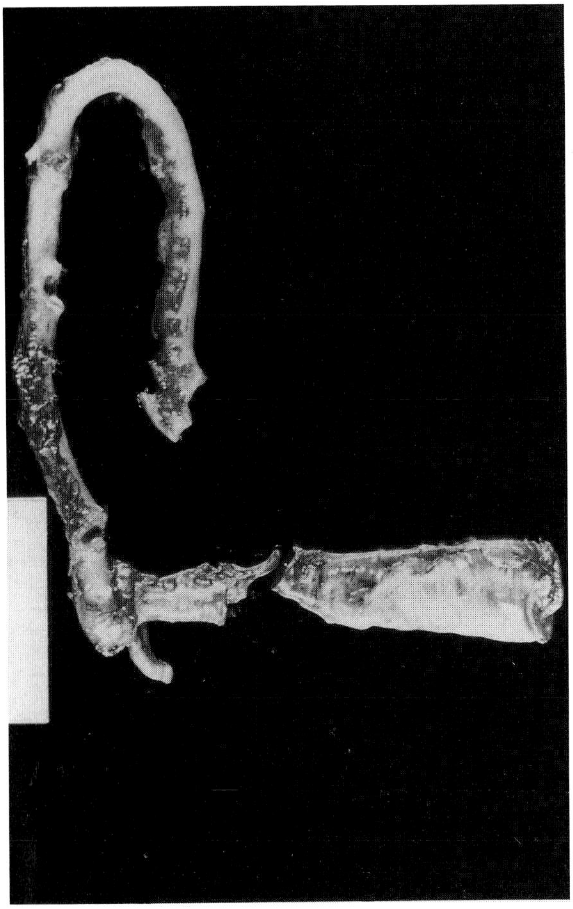

FIGURE 7-17. Total colonic aganglionosis with extension to terminal ileum. Note the narrow colon and terminal ileum and dilated more proximal ileum.

of development the apolar neuroblasts mature into multipolar ganglion cells. The characteristic morphologic features of ganglion cells described above in the section on normal enteric plexus are seen best from age of 2 years onward. The immature plexuses in the newborn and young infants show neural units that are to be distinguished from small blood vessels, inflammatory cells, groups of smooth muscle cells, and collections of lymphocytes. The neural units contain small cells in different stages of development. The cells form an ovoid or elongated organoid structure with central or eccentric bubbly mass surrounded by nuclei, one or two of which are bigger and less intensely stained than the others (Figures 7-19–7-21). A small nucleolus may be seen in these maturing nuclei. These are the immature ganglion cells. Mature ganglion cells may be present in some of these units.[17] However, presence of the immature neural units containing the immature ganglion cells described above is considered as presence of ganglion cells—thus ruling out HD. Lack of appreciation of the immature

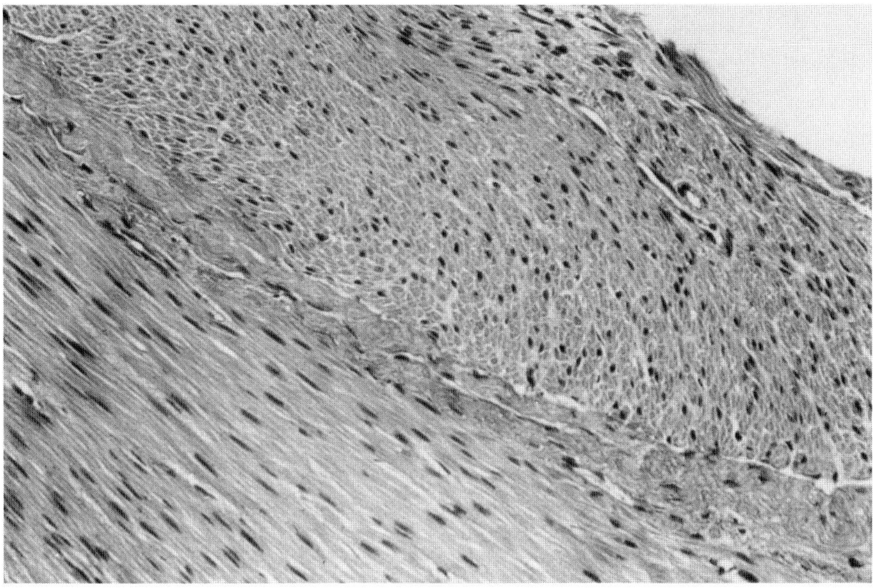

FIGURE 7-18. Note total absence of any nerve elements between the two layers of muscle of the colon in total colonic ganglionosis. No nerve elements were present in the multiple sections taken from involved colon and the terminal ileum. (H&E, ×250).

ganglion cells may lead to a false diagnosis of HD. Immunoperoxidase stain for NSE and S-100 may be helpful as outlined above.

Ultrashort-Segment HD

As indicated above, in this type of HD[18–20] the distal third of rectum and anal canal is involved. Chronic constipation is the main presenting feature. The diagnosis is usually made in an older child rather than in an infant. Anorectal myectomy is both a diagnostic and therapeutic procedure. In this procedure a 0.5–1-cm-wide × 5–10-cm-long strip, including anal sphincter and rectal muscle, is removed. The diagnosis may be missed if prior to myectomy, a rectal biopsy is done at the recommended level of 2–3 cm above the pectinate line since the ultrashort segment may not extend that far proximally. A low rectal biopsy and histochemical stain for acetylcholinesterase will enable the pathologist to make the diagnosis of ultrashort segment HD. Venugopal et al[7] have shown that in normal children rectal biopsies taken at a distance of 1–1.5 cm from the pectinate line, always show some ganglion cells. Therefore, a low rectal biopsy showing total absence of ganglion cells can be diagnostic of ultrashort HD. However, if one sees squamous epithelium (Figure 7-22) in such a low biopsy, the specimen should be considered inappropriate for evaluation.[7]

Inadequate Suction Biopsies

In some cases, there may not be a sufficient amount of submucosa in the suction biopsies. A diagnosis of HD is not possible on the basis of demonstration

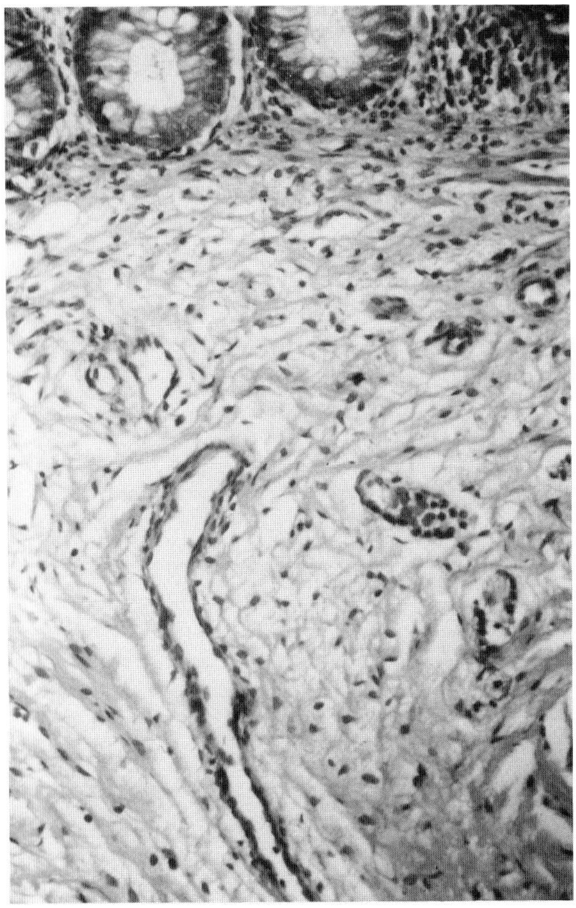

FIGURE 7-19. Rectal biopsy in a newborn infant who did not have Hirschsprung's disease; note the immature nerve plexuses in the submucosa (H&E, ×100).

of absence of ganglion cells on histologic assessment of such a specimen. AChE stain must be done. If there are no AChE-positive fibers in the mucosa of such a biopsy specimen, repeat biopsy may not always be necessary to confidently rule out the diagnosis of HD depending upon the clinical and radiologic findings.[13]

FROZEN SECTION IN HD

Primary diagnosis of HD on a frozen section is not recommended. Suction (or full-thickness) biopsies that are taken from beyond the normal hypoganglionic zone, which are properly oriented and from which multiple permanent sections after paraffin embedding are taken, are essential for the primary diagnosis. In an emergency situation when the patient has necrotizing enterocolitis, a *tentative* diagnosis may be made on frozen section and should be

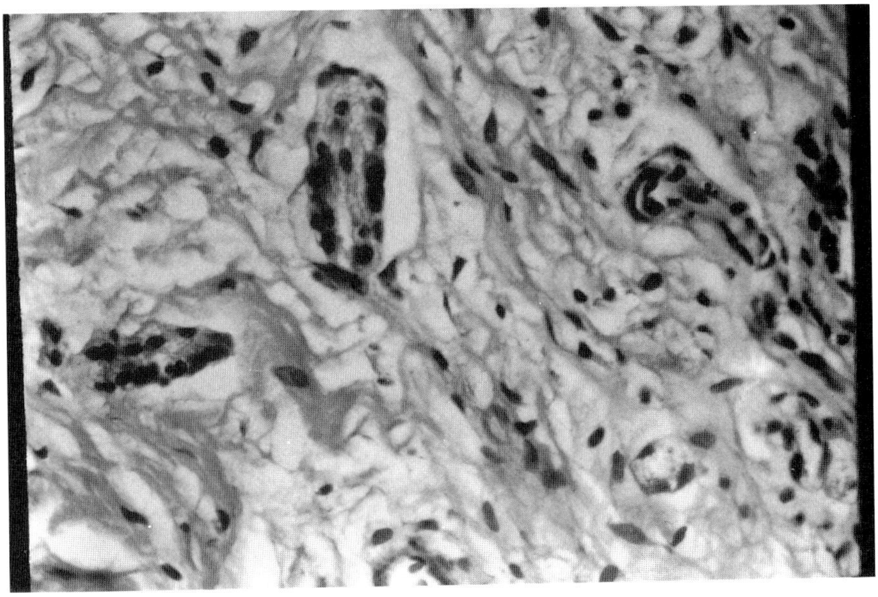

FIGURE 7-20. Immature nerve plexuses in the submucosa of rectal biopsy specimen from a normal newborn infant; note the small round cells with a moderate amount of cytoplasm (H&E, ×250).

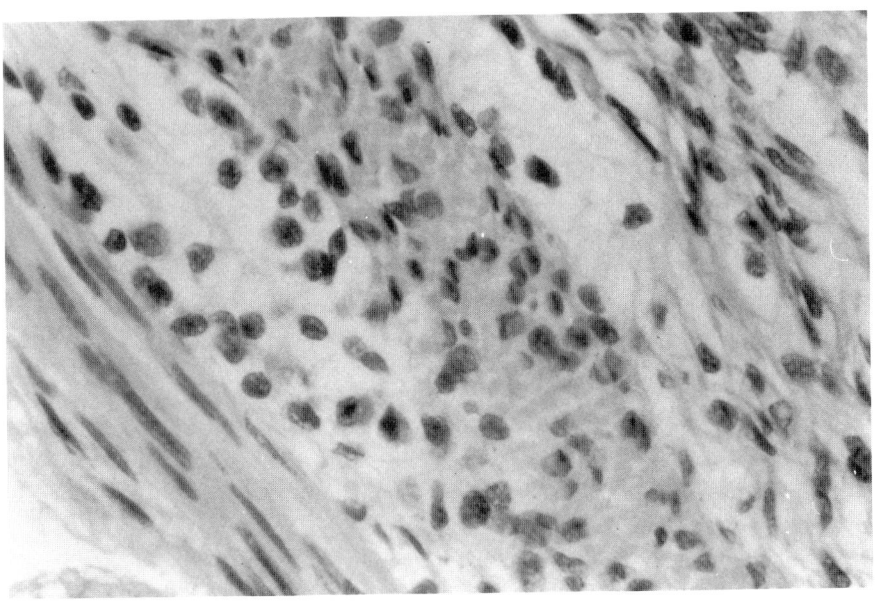

FIGURE 7-21. Myenteric nerve plexus in a normal newborn infant. Note the immature ganglion cells, which are small in size and have moderate amount of cytoplasm. In the nucleus of the ganglion cells a nucleolus is seen. (H&E, ×250.)

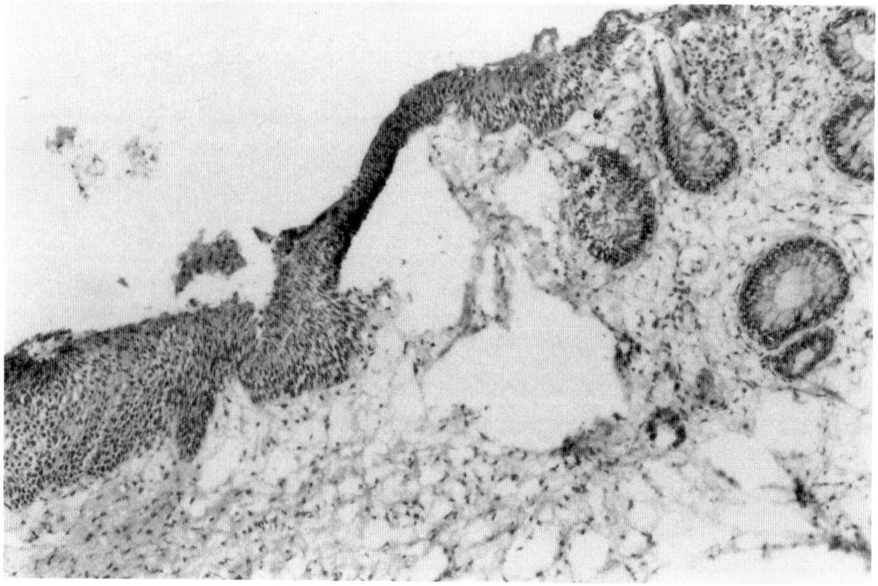

FIGURE 7-22. Biopsy showing squamous epithelial mucosa in one portion. This biopsy is considered as "too low" (it represents the normal hypoganglionic zone of the anal canal) and is inappropriate for diagnosis of Hirschsprung's disease (H&E, ×100).

confirmed by studying permanent sections of the frozen piece and of another piece taken at the same level as the frozen section. In most instances the diagnosis is suspected in the neonatal age group and a definitive surgical procedure is deferred till the infant is one year of age. Therefore there is usually no reason to insist on a primary diagnosis by frozen section. On occasion the surgeon might want to confirm that the biopsy is not too low (i.e., that it contains rectal and not squamous mucosa) by doing a frozen section. Such a request is rare. Some surgeons without experience of suction biopsies may ask for a primary diagnosis of HD on a frozen section done on a *full-thickness* rectal biopsy obtained under general anesthesia since they might prefer to do a colostomy at the same sitting. In such situations it may be advisable to ask the surgeon for another piece for permanent section from the same level as the frozen piece since freezing the biopsy may interfere with proper orientation. In the case in which a primary diagnosis is requested on frozen section of a full-thickness biopsy, it should be indicated that the diagnosis is to be confirmed on the multiple permanent sections of the frozen tissue itself (and the additional biopsy done at the same level as the frozen biopsy). Frozen section may also be requested for ascertaining that the proximal margin of anorectal myectomy in ultrashort HD contains ganglion cells. I prefer to obtain at least three sections from the block of frozen tissue before I render the primary diagnosis of HD on a frozen section.

Decompression by colostomy is usually performed in the newborn period after the diagnosis is established by studying carefully and systematically permanent sections from rectal biopsy. Frozen section will then be necessary to guide the surgeon for placement of colostomy in the normoganglionic zone. Seromuscular biopsies rather than full thickness biopsies may be taken by the surgeon during this procedure. Multiple frozen sections are required to reach the normal ganglionic zone in unsuspected cases of total colonic aganglionosis (which may also extend to variable length of small intestine).

HD IN ADULTS AND ACQUIRED HD

Occasionally the symptoms related to HD are minimal and the disease may go unrecognized for several years. McCready et al[21] have reported 50 cases of HD in adults (average age 21 years, oldest patient 59 years) with diagnosis established by histologic examination of a biopsy specimen in each case.

HD can occur as a result of destruction of ganglion cells in Chagas' disease (American trypanosomiasis) in South America. Rare cases of HD in premature infants with hypoxemia in whom ganglion cells were present in the initial rectal biopsy followed by their absence in a subsequent biopsy several weeks later have been reported.[22] Hypoxemia of a segment of intestine due to selective hypoperfusion has been implicated as the pathogenetic mechanism of destruction of ganglion cells in such cases. Similar mechanism is implicated in occurence of HD-like disease following an attack of neonatal necrotizing enterocolitis that is successfully treated medically (see Figure 4-19 of chapter on neonatal necrotizing enterocolitis). Acquired aganglionosis has also been described in the pulled-through bowel in rare cases of HD who have undergone definitive surgery (Swenson, Soave or Duhamel procedures). Cohen et al have recently reported 5 such cases.[23] Clinically the patients developed obstructive symptoms. The surgical margins of the pulled through bowel at the time of original surgery had shown normal ganglion cells in the plexuses. Submucosal biopsy specimens from the obstructed pulled-through bowel revealed the following histologic and histochemical findings: (1) absence of ganglion cells with presence of prominent nerves in the submucosa, (2) fibrosis of muscularis mucosae and submucosa, and (3) in some cases subendothelial and medial fibrosis of the submucosal blood vessels. The authors suggested that the acquired aganglionosis may be related to regional ischemia in some but not all cases of acquired HD.

COMPLICATIONS OF HD

The most serious complication is necrotizing enterocolitis. It involves the intestine proximal to the aganglionic segment. There is hemorrhagic necrosis of mucosa, which may extend to the small intestine. Pneumatosis, pseudomembrane formation, and transmural necrosis with perforation may be seen. Mucosal ischemia and *Clostridium difficile* have been implicated in the pathogenesis. Enterocolitis can appear before or after colostomy or definitive surgery. Perforation and septicemia may cause fatal outcome.

Teitelbaum et al[24] have described progressive mucosal changes in biopsies in children with HD. The changes were graded as follows: *grade 0*—no changes, *grade 1*—crypt dilatation and mucin retention, *grade 2*—cryptitis or two crypt abscesses, *grade 3*—multiple crypt abscesses, *grade 4*—fibrinopurulent debris and mucosal ulceration, *grade 5*—total thickness mucosal necrosis or perforation (Figures 7-23–7-27). Six of their seven patients with a histologic grade III or higher subsequently developed necrotizing enterocolitis. They indicated that the histologic grade of III or above should alert the clinician to the possibility of development of necrotizing enterocolitis irrespective of clinical history. These authors also detected enterocyte adhering organisms such as *E. coli*, *C. difficile*, and cryptosporidia in 39% of the biopsies. They considered this finding as further evidence of altered mucosal defense mechanism in necrotizing enterocolitis associated with Hirschsprung's disease. It is likely that the toxin released by these organisms which produce epithelial damage induce the necrotizing enterocolitis.

TYPES OF SPECIMEN RECEIVED AFTER DEFINITIVE SURGERY FOR HD

Three basic procedures are used for therapy of HD: (1) *Swenson procedure*—the entire abnormal segment is resected to enable the pathologist to get the entire full-thickness specimen of aganglionic segment; (2) *Duhamel procedure*—the abnormal colonic segment is resected, but the abnormal rectum is left behind; and (3) *Soave procedure*—mucosa of the rectum is peeled off from the muscle coat and resected. The normal colon is pulled through the abnormal rectal

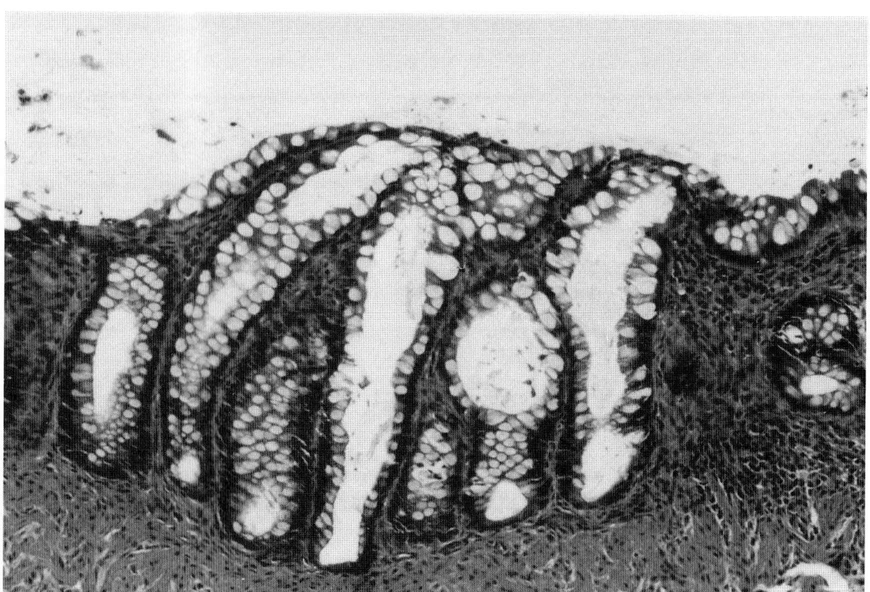

FIGURE 7-23. Colonic mucosa with dilatation of crypts (grade 1 changes) (H&E, ×90). (Courtesy of Dr. Stephen J. Qualman; reprinted from reference 18.)

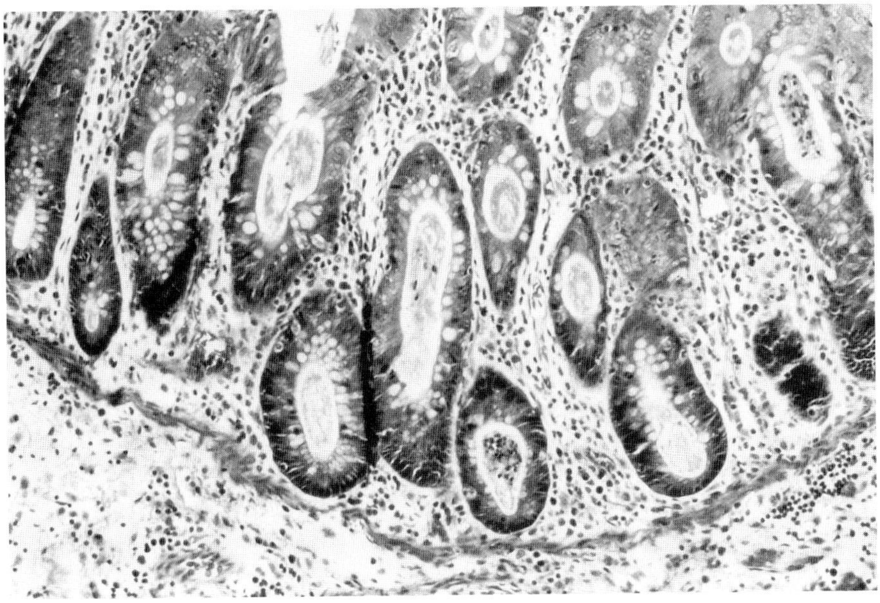

FIGURE 7-24. Colonic mucosa showing an isolated crypt abscess (grade 2 changes). Mucous retention and dilatation of crypts are also present (H&E, ×90). (Courtesy of Dr. Stephen J. Qualman; reprinted from reference 18.)

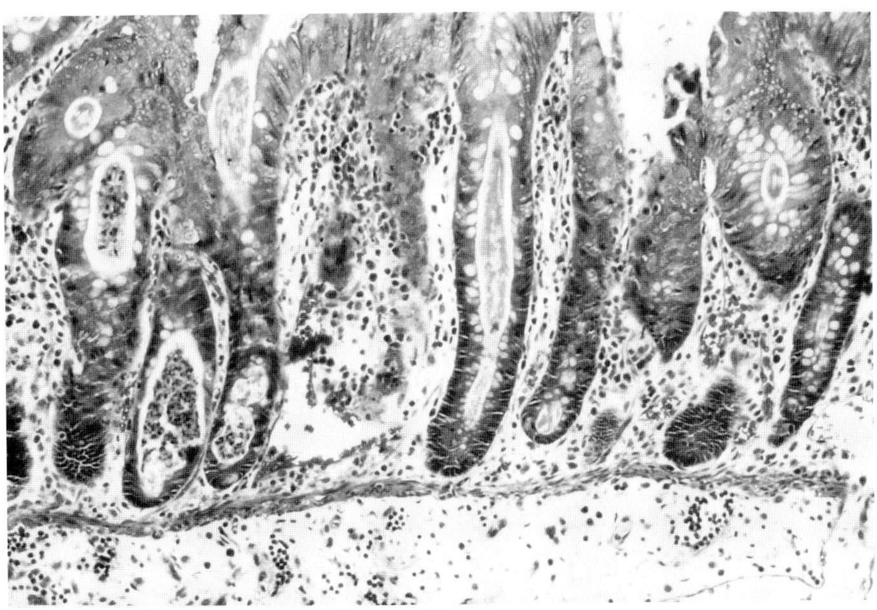

FIGURE 7-25. Colonic mucosa showing multiple crypt abscesses (grade 3 changes) (H&E, ×90). (Courtesy of Dr. Stephen J. Qualman; reprinted from reference 18.)

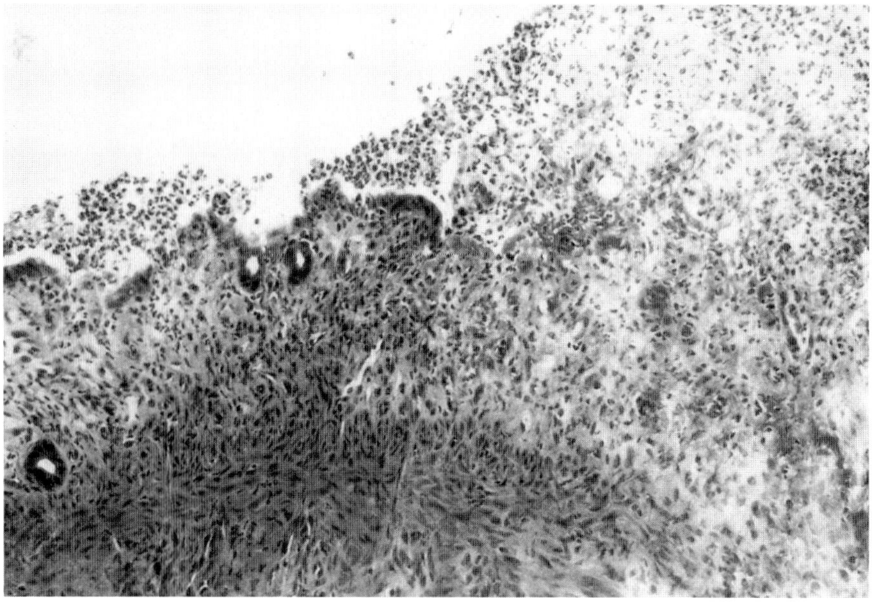

FIGURE 7-26. Colonic mucosa showing ulceration and fibrinous purulent exudate extending into the lumen (grade 4 changes) (H&E, ×90). (Courtesy of Dr. Stephen J. Qualman; reprinted from reference 18.)

muscle. The pathologist receives rectal mucosa with a small amount of attached submucosa.

In some cases arterial changes in the wall of the transitional zone of the resected specimen have been described.[25] These changes consist of marked thickening of adventitia due to smooth muscle proliferation [adventitial fibromuscular dysplasia (FMD)]. The authors suggested that the migration of ganglion cells might be interrupted by intestinal ischemia related to arterial FMD.

Diversion Colitis in Bypassed Segment

In HD, a colostomy is performed initially as a palliative procedure. Reanastomosis of the functioning bowel is done at the time of a definitive pull-through procedure subsequently after a variable period of few to several months. The bypassed segment may be resected partially or completely at the time of definitive surgery. Drut and Drut[26] and Haque et al[27] have recently reviewed the histologic features of the resected bypassed segment in patients with HD. Of these 37 patients reviewed by Haque et al,[27] 26 had diversion colitis characterized by hyperplastic mucosal lymphoid follicles, cryptitis, lymphoplasmacytic infiltration of lamina propria, and goblet cell depletion. In severe cases crypt abscesses, ulceration, slight distortion of crypt architecture, and Paneth cell hyperplasia were present. Haque et al suggested that the mucosal histologic changes may be related to deficiency of short-chain fatty acids in the lumen of the bypassed segment, which leads to nutritional deficiency of the colonic epithelium. There may also be a superimposed element of a low-grade pathogen

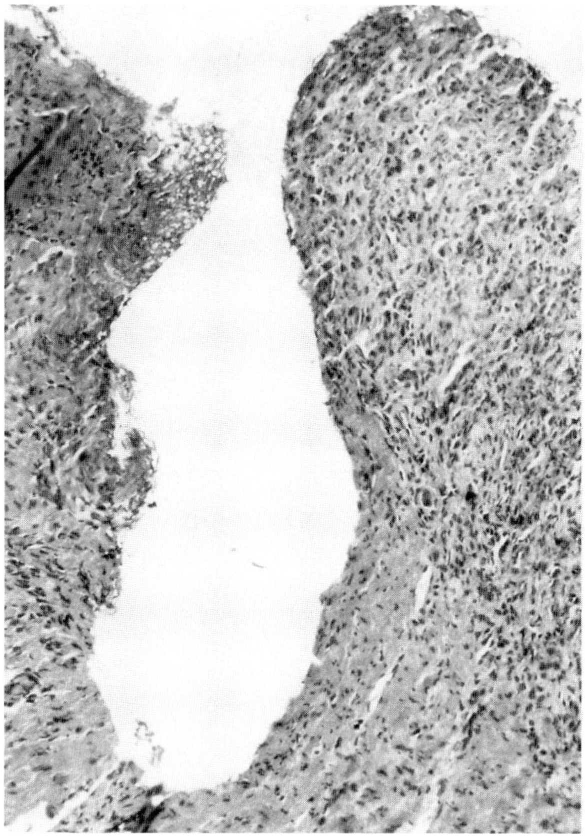

FIGURE 7-27. Colonic mucosa showing ulceration and necrosis involving its entire thickness (grade 5 changes) (H&E, ×90). (Courtesy of Dr. Stephen J. Qualman; reprinted from reference 18.)

in diversion colitis.[28] Diversion colitis may be asymptomatic or may be associated with abdominal pain or mucoid and/or bloody discharge.

HYPOGANGLIONOSIS

As outlined above, the diagnosis of HD requires demonstration of absence of ganglion cells (aganglionosis) by using a systematic and detailed method. Hypoganglionosis (HGS) is an entity which has not been delineated with certainty.

However, according to some authors,[29,30] HGS of the colon can occur. HGS has also been called "pseudo-HD."[31] In HGS, there is reduction in not only the ganglion cells but also in the nerve fibers in the plexuses and absence of AChE-positive nerve fibers in the muscularis mucosae and lamina propria. In HD the ganglion cells are absent and the nerves are hyperplastic with presence of AChE-positive nerve fibers in the muscularis mucosae and lamina propria.[30]

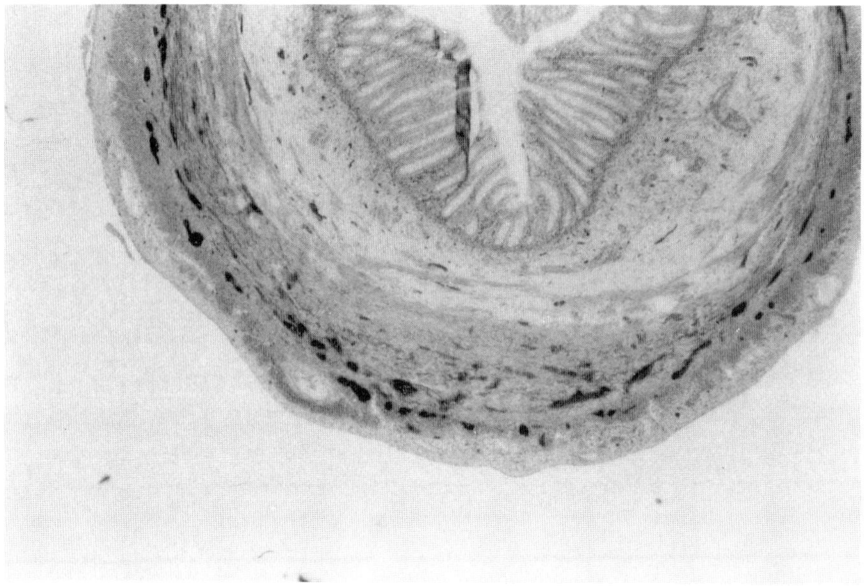

FIGURE 7-28. Marked hyperplasia of the myenteric plexus in a case of neuronal intestinal dysplasia (immunoperoxidase stain for S-100, ×40).

Morphometric studies done on rolled up sections of the entire resected specimen of affected segment of intestine have shown that in HGS the number of ganglion cells per unit length of intestine, the length of the plexus, and the number of ganglion cells per plexus differ by a factor of 3–10. Meier-Ruge[30] emphasizes that the definitive diagnosis of HGS can be made only (1) on a full-thickness biopsy containing at least three pieces, (2) by morphometric studies, *and* (3) by histochemical assessment of the AChE nerve fibers. From a practical point of view, the following points regarding HGS should be noted: (1) HGS is seen in the transition zone proximal to the involved segment of HD; (2) HGS is seen normally in the anal nerve plexuses up to ~2 cm proximal to the dentate line; (3) the cutoff point with respect to the number of ganglion cells per plexus, etc. for the diagnosis of hypoganglionic plexuses has not been established; and (4) primary HGS by itself, i.e., independently of HD, which occurs according to some investigators as a rare clinicopathologic entity, is still not established firmly and there is no practical routinely usable method for its definitive diagnosis.

DISORDERS RESEMBLING HD

In these disorders the clinical features resemble those of HD but tend to be less severe. Rectal biopsy is done with presumptive clinical diagnosis of HD. Histologically there is what has been labeled as myenteric hyperplasia (Figure 7-28).[32] Two types of abnormalities are noted: (1) intestinal neurofibromatosis associated with von Recklinghausen's disease in which markedly enlarged (sympathetic) nerve trunks are found in the submucosal and myenteric plexuses and (2) intestinal neuronal dysplasia (IND), also referred to as "hyperganglionosis," characterized by (a) hyperplasia of ganglion cells and nerve fibers of submucous plexus and myenteric plexus with formation of giant ganglia (Figures 7-28, 7-29), (b) isolated ganglion cells may be seen in the mucosal lamina propria or between the muscle layers of muscularis mucosae, (c) prominent parasympathetic nerve fibers in the muscularis mucosae and lamina propria demonstrated by acetylcholinesterase stain, and (d) hypoplasia or aplasia of sympathetic innervation of the myenteric plexus. IND may occur by itself or may be seen in the segment proximal to the aganglionic segment of HD. Localized (only colon) and disseminated (colon and small intestine) forms of IND are seen. IND has not been diagnosed in the United States with the same frequency as reported by the European authors.

Schofield and Yunis of Children's Hospital of Pittsburgh reviewed 38 cases of "isolated" IND, i.e., cases unassociated with HD.[33] They used the following criteria for diagnosis of IND for the suction biopsies (containing mucosa and submucosa only): slight to moderate increase in AChE-stained fibers in the lamina propria (and/or muscularis mucosae) and either >5 ganglion cell clusters per high-power field or clusters of ganglion cells containing >10 cells. Their 38 cases formed a heterogeneous group. The associated conditions include prematurity, small left colon/meconium plug syndrome, and obstructive anatomic gastrointestinal abnormalities. Lake et al[13] cautioned that the interpretation of hyperplasia of submucosal plexuses cannot be made with certainty since

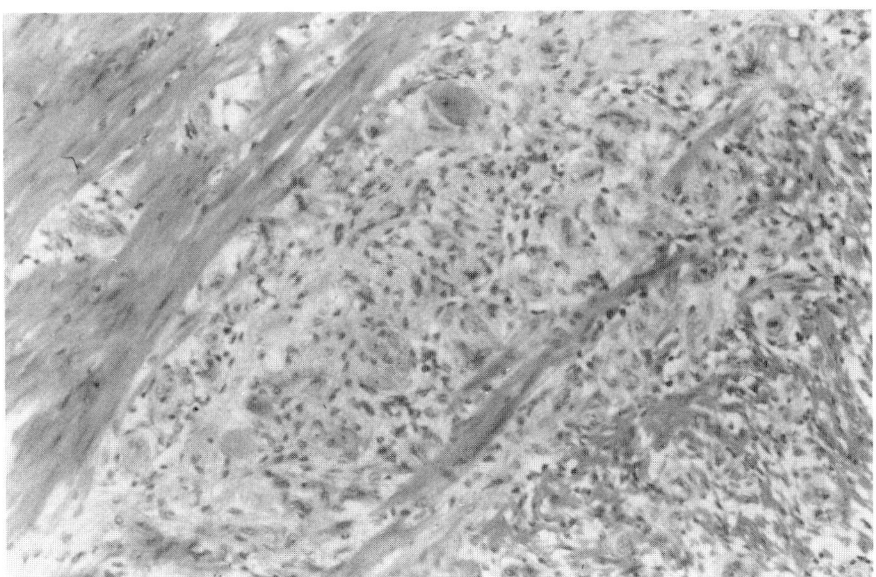

FIGURE 7-29. Hyperplasia of nerve fibers and ganglion cells in the myenteric nerve plexus in a case of neuronal intestinal dysplasia (H&E, ×400).

clusters of 10 or more ganglion cells can be found sometimes without other features of IND. Further, presence of ganglion cells in the lamina propria may be part of a normal spectrum, and the only abnormal feature seen in some cases of IND is the increase in AChE fibers (which are not coarse as in HD).[13] It appears that there is a need for formulation of minimum diagnostic criteria for IND.[33] A more extensive tissue sampling than a mere suction biopsy may be necessary to make the diagnosis.

The other group of heterogeneous disorders in which there is impaired intestinal propulsion is the chronic intestinal pseudoobstruction syndrome (CIPS) in which there may be involvement of segments of or entire gastrointestinal tract[34–38] with megaduodenum, megacolon, etc. These disorders are seen mainly in adults and less commonly in children. The syndrome is divided into myopathic and neuropathic groups. The histologic studies need to be done with great care, and special stains (trichrome, silver stain for ganglion cells and their processes) are required. In the pediatric series of CIPS by Vargas et al[34] such studies were lacking in many cases. In myopathic type there is vacuolar degeneration with dropout of smooth muscle, fibrosis of muscle coat, and variable thinning of the bowel wall. The vacuolar degenerative change in the muscle may not be appreciated on H&E stain but is well delineated in the trichrome stain. A myopathic form of CIPS has also been described in indigenous African children.[39] The following features were seen in the colon and small intestine in these cases of degenerative leiomyopathy (DL): cellular and interstitial edema of muscularis propria, degenerative changes in the smooth muscle characterized by deeply eosinophilic cytoplasm, and pyknotic nuclei. The muscle fibers were eventually replaced by fibrous tissue. The etiology and pathogenesis of DL is not known. Infectious agents do not appear to be involved.

In neuropathic-form degeneration of neurons and/or axons with marked Schwann cell proliferation or eosinophilic intranuclear inclusions in neurons has been described. Sections cut in the plane of the myenteric plexus and stained by special silver impregnation methods are recommended.[36] The familial type with variable mode of inheritance and the sporadic type are described in both myopathic and neuropathic forms of CIPS. Other organs besides the GI tract may be involved. Full-thickness biopsy of the involved segment of the GI tract is required for the demonstration of pathologic lesions. The reader is referred to the articles for details.

RECTAL BIOPSY IN METABOLIC DISEASES

For the sake of completeness it may be mentioned that suction or full-thickness rectal biopsy may be done in a child for demonstration of characteristic ultrastructural features in metabolic diseases (gangliosidosis, mucopolysaccharidoses, neuronal ceroid lipofuscinosis, etc.).[40] Macrophages in the mucosa or neurons of the myenteric plexuses are examined. It is important to note that the rectal biopsy should be fixed in glutaraldehyde and embedded with proper orientation of mucosa, submucosa and muscle coat. For certain metabolic diseases such biopsies containing mucosa and submucosa are sufficient.[41] Since in recent years enzyme assay can be performed in leukocytes and fibroblasts in some of the metabolic disorders, the need for an invasive procedure such as rectal biopsy has diminished.[40]

REFERENCES

1. Sieber WK: Hirschsprung's disease. In *Pediatric surgery* (Welch KJ, Randolph JG, Ravitch MM, et al, Eds). Mosby, St. Louis, 1986, Chap 106, pp 995–1016.
2. Holschneider AM, Kraeft H: The value and reliability of ano-rectal electromanometry. *Z Kinderchir* 33:25–38, 1981.
3. Okamoto E, Ueda T: Embryogenesis of intramural ganglia of gut and its relation to Hirschsprung's disease. *J Pediatr Surg* 2:437–443, 1967.
4. Weinberg AG: Hirschsprung's disease—a pathologist's view. *Perspect Pediatr Pathol* 2:207–239, 1975.
5. Aldridge RT, Campbell PE: Ganglion cell distribution in the normal rectum and anal canal. A basis for the diagnosis of Hirschsprung's disease by anorectal biopsy. *J Pediatr Surg* 3:475–490, 1968.
6. Weinberg AG: The anorectal myenteric plexus: Its relation to hypoganglionosis of the colon. *Am J Clin Pathol* 54:637–642, 1970.
7. Venugopal S, Mancer K, Shandling B: The validity of rectal biopsy in relation to morphology and distribution of ganglion cells. *J Pediatr Surg* 16:433–437, 1981.
8. Jacobs-Cohen RJ, Payette RF, Gershon MD, et al: Inability of neural crest cells to colonize the presumptive aganglionic bowel of *ls/ls* mutant mice: Requirement for a permissive microenvironment. *J Comp Neurol* 255:425–438, 1987.
9. Payette RF, Tennyson VM, Pomeranz HD, et al: Accumulation of components of basal laminae: Association with the failure of neural crest cells to colonize the presumptive aganglionic bowel of *ls/ls* mutant mice. *Dev Biol* 125:341–360, 1988.
10. Parikh DH, Tam PK, Van Velzen D, et al: Abnormalities in the distribution of laminin and collagen type IV in Hirschsprung's disease. *Gastroenterology* 102:1236–1241, 1992.
11. Lake BD, Puri P, Nixon HH, et al: Hirschsprung's disease: An appraisal of histochemically demonstrated acetylcholinesterase activity in suction rectal biopsy specimens as an aid to diagnosis. *Arch Pathol Lab Med* 102:244–247, 1978.
12. Challa VR, Moran JR, Turner CS, et al: Histologic diagnosis of Hirschsprung's disease: The value of concurrent hematoxylin and eosin and cholinesterase staining of rectal biopsies. *Am J Clin Pathol* 88:324–328, 1987.
13. Lake BD, Malone MT, Risdon RA: The use of acetylcholinesterase (AChE) in the diagnosis of Hirschsprung's disease and intestinal neuronal dysplasia. *Pediatr Pathol* 9:351–354, 1989.
14. Robey SS, Kuhajda FP, Yardley JH: Immunoperoxidase stains of ganglion cells and abnormal mucosal nerve proliferations in Hirschsprung's disease. *Hum Pathol* 19:432–437, 1988.
15. Tam PKH, Owen G: An immunoshistochemical study of neuronal microtubule-associated proteins in Hirschsprung's disease. *Hum Pathol* 24:424–431, 1993.
16. Kluck P, Van-Muijen GNP, Van-der-Kamp AWM, et al: Hirschsprung's disease studied with monoclonal antineurofilament antibodies on tissue sections. *Lancet* 1:652–654, 1984.
17. Yunis EJ, Dibbin AW, Sherman FE: Rectal suction biopsy in the diagnosis of Hirschsprung's disease in infants. *Arch Pathol Lab Med* 100:329–333, 1976.
18. Chow CW, Campbell PE: Short segment Hirschsprung's disease as a cause of discrepancy between histologic, histochemical and clinical features. *J Pediatr Surg* 18:167–171, 1983.

19. Lynn HB, Van Heerden JA: Rectal myectomy in Hirschsprung's disease. *Arch Surg* 110:991–994, 1975.
20. Bentley JFR: Posterior excisional anorectal myotomy in management of chronic fecal accumulation. *Arch Dis Child* 41:144–147, 1966.
21. McCready RA, Beart Jr RW: Adult Hirschsprung's disease: Results of surgical treatment at Mayo Clinic. *Dis Col Rect* 23:401–407, 1980.
22. Dimler M: Acquired Hirschsprung's disease. *J Pediatr Surg* 16:844–845, 1981.
23. Cohen MC, Moore SW, Neveling U, et al: Acquired aganglionosis following surgery for Hirschsprung's disease: A report of five cases during a 33 year experience with pull-through procedures. *Histopathology* 22:163–168, 1993.
24. Teitelbaum DH, Caniano DA, Qualman SJ: The pathiophysiology of Hirschsprung's-associated enterocolitis: Importance of histologic correlates. *J Pediatr Surg* 24:1271–1277, 1989.
25. Taguchi T, Tanaka K, Ikeda K: Fibromuscular dysplasia of arteries in Hirschsprung's disease. *Gastroenterology* 88:1099–1103, 1985.
26. Drut R, Drut R: Hyperplasia of lymphoglandular complexes in colon segments in Hirschsprung's disease. A form of diversion colitis. *Pediatr Pathol* 12:575–581, 1992.
27. Haque S, Eisen RN, West AB: The morphologic features of diversion colitis: Studies of a pediatric population with no other disease of the intestinal mucosa. *Hum Pathol* 24:211–219, 1993.
28. Neut C, Colombel JF, Guillemot F, et al: Impaired bacterial flora in human excluded colon. *Gut* 30:1094–1098, 1989.
29. Ehrenpreis T: Some newer aspects of Hirschsprung's disease and allied disorders. *J Pediatr Surg* 1:329–337, 1966.
30. Meier-Ruge W: Hirschsprung's disease: Its aetiology, pathogenesis and differential diagnosis. *Curr Top Pathol* 59:131–179, 1974.
31. Ehrenpreis T: Pseudo-Hirschsprung's disease. *Arch Dis Child* 40:177–179, 1965.
32. Scharli AF, Meier-Ruge W: Localized and disseminated forms of neuronal intestinal dysplasia mimicking Hirschsprung's disease. *J Pediatr Surg* 16:164–169, 1981.
33. Schofield DE, Yunis EJ: Intestinal neuronal dysplasia. *J Pediatr Gastroenterol Nutr* 12:182–189, 1991.
34. Vargas JH, Sachs P, Ament ME: Chronic intestinal pseudoobstruction syndrome in pediatrics. Results of national survey by members of North American Society of Pediatric Gastroenterology and Nutrition. *J Pediatr Gastroenterol Nutr* 7:323–332, 1988.
35. Christensen J: The syndromes of intestinal pseudoobstruction (editorial). *J Pediatr Gastroenterol Nutr* 7:319–321, 1988.
36. Schuffler MD: Chronic intestinal psuedoobstruction syndromes. *Med Clin N Am* 65:1331–1358, 1981.
37. Mitros F, Schuffler MD, Teja K, et al: Pathology of familial visceral myopathy. *Hum Pathol* 13:825–833, 1981.
38. Rohrmann CA, Ricci MT, Krishnamurthy S, et al: Radiologic and histologic differentiation of neuromuscular disorder of the gastrointestinal tract. Visceral myopathies, visceral neuropathies and progressive systemic sclerosis. *Am J Roentgenol* 143:933–941, 1984.
39. Kaschula ROC, Cywes S, Katz A, et al: Degenerative leiomyopathy with massive megacolon. Myopathic form of chronic idiopathic intestinal pseudo-obstruction occurring in indigenous Africans. *Persp Pediatr Pathol* 11:193–213, 1987.
40. Brett EM, Lake BD: Reassessment of rectal approach to neuropathology in childhood. *Arch Dis Child* 50:753–762, 1975.
41. Rapola J, Santavuori P, Savilahti E: Suction biopsy of rectal mucosa in the diagnosis of infantile and juvenile types of neuronal ceroid lipofuscinoses. *Hum Pathol* 15:352–360, 1984.

8 BRONCHOPULMONARY VASCULAR AND FOREGUT MALFORMATIONS AND LOCALIZED ACQUIRED CYSTIC LESIONS OF THE LUNG

INTRODUCTION

A number of "cystic" lesions occur in the mediastinum and the lungs. On the basis of embryologic consideration, these lesions have been grouped as bronchopulmonary foregut malformations or bronchopulmonary vascular malformations.[1,2] The term "cyst" is used in a broad sense to include not only the conventional primary cystic lesions such as bronchogenic cyst but also certain examples of infantile lobar emphysema that show microcystically overdistended alveoli. Some variants of "cystic" lesions of the lungs such as the type III congenital cystic adenomatoid malformation may be mostly solid on gross examination, while others may simply contain increased numbers of normal alveoli (infantile lobar emphysema of "polyalveolar" type). Both congenital and acquired cystic lesions occur. The lesion may manifest clinically in a neonate, young infant, or child. Occasionally a congenital cystic lesion may be detected in the adult as an incidental finding on a chest x-ray. Respiratory distress due to compression of surrounding lung parenchyma, pneumothorax due to rupture, infection of stagnated secretions, and hemorrhage constitute the clinical manifestations. Congestive heart failure and ulceration and erosion of the cyst wall are seen in cystic lesions with anomalous vascular connections and acid-secreting gastric-type mucosal lining, respectively. Most of the localized lesions, if diagnosed early, are amenable to surgical cure. However, some of the lesions, if not diagnosed or treated early, may develop life threatening complications or prove fatal. In rare instances, the neoplastic potential of the mesenchyme in the septa of the cysts may be expressed.

Knowledge of the pathogenesis of these cystic lesions is essential for the understanding of the terminology and of the differences in the epithelial lining, structure of the wall and blood supply of the different types of lesions, and also the subtypes of individual cystic lesions. The precise incidence of these lesions is not known, but these are not uncommon lesions. Most of the lesions are intrathoracic, but abdominal location has also been described. In rare cases two different types of cystic lesions may be present in a child.[3] The various cystic lesions may not communicate with the respiratory tract or esophagus. Thus these cystic lesions present a fascinating array of clinical features, complications, pathologic features, locations, and prognosis. Most of these lesions are treated by surgical resection. Hence the surgical pathologist encounters them in his/her practice, although some of these lesions may be encountered at autopsy.

The pulmonary cystic lesions may be localized with presence of a single mass or involvement of a single lobe (with single or multiple cysts within it) or may show multifocal, diffuse, or generalized involvement of one or both the lungs. The lesions may be congenital or acquired. The various congenital localized lesions in Table 8-1 are described and illustrated in this chapter. Acquired lesions which need to be considered in the differential diagnosis are also described briefly.

CONGENITAL LOCALIZED CYSTIC LESIONS

Bronchogenic Cyst

The term "bronchogenic cyst" (BC) implies that the gross and microscopic features of the cyst wall are similar to the bronchus. BC is most commonly located along the midline in the mediastinum in relation to carina, trachea, or

TABLE 8-1 Bronchopulmonary Vascular and Foregut Malformations and Acquired Cystic Lesions of the Lung

Localized lesions	Multifocal lesion
Congenital origin	Congenital origin
Bronchogenic cyst	Congenital cystic bronchiectasis
Congenital cystic adenomatoid malformation (CCAM)	Congenital pulmonary lymphagiectasis
Infantile lobar emphysema	
Extralobar pulmonary sequestration and its variants	
Simple cyst	
Esophageal/gastric/enteric cyst	
Segment or lobe of lung or CCAM with systemic arterial supply	
Acquired origin	Acquired origin
Localized persistent interstitial pulmonary emphysema	Cystic lung disease is Down's syndrome
Intralobar pulmonary sequestration	Postinfarction pulmonary cysts
Posttraumatic pulmonary pseudocyst	Multifocal acute interstitial pulmonary emphysema
Mesenchymal cystic hamartoma	Diffuse persistent interstitial pulmonary emphysema
Healed abscess	

main-stem bronchi. Intrapulmonary location may be seen in occasional cases (Figure 8-1). Rare subcutaneous BC may occur along the midline of the chest.[4] In adults, BC may be seen in the posterior mediastinum, within the diaphragm or along the esophagus.[5]

BC is seen most frequently as an asymptomatic incidental finding on chest x-ray in children and young adults. Prenatal diagnosis can be made by sonographic examination.[6] Definitive diagnosis of an asymptomatic hilar BC found incidentally in adults can be made by transbronchial fine-needle aspiration.[7] Secondary infection and hemorrhage occurring in the cyst are associated with clinical manifestations such as fever and pain. Respiratory distress may occur from compression of an airway. Perforation is a rare complication seen in infected BC. The surgical excision is curative. The surgically resected specimen, which measures ≤5 cm in diameter, may show grossly demonstrable cartilage in the wall (Figure 8-2). BC forms a spheroidal mass that does not usually communicate with the respiratory tract. The cyst contents vary from serous fluid to turbid, viscous, mucinous, or hemorrhagic fluid (Figure 8-1). Histologic examination reveals a ciliated and nonciliated columnar epithelial lining (Figure 8-3). The epithelial lining may show squamous metaplasia or ulceration creating difficulties in the diagnosis of BC. The wall of BC is composed of fibrous tissue. Mucous gland and spicules of cartilage are found in the wall of the cyst. Smooth muscle is also present (Figure 8-3). Compressed surrounding pulmonary parenchyma is seen in the intrapulmonary BC. Pulmonary parenchyma is not seen in the extrapulmonary mediastinal BC. Chronic infection of the BC may occur. Histologically chronic inflammatory infiltrate is present in the wall of the cyst in such cases (Figure 8-4).

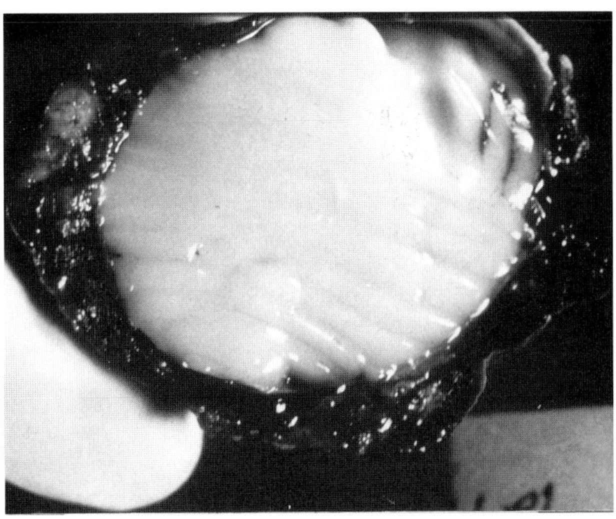

FIGURE 8-1. Intrapulmonary bronchogenic cyst (diagnosed as such on microscopic examination; see Figure 9-3) containing mucoid secretion. The cyst is surrounded by compressed lung parenchyma of the lobe in which it occurred.

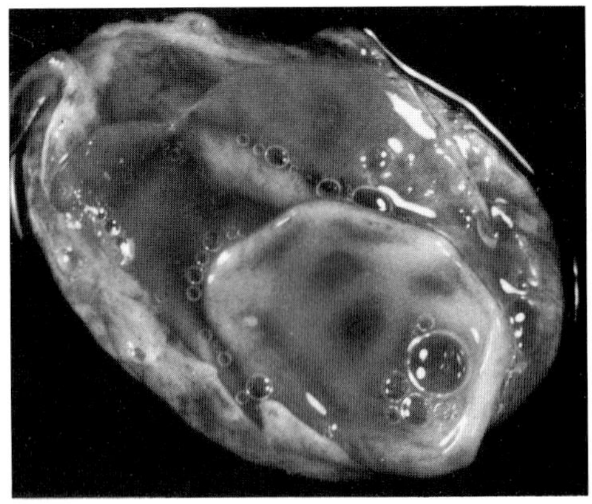

FIGURE 8-2. Extrapulmonary bronchogenic cyst showing grossly identifiable cartilage in the wall.

Congenital Cystic Adenomatoid Malformation (CCAM)

CCAM is an intrapulmonary lesion involving a segment, or a lobe or rarely almost an entire lung. CCAM is one of the more common cystic lesions of the lung. Antenatally diagnosed CCAM may be resected from a fetus to prevent pulmonary hypoplasia and hydrops fetalis.[8] Most specimens of CCAM show grossly demonstrable cysts; however, in what is labeled as type III CCAM, the lesion may be solid with virtually no grossly demonstrable cysts in the speci-

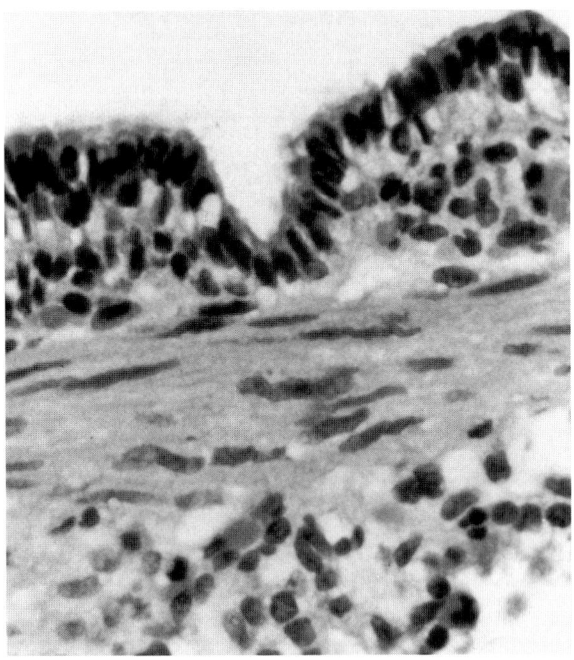

FIGURE 8-3. Nonciliated and ciliated columnar epithelial lining and smooth muscle in the wall of a bronchogenic cyst (H&E, ×250).

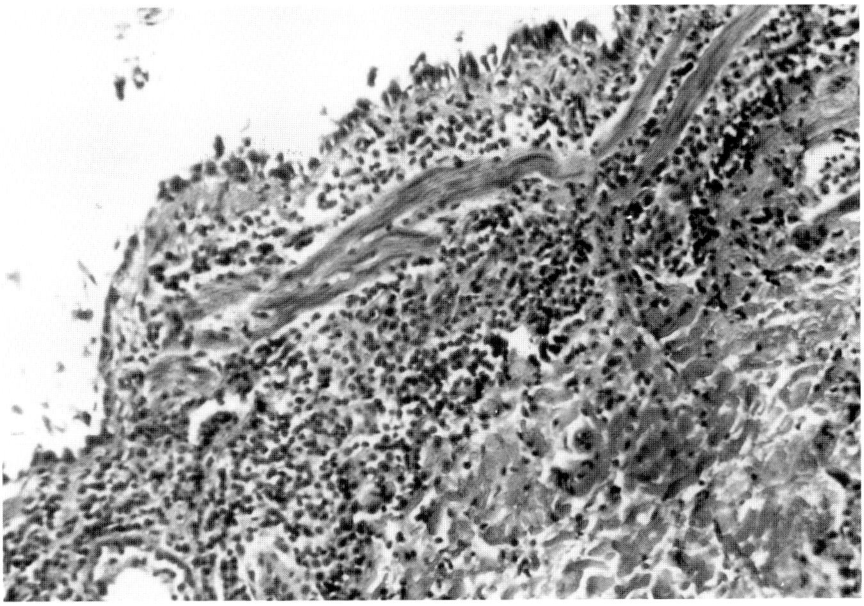

FIGURE 8-4. Chronic inflammatory infiltrate with disruption of the smooth muscle in the wall of bronchogenic cyst secondary to repeated infection (H&E, ×100).

men. Cartilage which is present in the cyst walls in rare cases of CCAM types I and II[9] may not be recognizable on gross examination.

Three types of CCAM are recognized.[10] Type I lesion has a single or multiple cysts measuring 3–10 cm in diameter (Figure 8-5). Type II lesion, which is smaller than types I and III, consists of multiple cysts varying from 0.5 to 2.0 cm (Figure 8-6). Type III lesion is the least common. It may involve an entire lung. On gross examination the lesion presents grayish-tan solid appearance on the cut surface (Figure 8-7). A few small grossly demonstrable 0.2-cm cysts may be present. Mucoid secretion may be seen oozing out from the cut surface.

On histologic examination large cysts or serpentine microcystic structures are seen. These cystic structures resemble bronchioles and are lined by ciliated and nonciliated columnar epithelium (Figure 8-8). The epithelium with the underlying connective tissue tends to be thrown into microscopic papillary folds. Mucous secreting epithelium is seen in some cases of types I and III lesions (Figure 8-9). The papillary projections may be large with the core formed by loose mesenchyme.[11] Smooth muscle is present in the cyst walls. Cartilage spicules have been described in the cyst walls in type I and type III lesions[8] (Figure 8-10). Skeletal muscle fibers may be present in the walls of the cysts particularly in type II CCAM. In type III lesion, the "bronchiolar" cystic structures are admixed with "alveolus"-like structures lined by cuboidal epithelium (Figure 8-9).

Occurrence of neoplasia has been reported in rare instances of CCAM. The neoplastic potential of the congenital cystic lesions of the lung is discussed in a separate section below.

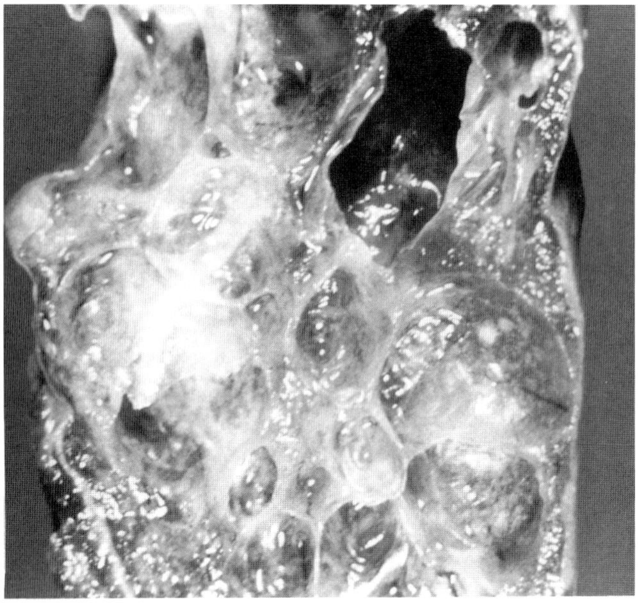

FIGURE 8-5. Type I congenital cystic adenomatoid malformation. Note multiple large cysts in the lesion. (Courtesy of Dr. Timothy Benning.)

Infantile Lobar Emphysema (ILE)

Certain cases of ILE may be acquired in origin. However, most are congenital. ILE may manifest itself shortly after birth or in early infancy. The upper lobe of left lung is most frequently affected. Rarely there may be involvement of two lobes. ILE is due to three different types of abnormality:[12] (1) intrinsic bronchial

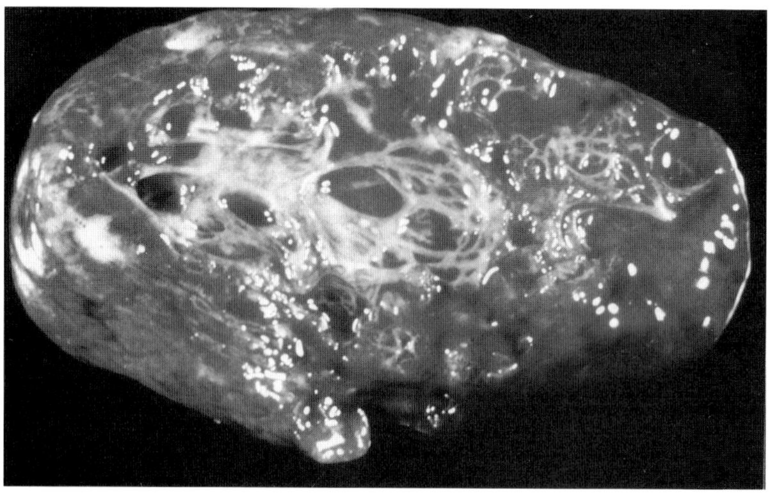

FIGURE 8-6. Type II congenital cystic adenomatoid malformation. Note admixture of small and large cysts.

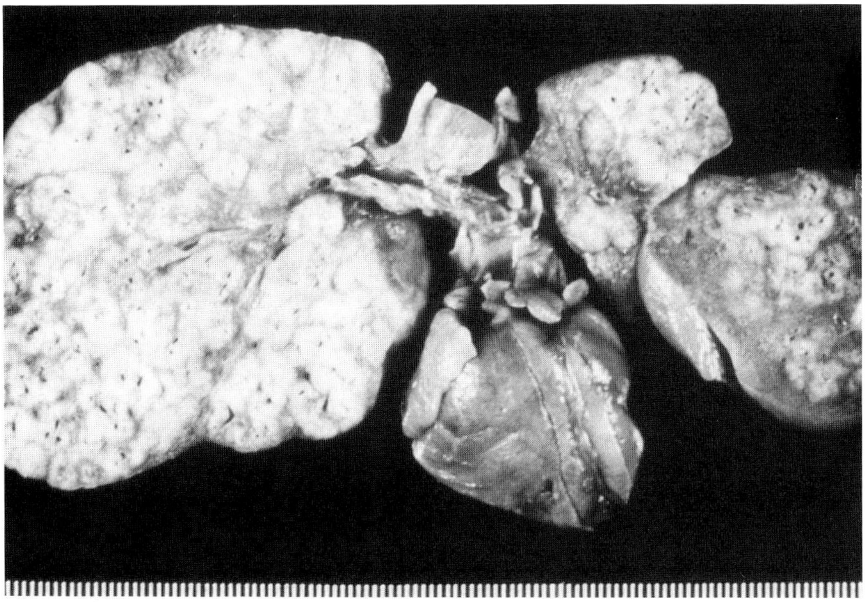

FIGURE 8-7. Type III congenital cystic adenomatoid malformation. Note virtually complete solid appearance of the lesion. A few scattered pinpoint cysts are present. There is involvement of the entire lung. (Courtesy of Dr. Timothy Benning.)

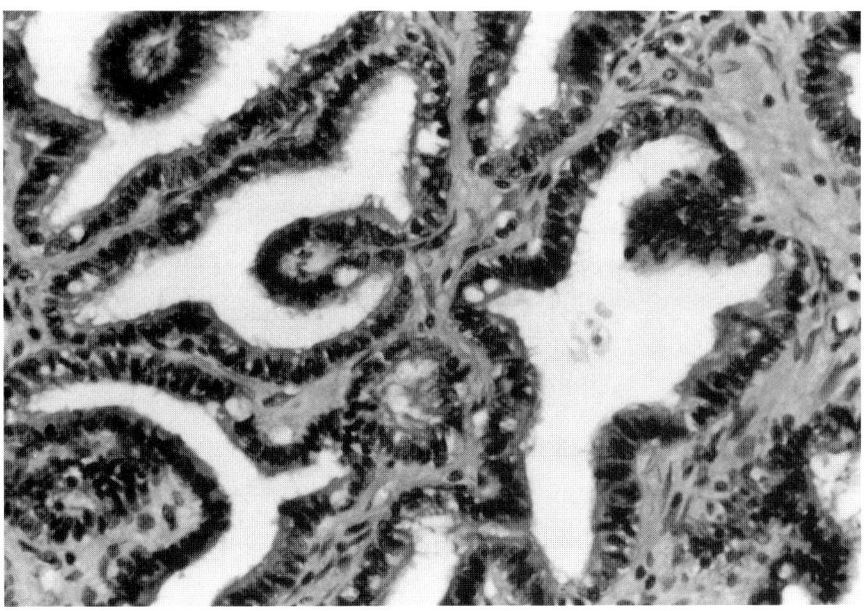

FIGURE 8-8. Congenital cystic adenomatoid malformation. Microcystic structures lined by ciliated and nonciliated columnar epithelium. Note the focal papillary folding and tufting of the lining epithelium. (H&E, ×250.)

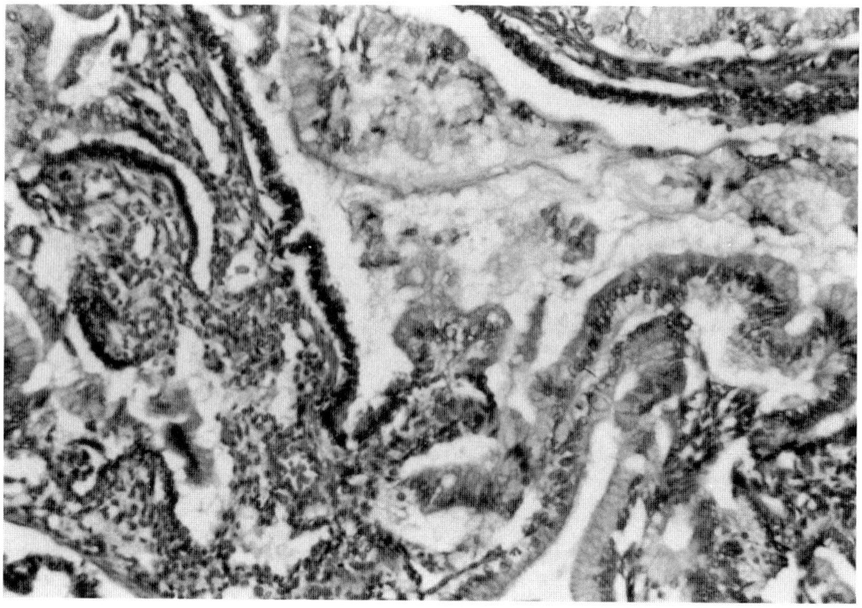

FIGURE 8-9. Congenital cystic adenomatoid malformation showing mucin secreting epithelium; note the admixture of "alveolus"-like structures (H&E, ×100).

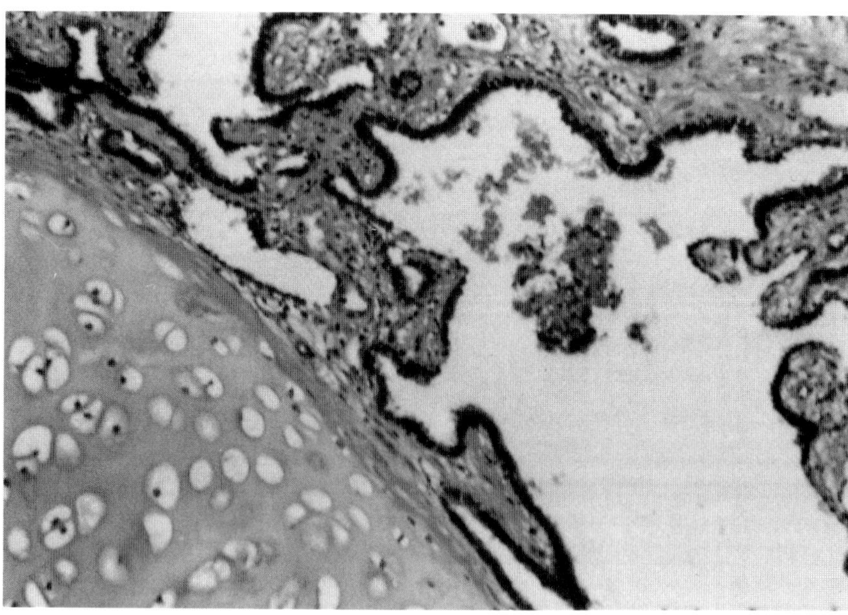

FIGURE 8-10. Congenital cystic adenomatoid malformation showing cartilage in the wall (H&E, ×100) (courtesy of Dr. Timothy Benning).

obstruction associated with bronchial stenosis, obstructing mucosal folds, mucous plug, granulation tissue, or abnormalities of bronchial cartilage such as hypoplasia or fragmentation (Figure 8-11); (2) extrinsic bronchial obstruction associated with enlarged lymph nodes, aberrant artery or vein, including ductus arteriosus, abnormal origin of bronchus (tracheal, eparterial), mediastinal mass (e.g., bronchogenic cyst); and (3) polyalveolar lobe in which the absolute number of alveoli is increased three to five times the normal number.[13] Thus ILE can be a congenital or an acquired lesion. The mucous plug, granulation tissue, or bronchomalacia producing luminal obstruction during expiration (ball valve obstruction) may be related to infection or to endotracheal intubation in an infant with BPD.[14] The lymphadenopathy secondary to infection resulting in bronchial compression is an acquired lesion. The aberrant artery and mucosal fold are congenital lesions.

The gross and microscopic features are related to the type of abnormality resulting in ILE. It is essential that the clinical, radiologic, and surgical findings be available to the pathologist. The bronchus of the resected lobe should be examined closely for presence of stenosis, mucosal folds, and granulation tissue. The deficiency or fragmentation of bronchial cartilage may be appreciated on gross examination if that portion of the bronchus is present in the resected specimen. Abnormal origin of the bronchus or compression by an aberrant artery or by a mediastinal mass cannot be demonstrated in the grossly resected specimen. Enlarged lymph nodes causing bronchial obstruction may be present in the resected specimen.

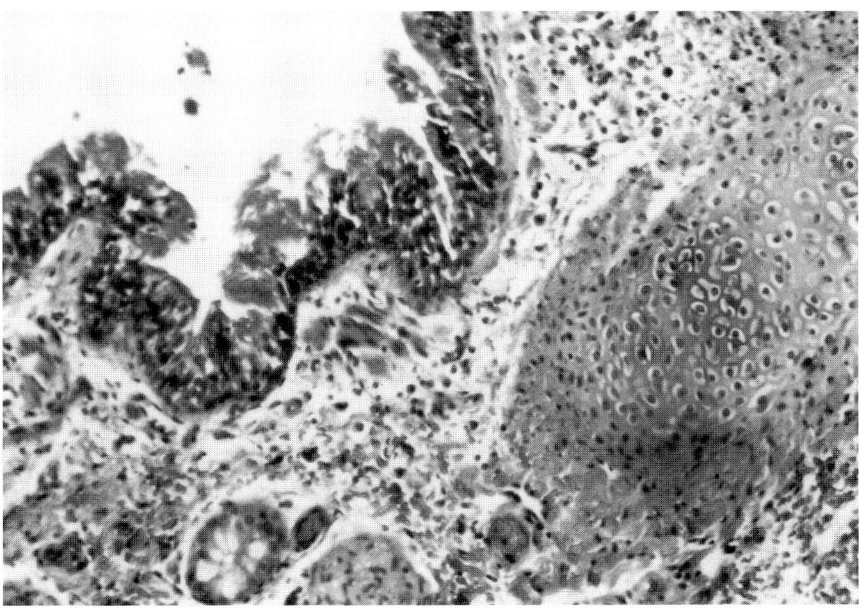

FIGURE 8-11. Bronchus of a lobe showing infantile lobar emphysema. Note the hypoplastic cartilage. This was the only cartilage present in the wall of the lobar bronchus. (H&E, ×100.)

On cut surface the resected lobe that is enlarged in size shows spongy appearance due to overdistended alveoli when intrinsic or extrinsic obstruction is the cause of ILE (Figure 8-12). Sections for histologic examination should be taken from the lung, the bronchus, and the lymph nodes if they are present. Histologic examination in the obstructive ILE reveals overdistended alveoli. The alveolar septa are not disrupted. Hence the term "emphysema" may be considered as incorrect, if the definition of the term is strictly applied.

In the polyalveolar lobe the resected lobe is enlarged in size, but the overdistension of alveoli is not seen on gross or microscopic examination. The gross volume of the lobe may be increased up to five times the normal size. The absolute of number of alveoli is increased by as much as three to five times the normal.[13] The terminal airways are absent in the peripheral portions of the lung. The increase in the number of alveoli can be demonstrated by the radial alveolar count.[15] In this method a line perpendicular to the pleura is extended up to the terminal bronchiole and the number of alveoli transected by the line between the pleura and the terminal bronchiole is counted. The normal counts are 2–5 for fetuses, 5–10 for infants and 10–12 for young children. In polyalveolar lobe the alveolar count is >20.[16] The alveoli in the polyalveolar lobe are not overdistended, nor is there disruption of alveolar septa.

Pulmonary Sequestration (PS)

The term sequestration introduced by Pryce[17] denotes a segment of lung tissue having systemic arterial supply and absence of connection with the tracheobronchial tree (i.e., sequestered from tracheobronchial tree or having lack of continuity with the tracheobronchial tree). However, four of Pryce's original seven cases deviated from his own definition since in these cases there was an abnormal artery supplying a segment of lung with normal bronchial connection as illustrated in Figure 8-13. Therefore the concept of sequestration spectrum has been introduced to include these "atypical" or "pseudo"-PS and the originally described classical PS. Systemic arterial supply is generally considered as an essential criterion of PS (Figure 8-14). PS may be associated with other types of

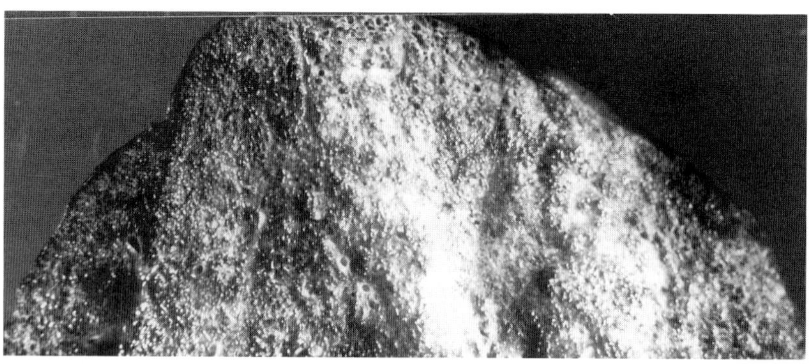

FIGURE 8-12. Infantile lobar emphysema showing grossly visible overdistended alveoli.

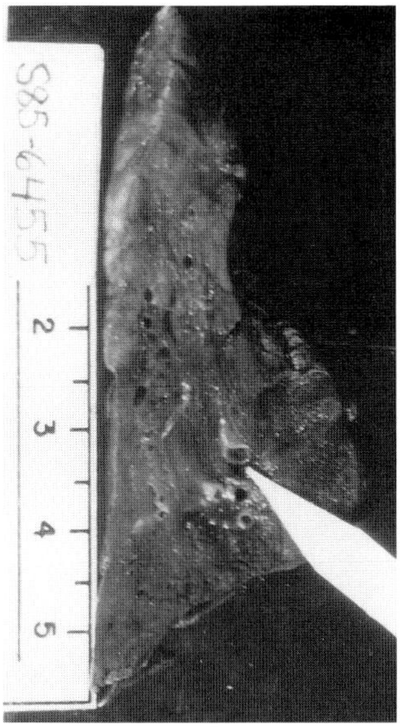

FIGURE 8-13. Normal lobe of the left lung showing a bronchial communication (above the arrow) and two systemic artery (below the arrow).

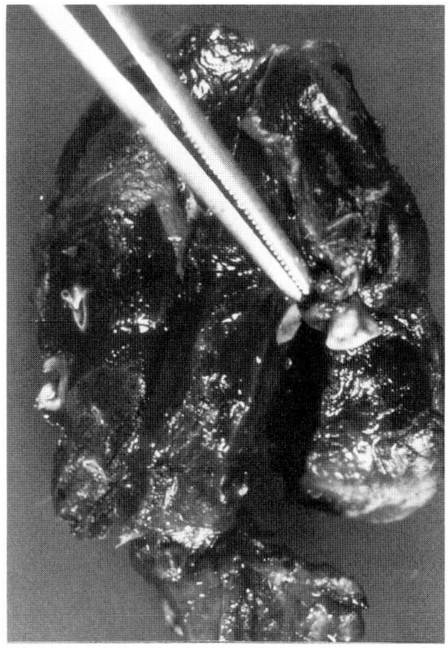

FIGURE 8-14. Extralobar pulmonary sequestration supplied by a large systemic artery. Note the dark (congested and hemorrhagic) appearance of the sequestered lobe. No bronchial communication was present.

cystic lesions such as CCAM, bronchogenic cyst, and bronchopulmonary foregut malformation such as gastric-type cyst.

Types of PS

On the basis of location PS is divided into two major types: Intralobar PS (IPS) and extralobar PS (EPS). Stocker[18] defines EPS as a segment of pulmonary parenchyma with systemic arterial supply and no connection to the tracheobronchial tree and that lies outside the normal investment of the visceral pleura (the majority are present between the lower lobe and diaphragm but may be found anywhere in thorax). Rarely EPS is infradiaphragmatic. IPS represents a segment of pulmonary parenchyma enclosed by normal visceral pleura (and surrounded by or adjacent to normal lung parenchyma). IPS, like EPS, has systemic arterial supply and absence of bronchial connection.

Pathologic Features of PS

Although there is no bronchial connection in classical PS, small bronchi are found within the lesion. PS may also have anomalous or mismatched venous drainage. The pulmonary parenchyma within the lesion usually consists of dilated but otherwise normal alveoli, alveolar ducts, and bronchioles. Intraalveolar recent and old hemorrhage (hemosiderin laden histiocytes) is seen frequently. Nodular aggregates of lymphoid cells and fibrosis secondary to previous infections may be present. The small bronchi within the lesion may be dilated and show mucous plugging (Figure 8-15). The lesion shows prominent branches of the systemic artery (Figure 8-16). In rare instances cystic adenomatoid-type change (dilated or nondilated bronchiolar spaces lined by ciliated cuboidal or columnar epithelium) may be seen within the lesion (Figure 8-17). This last lesion can be labeled as CCAM with systemic arterial supply (see recommendations for terminology below). In rare instances PS may have a communication with the esophagus or stomach.

Spectrum of PS

Thus from the foregoing it is obvious that lesions with variable features are included under the broad category of PS. Using the term in this broad sense can be confusing. I would recommend that the term "PS" be restricted to those lesions that fulfill both the original criteria, i.e., systemic arterial supply and lack of bronchial connection. Pulmonary lesions having systemic arterial supply but with bronchial connection should not be labeled as pseudo- or atypical PS. These lesions should be given a descriptive diagnosis such as segment of lung showing systemic arterial supply (Figure 8-13), or as in the case illustrated in Figure 8-17, the lesion should be designated as a CCAM with systemic artery rather than atypical or pseudo-PS with arterial supply and bronchial connection showing cystic adenomatoid change. A lesion which shows features such as communication with esophagus–stomach or anomalous or mismatched venous drainage in addition to systemic arterial supply and lack of bronchial connection qualifies for the diagnosis of "PS" with esophageal–gastric connection or

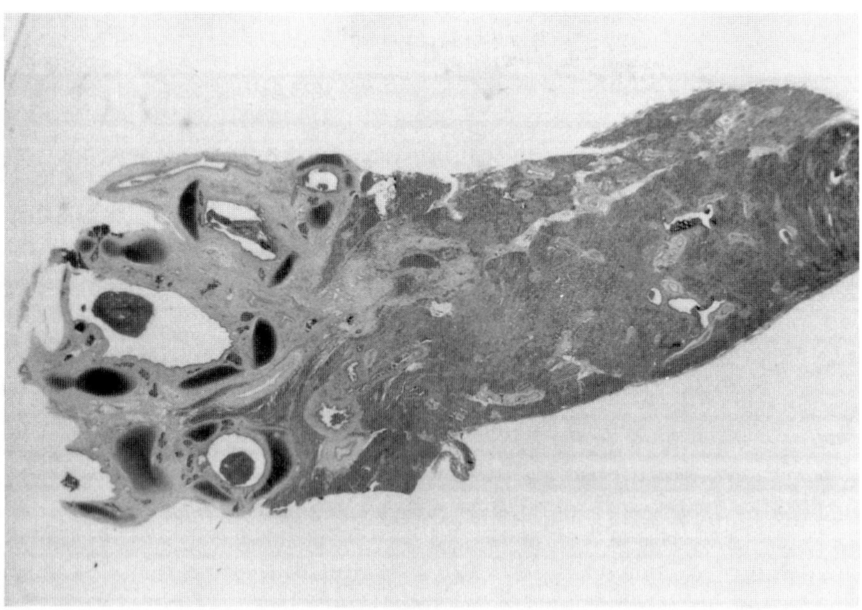

FIGURE 8-15. Intralobar pulmonary sequestration with dilatation of bronchi and bronchioles within the sequestered lobe (H&E, ×2).

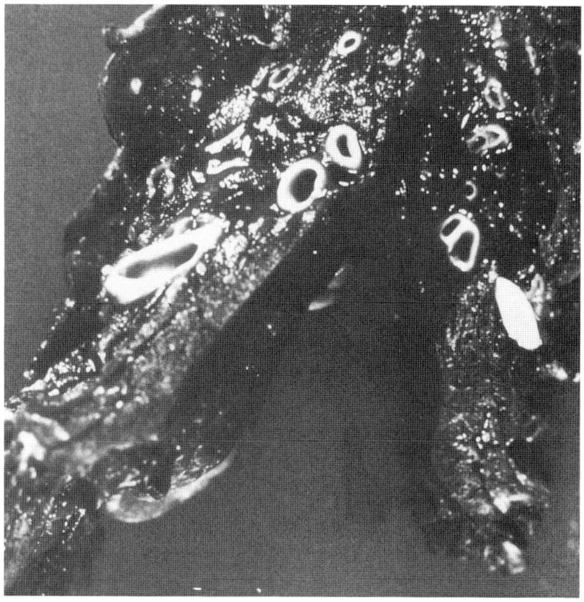

FIGURE 8-16. Extralobar pulmonary sequestration. Note the prominant branches of the systemic pulmonary artery shown in Figure 8-14.

anomalous or mismatched venous drainage. (Tables 8-1, 8-2). The terms "atypical" or "pseudo-PS," "atypical PS with cystic adenomatoid change," etc. should be avoided.

Besides the abnormalities of bronchial communication and arterial supply, anomalous or mismatched venous drainage can also occur in these lesions.[19] Scimitar syndrome in which the pulmonary lesion belongs to the spectrum of PS

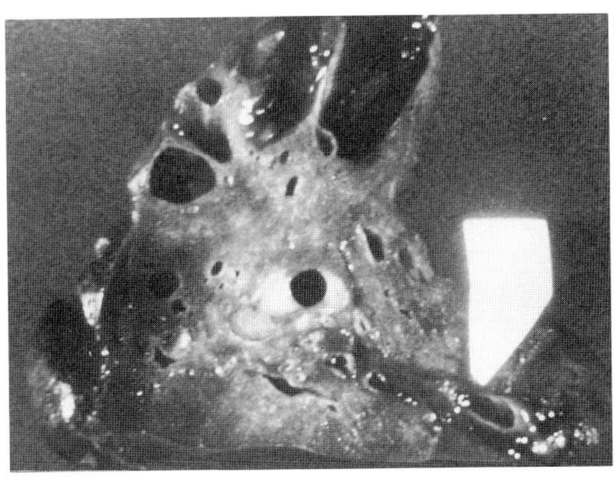

FIGURE 8-17. Congenital cystic adenomatoid change in an extralobar sequestration or congenital adenomatoid malformation with systemic arterial supply (the white pointer) and no bronchial connection.

TABLE 8-2 Recommended Terminology of Pulmonary Sequestration

Variation	Recommended terminology
Atypical PS[a] with bronchial connection	Segment of lung with systemic artery
Atypical PS with bronchial connection and cystic adenomatoid change	CCAM[b] with systemic artery
Atypical PS with esohageal–gastric communication	PS with esophageal–gastric communication
Atypical PS with anomalous or mismatched venous drainage	PS with anomalous or mismatched venous drainage

[a]Pulmonary sequestration.
[b]Congenital cystic adenomatoid malformation.

serves as an example of this phenomenon. In this syndrome systemic arterial supply is limited to the lower zone of a hypoplastic right lung while the anomalous vein or veins drain the major part of or entire right lung into the right atrium or the major thoracic or abdominal veins. This is considered as a mismatched or anomalous venous drainage. The name of the syndrome is derived from the convex shadow of the anomalous vein in the chest x-ray resembling a curved Turkish saber. The child with this syndrome may be asymptomatic. However, repeated infection of the involved lung may necessitate resection of the right lung. The surgical pathologist should verify from the surgeon the anomalous artery and the veins of the resected lung and describe these specifically in the report on gross examination. Histologic examination of the lung shows chronic inflammatory changes involving the bronchi and the parenchyma due to repeated infection.

Pathogenesis of IPS

There is controversy regarding the very existence of IPS as an entity and its nature (i.e., whether it is a congenital or acquired lesion). According to Holder and Langston,[20] IPS either represents CCAM recognized clinically after the lesion becomes infected or a segment of lung with developmentally normal parenchyma having systemic arterial supply. Stocker[18] supports the contention by Gebauer and Mason[21] that IPS is an acquired lesion resulting from obstructive bronchopulmonary disease. The following sequence is suggested:[18] obstruction of lower lobe bronchus due to aspiration, e.g., of foreign body or due to inflammatory process in a segment of normal lung parenchyma—persistence of obstruction with chronic pneumonia—partial or complete interruption of pulmonary artery supply (thrombotic occlusion) due to the infectious pneumonic process—formation of richly vascular granulation tissue deriving its blood supply from the arteries in the pulmonary ligament (vertical pleural folds extending from the hilus to the base on the medial pulmonary surface) or diaphragmatic arteries (the arteries in the pulmonary ligament and diaphragmatic arteries are systemic arteries)—persistence of one or more of these systemic arteries supplying the chronically infected segment of lung. The endpoint is a "sequestered" portion of lung parenchyma enclosed within the pleura that derives its blood supply from the systemic arteries, thus fulfilling the criteria for the diagnosis of PS.

The pathologic features of IPS (thickened pleura with adhesions, dense fibrous changes in the parenchyma with cystically dilated bronchi filled with mucus, or inflammatory exudate, lymphoid aggregates around bronchioles and in alveolar septa, etc.), the age of the patients (older children and adults), and location (frequent involvement of lower lobes) support the theory of acquired origin of IPS.

Esophageal, Gastric, and Enteric Cyst

These cysts, which are located in the mediastinum, are also called "reduplication cysts of the alimentary tract" or "of the foregut." Bronchogenic cysts belong to this spectrum of foregut cysts. These cysts may communicate with the esophagus, trachea or bronchus. On gross examination the cysts are spheroidal or oval masses with a relatively thick wall. The gastric cyst may show rugal folds of the inner surface (Figure 8-18). The esophageal cyst is lined by nonkeratinizing squamous or ciliated columnar epithelium and has two layers of smooth muscle in the wall. The gastric cyst is partly or completely lined by epithelium containing chief and parietal cells. The gastric cyst is frequently associated with ulceration (Figure 8-19) and perforation with adhesions, fistula formation, and/or erosion of the surrounding structures. Tracheal and bronchial perforation leads to aspiration pneumonia. These complications can be avoided by early diagnosis and surgical resection of the cysts.

The gastric cyst also has a well-developed muscle coat consisting of two layers with myenteric plexuses[22] (Figure 8-20). The enteric cysts are lined by small intestinal-type mucus-secreting epithelium. Occasionally a cyst may show a combination of various epithelial linings. A diagnosis of foregut cyst is warranted in such instances. In such a cyst the gastric epithelium is the most significant from the functional and therefore clinical point of view.

PATHOGENESIS

Theories of Pathogenesis of EPS and Related Malformations

At 5 weeks of gestation the lung bud develops from the ventral wall of the cephalic end of the foregut (pharynx). There is bifurcation of the lung bud by 7

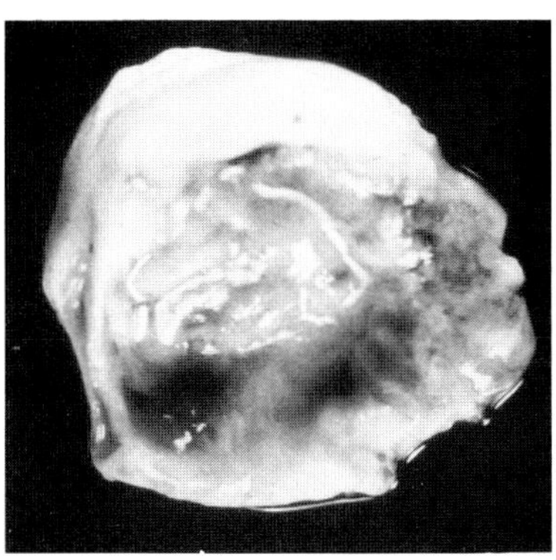

FIGURE 8-18. Gastric cyst of posterior mediastinum. Note the mucosal folds resembling gastric rugae.

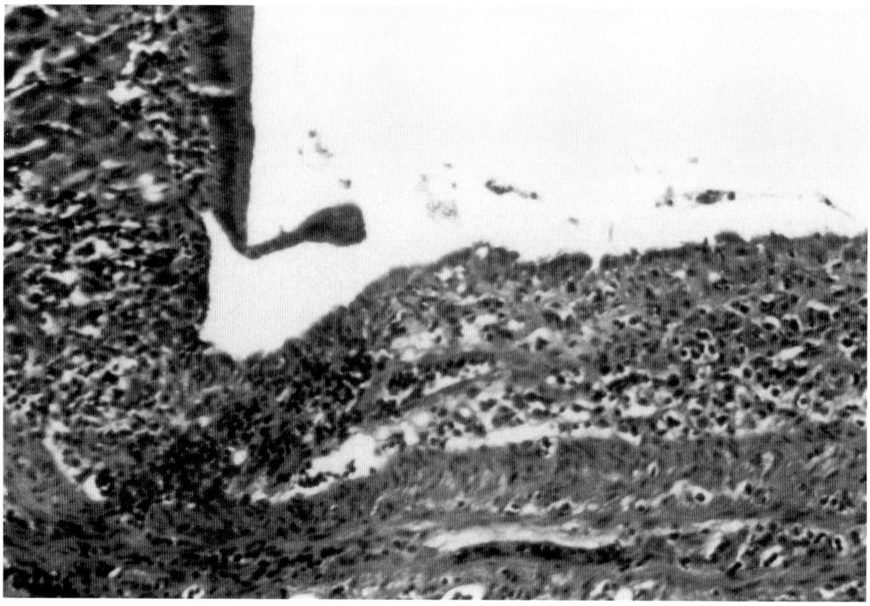

FIGURE 8-19. Ulceration of gastric cyst. Note the chronic inflammatory infiltrate in the base of the ulcer. A portion of the lining of the cyst consisting of columnar epithelial cells and mucous glands is seen. Chief and parietal cells were noted in the epithelial lining elsewhere (H&E, ×250).

weeks. Eventually the lungs develop from the bifurcation. The various cystic, solid, or mixed cystic–solid malformations involving the bronchi, lungs, and foregut are included under the broad term "bronchopulmonary foregut malformations" (BPFM).[1] The term is sometimes used in a more restricted sense to describe those anomalies which retain a connection with foregut (esophagus, stomach). More recently another term has been suggested: "bronchopulmonary vascular malformation" (BPVM).[2] A brief consideration of theories of pathogenesis will be helpful in conceptualizing the possible embryologic processes involved in the origin of these lesions and their typical and atypical features.

Theory of Accessory or Supernumerary Bud

The spectrum of BPFM includes PS (and its variants), bronchogenic cyst, enteric cyst, and true diverticulum. According to this theory, each of these malformations arises from an abnormal accessory or supernumerary lung bud (Figure 8-21). The location and type of malformation are determined by (1) the timing of the accessory bud, (2) the type of differentiation it shows, (3) the type of blood supply it receives, (4) the degree and route of migration of the bud or lack of it, and (5) whether it maintains its connection to the foregut–respiratory tract. Thus, for example, an abnormal accessory lung bud, which arises before the development of pleura, derives systemic arterial supply, severs its respiratory

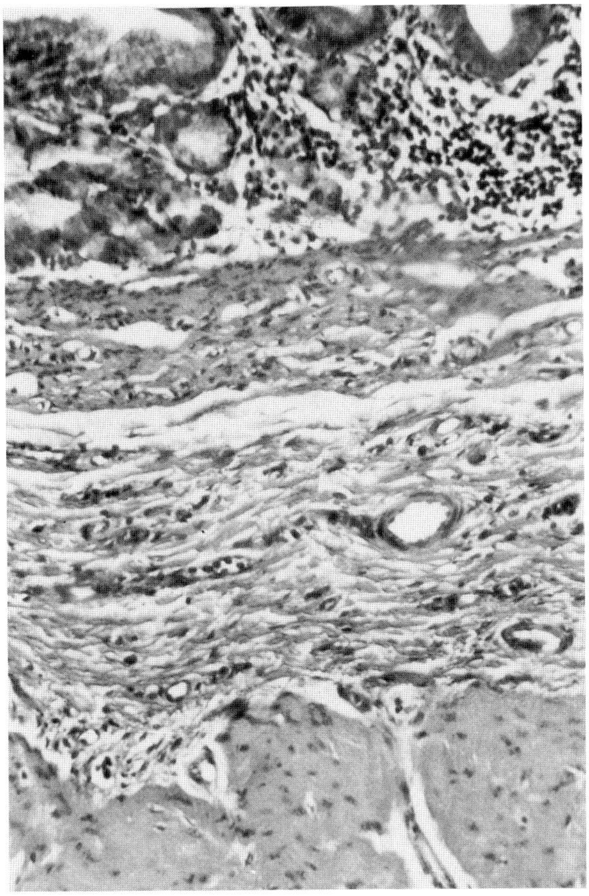

FIGURE 8-20. Gastric cyst with gastric mucosal lining containing chief and parietal cells and well-developed submucosa and internal and external muscle layers (the latter is not shown in the photomicrograph) (H&E, ×250).

tract connection, differentiates into lung parenchyma, and migrates to extrapulmonary location will form an extralobar PS.

Theory of Bronchopulmonary Vascular Malformations

In the spectrum of BPVM, infantile lobar emphysema, CCAM, scimitar syndrome, and all the lesions in the spectrum of BPFM are included. There are four basic components in the normal development of the lung:[2] airway, arterial supply, venous drainage, and lung parenchyma (Figure 8-22). The development of pulmonary segments from the lung bud normally shows the following features and sequence: (1) completion of bronchial branching at 16 weeks' gestation, (2) pulmonary artery branching similar to the pattern of bronchial branching except that it follows slightly later, (3) alveolar development following that of terminal and respiratory bronchioles and sacules, (4) differing rates of growth in various

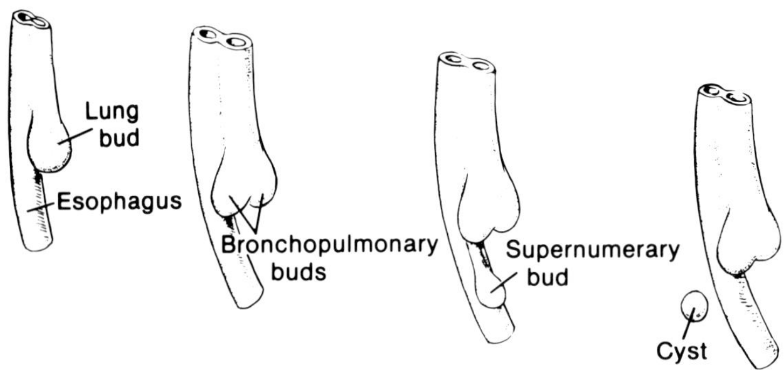

FIGURE 8-21. Diagrammatic representation of supernumerary bud arising from the foregut.

tissues of the lung, (5) regression of systemic capillary plexus of the tips of branching bronchial buds with progressive development of lung parenchyma and of its pulmonary arterial supply, and (6) the development of venous drainage (which is poorly understood).

Following an insult of undetermined etiology or as a result of localized trauma, ischemia, infection, adhesions, or any nonspecific injury, abnormalities can occur in *one or more* of these components of normal development: airway, arterial supply, venous drainage and lung parenchyma. All combinations of malformations and abnormal vascular connections can occur.

The timing and severity of injury, the particular developmental process in the sequence that is disturbed, and the type of differentiation will determine the type of malformation seen. Thus, for example, minor insult to the airway may

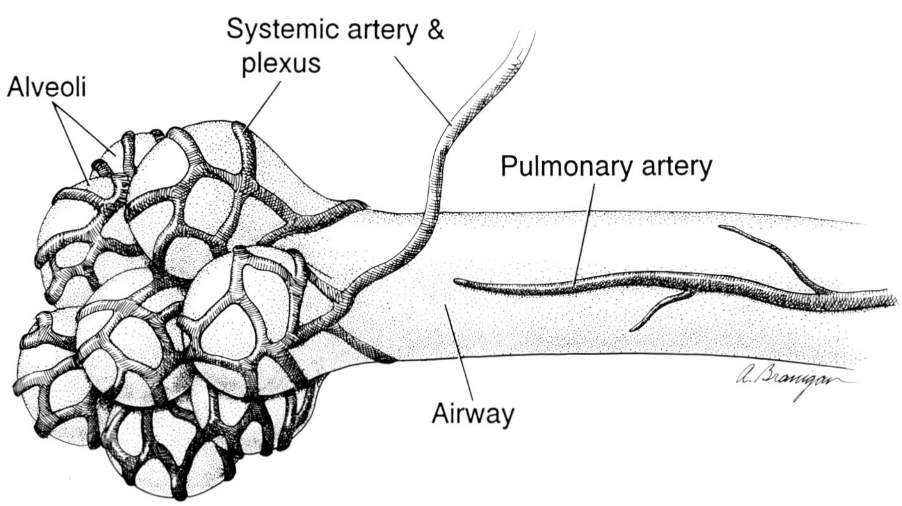

FIGURE 8-22. Diagrammatic representation of the four components of pulmonary development (airway, pulmonary artery, systemic arterial supply, and parenchyma).

result in a localized abnormality such as bronchogenic cyst. On the other hand, the injury may be severe enough to produce complete arrest of development of the bronchus and of pulmonary artery supply, resulting in agenesis of a segment or lobe or entire lung. An injury of intermediate severity, occurring later in the sequence, may disrupt the development of bronchus and pulmonary artery of a segment of lung. The systemic arterial supply does not regress in these circumstances, and the segment of lung parenchyma that develops subsequently has the classical features of PS. The development of the remaining bronchial tree and the lung proceeds normally in such an instance. The probable pathogenesis of various pulmonary malformations according to this theory is given in Table 8-3.

DIFFERENTIAL DIAGNOSIS

Mediastinal BC must be differentiated from esophageal, gastric, and enteric cyst. The esophageal, gastric and enteric cysts are lined by squamous epithelium, parietal and chief cells, and mucus-secreting columnar epithelium, respectively. Well-developed layers of smooth muscle are present in the walls of these cysts. Cartilage is absent. The esophageal cyst may also contain skeletal muscle in its wall. Infection of BC may result in ulceration and/or squamous metaplasia in the lining epithelium. The precise diagnosis of the type of cyst will depend on demonstration of cartilage in the wall of the cyst. The intrapulmonary BC must be differentiated from type I CCAM. Cartilage is rarely present in type I and type II CCAM.[8]

Localized persistent interstitial pulmonary emphysema (PIPE),[23] an acquired localized cystic lesion and occasionally diffuse cystic lung disease may also have to be considered in the differential diagnosis. PIPE, which has characteristic multinucleated giant cells lining the cyst, is described in the chapter on perinatal iatrogenic lesions. There are multiple small cysts in both the lungs in Down's syndrome.[24] The cysts are often prominent in the subpleural region (Figure 8-23). The 0.1–0.4-cm cysts represent dilated alveoli lined by cuboidal epithelium (Figure 8-24). Cholesterol granulomas may be present within the cysts.

Other conditions in multifocal cystic pulmonary disease in which a biopsy may be performed occasionally include postinfarction pulmonary cysts and congenital pulmonary lymphangiectasis. In the former condition, there are subpleural cysts measuring up to 1 cm in diameter having connective tissue wall derived from interlobular septa. No epithelial lining is present, and the lumen contains necrotic debris.[25] In the latter condition dilated lymphatic channels are present in the interlobular septa and the pleura. The channels have thin walls and are lined by endothelium.[26,27] The cytokeratin stain is helpful in distinguishing between the endothelial lining of the cysts of congenital pulmonary lymphangiectasis and epithelial lining of other pulmonary cysts described above.

NEOPLASTIC POTENTIAL OF MESENCHYMAL COMPONENT OF CYSTIC LESIONS

The cyst walls in the lesions described in this chapter consist of mesenchymal tissue containing fibroblasts, smooth muscle, cartilage, and in the rare cases

TABLE 8-3 Pathogenesis of Bronchopulmonary Vascular Malformations[a]

Component of development and type of lesion	Possible pathogenesis	Type of differentiation within the lesion	Location
Abnormality of airway			
Bronchogenic cyst	Localized abnormality of bronchial development	Bronchial epithelium, smooth muscle, cartilage	Mediastinum, hilum, occasionally intrapulmonary (peripheral lung cysts)
Abnormality of airway and arterial supply			
Classical extrapulmonary sequestration	Disruption of bronchial and pulmonary artery development resulting in persistence of systemic arterial supply	Normal alveolar development (with secondary changes due to obstruction and infection)	Extrapulmonary—thoracic or uncommonly abdominal
Abnormality of arterial supply			
Otherwise normal lung segment with systemic artery	Disruption of pulmonary artery development resulting in persistence of systemic arterial supply	Normal alveolar development	Part of normal lung parenchyma
Abnormality of arterial supply and pulmonary parenchyma			
Congenital cystic adenomatoid malformation (CCAM) with systemic artery	Same as above plus abnormal differentiation	Spaces lined by ciliated epithelium (bronchiolar type differentiation)	Within the lung
Abnormality of pulmonary parenchyma			
CCAM	Abnormal differentiation	Spaces lined by ciliated epithelium	Within the lung
Infantile lobar emphysema	Abnormal lung parenchyma	Polyaveolar lobe	Within the lung
Abnormality of venous drainage			
Scimitar syndrome[b]	Anomalous venous drainage into inferior vena cava	Alveolar differentiation	Within the lung

[a] Abnormalities of one or more of the following can occur (airway, arterial supply, venous drainage and pulmonary parenchyma)

[b] Scimitar syndrome-Complete or partial venous drainage of usually hypoplastic right lung into inferior vena cava (the convex shadow of the anomalous vein resembles scimitar [short curved sword)

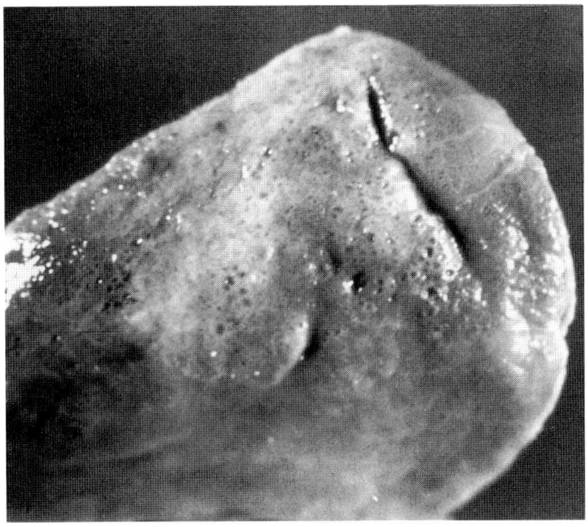

FIGURE 8-23. Subpleural cysts in a case of Down's syndrome.

of type II CCAM, skeletal muscle. It appears that this mesenchymal tissue has a neoplastic potential, which may be expressed during childhood in rare instances. Four types of neoplasms arising in previously diagnosed pulmonary cystic lesions have been described. These include rhabdomyosarcoma, malignant mesenchymoma (with fibrous tissue, cartilage, and skeletal muscle), sarcoma (not otherwise specified), and the biphasic pulmonary blastoma.[28–34]

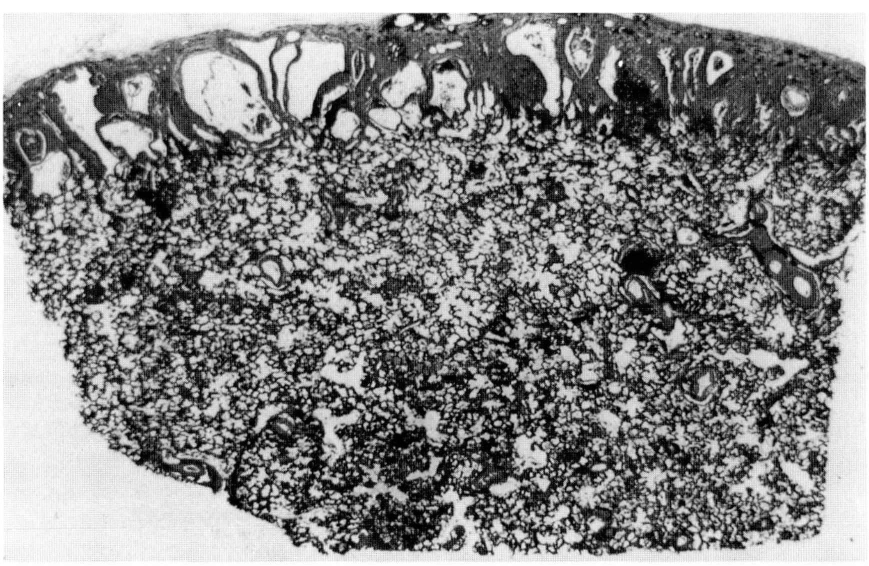

FIGURE 8-24. Subpleural cysts in a case of Down's syndrome (H&E, ×5).

Weinberg et al[29] suggested that the prominent hyperplastic epithelial component of the congenital cystic lesion within what is basically a sarcoma may mimic neoplastic epithelium leading to a diagnosis of pulmonary blastoma. Bove[32] pointed out that the metastatic lesions arising from these neoplasms contain only mesenchymal element. Therefore, it appears that many of the cases of "pulmonary blastoma" arising in these cystic lesions may in fact represent sarcomas. The commonest original cystic lesion in which the malignancy arose was CCAM.[27,28] In one case the sarcomatous change was diagnosed only after microscopic examination of the cystic lesion.[32] For this reason, the pulmonary cystic lesions should be adequately sampled for histologic examination. The risk of malignant change in pulmonary cystic lesion is low. However, the sarcomas arising in these lesions may take an aggressive course, metastasize, and prove to be fatal.[30,33] It is therefore advisable to resect a pulmonary cystic lesion, although the lesion may be asymptomatic at the time of diagnosis. Subsequent infection and compression of surrounding structures may also occur.

Another rare neoplastic lesion with cystic change occurring in the lung in children is the mesenchymal cystic hamartoma.[35] One of the five cases reported by Mark[35] was seen in a 1½-year-old child. Interestingly, systemic arterial supply may be present in mesenchymal cystic hamartoma. The mesenchymal cells of this lesion have hyperchromatic nuclei. Rare mitoses are present. Mark suggested that the lesion arises as a solid mass due to mesenchymal proliferation. The entrapped air passages, which become focally dilated, give the characteristic mixed cystic and solid appearance of the lesion. It is also possible that the mesenchymal proliferation occurs in a preexisting cystic lesion of the lung of a child. Thus mesenchymal cystic hamartoma, which takes an indolent course, may belong to the spectrum of neoplastic change in the congenital pulmonary cystic lesions.

EXAMINATION OF RESECTED SPECIMENS

The diagnosis of the precise type of pulmonary cystic lesion can be readily made in most of the cases. Details of clinical, radiologic, and operative findings should be available to the pathologist. In the gross examination the following features should be specifically looked for:

1. *Bronchial communication.* In the bronchus of the resected segment abnormalities such as stenosis, narrowing due to intrinsic factors such as granulation tissue or to extrinsic factors such as enlarged lymph nodes may be present on gross examination. Hypoplastic fragmented cartilage in the wall of the bronchus should be specifically looked for. These bronchial abnormalities will provide clues regarding the type of lesion. There may not be any bronchial connection with the resected lesion, or the portion of the bronchus showing the obstructive lesion may be left in the bronchial stump in the infant.
2. *Systemic arterial supply.* The surgeon will have ligated the systemic artery supplying the lesion. There may be more than one artery in rare instances. If there is any doubt about the identification of the systemic artery, the surgeon or the surgical resident should be consulted. Identification and histologic

documentation of the systemic arterial supply when present are essential aspects of pathologic study of these lesions.

3. It is recommended that formalin be injected in the cyst cavity after aspirating the cyst contents and the specimen fixed for several hours.
4. The number and size of cyst(s) present in the lesion should be described in the report. The classification of CCAM depends on the size and variations in the cysts.
5. Gross photographs to document the findings described above are recommended.
6. The septa of cysts should be examined carefully to see if there are any mural nodules.
7. Sections for histologic examination should be taken from the bronchus (e.g., to demonstrate abnormalities of the bronchial cartilage), from peribronchial lymph nodes when present, the artery supplying the lesion and the walls of the cyst(s) in the lesion. Multiple sections from different areas of the wall of the cyst(s) are recommended. Adequate sampling will ensure recognition of early neoplastic changes in the mesenchyme of the septum and presence of skeletal muscle in the cyst walls, e.g., in CCAM.
8. Radial alveolar count as outlined above should be done in cases of ILE due to polyalveolar lobe.

COMMENT

The cystic lesions described in this chapter may be encountered at autopsy or surgical pathology specimens. At autopsy, congenital anomalies of other organs that may be associated with these cystic lesions should be looked for. Anomalies of cardiovascular system (tetralogy of Fallot, ventricular septal defect, tricuspid atresia, etc.) have been reported in association with ILE.[36] Asplenia, cardiovascular anomalies (total anomalous pulmonary venous connection, aortic arch malformation, etc.), and renal malformation occur in association with congenital pulmonary lymphangiectasis. Strong association between CCAM type II and other congenital anomalies such as renal malformation and cardiac anomalies, etc. has been described.[36]

In rare instances advanced secondary changes such as infection, ulceration, and/or metaplasia occur in the lining epithelium and the wall of the cyst. The epithelium may be of nondescript cuboidal or flattened type. Thus, the original diagnostic features of the lesion may be obscured. Findings noted by the surgeon at the time of operation and radiologic studies may be helpful in the diagnosis. A diagnosis of pulmonary cystic lesion of undetermined type may have to be rendered in such instances if additional sections and surgical and radiologic findings also fail to reveal the identity of the lesion.

The terminology of and variations in PS can be confusing. The variations of PS and the recommended terminology are given in Table 8-2.

REFERENCES

1. Heithoff KB, Sane SM, Williams HJ, et al: Bronchopulmonary foregut malformations: A unifying etiological concept. *Am J Roentgenol* 126:46–55, 1976.

2. Clements BS, Warner JO: Pulmonary sequestration and related congenital bronchopulmonary vascular malformations: Nomenclature and classification based on anatomical and embryological considerations. *Thorax* 42:401–408, 1987.
3. Black TL, Fernandes ET, Wrenn EL Jr, et al: Extralobar pulmonary sequestration and mediastinal bronchogenic cyst. *J Pediatr Surg* 23:999–1001, 1988.
4. Bagwell CE, Schiffman RJ: Subcutaneous bronchogenic cysts. *J Pediatr Surg* 23:993–995, 1988.
5. Harmand D, Grosdidier J, Hoeffel JC: Multiple bronchogenic cysts of the esophagus. *Am J Gastroenterol* 75:321–323, 1981.
6. Young G, LHeureux PR, Krueckeberg ST, et al: Mediastinal bronchogenic cyst: Prenatal sonographic diagnosis. *Am J Roentgenol* 152:125–127, 1989.
7. Schwartz DB, Beals TF, Wimbish KJ, et al: Transbronchial fine needle aspiration of bronchogenic cysts. *Chest* 88:573–575, 1985.
8. Harrison MR, Adzick NS, Jennings RW, et al: Antenatal intervention for congenital cystic adenomatoid malformation. *Lancet* 336:965–968, 1990.
9. Benning TL, Godwin JD, Roggli VL, et al: Cartilaginous variant of congenital adenomatoid malformation of the lung. *Chest* 92:514–516, 1987.
10. Stocker JT, Madewell JE, Drake RM: Congenital cystic adenomatoid malformation of the lung. Classification and morphologic spectrum. *Hum Pathol* 8:155–171, 1977.
11. Fisher JE, Nelson SJ, Allen JE, et al: Congenital cystic adenomatoid malformation of the lung. A unique variant. *Am J Dis Child* 136:1071–1074, 1982.
12. Iancu T, Elian E, Lerner MA: Case report: Infantile sublobar emphysema and tracheal bronchus. *Acta Paediatr Scand* 64:551–554, 1975.
13. Hislop A, Reid L: New pathological findings in emphysema of childhood: 1. Polyalveolar lobe with emphysema. *Thorax* 25:682–690, 1970.
14. Azizkhan RG, Grimmer DL, Askin FB, et al: Acquired lobar emphysema (overinflation): Clinical and pathological evaluation of infants requiring lobectomy. *J Pediatr Surg* 27:1145–1152, 1992.
15. Emery JL, Mitual A: The number of alveoli in the terminal respiratory unit of man during late intrauterine life and childhood. *Arch Dis Child* 35:544–547, 1960.
16. Case Records of the Massachusetts General Hospital. Case 32-1990. *N Engl J Med* 33:398–408, 1989.
17. Pryce DM: Lower accessory pulmonary artery with intralobar sequestration of lung: A report of seven cases. *J Pathol* 58:457–467, 1946.
18. Stocker JT: Sequestrations of the lung. *Semin Diagn Pathol* 3:106–121, 1986.
19. Thilenius OG, Ruschhaupt DG, Replogle RL, et al: Spectrum of pulmonary sequestration: Association with anomalous pulmonary venous drainage in infants. *Pediatr Cardiol* 4:97–103, 1983.
20. Holder PD, Langston C: Intralobar pulmonary sequestration (a nonentity?). *Pediatr Pulmonol* 2:147–153, 1986.
21. Gebauer PW, Mason CB: Intralobar pulmonary sequestration associated with anomalous pulmonary vessels. A nonentity. *Dis Chest* 35:282–288, 1959.
22. Chitale AR: Gastric cyst of the mediastinum. A distinct clinicopathological entity. *J Pediatr* 75:104–110, 1969.
23. Stocker JT, Madewell JE: Persistent interstitial pulmonary emphysema: Another complication of the respiratory distress syndrome. *Pediatrics* 59:847–857, 1977.
24. Joshi VV, Kasznica J, Khan MAA, et al: Cystic lung disease in Down's syndrome: A report of two cases. *Pediatr Pathol* 5:79–86, 1986.
25. Stocker JT, McGill LC, Orsini EN: Postinfarction peripheral cysts of the lung in pediatric patients: A possible cause of idiopathic spontaneous pneumothorax. *Pediatr Pulmonol* 1:7–18, 1985.
26. Lawrence KM: Congenital pulmonary lymphangiectasis. *J Clin Pathol* 12:62–69, 1959.

27. Case Records of the Massachusetts General Hospital. Case 31-1989. *N Engl J Med* 321:309–316, 1989.
28. Ueda K, Gruppo R, Unger F, et al: Rhabdomyosarcoma of lung arising in congenital cystic adenomatoid malformation. *Cancer* 40:383–388, 1977.
29. Weinberg AG, Currarino G, Moore GC, et al: Mesenchymal neoplasia and congenital pulmonary cysts. *Pediatr Radiol* 9:179–182, 1980.
30. Krous HF, Senauer CL: Embryonal rhabdomyosarcoma arising within a congenital bronchogenic cyst. *J Pediatr Surg* 16:506–508, 1981.
31. Becroft D, Jagusch MF: Pulmonary sarcomas arising in mesenchymal cystic hamartomas. *Pediatr Pathol* 7:478, 1987.
32. Bove KE: Case 6: Sarcoma arising in pulmonary mesenchymal cystic hamartoma. *Pediatr Pathol* 9:785–792, 1989.
33. Holland-Moritt RM, Heyn RM: Pulmonary blastoma associated with cystic lesions in children. *Med Pediatr Oncol* 12:85–88, 1984.
34. Domizio P, Liesner RJ, Dicks-Mireaux C, et al: Malignant mesenchymoma associated with a congenital lung cyst in a child. Case report and review of the literature. *Pediatr Pathol* 10:785–797, 1990.
35. Mark EJ: Mesenchymal cystic hamartoma of the lung. *N Engl J Med* 315:1255–1259, 1986.
36. Stocker JT, Drake RM, Madewell JE: Cystic and congenital lung disease in the newborn. *Persp Pediatr Pathol* 4:93–154, 1978.

9 GLYCOGEN STORAGE DISEASE

INTRODUCTION

Glycogen storage disease (GSD) was first recognized in 1929 by von Gierke. The glycogen concentration of the tissues is increased in these disorders of metabolism. There may be a prominent involvement of liver and/or other tissues (e.g., muscle).[1,2] In 1952 the Coris detected glucose-6-phosphatase deficiency as the basic biochemical abnormality in one of the types of GSD.[1] Since until now about 20 different types of GSD have been recognized on the basis of defective enzymatic steps in the glycogen metabolism, the numerical designation originally based on chronologic sequence of enzyme identification is not feasible. Subtypes of certain types (e.g., six subtypes of type III) are also recognized. Numerous conflicting numbering systems have been used, which further adds to the confusion. For example, the numbering systems used by McAdams et al[4] and Greene[3] are different. GSD designated as type X by McAdams et al[4] is designated as type XI by Greene.[3] Therefore designation by the specific enzyme defect or by eponym is recommended (e.g., glucose-6-phosphatase deficiency for type I GSD). However, the terminology according to numerical types is still being used. The numerical system given by McAdams, et al[4] is used in this chapter for the sake of brevity and comparability with this definitive article in the pathology literature on GSD. The specific enzyme defect for each type is given in Table 10-1. GSD results from defects in the enzymes involved in glycogen metabolism. Most of these defects are located in the sequence that degrades glycogen to glucose-6-phosphate (G-6-P) or G-6-P to glucose. This results in excess of glycogen in liver and other tissues depending upon the type of GSD (Table 9-1). Most of the types manifest during infancy or childhood. Some may manifest in childhood or adulthood (e.g., type II and III) or usually in adulthood (e.g., type V). Most types of GSD are autosomal recessive conditions (a few subtypes are cross-linked recessive, e.g., GSD type IX-b).[2] The different types of GSD can be conveniently divided into liver types and muscle types.[2] The liver types include type O (due to glycogen synthetase deficiency), I (von Gierke's disease), III, IV, VI, VIII, and IX.

In the liver types hepatomegaly and hypoglycemia are the prominent clinical features. There may be progression to hepatic fibrosis or cirrhosis in some of these types. The muscle types in which cardiac and/or skeletal muscle are involved include types II (Pompe's disease), V and VII. In some of the types both liver and muscle are affected (types III, VII, etc.).

The clinical features and enzymatic defect in the better known types of GSD are given in Table 9-1.[3,4] Type I GSD, due to glucose-6-phosphatase deficiency (van Gierke's disease), is the most common type, accounting for about 25% of the

TABLE 9-1 Glycogen Storage Diseases Clinical and Biochemical Aspects

Type	Enzyme affected	Primary organs affected	Manifestations	Comment
0	Glycogen synthetase	Liver	Hypoglycemia, failure to thrive	Hepatic fibrosis occurs; prognosis is uncertain
I (von Gierke)	Glycose-6-phosphatase	Liver, kidney, intestine	↑ Liver and kidney, growth failure, hypoglycemia, lipemia, acidosis	Prototype of GSD; present in about 25% of cases of GSD
II (Pompe)	Lysosomal acid α-glucosidase	Skeletal muscle, heart, ↑ glycogen in all organs (e.g., brain)	Muscle weakness, cardiomegaly, ↑ liver, no hypoglycemia, hypoglycemia, CNS involvement	Death usually by 2 years
III	Amylo-1, 6-glucosidase (debrancher enzyme)	Liver, (muscle may be involved), WBCs	Marked ↑ liver, variable muscle weakness	Hepatic fibrosis and splenomegaly may occur
IV (Andersen)	Amylo-1, 4-1, 6-transglucosidase (branching enzyme)	Liver and other organs (e.g., brain)	↑ Liver, spleen, CNS involvement	Cirrhosis with death in childhood
V (McArdle)	Muscle phosphorylase	Skeletal muscle	Weakness after exercise	Good prognosis
VI	Liver phosphorylase	Liver, WBCs	Marked ↑ liver, mild hypo-glycemia	Good prognosis
VII	Phosphofructo-kinase	Muscle	Muscle weakness	Good prognosis
VIII	Liver phosphorylase	Liver, brain	↑ Liver, neurologic deterioration	Progression of neurologic deterioration
IX	Liver phosphorylase kinase	Liver, WBCs, RBCs	Marked ↑ liver, mild hypo-glycemia	Good prognosis
X	Cyclic AMP dependent kinase	Liver, muscle	↑ Liver	Good prognosis

Adapted from Green HL: *Sem Liver Dis* 2:291, 1982.

patients. It serves as the prototype of hepatic GSD. It is described in some detail below. Despite various enzyme defects, most patients with GSD do well when increased frequency of feedings is instituted to avoid hypoglycemia. Notable exceptions to this rule are patients with type IV GSD due to branching enzyme deficiency who develop cirrhosis and liver failure, type II GSD with severe cardiac involvement and patients with type I GSD who develop hepatic adenomas and adenocarcinomas.[3]

DIAGNOSIS OF GSD

Glycogen Content of Human Tissues

Limited data are available.[1] Usually the concentration of glycogen in the liver is less than 5–7 g per 100 g wet weight and in the muscle it is less than 2 g per 100 g wet weight. Accumulation of glycogen in the fetal liver commences in the last trimester of pregnancy. There is rapid fall in the neonatal period with increasing phosphorylase activity. Adult levels are reached by 2–3 weeks of age.

Tissue glycogen is affected by various conditions (e.g., fasting, exercise, glucose infusion, general nutritional status). Hyperalimentation alone cannot result in abnormally excessive deposition of liver glycogen.

Because of these variations, measurement of tissue glycogen content alone may not establish or rule out GSD except when abnormally high concentrations (or abnormal glycogen structure) are found. In certain types of GSD excessive glycogen is not present (e.g., type IV GSD). Demonstration of enzyme defect is essential for definitive diagnosis.

Morphologic Methods

The two main tissues that are used for diagnosis are liver and muscle. Although needle biopsy of liver can show characteristic morphologic changes, and certain biochemical assays can be done on a small sample of liver tissue by microtechnique,[5] an open-wedge biopsy is advisable since it gives adequate tissue for both morphologic (light microscopy in frozen section for fat stain, paraffin sections for other stains, and electron microscopy) and biochemical studies by the established method. At the time of open biopsy abdominal muscle can be biopsied through the same incision.

Liver Biopsy

The morphologic features of different types of GSD are given in Table 9-2.[4] Although morphologic features described by McAdams et al[4] are well established and can be helpful in distinguishing between different types of GSD and some degree of overlap of features such as nuclear glycogen, mosaic pattern, fatty change, and structure of glycogen by electron microscopy is seen in the different types.[6] Abundant amount of glycogen is demonstrated by PAS stains with and without diastase digestion (Figures 9-1–9-3). It should be noted that in type IV GSD there is accumulation of amylopectin, which is PAS-positive even after diastase digestion. Glycogen content in type IV is normal or reduced (Table 9-2). It is preferable to fix the liver biopsy specimen in alcohol for better preservation of glycogen. Frozen section should be done on a portion of the biopsy for fat stain if sufficient tissue is available. Electron-microscopic studies should be done. The mosaic pattern which is seen in a number of subtypes of GSD is produced by presence of distension of hepatocytes due to glycogen accumulation, distinctive cell borders, and collapse of sinusoids (Figure 9-1). The nuclear glycogenation produces a ground glass appearance of nuclei (Figure 9-4). PAS stain demonstrates diastase sensitive PAS-positive granules in the nuclei. Fatty change is seen as small vacuoles on the routine paraffin-embedded H&E-stained H&E-

TABLE 9-2 Glycogen Storage Diseases Pathologic Aspects

	Liver		Muscle	
Type	Light microscopy	Electron microscopy	Light microscopy	Electron microscopy
0	Glycogen is present (0.5% after meal)	—	—	—
I	Uniform distribution of glycogen with distention of liver cells, mosaic pattern, small and large fat vacuoles, nuclear glycogenation	Uniform increase in normal appearing glycogen, lipid droplets with glycogen particles within them	Normal	Normal
II	Uniform slight distention of liver cells, microvacuolation due to glycogen accumulation, nonmosaic pattern, fat absent	Glycogen vesicles surrounded by membranes (so-called lysosomes)	Marked glycogen deposition	Excessive glycogen (free and in vesicles), loss of myofibrils
III	Uniform distension of liver cells due to glycogen, mosaic pattern, nuclear glycogenation, fibrous septa formation, small droplets of fat	Same as type I (lipid vacuoles less frequent)	Normal or subsarcolemmal glycogen	Glycogen (subsarcolemmal and between myofibrils)
IV	Pale, amphophilic, hyaline or vacuolated, PAS-positive, diastase-resistant, material (amylopectin) particularly in periportal hepatocytes, variable, large lipid vacuoles, prominent septa formation progressing to cirrhosis	Fibrillar appearance of amylopectin	Amylopectin deposits	—
V	Normal	Normal	Subsarcolemmal glycogen	Same as in light microscopy

TABLE 9-2 Continued

	Liver		Muscle	
Type	Light microscopy	Electron microscopy	Light microscopy	Electron microscopy
VI	Nonuniform distention of hepatocytes due to glycogen, mosaic pattern, septa formation, small fat droplets	Burst appearance of glycogen, rosettes, lipid vacuoles with glycogen in them	Normal	Normal
VII	Not known	Not known	Subsarcolemmal glycogen	Same as in light microscopy
VIII	Nonuniform distention of hepatocytes due to glycogen, mosaic pattern	Same as in type VI, less frequent lipid vacuoles with glycogen in them	Normal	Normal
IX	Nonuniform distention of hepatocytes due to glycogen, mosaic pattern, septa formation, small lipid droplets	Same as in type VI, frequent lipid vacuoles with glycogen in them	Normal	Normal
X	Nonuniform distention of hepatocytes due to glycogen, mosaic pattern, septa formation, small lipid droplets	Same as in type VI	Subsarcolemmal glycogen	Same as in light microscopy

Adapted from McAdams AJ, et al: *Hum Pathol* 4:463, 1974.

stained sections (Figure 9-4) and small globules on the fat stain (Oil-Red-O, etc.) done on the frozen section. Fibrous septa formation with or without cirrhosis can be demonstrated effectively by the trichrome stain (Figure 9-5).

On electron microscopy the main finding is the presence of overabundant amount of glycogen displacing the organelles in the cytoplasm. The glycogen is in the form of rosettes (alpha particles). These glycogen particles show a frayed or burst appearance in certain types of GSD (Table 9-2). In type II GSD, the glycogen is present in the form of vesicles lined by membranes (so-called lysosomes). Lipid droplets are seen in some types of GSD. Glycogen may be present within the lipid droplets (Figure 9-6).

In the presence of characteristic morphologic features (Table 9-2, Figures 9-1–9-6), diagnosis of GSD and even the possible type can be suggested or strongly suspected. However, a definitive diagnosis cannot be made on morphologic grounds alone. The only possible exceptions are the electron microscopic

TABLE 9-3 Ultrastructural Changes in Metabolic Diseases

Abnormal quantities of normal metabolites
Glycogen storage diseases
High-density lipoprotein deficiency (Tangier's disease)—deposition of cholesterol ester and triglycerides
Various types of familial hyperlipoproteinemias with deposition of triglycerides, cholesterol
Abnormal quantities and abnormal location of normal metabolite
Glycogen storage disease (type II: lysosomal glycogen deposition)
Wolman's disease (accumulation of triglycerides and cholesterol in Kupffer cells and liver cells and macrophages in bone marrow)
Cholesterol ester storage disease (foam cells in the interstinal mucosa)
Ceroid lipofuscinosis (ceroid pigment, curvilinear bodies, or fingerprint pattern in various organs)
Hemochromatosis
Wilson's disease
Cystinosis
Accumulation of normal intermediate metabolites in abnormal amounts due to enzyme block
Diseases resulting from block in catabolism of sphingosides (gangliosidoses, Fabry's disease, metachromatic leukodystrophy, Gaucher's disease, Niemann–Pick's disease, etc.)
Accumulation of abnormal metabolites
Glycogen storage disease type IV (Amylopectinosis)
Amyloidosis
Ochronosis (alkaptonuria)
Adrenoleukodystrophy

Adapted from reference 28.

demonstration of characteristic lysosomal vacuoles containing glycogen in the uncultured amniotic cells in fetuses with type II GSD[7] and the characteristic morphologic features in type IV GSD (Table 9-2). But even in these cases, the diagnosis should be confirmed by biochemical studies on appropriate tissues (cultured amniotic cells and fetal liver if the pregnancy is terminated in type II and liver and/or muscle in type IV GSD). Fetal liver biopsy has also been used for prenatal diagnosis of GSD.[8]

MUSCLE BIOPSY

In certain types of GSD only the muscle is involved (e.g., types V and VII—Tables 9-1 and 9-2). The muscle biopsy fixed in alcohol shows abundant glycogen on PAS stain with and without diastase digestion (Figures 9-7, 9-8). Electron-microscopic examination shows abundant intermyofibrillar and/or subsarcolemmal glycogen (Figure 9-9). In type II GSD glycogen is present in the lysosomal vacuoles (Figure 9-10, Table 9-2). A portion of the muscle should be analyzed in the fresh or frozen state (depending on local availability of biochemical assays) for enzymatic activity.

Histochemical methods for demonstrating absence of phosphorylase activity in type V and phosphofructokinase activity in type VII by using frozen

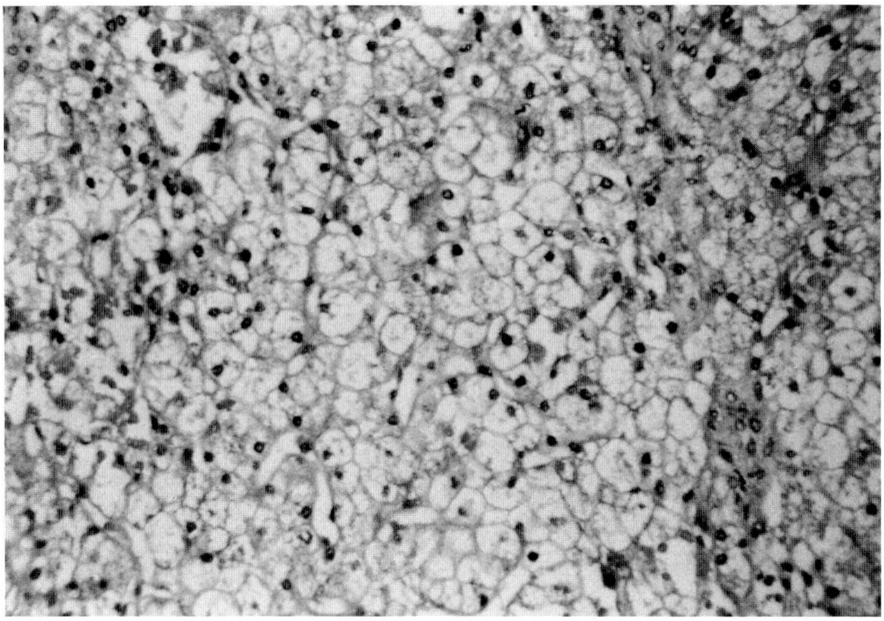

FIGURE 9-1. Note the swelling of hepatocytes with vacuolated and granular cytoplasm, distinct cell borders and collapse of sinusoids producing a mosaic pattern in type I GSD (H&E after alcohol fixation, ×100).

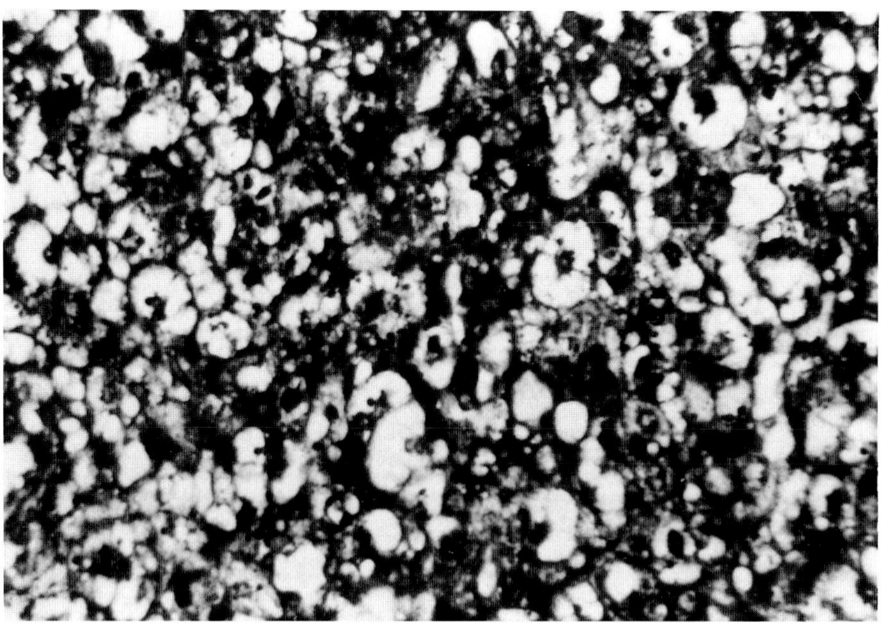

FIGURE 9-2. Note abundant amount of glycogen characterized by granular and diffuse darkly staining cytoplasm of hepatocytes in type I GSD (PAS stain without diastase digestion, ×250).

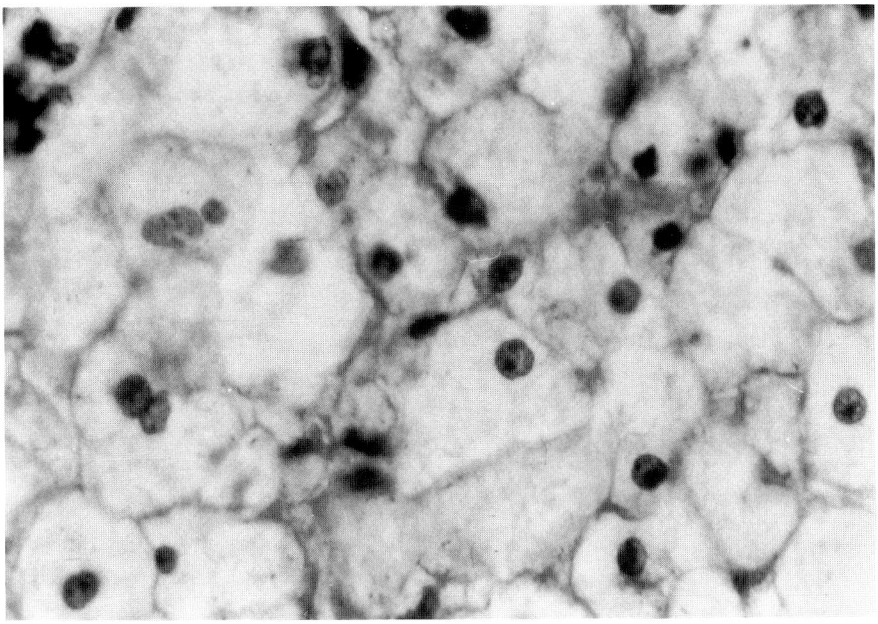

FIGURE 9-3. Same biopsy specimen as in Figure 10-2 showing total absence of the dark granular and diffuse staining of the hepatocytes (PAS stain after diastase digestion, ×400).

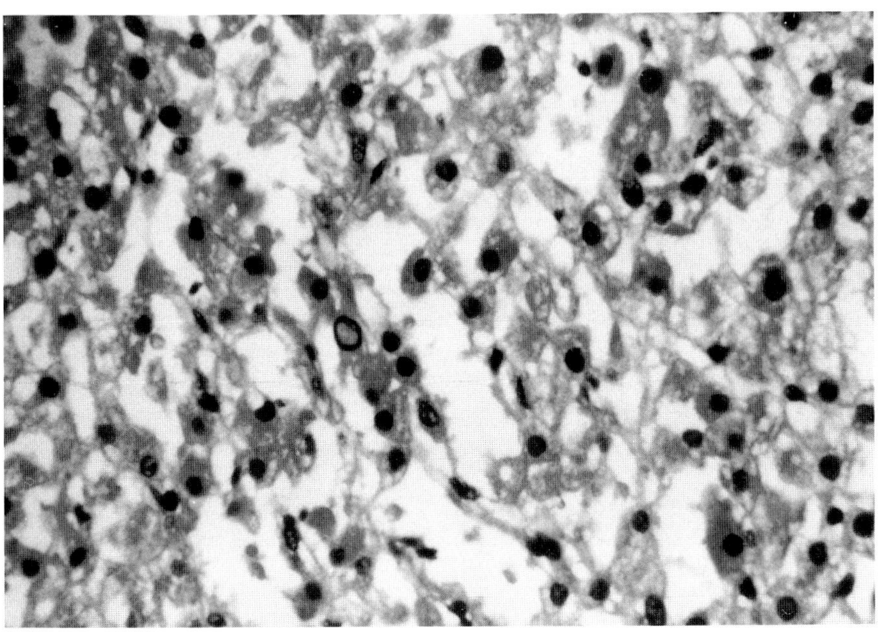

FIGURE 9-4. Nuclear glycogenation in type III GSD. Note the ground glass appearance of one of the nuclei. There are small (fat) vacuoles in the cytoplasm (H&E, ×100).

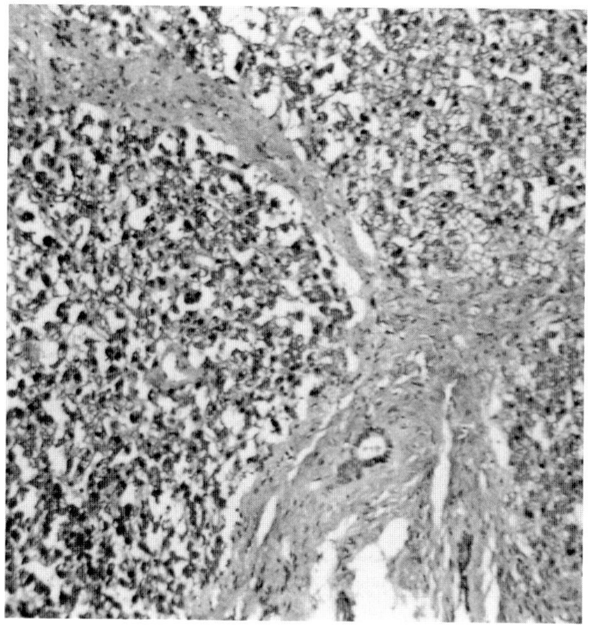

FIGURE 9-5. Fibrous septa formation in type IX GSD (trichrome stain, ×100).

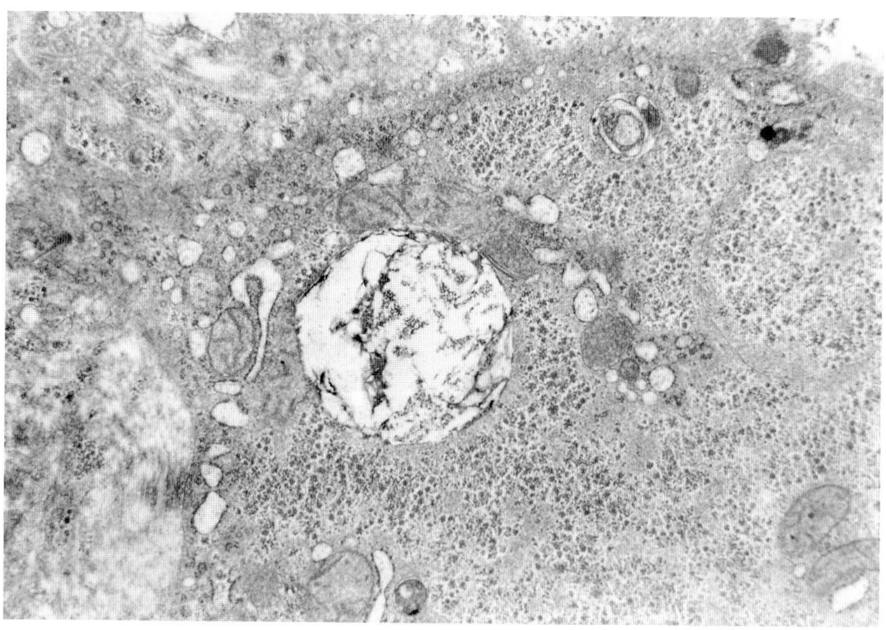

FIGURE 9-6. Abundant cytoplasmic glycogen in the form of rosettes (alpha particles) in the hepatocyte seen on ultrastructural examination of liver biopsy in type I GSD. Note also a lipid vacuole with glycogen within it (uranyl acetate and lead citrate, ×7100).

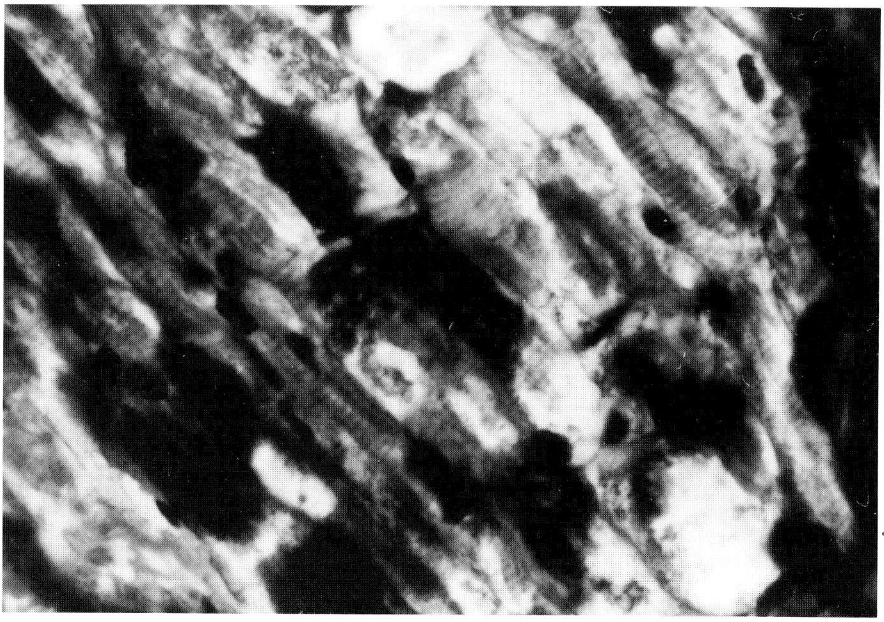

FIGURE 9-7. Muscle biopsy showing abundant glycogen seen as areas of dark staining in the cytoplasm of the muscle fibers in type II GSD (PAS stain without diastase digestion, ×400).

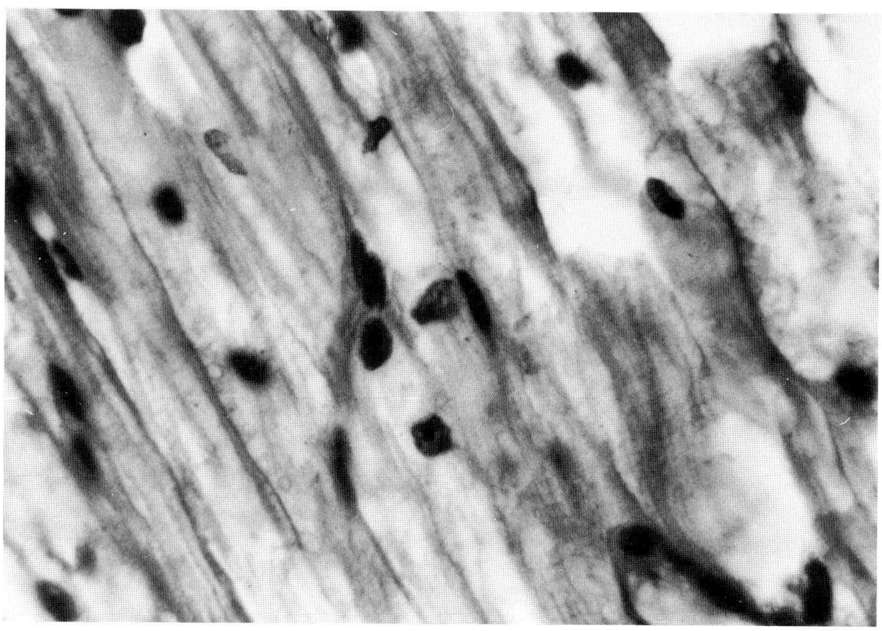

FIGURE 9-8. Same muscle biopsy as in Figure 9-7 showing absence of dark staining of the cytoplasm (PAS stain after diastase digestion, ×400).

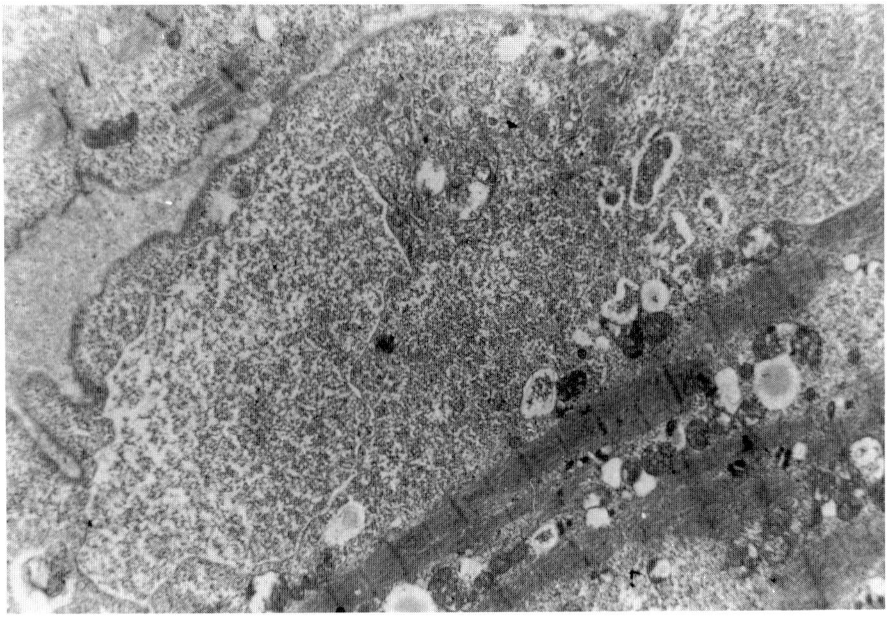

FIGURE 9-9. Muscle biopsy in type III GSD showing abundant subsarcolemmal free glycogen on ultrastructural examination (uranyl acetate and lead citrate, ×7100).

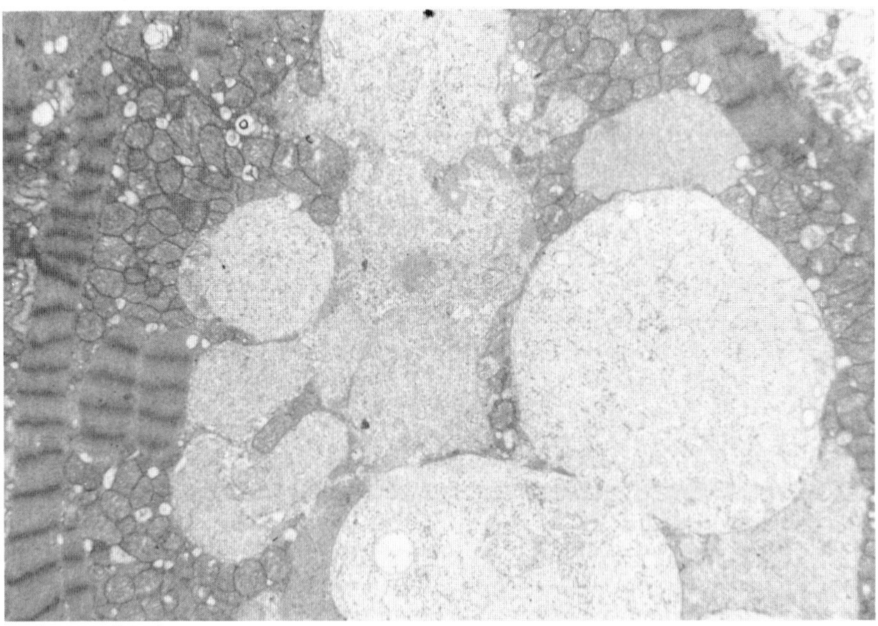

FIGURE 9-10. Muscle biopsy in type II GSD showing lysosomal vacuoles containing glycogen (uranyl acetate and lead citrate, ×7100).

sections of muscle biopsy have been described.[9,10] However, the final diagnosis is made by biochemical assays of the tissues.

BIOCHEMICAL METHODS

Final diagnosis of GSD is established by quantitative biochemical analysis of glycogen content and assays of various enzymes involved in glycogen metabolism demonstrating abnormally high concentrations of glycogen and deficiency of enzyme activity. The glycogen structure is also analyzed. Although ideally enzyme assays should be done on fresh, unfrozen, unfixed tissue, such conditions are not feasible when the assays are not available in the local institutions. A 1-cm^3 portion of fresh liver tissue is wrapped in aluminum foil and snap-frozen in liquid nitrogen. The biochemists recommend that OCT compound should not be used in the process of snap-freezing. A $1 \times 0.5 \times 0.5$ cm portion of fresh muscle tissue is snap-frozen in a similar manner. The snap-frozen specimens are then transported on dry ice to the reference laboratory by overnight mail.

OTHER MATERIALS USED FOR DIAGNOSIS

Peripheral leukocytes and skin fibroblasts can be used for biochemical assays in certain types of GSD (e.g., type II). As mentioned above, prenatal diagnosis can be made by biochemical assays on amniotic fluid cells in type II GSD. It is recommended that at least one confluent T75 flank along with a control culture be sent to the reference laboratory. The shipping of these samples should be at room temperature. Care should be taken to avoid freezing or overheating during transport.

GLYCOGEN STORAGE DISEASES OF VARIOUS TYPES

The clinical and laboratory and pathologic features and the diagnostic methods of various types of GSD are described below. They are summarized in Tables 9-1 and 9-2.

Type 0 GSD[11]

Clinical and Laboratory Features

Type 0 GSD is caused by deficiency of glycogen synthetase. Failure to grow and fasting hypoglycemia are the main features. Postprandial hyperglycemia and hyperlacticacidemia occur. Glycagon has no effect on fasting hypoglycemia.

Pathologic Features

Histologic features of liver biopsy in one of the two cases described by Lewis et al[12] were as follows. Despite the complete inactivity of glycogen synthetase in the liver, a small amount of glycogen was present in the liver. There was no evidence of necrosis or fibrosis. Quantitative determination of glycogen showed it to be 0.5% in the liver. The muscle glycogen was normal.

Diagnosis

It is established by demonstrating the enzyme deficiency in liver, muscle, and red blood cells.

Type I GSD

There is glucose-6-phosphatase (GSPS) deficiency in type I GSD. GSPS is an enzyme complex consisting of five different polypeptides: GSPS with its active site on the luminal aspect of the endoplasmic reticulum, a regulatory stabilizing calcium-binding protein, and three transport proteins T1, T2, and T3, which enable G-6-P, phosphate, and glucose respectively to get across the endoplasmic reticulum.[13] Deficiency of GSPS itself is labeled as type Ia, that of T1 as type Ib, and that of T2 as type Ic. T3 deficiency has not been described yet. It is presumptively labeled as type Id.[13] The clinical outcome in all these subtypes is similar.

The child presents with hepatomegaly, fasting hypoglycemia, lactic acidosis, short stature, hyperlipidemia, hyperuricemia, and renal enlargement. These metabolic abnormalities explain the occurrence of xanthomas on the skin of extensor surfaces of the skin and gouty tophi in these patients. It is of interest that in a series of 38 cases of sudden infant death syndrome, raised hepatic glycogen and deficiency of GSPS or of transport protein T2 was found in 10 infants.[13]

Mechanism of Hyperlacticacidemia[11]

The liver, which normally converts lactic acid produced mainly by muscle and red blood cells to glucose, cannot do so. On the other hand, the liver itself produces large amounts of lactic acid because glycogen, galactose, fructose, and gluconeogenic amino acids, which are normally converted to glucose, are converted to lactic acid. Glucose itself is also converted to lactic acid because of the interruption of the reaction glucose to glucose-6-phosphate.

Mechanism of Lipid Abnormalities[11]

Because of hypoglycemia, the peripheral tissues are in a "fasting" state. Therefore there is release of large amounts free fatty acids and glycerol from the fatty tissue. Esterification of these free fatty acids to triglycerides occurs in the liver. These triglycerides are exported as very-low-density lipoproteins (VLDL). The increased VLDL formation explains the high levels of triglycerides, phospholipids, and cholesterol.

Mechanism of Hyperuricemia[11]

There is competitive inhibition of renal tubular secretion of urate by lactate, which is present in large amounts type I GSD. Increase in purine synthesis is also a factor in hyperuricemia.

Therapy

Continuous nocturnal nasogastric feeding with high glucose formula and use of uncooked starch during daytime have given remarkable therapeutic results.

Morphologic Lesions in GSD—Type I

Besides the glycogen accumulations in the liver and other organs (kidneys), xanthomas of the skin, and gouty tophi, the following lesions have been reported in GSD:

1. *Hepatic adenomas.* Patients with GSD type I are prone to develop hepatic adenomas. These lesions are detected on ultrasound, CT, or radioisotope scans. Biopsies may be obtained for diagnosis. Poe and Snover[14] have described histologic features in adenomas seen in two patients (27- and 26-year-old males) in whom the livers were resected before hepatic transplantation was done. Multiple nodules were present in the liver. Histologically fatty change, Mallory's hyaline and lamellar fibrosis were present in the adenomas.
2. *Hepatocellular carcinoma.* Malignant transformation of hepatic adenomas has been described.[1,15] On the other hand regression of hepatic "adenomas" can occur with institution of intensive dietary therapy.[16] The diagnosis of hepatic "adenomas" in such instances was made by radioisotope scan and not by pathologic methods. The hepatic filling defects may have been areas of focal nodular hyperplasia. Early institution of dietary therapy may also be effective in prevention of these hepatic lesions.
3. *Renal lesions in type I GSD.* Renal enlargement occurs due to glycogen accumulation. However normal renal function is found in these patients during childhood. Chen et al[17] found that in older patients 13–47 years of age) renal dysfunction may be present (proteinuria, hematuria, hypertension, altered creatinine clearance). Renal biopsies done in three patients after an average of 10 years of proteinuria showed focal segmental glomerulosclerosis (Figure 9-11) in various stages of progression. The pathogenesis of the glomerulosclerosis is probably related to the glomerular hyperfiltration.[18]

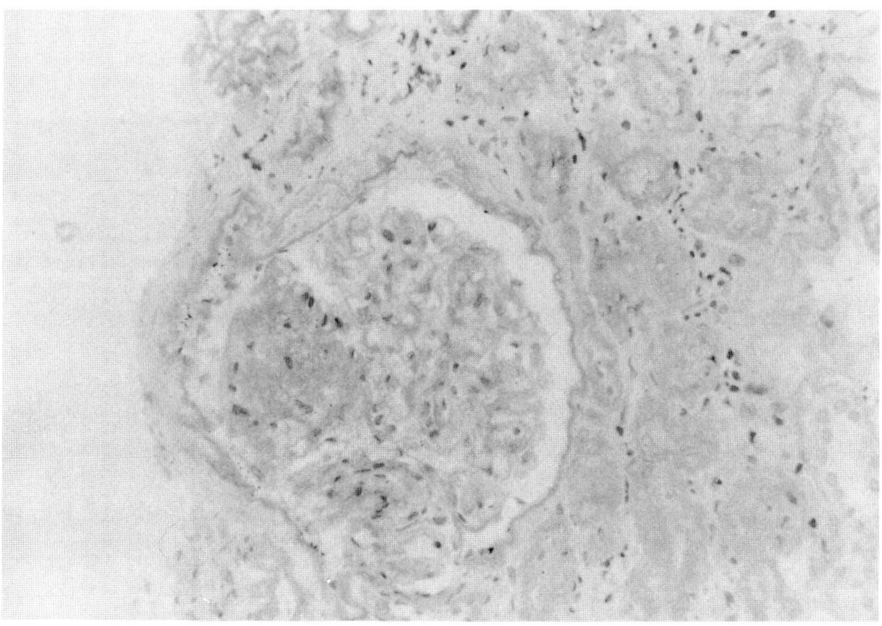

FIGURE 9-11. Renal biopsy in type I GSD showing focal glomerulosclerosis (PAS stain, ×250).

Type II GSD (Pompe's Disease)[11]

Clinical Features

Type II GSD is caused by lysosomal acid α-glucosidase. Functional impairment is seen primarily in the heart, skeletal muscle, and nervous system. The infantile form is characterized by defective motor activity, respiratory difficulty, and cardiac failure. Cardiomegaly and progressive general muscular weakness (in the face of a large muscle mass) are characteristically seen. There is hepatomegaly without liver dysfunction. Death from cardiac failure is seen in the first year of life. Difficulty in walking is usually the first manifestation in the late infantile or juvenile forms. The adult form of disease is seen in the second or third decade. There is girdle myopathy beginning at the lower limbs.

Pathologic Features

Cardiomegaly (≤10 times normal) with thickened ventricular walls is the major finding. Increased amount of glycogen is freely dispersed in the cytoplasm of the affected cells (liver, skeletal and cardiac muscle, kidney, skin, cultured fibroblasts, and nervous system) and is also present in the lysosomal vacuoles (Figure 9-10).

Diagnosis

Determination of acid-α-glucosidase in the muscle, liver, or leukocytes establishes the diagnosis. As mentioned above, prenatal diagnosis by ultrastructural demonstration of glycogen containing lysosomal vacuoles in the amniotic cells, followed by the demonstration of the specific enzyme deficiency, has been reported.[7]

Type III GSD (Forbes Disease)[11]

Clinical and Laboratory Features

Type III GSD is caused by deficiency of amylo-1, 6-glucosidase deficiency. The onset is usually between one month and one year of age. Hepatomegaly is a constant feature. Muscle weakness appears in adult life in some patients. The heart may be affected clinically and cardiac failure with death may occur. Low fasting glycemia, hypertriglyceridemia, and hypercholesterolemia are frequently present. The liver function tests are abnormal.

Diagnosis

Abnormally high glycogen content and deficiency of amylo-1, 6-glucosidase can be demonstrated in red blood cells, liver, or muscle. Abnormal structure of glycogen (short outer branch points) is also characteristic of the disease. Two subtypes are recognized: (1) IIIA with deficiency of enzyme in both the liver and muscle and (2) IIIB with deficiency in either liver or muscle.

Pathologic Features

The fibrous septa formation seen in the liver (Table 9-2) may progress to liver cirrhosis.[4] The lipid vacuoles seen in the liver on electron microscopy are smaller and less numerous as compared to these in GSD type I.

Type IV GSD (Amylopectinosis, Andersen Disease)[11]

Clinical and Laboratory Features

Type IV GSD is caused by deficiency of branching enzyme. The onset of the disease is usually at a few months of age. There is progressive hepatosplenomegaly, which subsequently leads to cirrhosis and its sequelae. Poor neuromuscular development and hypotonia are present. An abnormally low blood level of glucose is rarely seen. The disease proves to be fatal usually in early childhood.

Pathologic Features

Diastase-resistant periodic acid-Schiff-positive amylopectin-like material is present in the hepatocytes and peripheral lymphocytes.[19] The glycogen concentration of liver is ≤5%. Ultrastructural studies reveal fibrillar configuration of the amylopectin-like material. The diagnosis can be strongly suspected on the basis of morphologic features.

Diagnosis

Demonstration of abnormal glycogen structure and of deficiency of branching enzyme in muscle, leukocytes, and cultured fibroblasts establishes the diagnosis. Prenatal diagnosis can be made by studying the amniotic cells.

Type V GSD (McArdle Disease)[11]

Clinical Features

Type V GSD is caused by deficiency of skeletal muscle phosphorylase. The disease has its onset usually in second or third decade. Exercise intolerance is the main symptom.

Pathologic Features

There is excessive amount of glycogen in the muscle. Excess of glycogen in the subsarolemmal and interfibrillar spaces can be demonstrated by electron microscopy. Myofibrillar disorganization is also present.

Diagnosis

The diagnosis is established by demonstrating the enzymatic defect by histochemical[9] and biochemical methods.

Type VI GSD (Hers' Disease)[11]

Clinical Features

Type VI GSD is caused by liver phosphorylase deficiency. There is mild hepatomegaly without hyperlacticacidemia and hyperurecemia.

Pathologic Features

Fibrous septa formation may lead to cirrhosis. Adenomas and hepatocellular carcinomas have been described as sequelae.

Diagnosis

Deficiency of the enzyme can be demonstrated in liver biopsy, leukocytes, or erythrocytes.

Type VII GSD (Tarui Disease)[11]

Clinical Features

Type VII GSD is caused by deficiency of muscle phosphofructokinase. Easy fatigability is the main clinical feature. The disease has its onset during childhood. Recurrent jaundice may occur.

Pathologic Features

There is increased amount of subsarcolemmal and intermyofibrillar glycogen. Diastase-resistant PAS-positive material having a filamentous ultrastructure similar to that seen in type IV GSD may be present in muscle fibers.[20] It is not known whether this abnormal polysaccharide represents an undetected additional enzyme deficiency.

Diagnosis

The enzyme deficiency can be demonstrated in the muscle by biochemical and histochemical methods. Leukocytes and fibroblasts also lack the enzyme.

Type VIII GSD[3]

Clinical and Laboratory Features

Type VIII GSD is caused by deficiency of liver phosphorylase. Hepatomegaly and progressive neurologic deterioration (ataxia, hypotonia followed by spasticity, decerebration) are seen from early childhood. Blood glucose level and response to glucagon are normal.

Pathologic Features

The distension of hepatocytes by glycogen accumulation is uneven, resulting in "localized mosaics."[3] There is excessive amount of glycogen in the giant alpha form in the axon cylinders and synaptic vesicles. Brain biopsy findings can be considered as strongly suspicious of GSD type VIII since alpha particles of glycogen are not normally present in the central nervous system.

Diagnosis

The diagnosis is established by demonstration of the enzyme deficiency in the liver tissue by biochemical methods.

Type IX GSD[3]

Clinical and Laboratory Data

Type IX GSD is caused by deficiency of liver phosphorylase kinase. Marked hepatomegaly is present. There is a tendency to mild hypoglycemia. Prognosis is good.

Pathologic Features

Unevenness in the hepatocellular distension, due to variable glycogen deposition, is seen as in type VIII. There is septa formation. On electron microscopy the lipid vacuoles with glycogen inclusion tend to be more frequent than in type VI and X GSD.[3]

Diagnosis

The diagnosis is established by the deficiency of the enzyme in the liver tissue.

Type X GSD[3]

Clinical and Laboratory Features

Type X GSD is caused by deficiency of cyclic-AMP-dependent kinase. Hepatomegaly is the main clinical feature. Hypoglycemia is not seen. But response to glucagon administration is defective.

Pathologic Features

Irregularity of hepatocellular distension due to glycogen accumulation is seen.[3] There is also an increased amount of subsarcolemmal and intermyofibrillar glycogen in the muscle.

Diagnosis

The diagnosis is established by demonstration of deficient activity of cyclic-AMP-dependent kinase in liver or muscle.

CEREBRAL GLYCOGENOSIS

The central nervous system (CNS) may be involved in type II (Pompe's disease), type IV (Andersen's disease), and type VIII GSD (Table 9-1). Increased amount of lysosomal glycogen and intracytoplasmic amylopectin can be demonstrated in the brain in types II and IV GSD, respectively. In addition to these two well-defined types of GSD, CNS is also involved in an ill-defined type of presumed GSD labeled as cerebral glycogenosis.[21] The glycogen that is present in the neurites and astrocytic processes produces a vacuolated appearance. Cerebral cortex, deep nuclei, and cerebellar cortex are primarily involved. PAS stain with and without diastase confirms the presence of glycogen in the CNS. Ultrastructural examination shows that the glycogen is in the form of alpha particles (rosettes). A vast amount of glycogen (as much as 100 times the normal amount) can be demonstrated on biochemical analysis of the brain. The enzyme analysis was not done in the reported cases of cerebral glycogenesis. It is presumed that there was deficiency of brain glycogen phosphorylase.[21] The heart showed increased glycogen content. The glycogen content of liver, muscle and kidney was normal.

LIVER BIOPSY IN METABOLIC DISORDERS OTHER THAN GSD

Although biochemical analysis of tissue or blood cells to demonstrate the accumulated metabolite and/or the specific enzyme deficiency gives the definitive final diagnosis, light and electron microscopic study of liver biopsy can be used to obtain supportive evidence in various metabolic disorders besides GSD. Pathologic changes in the liver occur in a large variety of metabolic disorders involving porphyrin, carbohydrates (e.g., galactosemia), glycoprotein (e.g., mucolipidoses, α-antitrypsin deficiency), aminoacid (e.g., tyrosinemia), lipid (e.g., Gaucher's disease), and metals (e.g., Wilson's disease) and in miscellaneous conditions such as peroxisomal disorders (e.g., Zellweger's syndrome). The reader is referred to reference 22 for a detailed discussion of the different disorders, but the more important ones in children are sphingolipidoses (Gaucher's disease, etc.), gangliosidoses (Sandoff's disease), Wolman's disease, mucopolysaccharidoses (Hurler's syndrome, etc.), mucolipidoses, neonatal iron storage disease, α-antitrypsin deficiency, galactosemia, and cystic fibrosis.

OTHER TISSUES USED FOR DIAGNOSIS OF METABOLIC DISEASES

Light- and electron-microscopic studies and biochemical assays can also be done on a variety of other tissues besides liver. Brief outline is given below since detailed discussion is outside the scope of this chapter. The reader is referred to the articles given in the list of references.

1. *Skin.* Ultrastructural abnormalities are seen in the fibroblasts, histiocytes, and endothelial cells in a number of lysosomal storage disorders.[23]
2. *Conjunctiva.* Biopsy of upper bulbar conjunctiva can be relatively readily done under local anesthesia. It is used in a number of lysosomal storage disorders as the skin biopsy.[24]
3. *Intestine.* Rectal biopsy to demonstrate changes in neurons of nerve plexuses used for diagnosis of neurometabolic diseases in childhood (gangliosidoses, Batten's disease, etc.) may be a good alternative to brain biopsy.[25]
4. *Peripheral nerve biopsy.* This may be useful in the diagnosis of leukodystrophies, in Fabry and Niemann-Pick diseases and in ceroid lipofuscinosis.
5. *Muscle biopsy.* This has been used in the diagnosis of some lipodoses and ceroid lipofuscinosis.
6. *Peripheral lymphocytes.* These have been used for ultrastructural studies for the diagnosis of neuronal ceroid lipofuscinosis.[26] It is of interest to note that enzyme assays in WBCs have been used in the diagnosis of disorders such as Maple syrup urine disease, methylmalonic aciduria, some types of GSD, etc. Enzymatic or phenotypic abnormalities are seen in WBCs and RBCs in about 35 different metabolic disorders.
7. *Bone marrow biopsy.* This may also be used since many different types of cells are available for examination.
8. *Brain biopsy.* This is used only when there is severe neurologic deterioration and no other method of diagnosis is available.
9. *Amniotic cells.* Ultrastructural observations can be made on cultured amniotic cells besides enzymatic assay and chromosomal studies for prenatal diagnosis. Antenatal diagnosis has been made by using the approach in GSD types I and II, Gaucher's disease, mucopolysaccharidoses, etc. Electron microscopic studies on tissues of fetuses can also be rewarding in some of the metabolic disorders (e.g., Niemann–Pick disease).
10. *Cartilage–bone biopsy.* This has been used for light and microscopic studies and biochemical analysis for diagnosis of disorders of skeletal development such as osteogenesis imperfecta, mucopolysaccharidosis, and metaphyseal chondrodysplasia.[27]

Additional general articles on pathology and laboratory detection of metabolic diseases are given in references 28–32.

REFERENCES

1. Howell RR, Williams JC: The glycogen storage diseases. In *The metabolic basis of inherited disease*, 5th ed. (Stanbury JB, Wyndgarden JB, Fredrickson DS, et al, Eds). McGraw-Hill, New York, 1983, Chap 6, pp 141–166.
2. Sidbury JB: The glycogenosis. In *Pediatrics*, 18th ed. (Rudolph AM, Ed). Appleton & Lange, Norwalk, CT, 1987, pp 270–273.
3. Greene HL: Glycogen storage disease. *Sem Liver Dis* 2:291–301, 1982.
4. McAdams AJ, Hug G, Bove KE: Glycogen storage disease. Types I to X. *Hum Pathol* 4:463–487, 1974.
5. Burchell A, Hume R, Burchell B: A new microtechnique for the analysis of the human hepatic microsomal glucose-6-phosphatase system. *Clin Chem Acta* 173:183–192, 1988.
6. Jevon GP, Finegold MJ: Glycogen storage diseases of the liver: Reliability of diagnostic criteria. *Mod Pathol* 5:6P, 1992 (abstract).
7. Hug G, Soukup S, Ryan M, et al: Rapid prenatal diagnosis of glycogen storage disease type II by electron microscopy of uncultured amniotic cells. *N Engl J Med* 310:1018–1022, 1984.
8. Golbus MS, Simpson TJ, Koresawa M, et al: The prenatal determination of glycose-6-phosphatase activity by fetal liver biopsy. *Prenat Diagn* 8:401–404, 1988.
9. Takeuchi T: Histochemical detection of phosphorylase in animal tissues. *J Histochem Cytochem* 3:153–160, 1955.
10. Bonilla E, Shotland DL: The histochemical diagnosis of muscle phosphofructokinase deficiency. *Arch Neurol* 22:8–12, 1970.
11. Hers HG, Van Hoof F, de Barsy T: Glycogen storage disease. In *The metabolic basis of inherited disease*, 6th ed (Scriver CR, Beaudet AL, Sly WS, Eds). McGraw-Hill, New York, 1989, Chap 12, pp 425–452.
12. Lewis GM, Spencer-Peet J, Stewart KM: Infantile hypoglycemia due to inherited deficiency of glycogen synthetase in liver. *Arch Dis Child* 38:40–48, 1963.
13. Burchell A, Bell JE, Busuttil A, et al: Hepatic microsomal glycose-6-phophatase system and sudden infant death syndrome. *Lancet* 2:291–294, 1989.
14. Poe R, Snover DE: Adenomas in glycogen storage disease type I: Two cases with unusual histologic features. *Am J Surg Pathol* 12:477–483, 1988.
15. Zangeneh F, Limbeck GA, Brown BI, et al: Hepatorenal glycogenosis (type I glycogenosis) and carcinoma of the liver. *J Pediatr* 74:73–78, 1969.
16. Parker P, Burr I, Slonim A, et al: Regression of hepatic adenomas in type I a glycogen storage disease with dietary therapy. *Gastroenterol* 81:534–536, 1981.
17. Chen YT, Coleman RA, Scheinman JI, et al: Renal disease in type I glycogen storage disease. *N Engl J Med* 318:7–11, 1988.
18. Baker L, Dahlem S, Goldfarb S, et al: Hyperfiltration and renal disease in glycogen storage disease, type I. *Kidney Int* 35:1345–1350, 1989.
19. Penchansky L, Agostini RM, Jaffe R: Leukocyte inclusions in glycogen storage disease, type IV. *Pediatr Pathol* 12:903–905, 1992.
20. Agamanolis DP, Askavi AD, Mauro SD, et al: Muscle phosphofructokinase deficiency: Two cases with unusual polysaccharide accumulation and immunologically active enzyme protein. *Musc Nerve* 3:456–467, 1980.
21. Towfighi T, Yoss BS, Wasiewski WW, et al: Cerebral glycogenosis, alpha particle type: Morphologic and biochemical observations in an infant. *Hum Pathol* 20:1210–1215, 1989.
22. Ishak KG, Sharp HL: In *Metabolic errors and liver disease in pathology of liver*, 2nd ed (MacSween RNM, Anthony PP, Scheuer PJ, Eds). Churchill Livingstone, Edinburgh, 1987, pp 99–180.

23. O'Brien JS, Bernett J, Veath ML, et al: Lysosomal storage disorder diagnosis by ultrastructural examination by skin biopsy specimens. *Arch Neurol* 32:592–599, 1975.
24. Libert J: Diagnosis of lysosomal storage diseases by the ultrastructural study of conjunctival biopsies. *Pathol Annu* 15:37–66, 1980.
25. Brett EM, Lake BD: Reassessment of rectal approach to neuropathology in childhood. *Arch Dis Child* 50:753–762, 1975.
26. Baumann RJ, Markesbery WR: Juvenile amaurotic idiocy (neuronal ceroid lipofuscinosis) and lymphocyte fingerprint profiles. *Ann Neurol* 4:531–536, 1978.
27. Engfeldt B, Hjerpe A, Mengarelli S, et al: Morphologic and biochemical analysis of biopsy specimens in disorders of skeletal development. *Acta Pediatr Scand* 71:353–363, 1982.
28. Applegarth DA, Dimmick JE, Toone JR: Laboratory detection of metabolic disease. *Pediatr Clin N Am* 36:49–65, 1989.
29. Byers PH, Barsh GS, Holbrook KA: Molecular pathology in inherited disorders of collagen metabolism. *Hum Pathol* 13:89–95, 1982.
30. Volk BW, Adachi M, Schneck L: The pathology of sphingolipidoses. *Semin Hematol* 9:317–348, 1972.
31. Goldfischer S, Reddy JK: Peroxisomes (microbodies) in cell pathology. *Int Rev Exp Pathol* 26:46–84, 1984.
32. Johannessen JV: *Electron microscopy in human medicine.* Vol 2; *Cellular physiology, metabolic and storage diseases.* McGraw-Hill, New York, 1978, Chap 8, pp 159–214.

10 PATHOLOGY OF TUMORS IN CHILDREN: GENERAL ASPECTS

INTRODUCTION

In the lecture "The Challenge to Man of the Neoplastic Cell" that Dr. Peyton Rous presented when he was awarded the Nobel prize in medicine in 1966, he said: "Tumors destroy man in a unique and appalling way, as flesh of his own flesh, which has somehow been rendered proliferative, rampant, predatory, and ungovernable. They are the most concrete and formidable of human maladies, yet despite more than 70 years of experimental study they remain the least understood. This is all the more remarkable because they can be evoked at will for scrutiny by any one of the myriad chemical and physical means which are left behind as the tumors grow. These had acted merely as initiators. Few situations are more exasperating to the inquirer than to watch a tiny nodule form on a rabbit's skin at a spot from which the chemical agent inducing it has long since been gone, and to follow the nodule as it grows, and only too often becomes a destructive, epidermal cancer. What can be the reason for these happendings?" In recent times, the Rous sarcoma virus has been characterized as a retrovirus and significant progress has been made in the understanding of mechanism of cancer. Discovery of oncogenes has started a new era. Investigations concerning the tumor suppressor gene, Rb in retinoblastomas and the oncogene, N-myc in neuroblastomas have contributed to our understanding of pediatric cancer with respect to oncogenesis and prognosis.

Dramatic progress has also been made in the therapy of pediatric malignancies. It is a matter of particular pride to pediatric pathologists that the modern era of chemotherapy of cancer and of pediatric oncology was ushered in by Dr. Sidney Farber, Pathologist-in-Chief at the Children's Hospital in Boston. In 1948 Dr. Farber and his colleagues reported temporary remission in children with acute leukemia by treatment with the folic acid antagonist—aminopterin.[1] Earlier Dr. Farber and his colleagues had observed an acceleration of leukemic process in bone marrow and different organs in children with leukemia who were given folic acid conjugates.[2] Therefore, it appeared logical to him to explore the possible beneficial effect of the folic acid antagonists made available through the research effort of Dr. Subbarow and his colleagues. Farber and his colleagues took further steps in chemotherapy of cancer by administering actinomycin D to children with Wilms' tumor.[3] Actinomycin D was discovered by Dr. Selman Waksman, who won the Nobel prize for the discovery of streptomycin. (The person who first isolated streptomycin was his graduate student, Allbert Schatz, who won an out-of-court settlement over rights to royalties on streptomycin.)

Since these initial observations, tremendous progress has been made in therapy of cancer in children. The improvement in survival in children with cancer in 1990s is in the range of 60–90% as compared with the preceding era for different types of cancers. Through 1965–1979 the decline in mortality rates compared with those expected in 1950 from cancer of various types in children is as follows: 50% for leukemia and bone tumors and 32%, 68%, and 80% for non-Hodgkin's lymphoma, renal tumors, and Hodgkin's disease, respectively.[4] Thus about 60% of all children who are diagnosed to have cancer can expect to be cured of their disease.[5] This improvement in survival is due primarily to a systematic multidisciplinary multiinstitutional approach to development of optimally effective therapeutic protocols employing surgery, chemotherapy, and radiation therapy. However, it needs to be recognized that a systematic and detailed pathologic study of pediatric tumors with emergence of prognostic morphologic classification (e.g., for rhabdomyosarcoma and Wilms' tumor), recognition of new entities requiring less or more aggressive therapy (e.g., conventional type of mesoblastic nephroma and clear cell sarcoma of kidney, respectively), and accurate pathologic staging have also contributed significantly to the improved survival.

The novel cooperative and coordinated multiinstitutional and multidisciplinary approach to study and management of human cancer was pioneered in 1955 by pediatric oncologists with the establishment of Children's Cancer Study Group A, currently known as Children's Cancer Study Group (CCG). The other major national study groups for pediatric tumors include Pediatric Oncology Group (POG), National Wilms' Tumor Study (NWTS), Intergroup Rhabdomyosarcoma Study (IRS), and Intergroup Ewing's Sarcoma Study (IESS). In Europe, the Societe Internationale d'Oncologie Pediatrique (SIOP) was established.[6]

These national studies involve several institutions from North America (and some from Europe). Medical personnel of various disciplines include pediatrician, pediatric oncologist, pediatric surgeon (general, urologic, neurologic, and orthopedic surgeons), pediatric pathologist, radiation therapist, geneticist, oncology nurse, psychologist, and rehabilitationist. The national studies mentioned above have accomplished systematic collection of data on various aspects of a large number of cases of pediatric cancer. Conscientious participation of the pathologists in these studies and their cooperation in sending pathologic materials to the pathology centers for various childhood tumors made the systematic collection of pathologic data possible. The large number of cases have enabled meaningful statistical analysis of effectiveness of one therapeutic protocol versus another or of prognostic significance of clinical, pathologic, and biologic markers. Thus the national studies have made possible something that no single investigator or a small group of investigators of pediatric cancer would ever have achieved. The multidisciplinary team approach has also played a vital role in the successful therapy of pediatric cancer.[7] With current therapy it is estimated that in 1990s one of every 1000 children reaching the age of 20 in United States will be a survivor of childhood cancer. In recent years, these national groups have also initiated basic scientific research in pediatric oncology.

INCIDENCE

The incidence of cancer in children less than 15 years of age is 124.5 per million children per year for whites and 97.8 for blacks.[8] Thus there are about 6600 new cases of pediatric cancer every year in the United States. This number, which is small when compared with about 900,000 new cases of cancer in adults every year, reflects the necessity of a national cooperative approach for collecting data on large numbers of pediatric cancer cases for meaningful statistical analysis. Cancer, despite the relatively low incidence as compared with other childhood diseases, is the second most common cause of death in children between 1 and 15 years of age.

Since malnutrition, diarrheal diseases, and infections take a heavy toll on the lives of children in the developing countries, the incidence of cancer in children is relatively low. In one study published from India, lymphomas and retinoblastomas were relatively more frequent while tumors of the central nervous system and kidney and neuroblastomas were relatively less frequent as compared with the incidence of these tumors in developed countries.[9]

TYPES OF NEOPLASTIC DISORDERS IN CHILDREN

The different types of neoplastic disorders seen in children and their incidence are given in Table 10-1.[8] The following tumors are relatively more common in the miscellaneous group in Table 10-1: carcinomas (thyroid, nasopharynx, adrenal, etc.), malignant carcinoid tumors, and thymomas. In a registry-based study published from Great Britain, carcinomas of thyroid, nasopharynx, adrenals, liver, salivary gland, kidney, gastrointestinal tract, female genital tract, bronchus, lungs, etc. represented 2% of all childhood malignant disease during the 10-year period 1971–1980.[10]

TABLE 10-1 Frequency of Different Types of Tumors in Children

Tumor type	Incidence[a]
Leukemia (all cell types including granulocytic sarcoma)	42.1
Central nervous system tumors	23.9
Lymphoma (all types including Hodgkin's disease)	13.2
Sympathetic nervous system tumors (including pheochromocytoma)	9.6
Soft tissue tumors	8.4
Renal tumors	7.8
Bone tumors	5.6
Retinoblastoma	3.4
Gonadal germ cell tumors	2.2
Liver tumors	1.9
Melanoma	0.7
Extragonadal teratoma	0.3
Miscellaneous (including carcinomas of various sites)	5.4

* Incidence is expressed as number of cases per million children per year.

Source: Adapted from Young JL, Miller RW: *J Pediatr* 86:254, 1975.

The frequencies of specific neoplastic disorders in 16,717 children registered with the CCG between 1974 and 1981 were as follows: leukemias (41% of all pediatric malignancies) with acute lymphoblastic leukemia being the predominant type, lymphomas including Hodgkin's disease (10%), brain tumors (10%), neuroblastoma (8%), Wilms' tumor (7%), bone tumors (6%), rhabdomyosarcoma (5%), retinoblastoma (3%), and other tumors including soft tissue tumors other than rhabdomyosarcoma, teratomas, etc. (10%). Brain tumors are probably underrepresented in these data. The neoplastic disorders other than leukemias are often referred to as *solid tumors*. In contrast, the different types of solid tumors occurring most frequently in adults are carcinomas involving lungs, colon, breast, and genital tract. Among the leukemias, acute and chronic myeloid leukemia and chronic lymphatic leukemia are more frequent in adults than in children.

Malignant neoplastic disorders are seen in all pediatric age groups extending from the neonatal period to adolescence. Tumors, particularly sacrococcygeal teratomas and to some extent neuroblastomas, are being diagnosed with increasing frequency by ultrasonography in the fetus.[11] Certain tumors are more frequent in the specific age groups. Thus the soft tissue and bone sarcomas are more frequent in older children. The embryonal tumors (e.g., neuroblastoma, Wilms' tumor, certain brain tumors) are more frequent in infants and young children. In the neonate neuroblastoma, acute lymphoblastic and myeloid leukemias, teratomas, Wilms' tumor, melanoma, retinoblastoma, liver tumors, and congenital/infantile fibrosarcomas are the most frequently occurring malignancies.[12,13]

ASSOCIATED CONGENITAL ANOMALIES

The incidence of congenital anomalies is higher in children with cancer as compared with normal children. For example, the incidence of aniridia (absence of iris) in children with Wilms' tumor is about 1 in 75 as compared with 1 in 75,000 in general population. This association is indicative of intimate relationship between teratogenesis and oncogenesis.[14–16] Bolande[14] suggested that teratogenesis may be a more primitive reaction than oncogenesis induced by mutagens. Certain congenital anomalies and syndromes are associated with or predispose to certain types of malignancies in children (Table 10-2). Thus, for example, leukemias are associated with preexisting chromosomal abnormality, lymphoma with congenital immunodeficiency, and Wilms' tumor with growth abnormalities. The risk of developing a malignancy in children with these anomalies or syndromes is variable. The probability that a child with Down syndrome will develop leukemia is 1 in 200 (i.e., about 15 times the normal rate), whereas that in a child with Fanconi's aplastic anemia or Bloom's syndrome (both characterized by chromosomal instability) it is 1 in 10, and the frequency of Wilms' tumor in children with aniridia is as high as 1 in 3. The knowledge of association between neoplastic disorders in children and congenital anomalies is of both theoretical and practical importance. These associations provide theoretical clues to the relationship between teratogenesis and oncogenesis. In practice, these observations can be useful in identifying children at high risk for development of specific neoplastic disorders.

TABLE 10-2 Neoplastic Disorders and Associated Congenital Anomalies or Syndromes in Children

Neoplastic disorder	Congenital anomaly or syndrome
Acute lymphoblastic leukemia	Down syndrome
Acute nonlymphoblastic leukemia	Down syndrome, Bloom's syndrome, Fanconi's anemia, Schwachman syndrome, Klinefelter's syndrome, congenital aplastic anemia, neurofibromatosis
Hodgkin's disease	Ataxia telangiectasia, congenial immunmodeficiency syndromes
Non-Hodgkin's lympoma	Congenital immunodeficiency syndrome
Central nervous system tumors	Neurofibromatosis, tuberous sclerosis, congenital immunodeficiency syndromes
Neuroblastoma	Neurofibromatosis, congenital immunodeficiency syndromes
Wilms' tumors	Aniridia, hemihypertrophy (hemihyperplasia), genitourinary malformations, Beckwith-Wiedemann syndrome, pseudohermaphroditism
Osteogenic sarcoma	Multiple exostosis, fibroosseous dysplasia
Rhabdomyosarcoma	Anomalies of: central nervous system (diffuse microgyria, congenital hydorcephalus, etc.), genitourinary system (renal cystic dysplasia, horseshoe kidney, etc.), cardiovascular system (tetracuspid pulmonary valve), and gastrointestinal tract (Meckel's diverticulum, ectopic pancreas, etc.)
Sacrococcygeal teratoma	Sacral agenesis, imperforate anus, duplication of lower intestinal and urogenital region
Other germ cell tumors	Anomalies of central nervous system and genitourinary tract

CHROMOSOMAL ABNORMALITIES

Technical advances in tissue culture and differential staining of chromosomes with improved resolution of chromosome structure have permitted recognition of small chromosomal abnormalities that were undetected previously. Another new, increasingly utilized technique is the fluorescence in situ hybridization (FISH) with chromosome-specific probes (see below).

Two basic types of chromosomal abnormalities can occur in pediatric neoplastic disorders: constitutional and acquired abnormalities. The former are seen in all the cells of the body and the latter, only in the neoplastic tissue, closely related tissue, or cell lines derived from the tumor.[17] These abnormalities, which are listed in Tables 10-3 and 10-4, can be demonstrated by obtaining

TABLE 10-3 Neoplastic Disorders in Children and Constitutional Chromosomal Abnormalities

Neoplastic disorder	Chromosomal abnormality
Wilms' tumor in children with aniridia	Deletion of *p*13 of chromosome 11
Sporadic retinoblastoma	Deletion of *q*14 of chromosome 13
Leukemia in Down's syndrome	Trisomy 21
Preleukemia	Trisomy 8

a karyotype from a metaphase spread combined with the banding technique. Recently FISH which uses DNA probes labeled with reporter molecules and broken into 200–400 bp (base pair) fragments to maximize the specificity and minimize background fluorescence has been introduced.[18] FISH can be employed in both metaphase and interphase nuclei to detect chromosomal abnormalities, gene amplification, and gene mapping.

Chromosomal abnormalities noted in pediatric tumors are of both theoretical and practical importance. The specific chromosomal abnormality occurring in a specific neoplastic disorder may provide clues to the relationship between chromosomal imbalance and oncogenesis. In practice, the chromosomal markers can be of diagnostic and prognostic significance. For example, a small round cell tumor showing *t*(11;22) (*q*24;*q*12) can be diagnosed as Ewing's sarcoma or peripheral primitive neuroectodermal tumor. Chromosomal abnormality characterized by *t*(2;13) (*q*35;*q*14) in a rhabdomyosarcoma is likely to be a marker of more aggressive behavior,[19] and cases of acute lymphoblastic leukemia with lymphoblasts showing hyperdiploidy (>50 chromosomes per cell or a DNA index of ≥1.6) have a better prognosis.[20] Structural abnormalities of chromosome 1 (trisomy of 1q and breakpoints of 1p) are found in various pediatric

TABLE 10-4 Acquired Chromosomal Abnormalities in Childhood Neoplastic Disorders

Malignancy	Chromosomal abnormality
Neuroblastoma	Deletion of p32 p36 of chromosome 1
Rhabdomyosarcoma (particularly alveolar subtype)	4(2;13)(q35;q14)
Ewing's sarcoma, peripheral primitive neuroectodermal tumor	t(11;22)(q24;q12)
Burkitt's lymphoma	t(2;8)(p12;q24) or t(8;22)(q24;q11) or t(2;14)(p13;q32.3)
Actue lymphoblastic leukemia	Hyperdiploidy or hypodiploidy
Germ cell tumors exept infantile YSC[a]	Isochromosome 12p
Snovial sarcoma	t(x;11)(p11.2;q11.2)
Meningioma	Monosomy 22, deletion q

[a] Yolk sac carcinoma.

tumors such as Wilms' tumor, Ewing's sarcoma, primitive neuroectodermal tumor, rhabdomyosarcoma, and hepatoblastoma.[21]

GENETIC AND ENVIRONMENTAL FACTORS IN CHILDHOOD ONCOGENESIS

While environmental exposure has been implicated in the etiology of certain pediatric cancers such as leukemia and carcinoma of skin and thyroid following radiation exposure, the latent period generally required for the development of tumor is so long that the patient reaches adulthood and goes out of the purview of the pediatric oncologist by the time the malignancy becomes clinically manifest. Therefore genetic factors are of greater importance in pediatric oncology. Furthermore, longer survival of children with cancer in recent years has enabled them to reach reproductive age, and the parents of and survivors among childhood cancer patients have become incrasingly aware of the greater importance of genetic factors in malignancies in children. The association with congenital anomalies, increased risk of development of malignancy in children with certain genetic syndromes (Table 10-2), and familial occurrence (e.g., Wilms' tumor) also vouch for the role of genetic factors in childhood malignancies. Survivors and relatives are likely to ask specific questions regarding the role of genetic factors in the causation of cancer, risk of development of second cancer in the survivor, and risk of cancer in the siblings, relatives, and eventually offspring of the survivor. The risk estimates for Wilms' tumor are given below to serve as an example. Only 1–2% of Wilms' tumor (WT) cases have a family history of WT. These cases are considered to be representative of the hereditary form of the disease with an autosomal dominant pattern of inheritance and a penetrance of 63%. If there is no family history of WT, the risk of developing WT in a sibling is $<1\%$ and the risk for the offspring is 5%. On the other hand, in the presence of family history of WT, the risk for the sibling and offspring is about 1–2% and 32%, respectively.[22]

The molecular genetic factors (oncogenes) related to pediatric tumors are discussed in the section on prognostic factors since the prime example of oncogene in pediatric tumors, viz., N-myc in neuroblastoma, is of primarily prognostic significance.

TRANSPLACENTAL CARCINOGENESIS

Besides the genetic factors and the postnatal environmental exposure, another factor—in utero exposure to various drugs and viruses—can result in increased incidence of certain childhood malignancies. The best examples of this phenomenon of transplacental carcinogenesis is the occurrence of clear cell adenocarcinoma of the vagina in women younger than 30 years of age who were exposed to diethylstilbestrol (DES) given to their mothers during pregnancy to prevent miscarriage (Figure 10-1). Melnick et al[23] have reviewed 519 cases of clear cell carcinoma of the vagina and cervix. In 60% of these cases the mothers had received DES during pregnancy. An additional 12% gave history of treat-

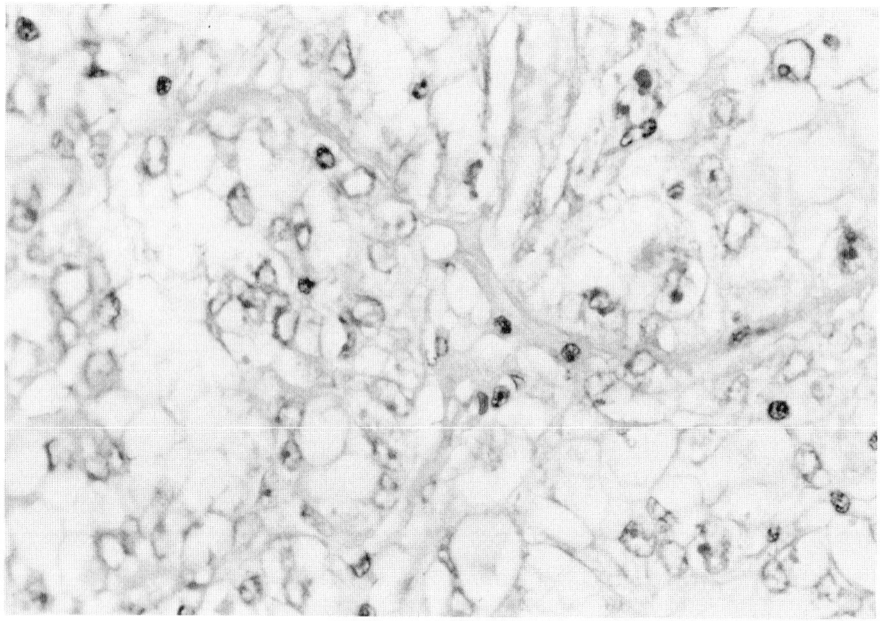

FIGURE 10-1. Clear cell adenocarcinoma of vagina. Note the large tumor cells with vesicular nuclei and clear cytoplasm (H&E, ×400). (Courtesy of Dr. James L. Finley.)

ment with another hormone or an unidentified medication. The median age and age range in patients with intrauterine exposure to stilbestrol were 19 years and 15–27 years, respectively. However, clear cell carcinoma can occur as early as 7 years of age.[24] Besides clear cell carcinoma, these patients also show the following genital lesions: (1) *nonneoplastic lesions*—vaginal ridge composed of fibrous tissue, hypoplasia of the cervix, obliteration of vaginal fornices, and pseudopolyp of the cervic are visible on colposcopic examination, and on microscopic examination vaginal adenosis with or without squamous metaplasia is seen (Figure 10-2); (2) *preneoplastic lesions*—these include atypical vaginal adenosis (nuclear pleomorphism and hyperchromasia and stratification of the lining cells) and squamous dysplasia of cervix and vagina.[24,25] Increased incidence of childhood malignancies has also been observed in fetal hydantoin syndrome resulting from intrauterine exposure to the drug taken by the mother for epilepsy. Neuroblastoma is the commonest among the tumors reported to occur in these children.[26]

BIOLOGIC MARKERS OF PEDIATRIC TUMORS

Tumor cells may synthesize a variety of substances such as hormones, enzymes, proteins, mucopolysaccharides, and humoral regulators of hematopoiesis. Oncogenes (see below) can also be considered as biologic markers

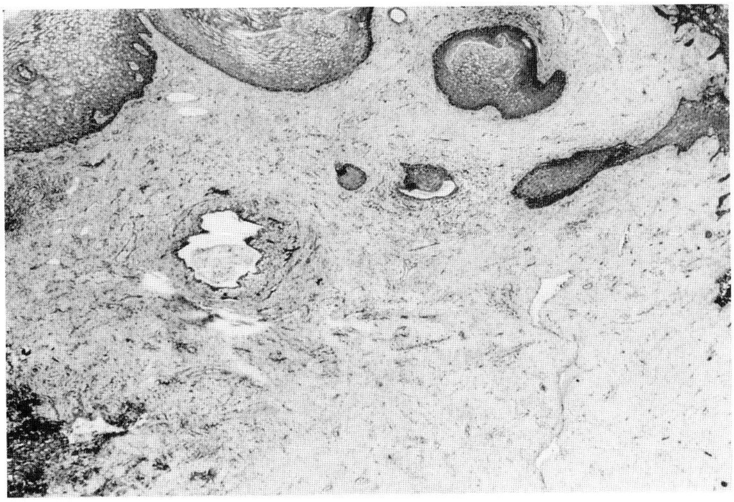

FIGURE 10-2. Vaginal adenosis with squamous metaplasia (H&E, ×100). (Courtesy of Dr. James L. Finley.)

of certain tumors. The synthesized substances may be released in the blood or body fluids (Table 10-5). Measurement of these biologic markers can be useful in the diagnosis, prognosis, and monitoring for relapse. The value of biological markers for diagnosis and monitoring for relapse is well established in neuroblastoma, germ cell tumors, and hepatoblastoma but is doubtful or yet to be established for other tumors (Table 10-5). The biologic markers can also be demonstrated in the histologic sections by immunocytochemical stain on paraffin sections.

TABLE 10-5 Biological Markers for Childhood Tumors

Tumor	Biological marker(s)
Neuroblastoma	Catecholamines[a], serum neuron-specific enolase, lactate dehydrogenase (LDH), and ferritin, N-myc amplification
Germ cell tumors	Serum hCG,[b] AFP,[c] CEA,[d] and LDH
Hepatoblastoma	AFP, hCG[b,e]
Wilms' tumor	Serum hyaluronic acid, erythropoietin, renin, hyaluronic acid
Hepatocellular carcinoma	Serum ferritin
Osteogenic sarcoma	Serum alkaline phosphatase

[a] Vanillylmandelic acid (VMA) and homovanillic acid (HVA) are the two most commonly assayed catabolites in urine/serum.
[b] Human chorionic gonadotropin.
[c] α-Fetoprotein.
[d] Carcinoembryonic antigen.
[e] Useful in cases with precocious puberty.

NEOPLASTIC DISORDERS IN CONGENITAL AND ACQUIRED IMMUNODEFICIENCY SYNDROMES

It is well recognized that the incidence of lymphoproliferative disorders is higher in children with congenital and acquired immunodeficiency syndromes. The former category includes severe combined immunodeficiency, complete DiGeorge syndrome, Wiskott-Aldrich syndrome, X-linked lymphoproliferative syndrome, ataxia telangiectasia, and common variable immunodeficiency. The latter include HIV-associated acquired immunodeficiency syndrome (AIDS) and organ transplant patients given immunosuppressive therapy. Patients belonging to both these categories have defective cellular immunity with or without defective humoral immunity. The risk of death from malignancy in children with congenital immunodeficiency is about 100 times that of normal children.[27] The most common neoplastic disorders are lymphomas, leukemias, and undefined diffuse lymphoproliferation in lymph nodes.[28] All these disorders are of B-cell origin. Hodgkin's disease also has increased incidence in these children. Similar spectrum of lymphoproliferative disorders is seen in children with AIDS (see Chapter 2, Table 6) and in patients with organ transplants.[29,30] It appears that immunodeficiency particularly related to T-cells response plays a role in the pathogenesis of lymphoproliferative disorders in both congenital and acquired immunodeficiencies. Epstein-Barr virus (EBV) DNA can be identified in many of these lymphoproliferative disorders.[31–33] The occurrence of EBV-related B lymphocyte proliferations in these patients is indicative of loss of normal immunologic control of EBV-infected B lymphocytes by T-cell response. EBV-related neoplasms have been shown to possess tumor-specific transplantation antigens (TSTA). The T-cell defect in the congenital and acquired immunodeficiencies results in increased incidence of these TSTA-expressing tumors.[34] It is of interest to note that the lymphoproliferative disorders occur more frequently in extranodal sites including brain and that the incidence of these disorders is significantly increased in patients in whom cyclosporine is used in the post-transplantation immunosuppressive therapy.[30] The lymphoproliferative lesions may regress following reduction or cessation of cyclosporine therapy.[35]

Besides the lymphoproliferative disorders, which are the commonest neoplastic disorders in children with AIDS, smooth muscle tumors (leiomyosarcoma and leiomyoma) have emerged as one of the commonest neoplastic processes in children with AIDS (Chapter 2, Table 7).[36] Leiomyosarcomas have also been reported in children with organ transplants.[37,38] It is of interest to note that the smooth muscle tumors in children with liver transplant reported by Lee et al[37] were associated with EBV as evidenced by the nuclear positivity of the tumor cells on in situ hybridization with EBER probe.

CLINICAL FEATURES OF PEDIATRIC MALIGNANCIES

The common clinical features include fever, lymphadenopathy (e.g., Hodgkin's disease, non-Hodgkin's lymphoma, and metastatic tumors such as neuroblastoma and nasopharyngeal carcinoma), rapidly and progressively growing subcutaneous or deeper masses with or without ulceration of overlying skin, pain (e.g., bone pain in primary and metastatic bone tumors and leukemia, abdominal pain in abdominal malignancies), headache and neurologic abnormalities (primarily in brain tumors), irritability and abnormalities of eyes (yellow white reflection seen through the pupil in retinoblastomas, and exophthalmos in primary and metastatic tumors of the orbital soft tissue or bones).[39] In some cases, the tumor may be totally asymptomatic. Thus abdominal neuroblastoma and Wilms' tumor may be palpated by the mother during routine handling of her child or the physician during a routine office visit. Alternatively, a thoracic neuroblastoma may be detected on a chest x-ray taken for some other reason.

SCREENING FOR EARLY DETECTION

Screening methods such as self-examination and mammography for breast cancer, blood in stools and colonoscopy for colon cancer, and Pap smear for cervical cancer have been used successfully for early detection of cancer in adults. The only pediatric malignancies in which screening can be used are neuroblastoma and to some extent fetal tumors. However, reduction in mortality due to mass screening of urine for raised catecholamines at 6 months of age has not been shown to occur in neuroblastomas.[40] Fetal tumors such as sacrococcygeal teratomas and neuroblastomas are being recognized with increasing frequency with routine ultrasound examination during pregnancy.[11]

PATHOLOGIC FEATURES OF TUMORS IN CHILDREN

Histogenesis and Line(s) of Differentiation

Histogenesis refers to the cells of origin (progenitor cells) of the tumor. In most instances it is inferred from the characteristics of the tumor cells visualized by routine light microscopy. Other studies such as immunocytochemistry, electron microscopy, tissue culture, and gene expression (e.g., MyoD1 gene expression in rhabdomyosarcomas—see Chapter 13) are also used when the histogenesis of the tumor is not clear on the basis of routine histologic examination. It is generally presumed that the cells that constitute the tumor parenchyma and from which tumor arises are the same. However, in many of the pediatric malignancies the cells of origin are embryonal cells in which differentiation of variable degrees and lineages can occur and the cells from which the tumor arose and the cells comprising the tumor differ in the degree and type of differentiation. In certain tumors the embryonal cells may be totally arrested in their differentiation. The result is a tumor such as undifferentiated neuroblastoma composed of undifferentiated embryonal neuroblasts (Figure 10-3). Determination of biochemical markers (catecholamines) and morphological markers (neuron-specific enolase, neuroendocrine granules, etc.) is required for demonstration of the precise nature of such undifferentiated tumors. At the other extreme are tumors that represent cytodifferentiated variants of embryonal tumors. Congenital mesoblastic nephroma of the kidney that shows myofibroblastic or fibroblastic differentiation and ganglioneuroma serve as examples of this phenomenon. It is assumed that the cells of origin of these cytodifferentiated tumors

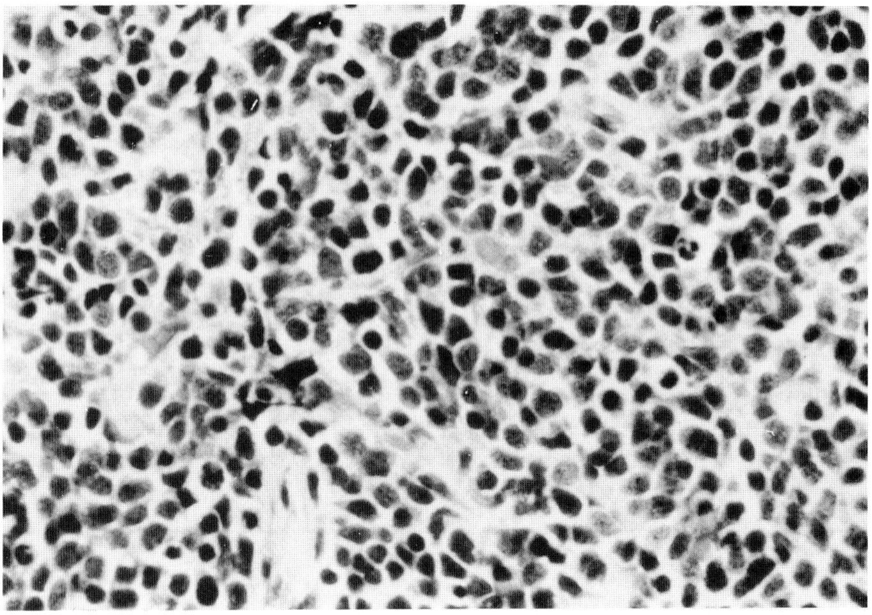

FIGURE 10-3. Undifferentiated neuroblastoma composed of undifferentiated neuroblasts. No neuropil is present (H&E, ×400).

are embryonal cells that have differentiated during the development of the tumor. There can be various gradations of differentiation exhibited by the embryonal tumor cells between these two extremes. Thus in a differentiating neuroblastoma or ganglioneuroblastoma, there is an admixture of undifferentiated neuroblasts, ganglion cells, and cells intermediate between the two (Figure 10-4). The various gradations in differentiation also result in a spectrum of related tumors with different morphologic features and potentially different biologic behavior. Congenital mesoblastic nephroma and its cellular variant (and possibly clear cell sarcoma of the kidney) serve as examples of this phenomenon. The spectrum may be well-defined in some instances but poorly defined, rare, gray-zone neoplastic lesions may occur (See section on cystic nephroma and cystic partially differentiated nephroblastoma in the Chapter on Pathology of Renal Tumors in Children). In rare instances, the tumor cells may show a different line of differentiation when there is relapse of the neoplastic process. For example, acute lymphoblastic leukemia of T-cell lineage may show myeloid differentiation when it relapses. It should also be recognized that tumors of diverse histogenesis may look alike and diverse tumor types in children may apparently have the same histogenesis. For example, while most of the extrarenal malignant rhabdoid tumors may be of neuroectodermal origin, a few may be of mesenchymal origin. Tumors of nephroblastic origin include such diverse types as Wilms' tumor and congenital mesoblastic nephroma. Tumors of neuroectodermal origin include neuroblastoma, peripheral primitive neuroectodermal tumors, and perhaps some examples of what are traditionally considered as Ewing's sarcoma.

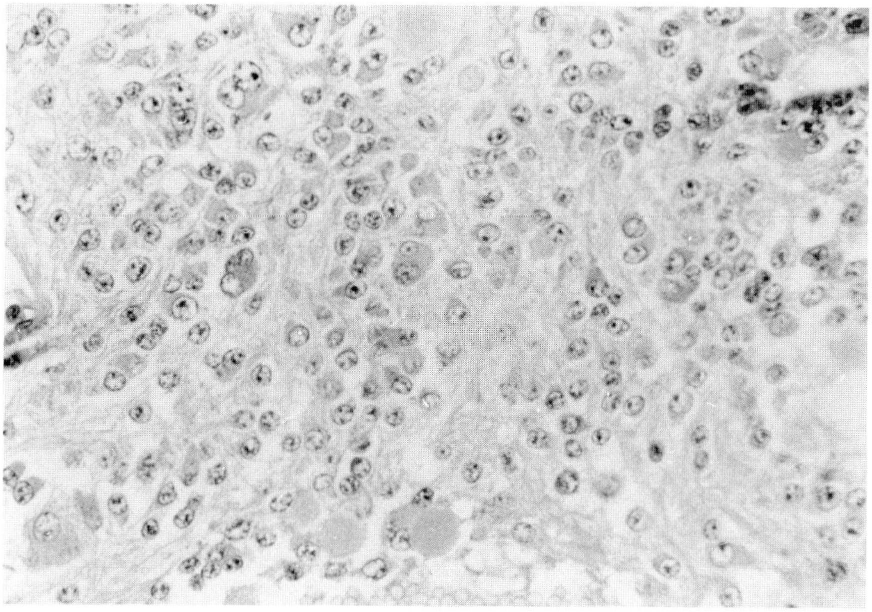

FIGURE 10-4. Differentiating neuroblastoma showing neuroblasts, ganglion cells, and intermediate cells (H&E, ×400).

The differentiation seen in the embryonal tumors may proceed along normal lineage or may be aberrant. Thus the differentiating or differentiated cells in an embryonal tumor may resemble the normal developmental counterparts during their early developmental stages. Therefore it can be said that oncogeny recapitulates ontogeny. For example, in rhabdomyosarcoma, the rhabdomyoblasts resemble similar cells in a fetus (Figure 10-5). In neuroblastoma, the formation of rosettes and ganglion cells represents recapitulation of similar structures in the developing sympathetic ganglion (Figures 10-4, 10-6, 10-7). On the other hand, aberrant differentiation is seen in Wilms' tumor as indicated by the presence of skeletal muscle, mucinous epithelium, cartilage, etc.[41] This type of aberrant differentiation also involves synthesis of certain enzymes and cell proteins not normally synthesized by the progenitor cells from which the tumor arises. Thus positive reaction on immunoperoxidase stain for cytokeratin in a rhabdomyosarcoma can be considered as an example of aberrant differentiation at the subcellular level.[42] Such aberrant differentiation cannot be detected at the ultrastructural level. Thus in the example of rhabdomyosarcoma showing positive reaction for cytokeratin, electron microscopic examination does not show tonofilaments.

Embryonal tumors can also arise from abnormal embryonal rest. Origin of Wilms' tumor from nephrogenic rests is an example of this phenomenon (Figures 10-8, 10-9). Another notable feature of histogenesis of tumors in children is that tumor can arise from the epithelial lining and mesenchyme in the wall of some of the congenital cystic lesions of different organs that have a neoplastic potential. The pulmonary blastoma and rhabdomyosarcoma arising

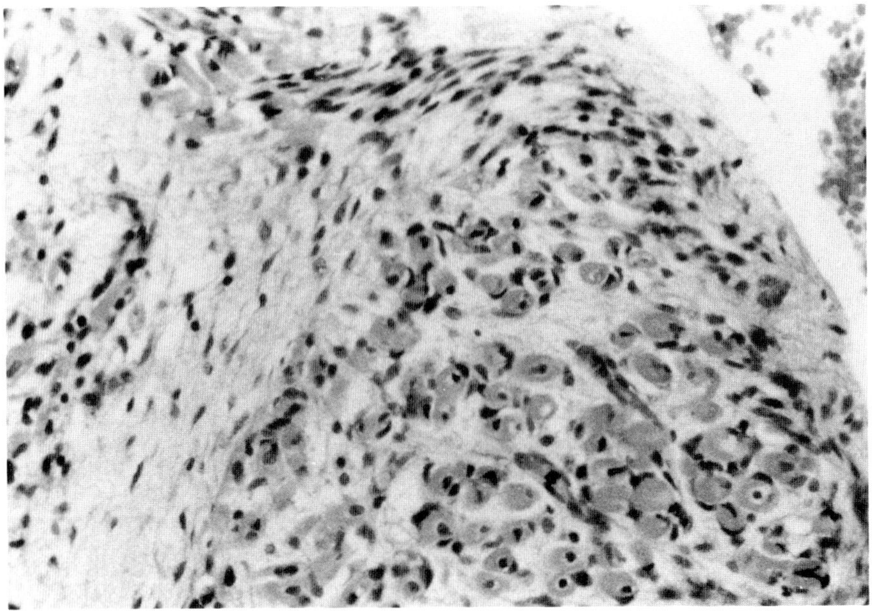

FIGURE 10-5. Skeletal muscle from a fetus showing round rhabdomyoblasts with abundant dense eosinophilic cytoplasm, spindle-shaped rhabdomyoblasts and loose myxoid background (H&E, ×400).

within pulmonary cystic lesions (congenital cystic adenomatoid malformation, etc.) serve as the best examples of this phenomenon.[43,44] Furthermore, embryonal tumors, e.g. neuroblastoma arise rarely within teratomas.

Pathologic Diagnosis of Pediatric Tumors

Before the definitive tissue diagnosis is attempted, the clinicians often start or even complete other investigations such as imaging procedures (ultrasound, CT scan, and/or MRI), biochemical markers, and bone marrow aspirates. The pathologist should have ready access to the results of all these investigations (see Chapter 12). For the pathologic diagnosis of tumors in children, it is conventional to take into consideration only the histologic features demonstrated on routine hematoxylin and eosin stain with or without the routine nonimmunocytochemical special stain(s) (e.g., trichrome, reticulin, PAS stains). Thus, for enrollment in all the national studies of tumors in children only routine histologic criteria are required for diagnosis. However, according to the current standard of practice of surgical pathology, it is essential to demonstrate the evidence of the nature of all "blastomas" by immunocytochemical stains and/or ultrastructural methods. Thus for the diagnosis of rhabdomyosarcoma, positive reaction on one or more of the immunocytochemical stains for the muscle proteins (myoglobin, muscle-specific actin, and desmin) and/or ultrastructural demonstration of thick and thin filaments and other rhabdomyoblastic features are required. In undifferentiated neuroblastoma either raised urinary excretion of catecholamine and neuron-specific enolase positivity on immunoperoxidase

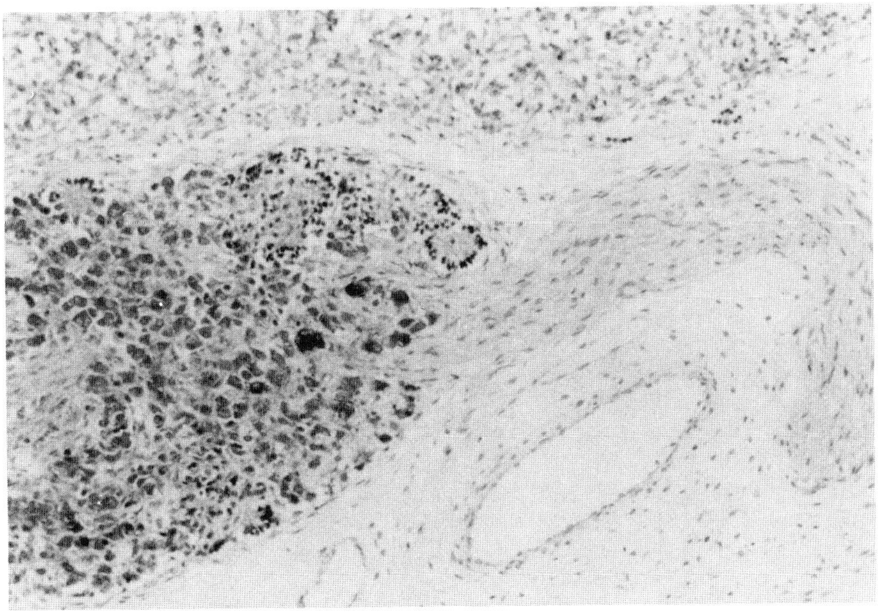

FIGURE 10-6. Sympathetic ganglion from a fetus showing neuroblasts forming rosettes. Note also the ganglion cells, intermediate cells, and neuritic processes accompanied by Schwann cells (H&E, ×250).

stain or ultrastructural features indicative of neuroblastic origin of the tumor are required for definitive diagnosis.

Gross Features of Pediatric Tumors

An important gross feature of practical significance in pediatric tumors is the cystic change. The cystic change seen on gross examination may represent on

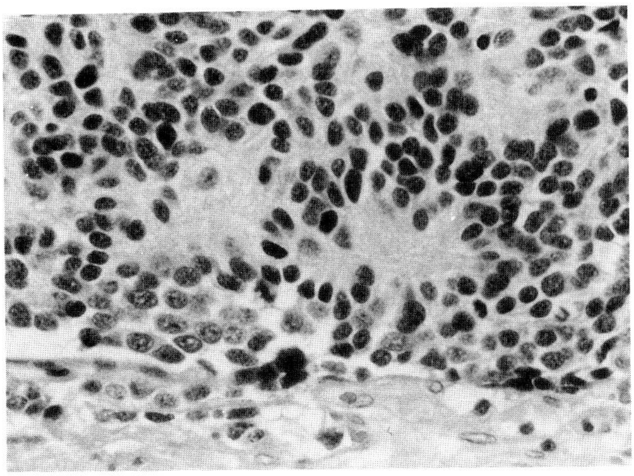

FIGURE 10-7. Neuroblastoma showing rosette formation (H&E, ×400).

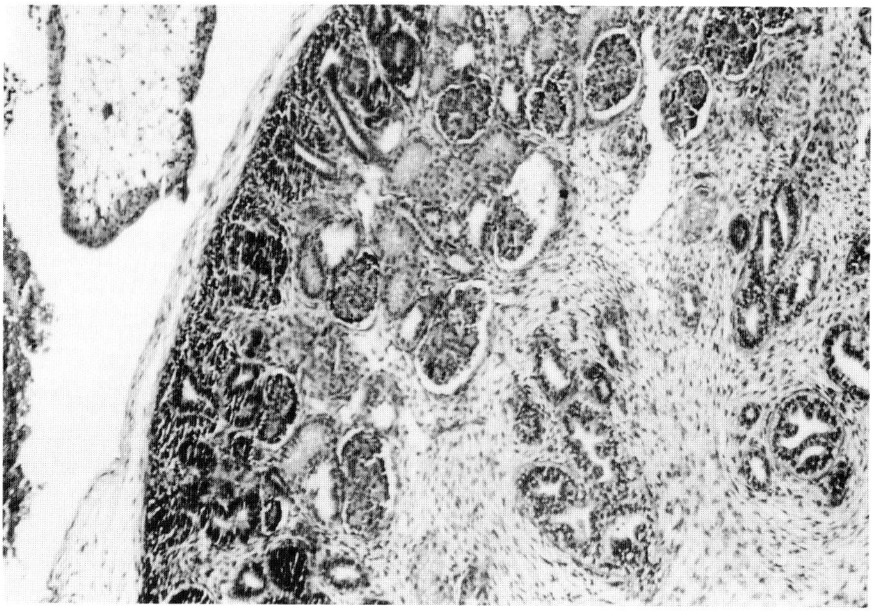

FIGURE 10-8. Normal subcapsular nephrogenic zone in the kidney of an 18-week fetus (H&E, ×100).

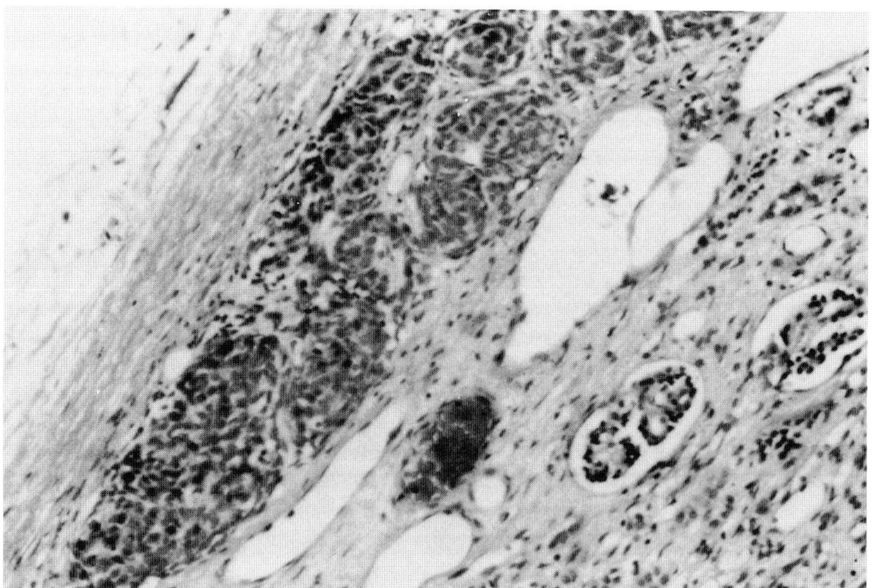

FIGURE 10-9. Abnormal persistent nephrogenic rest in the kidney with Wilms' tumor in a 3-year-old-child (H&E, ×250).

microscopic examination true epithelium-lined cysts or pseudocysts resulting from necrosis and hemorrhage. The cystic change may be focal, or the entire tumor may be composed of single or multiple cysts (e.g, cystic nephroma, cystic partially differentiated nephroblastoma, and mature cystic teratoma). The true cystic change, when it is present throughout a teratoma and certain renal tumors (e.g., cystic partially differentiated nephroblastoma), is indicative of good prognosis. It is necessary to examine the tumor showing cystic change thoroughly to make sure that there is no solid portion except the septa of the cysts in the tumor. "Bread loafing" of a previously adequately fixed tumor is an appropriate method of examination. Another important gross feature found in pediatric tumors is calcification. Calcification is particularly common in neuroblastoma and teratoma, although it may be seen rarely or occasionally in other pediatric tumors as well (e.g., Wilms' tumor). The calcification can be visualized or palpated on gross examination or detected by the gritty feel during serial slicing of the tumor (Figure 10-10). In neuroblastoma the calcification involves necrotic foci in the tumor, whereas in teratoma it is related to presence of bone, teeth, or calcified cartilage. Calcification in neuroblastoma is associated with better prognosis.

Degree of Differentiation

The degree of differentiation is variable from one tumor to another of the same type and also from one area to another area of the same tumor. For assessment of degree of differentiation, an attempt is made to get semiquantitative estimates of differentiating or differentiated cells. Differentiating cells are those that show partial development of some of the nuclear and/or cytoplasmic features of mature cells. Thus differentiating cells are intermediate between undifferentiated and differentiated cells. Thus in neuroblastoma the differentiating tumor cells show development of one or more of the following features: nucleolus, vesicular appearance of the nucleus, cytoplasmic rim, enlargement of size, and cell processes (Figure 10-4). Differentiated cells are the cells that have reached the normal endpoint(s) of differentiation (e.g., ganglion cells and Schwann cells in neuroblastic tumors). Rare or occasional cells of an embryonal and alveolar rhabdomyosarcoma composed largely of undifferentiated cells may

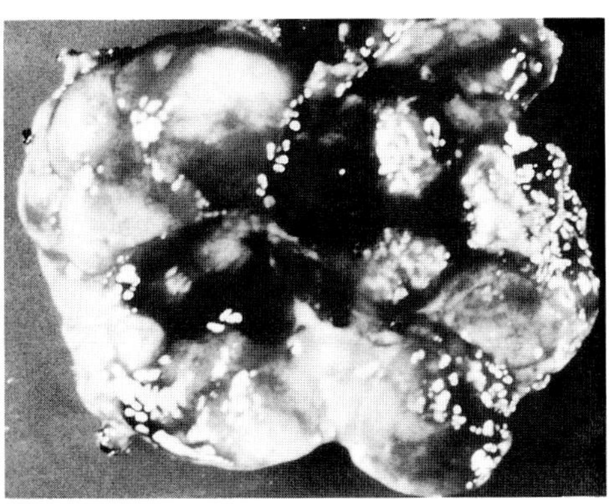

FIGURE 10-10. Gross photograph of neuroblastoma showing multiple foci of calcification.

show presence of bright eosinophilic cytoplasm or may become strap-shaped. Striations may or may not be present in these cells. Detection of the differentiating and differentiated cells is of diagnostic value in a small round cell tumor.

The degree of differentiation may be related to prognosis. Thus differentiating neuroblastomas have a better prognosis than do undifferentiated or poorly differentiated neuroblastomas.[45] The categorization into poorly differentiated or differentiating is based on the proportion of differentiating cells. Degree of differentiation is of prognostic value also in hepatoblastoma. Haas et al[46] have shown that hepatoblastomas consisting of "fetal" hepatocytes have better prognoses than do those showing "embryonal" hepatocytes.

Sampling of Tumors for Histologic Examination

Because of heterogeneity in terms of the variable cellularity, variable degree of differentiation in different areas of the tumor and focal presence of diagnostic features (e.g., rosettes in peripheral primitive neuroectodermal tumor, or rhabdomyoblasts in a rhabdomyosarcoma) and of prognostic features (e.g., anaplasia in Wilms' tumor, immaturity of tissues in a teratoma), adequate sampling of pediatric tumors for histologic examination is of great practical importance. The usual guideline is one block for each centimeter of the longest dimension of the tumor. However, with this guideline tumors with approximately similar volume may be sampled unequally (e.g., a tumor measuring $9 \times 6 \times 5$ cm, i.e., 270 cm^3 vs. another one measuring $7 \times 7 \times 6$ cm, i.e., 294 cm^3). Therefore, the guideline should be modified as follows: the number of blocks should be 1.5 times the mean of the total of three dimensions of the tumor (the mean and/or final figure should be rounded out to the next whole number). In the examples given above 11 blocks will be taken from both the tumors. In certain tumors such as teratomas showing solid components, even larger numbers of blocks may be taken.[47] There are no agreed-on guidelines for the size of each block. But considering the size of the standard plastic cassette used for embedding the tissues, the blocks should be about 6 cm in perimeter. The sites of sampling also are important. Blocks should be taken preferably from viable areas with additional blocks from areas showing hemorrhage, necrosis, calcification, cystic change, and any unusual gross feature(s). In tumors that are largely composed of single or multiple cysts with a minor solid component, the latter should be sampled extensively since it is more likely that if the features related to unfavorable outcome are present, those will be encountered in the solid component.

Anaplasia in Pediatric Tumors

Although the term *anaplasia* implies loss of structural (and functional) differentiation of normal cell (dedifferentiation), conventionally it is considered equivalent to lack of differentiation in reserve cells or embryonal cells of a particular tissue from which tumors arise. Furthermore, it also implies that the anaplastic tumor cells are markedly pleomorphic. Presence of totally undifferentiated small round cells has been labeled by some authors, including the present one, as anaplasia.[48] The term *undifferentiated* better describes these tumors. According to the definition of the term recommended for Wilms' tumor by Beckwith and colleagues,[41,49] the morphologic characteristics of anaplasia include not only the marked nuclear pleomorphism, enlargement (macronucleation), and hyperchromasia but also atypical multipolar mitotic figures. Macronucleation (nuclear enlargement at least three times in two dimensions as compared with the normal-size nuclei of adjacent tumor cells) should be distinguished from multinucleation. Anaplasia in Wilms' tumor, so defined, is of prognostic significance (see Chapter 13 for details). Anaplasia in neuroblastoma does not appear to be of prognostic value despite claims to the contrary.[50] Pleomorphism in embryonal rhabdomyosarcoma labeled as anaplasia by Kodet et al[51] and defined as presence of cells with markedly enlarged hyperchromatic lobated nuclei is associated with reduced survival when the pleomorphic tumor cells are present in clusters or sheets. The prognostic value of anaplasia in other pediatric tumors has not been defined yet.[52]

Tumor Heterogeneity

There are two types of tumor heterogeneity or variability: intertumor and intratumor.[53] *Intertumor heterogeneity* refers to the variability between different types of tumors or different tumors of the same type. The variability is related to cell of origin, organ or site in which the tumor arises, the age of the child, hormonal status of the child, etc. The differences in various tumors of the kidney and teratomas arising in different age groups and different sites illustrate this type of variability. *Intratumor heterogeneity* refers to the cellular differences within a single tumor. The regional differences in cell morphology, differentiation, mitotic rate, architectural patterns, vascularity, karyotype, antigen expression, membrane composition, hormonal responsiveness, response to chemotherapy, invasiveness, metastatic capacity, anaplasia, etc. within the same tumor illustrate intratumor variability. Some investigators use the term *tumor heterogeneity* only for tumor cell differences due to differences in cell lineage, i.e., presence of cell subpopulations capable of breeding true.[53] Pathologists are more familiar with the regional morphologic variability within the same tumor. Such morphologic variability is more common in pediatric tumors than in tumors in adults. The varying degrees and diverse types of differentiation in tumors such as Wilms' tumor, neuroblastoma, and hepatoblastoma serve as examples of this phenomenon. Other morphologic features such as cell size and shape, degree of nuclear enlargement and of hyperchromasia (large cell vs. small cell, pleomorphism, etc.), and mitotic rate also show variability. Morphologic heterogeneity may also be seen when primary tumor is compared with its recurrence or metastasis following surgical resection or following other additional modes of therapy for the primary tumor.

Foulds first recognized that growth of tumor is associated with emergence of greater heterogeneity.[54,55] He referred to this phenomenon as tumor progression, which was defined as "acquisition of permanent, irreversible, qualitative changes in one or more characteristics of a neoplasm." Progression may occur in certain pediatric tumors even prior to clinical detection and may be associated with emergence of subclones of tumor cells with high proclivity for producing metastases. Neuroblastomas that are stage C or D at the time of diagnosis serve as probable examples of this phenomenon.

Histologic Patterns in Pediatric Tumors

The histologic patterns characteristic of pediatric tumors include nesting (lobular), alveolar, starry sky and diffuse patterns, and rosette formation.

Nesting Pattern

The nesting or lobular pattern results from presence of fibrovascular septa that divide the tumor parenchyma into completely or partially formed lobules or nests. The nesting pattern may be present diffusely or focally. When the nests or lobules of tumor cells are completely surrounded by septa, they may be referred to as forming an *organoid pattern*. The nesting pattern tends to be replicated also in the tumor metastasis. Neuroblastoma shows all the aforementioned characteristics of the nesting pattern. The nesting pattern is also seen in germinomas, blastemal Wilms' tumor, and focally in peripheral primitive neuroectodermal tumor. In clear cell sarcoma of the kidney, fibrovascular septa are present diffusely but do not divide the tumor parenchyma into well-delineated nests or lobules.

Alveolar Pattern

The alveolar pattern is characteristically present in alveolar type of rhabdomyosarcoma and alveolar soft tissue sarcoma. A pseudoalveolar pattern may be seen in certain tumors due to artifact produced by degeneration, lysis, or autolysis of tumor cells at the periphery of the lobules. In the true alveolar pattern the fibrovascular septa divided the tumor into "alveoli" that are bounded by these septa. One or more layers of tumor cells line the inner aspect of the septa and an apparently loose collection of tumor cells fills the "alveolar" spaces partially (Chapter 12, Figures 26 and 27).[56]

Starry Sky Pattern

The starry sky pattern is characterized by a blue background of tumor cells with large nuclei and little cytoplasm and scattering of macrophages that have phagocytosed nuclear debris of dead tumor cells (tingible body macrophages). The tumor cells in the vicinity of the macrophages show increased mitotic activity.[57] In an active hyperplastic germinal center of a lymph node or Peyer's patches or in a thymus showing acute involuntionary changes, a similar pattern is observed. In pediatric tumors, the starry sky pattern is seen in a non-Hodgkin's lymphoma (NHL) of various types but particularly in small cell, non-cleaved Burkitt's type (Chapter 12, Figure 31). The relative sizes of the nuclei of tumor cells and those of the macrophages give a clue regarding the type of NHL (see Chapter 12 for details). The starry sky pattern may be seen focally in rare cses of neuroblastoma and medulloblastoma.

Diffuse Pattern

The diffuse pattern is characterized by the arrangement of tumor cells in sheets with few or no fibrovascular septa. NHL, Ewing's sarcoma, and PNET characteristically show diffuse patterns.

Rosette Formation

This is a distinctive pattern exhibited by certain pediatric tumors. There are two types of rosettes: (1) *Flexner rosettes*, seen in retinoblastoma, characterized by circular or spherical arrangement of tumor cells around a lumen (Figure 10-11); and (2) *Homer Wright rosettes*, seen in neuroblastoma and PNET, characterized by circular or spherical arrangement of tumor cells with tangled fine fibrillary processes in the center (Figure 10-7). Rare Flexner and Homer Wright rosettes may be seen in blastemal Wilms' tumor.

Semiquantitative Assessment of Histologic Features

In pediatric tumors certain features when assessed quantitatively assume prognostic significance. Thus in neuroblastic tumors, for example, the proportion of histologic components, extent of mitotic activity, mitosis karyorrhexis index, and proportion of differentiating neuroblasts are related to prognosis. Detailed and elaborate morphometric methods for quantification of these histologic features are not of practical use in diagnostic pediatric surgical pathology. Therefore, these features are assessed semiquantitatively.

Mitotic Karyorrhectic Cells in Pediatric Tumors

Many of the pediatric tumors show individual cell death characterized by pyknosis of nuclei (condensed chromatin), karyorrhexis (dispersed chromatin masses), and condensation of cytoplasm. It is possible that the individual cell death seen in these tumors represents apoptosis (programmed cell death) related to activation of endogenous endonuclease.[58] Interspersed in these cells, which are often referred to as *karyorrhectic cells*, are the mitotic figures. Although mitotic and karyorrhectic cells can be distinguished from each other by application of stringent criteria (Figure 10-12), some investigators refer to both types of cells as mitotic karyorrhectic cells (MKCs).[59] MKCs are seen most characteristically in neuroblastomas but are also present in the NHL (particularly in Burkitt's

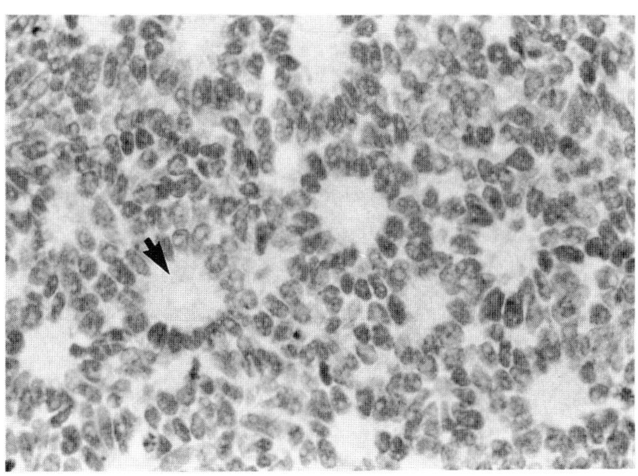

FIGURE 10-11. Retinoblastoma showing Flexner rosettes characterized by circular (spheroidal) arrangement of tumor cells around a central lumen (arrow) (H&E, ×400).

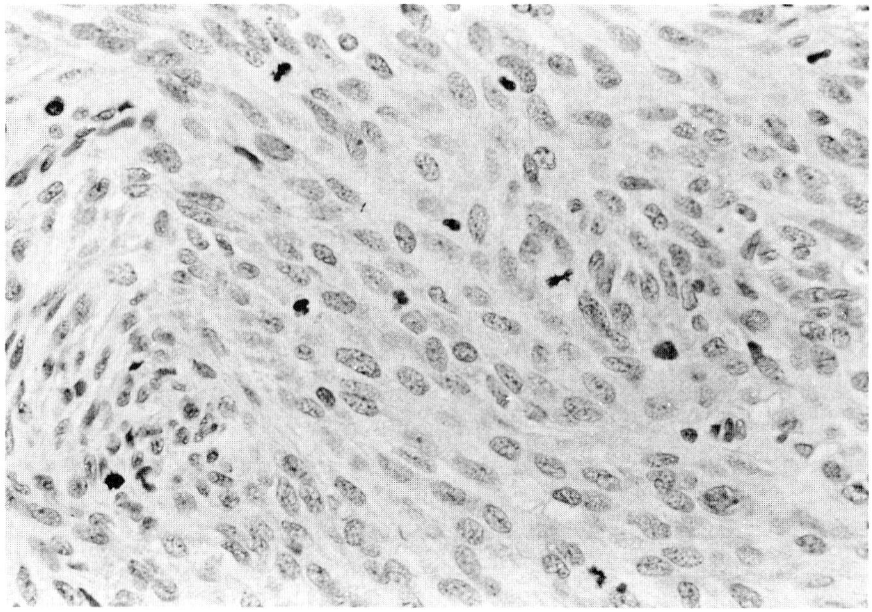

FIGURE 10-12. Miotic figures with spiky outline of nuclear material and clear cytoplasm and karyorrhectic cells with condensed lumpy nuclear material with lobulated, round, or oval outline in a leiomyosarcoma (H&E, ×400).

lymphoma), Wilms' tumor (particularly in its blastemal areas), etc. The proportion of MKCs in a tumor is referred to as *mitosis karyorrhexis index* (MKI). In the Shimada classification of neuroblastoma, MKI is the major morphologic feature taken into consideration for prognostic categorization.[59]

Prognostic Classification According to Histologic Features

Two histologic categories are recognized in many of the pediatric tumors: favorable histology (FH) and unfavorable histology (UFH).[60] The concept of FH and UFH was introduced in relation to Wilms' tumor by Beckwith and Palmer.[61] The category of FH within the same type of tumor includes cases that have relatively favorable prognosis in terms of relatively less malignant biologic behavior, and better eventual outcome (see different categories of outcome below). Category of UFH includes those tumors that take a more aggressive course of varying severity and require more intensive therapy. The histologic features associated with unfavorable prognosis for different types of tumors are given in Table 10-6. In some of the tumors the FH and UFH categories are well defined and even a different therapeutic approach is recommended (e.g., FH Wilms' vs. UFH Wilms'). In the following types of pediatric tumors the pathologic features show reliable correlation with prognosis: rhabdomyosarcoma, embryonal type, including sarcoma botryoides (FH) vs. alveolar type (UFH); Wilms' tumor with anaplasia (UFH), without anaplasia (FH); Hodgkin's lym-

TABLE 10-6 Histologic Features Associated with Unfavorable Prognosis in Pediatric Tumors

Tumor type	Histologic feature(s) associated with unfavorable prognosis
Wilm's tumor	Anaplasia
Neuroblastoma	High MKI,[a] lack of differentiation, high mitotic rate
Rhabdomyocsarcoma	Alveolar pattern, pleomorphism (anaplasia) in tumors with embryonal pattern
Hepatoblastoma	Predominantly embryonal hepatocytes, mitotic activity, undifferentiated small cell subtype
Hodgkin's disease	Lymphocytic depletion subtype

[a] Mitosis karyorrhexis index.

phoma (FH) lymphoblastic lymphoma (UFH); and hepatoblastoma with fetal pattern (FH) vs. embryonal pattern (UFH).[46,60] Comparable FH and UFH categories are also recognized in neuroblastic tumors.

It should be noted that the recent emergence of the FH and UFH prognostic subgroups is probably related to development of effective therapy for the pediatric malignancies and the availability of large statistically analyzable number of cases due to the establishment of the national cooperative studies. For example, it is possible that the poorer prognosis of anaplastic Wilms' tumor was not apparent in the past because many of the patients with Wilms' tumor had relatively poor outcome. Even if it were apparent, it would not have been statistically analyzable because of lack of a sufficiently large number of cases and their sufficiently long follow-up. With the availability of effective therapy for the "garden" (nonanaplastic) variety of Wilms' tumor, the difference between it and the anaplastic Wilms' tumor became apparent in terms of survival, and with the establishment of NWTS and centralized collection of pathologic material, a sufficiently large number of cases of this relatively rare variant of Wilms' tumor (only about 6% of Wilms' tumors) became available for appropriate statistical analysis. The same observations explain the definitive recognition of FH and UFH subgroups of rhabdomyosarcoma. Just as these tumor subtypes were recognized as UFH, some other subtypes that were conventionally thought to be associated with aggressive behavior and therefore poor outcome before the prechemotherapy era, lost their prognostic differences because these subtypes were responsive to the therapy. Thus the predominantly or exclusively blastemal subtype of Wilms' tumor, which, because of its primitive undifferentiated nature, would appear to be associated with poor prognosis, responds well to modern therapy and therefore is not included in the UFH subgroup of Wilms' tumor. Therefore response to currently available therapy is an important factor in the definition of pediatric tumors into FH and UFH.

Age-Linked Classification

This classification applies particularly to neuroblastoma. Cytologic features generally associated with aggressive biologic behavior may not have the same grave significance in a young infant as compared with an older child. This has been formalized and included into the histologic classification system of neuroblastoma introduced by Shimada et al.[59] Thus a differentiating neuroblastoma with MKI of 150 in a 2-year-old child will be classified as UFH, whereas the same type of neuroblastoma (i.e., differentiating) with the same MKI (i.e., 150) in a 1-year-old child would be considered FH. In the histologic grading system for neuroblastoma described by us, grade 2 tumors in children <1 year of age and ≥ 1 year of age were included in the low-risk and high-risk groups, respectively.[62] Similarly, atypical features in a mesoblastic nephroma occurring in an infant <3 months of age may not have the same prognostic significance as the same features in the same tumor occurring in an older infant or a child.

Importance of Autopsy Examination in Pediatric Malignancies

There has been a decline in the autopsy rate in recent years. Systematic autopsy studies have the potential of providing a great deal of information besides cause(s) of death. In malignancies, it can provide data regarding the extent of local relapse, distribution of metastases, histologic changes related to therapy in primary and metastatic tumors, extent of response to therapy, complications related to diagnostic and therapeutic procedures, drug toxicity, infections, second malignancies, etc.[63,64] In 49% of 161 autopsy cases of leukemia in children reported by Nigro et al,[64] a new diagnosis was made. The most common and significant contribution of the autopsy study was the demonstration of fungal infections that were totally unsuspected or were considered to be of bacterial origin during the clinical course. The results of this autopsy series led to increased use of antifungal therapy. Other diagnoses included splenic rupture, gastrointestinal hemorrhage, leukemic infiltration of upper respiratory tract, and bacterial and CMV infection. The lesions related to drug toxicity included interstitial pneumonia or fibrosis (associated with cyclophosphamide, radiation, carmustine), pancreatitis (associated with L-asparagine amidoyhydrolase), myocardial necrosis (associated with doxorubicin), etc. The study of leukemia has shown involvement of ovaries in 35–50% of autopsied fatal cases of acute lymphoblastic leukemia in girls.[65] There is another aspect of autopsy study of certain disease processes in which a high incidence of lymphoproliferative and/or other neoplastic disorders is expected. For example, autopsy study of fatal cases of acquired immunodeficiency syndrome (AIDS) in children has led to recognition of a lymphoproliferative disorder and has added to the number of cases of smooth muscle tumors.[66,67] Autopsy study may also confirm the presence of lesions that may have implications in genetic counseling.[68]

APPROACH TO PATHOLOGIC DIAGNOSIS OF PEDIATRIC TUMORS

Types of Pathology Specimens

The material submitted for diagnosis may be a fine-needle aspiration specimen, needle biopsy, incisional biopsy, or partial or complete excision of the tumor. In brain tumors, stereotactic biopsies may be done. Rarely, fluid from a pleural or peritoneal effusion may be submitted for diagnosis of a pediatric tumor. One problem with needle or small incisional biopsies is the crush artifact. Clinicians rarely sufficiently appreciate how the crush artifact can hinder the arrival at the pathologic diagnosis. If the amount of biopsy material is inadequate, it is advisable to offer only a tentative impression regarding the nature of the tumor or not offer any opinion at all rather than being pressured into making a definitive diagnosis. In most instances the biopsy material is obtained from the primary tumor. In occasional cases the biopsy material may represent metastasis of a known but pathologically undiagnosed, or of an unknown and unsuspected, primary tumor. When a tumor is found to be unresectable or disseminated, only an FNA (fine-needle aspiration) or needle biopsy of the tumor may be done for definitive diagnosis so that appropriate chemotherapy can be started immediately.

Triaging of the Pathologic Specimen

Since most of the major medical centers in this country are affiliated with one of national pediatric tumor study groups (POG, CCG, NWTS, IRS, IESS, etc.), it is imperative that the triaging of the pathology specimen follow the guidelines established by these national study groups for pathology protocols for each type of pediatric tumor. The specimen needs to be triaged for the following markers: oncogene determination, karyotype, immunophenotyping, and ploidy or DNA index. The tumor should be sent in a sterile container as soon after resection as possible to the attention of the pediatric pathologist or the general surgical pathologist who is specially assigned to sign out pediatric tumors in the department. Samples for the aforementioned markers should be taken from viable areas of the tumor. Most investigators determining these markers require 1 g of tumor tissue, i.e., about 1 × 1 × 1 cm fragment of tumor. The specimen for DNA index or karyotyping is collected under sterile conditions and is sent fresh in a tissue culture medium. A set of sterile instruments should be available in the surgical pathology laboratory for that purpose. The specimen for oncogene studies is snap-frozen and sent on dry ice. All specimens are sent by overnight mail to the appropriate laboratory.

The data manager of the Division of Pediatric Hematology/Oncology of each institution has the latest information on the triaging requirements for biologic and pathologic studies of each tumor. The pathology manuals put together by the national study groups give the requirements regarding pathologic material to be sent to the pathologist in charge of the pathologic study of that particular type of tumor.

Appropriate optimum triaging of the specimen and processing for pathologic studies can be achieved in every case by establishing ongoing communication and rapport between the pediatric oncologist and (general or pediatric) surgical pathologist. For smooth and efficient functioning of these procedures, it is advisable to assign one surgical pathologist to supervise and sign out *all* pediatric tumors. The advantages of such a system are: (1) the assigned individual gains experience and expertise in the triaging and diagnosis of pediatric tumors, (2) it is easier to establish rapport between pediatric oncology and surgical pathology if only a single individual is consistently involved in signing out pediatric tumors, and (3) lapses in sending certain types of specimens are eliminated (or minimized) when a single individual handles all cases of pediatric tumors. The clinicians should ideally inform the pathologist usually a day in advance of the anticipated biopsy or resection of a pediatric tumor so that the possible or probable diagnosis can be discussed and some idea regarding the triaging requirements can be obtained. Arrangements for appropriate triaging (a set of sterile instruments, sterile RPMI, equipment for snap-freezing) can then be made prior to the actual arrival of the biopsy or resected specimen in the department to avoid last-minute rush and lapses. The details of triaging vary for different tumors. The essential aspects are given in Chapter 12. I have learned by experience that pediatric tumors can arise in unusual primary sites (e.g., neuroblastoma of kidney, malignant lymphoma in pelvic "soft tissues"). Snap-freezing an appropriate portion of the biopsy of small round cell tumor for whatever additional studies (immunophenotyping of tumor cells, oncogene amplification or overexpression, etc.) may be required once the definitive diagnosis is established and is of great practical importance. When the size of the biopsy is small, the items for triaging will have to be prioritized (see Chapter 12). It is often more convenient to take sterile samples of tumor tissue in a frozen-section room when the pathologist is called for a frozen section. Although most surgeons ask for a frozen section on a biopsy or resection specimen, it is rarely for the primary diagnosis. In many cases of pediatric tumors, the primary site of the tumor, the age of the patient, biochemical markers (e.g., catecholamines in neuroblastic tumors), and/or fine-needle aspiration biopsy are helpful in formulating a preoperative diagnosis. In certain cases the diagnosis may not be known and only an undifferentiated small round cell tumor (SRCT) may be seen on frozen section. In certain instances when a superficial open biopsy of a large unresectable tumor is done, the surgeon wants to know whether the biopsy is representative of the tumor and is adequate for making the diagnosis (and for the essential items of triaging for other studies), and may ask for a frozen section on a small portion of the biopsy to answer that question.

The pediatric oncologist and the data manager in the Division of Pediatric Oncology should coordinate with the pathologist the appropriate dispersal of these specimens. If a specimen is sent to a reference laboratory for determination of markers on Friday (and as luck would have it, many of these specimens are received in the surgical pathology laboratory on a Friday afternoon), it should be ascertained that there are arrangements in place for receiving it in the reference laboratory on Saturday.

All surgical resections may not be elective or done during regular working hours. In such instances, the surgical pathologist on call should be conversant with the special needs of triaging of the specimen. It is helpful also to have a surgical pathology laboratory technologist or pathologist's assistant available to help with the triaging of the specimen. If that is not feasible, the surgical pathologist on call can seek help for specimen triaging from the laboratory staff working in other sections of the department in which 24-hour coverage is usually available (e.g., clinical chemistry, microbiology).

Besides triaging for the prognostic markers mentioned above, samples from viable areas of the tumor should be taken routinely for (1) immediate glutaraldehyde fixation for electron microscopy and (2) tumor bank (immediate snap-freezing). Several imprints should be made from the fresh specimen for demonstration of details of cytologic features of the tumor cells and for DNA analysis by image cytometry.

Diagnostic Methodology

Although for most of the tumors registered with the national study groups only routine hematoxylin- and eosin-stained sections are used for diagnosis of the type and subtype of the tumor, as indicated above, current standard of practice of surgical pathology requires the use of special procedures for establishing a definitive diagnosis of certain types of tumors. Special procedures are also indicated for determining certain biologic parameters related to the prognosis of tumors (e.g., DNA index by image or flow cytometry). Prompt fixation in buffered 10% neutral formalin (and B5 for lymphoid malignancies) is the most important first step. Delay in fixation will not only interfere with cytologic preservation but may also result in false mitotic counts. The following procedures should be used in pediatric tumors: imprints (for studying cytologic details, image cytometry, and certain special stains); routine histology, immunoperoxidase stain for one or more of the following markers: enzymes (e.g., neuron-specific enolase), cytoskeletal proteins (e.g., vimentin), neural markers (e.g., Leu7 or HNK-1), muscle markers (e.g., myoglobin, muscle specific actin); and surface markers in lymphoid cells and electron microscopy. New markers (e.g., MyoD1 gene expression in rhabdomyosarcoma) and new methods (e.g., FISH) are continuously evolving. However, many of these remain confined to specialized research laboratories. The practical use of any new methods or markers and their wide acceptance require repeated testing on a large number of cases by a number of investigators, standardization, and refinement of procedures and their adaptation to the surgical pathology laboratory. However, generally snap-frozen unfixed tissue is required for the newer methods, and it is advisable to have a couple of extra portions of snap-frozen tumor tissue in a tumor bank. The national tumor study groups have centralized tumor tissue banks, and surgical pathologists should be encouraged to send extra portions of fresh frozen tissue to these banks.

SURGICAL GUIDELINES

The POG, CCG, NWTS, IRS, and other national groups have recommended specific surgical guidelines for each tumor type. The pathologist should get a copy of the surgical guidelines from the pediatric oncologist in order to anticipate the types of specimens that will be sent from each type of tumor and the types of pathologic studies that are required to be done.

Surgical Procedures in Pediatric Tumors

The surgical procedures include
(1) incisional biopsy of primary or metastatic tumor,
(2) primary complete excision,
(3) debulking of primary and/or metastatic tumor (cytoreductive surgery),

(4) prophylactic lymph node dissection (e.g., retroperitoneal lymph node dissection in testicular germ cell tumors or paratesticular rhabdomyosarcomas),

(5) early secondary surgery for resection of residual tumor (known to be present because of previous pathologic report stating that surgical margins contain tumor) or to do a wider resection because the pathologic diagnosis of the primary resection indicates such a procedure,

(6) second-look surgery (SLS) (the objective of SLS is to assess the effects of chemotherapy of a previously unresectable tumor and to resect the residual tumor or remnant mass present at the original site of the tumor)[69]: SLS is done for neuroblastomas, rhabdomyosarcoma, malignant germ cell tumors, and malignant hepatic tumors, and in stages III and IV neuroblastoma patients, SLS is done after completion of induction (18–20 weeks of chemotherapy); in malignant teratomas and hepatoblastomas SLS may be done when recurrence is suspected on the basis of biochemical markers,

(7) surgery for local relapse suspected by clinical examination or imaging procedures (pathologic examination of the resected specimen will confirm the diagnosis of local relapse; however, in rare instances enlarged lymph node in or near the tumor bed showing nonspecific reactive changes may be mistakenly interpreted as tumor recurrence),

(8) surgery for metastatic disease—although chemotherapy may clear metastatic disease that develops during follow-up, in some cases areas of persistent metastatic disease (in the lungs, liver, etc.) may have to be treated by surgery.

It is of great practical importance to process optimally and appropriately the pathology specimens from each type of surgical procedure described above. The processing of biopsy or resection of primary tumor has been described above. The SLS specimen should be serially sliced during gross examination and all suspicious areas sampled for histology. If the SLS specimen is not too large, the entire specimen should be sent for histologic examination. The margins of the specimen should be inked. The SLS specimen may also include regional lymph nodes and, in case of abdominal tumor, also a liver biopsy. The specimen of resection of pulmonary metastasis should be inked and processed appropriately so that the margins can be assessed histologically for presence or absence of tumor. The SLS specimens and specimens of metastasis also provide an opportunity to study effects of chemotherapy on the tumor histology and prognostic significance of the latter.

STAGING OF PEDIATRIC TUMORS

Staging is assessed on the basis of findings on clinical examination, on imaging procedures, and on the basis of surgeon's findings at operation. The pathologist contributes to the determination of the stage by confirming these findings by gross and histologic examination of the resected tumors, lymph nodes, bone marrow, peritoneal fluid, etc. Pathologic findings may indicate a higher stage than originally diagnosed. Therapy is often based on the tumor stage. Therefore appropriate processing of the pathologic specimen to determine the stage is of great practical importance. Any area in the capsule suggestive of capsular invasion on gross examination should be sampled for histologic examination. All the lymph nodes found with the resected specimen or submitted separately should be sent for histologic examination. The staging criteria for different types of tumors differ but in general include the extent of the primary tumor (confined to the organ of origin, crossover beyond the contralateral border of the vertebral column, etc), completeness of resection, as judged by the surgeon and metastasis to lymph nodes and other tissues. Hodgkin's disease presents a special situation since laparotomy may be done with the express purpose of determining the stage.[70,71] Staging laparotomy with detailed pathologic examination of the spleen, liver biopsies, and various abdominal lymph nodes may move down or up the original clinical staging. Moving down the stage would result in contraction of the abdominal radiation fields.[70] Laparotomy with splenectomy followed by a systematic gross examination of the spleen (thin serial slicing) is the only reliable way to evaluate the spleen for involvement by Hodgkin's disease. In Wilms' tumor, besides confirming the stage, pathologic microsubstaging is also essential in stage I cases (see Chapter 13 for details). In neuroblastoma, the location of the lymph nodes (whether adherent to or distant from the primary tumor) influences the staging.

PROGNOSTIC FACTORS IN TUMORS

The prognostic outlook in pediatric malignancies has improved remarkably during the last several years. A number of factors such as age, biologic markers, and pathologic features have emerged as prognostic factors. New prognostic factors may emerge as a result of molecular biologic studies of the tumor and effective therapy being available for majority of the cases of a particular type of tumor. On the other hand, certain factors known to be of prognostic significance may be no more so because more effective therapy becomes available and a larger database enables detailed statistical analysis. Thus the known prognostic significance of age in Wilms' tumor has not held up in the NWTS II.[72] The various prognostic factors in pediatric tumors are discussed in this section.

Types of Survival in Children with Cancer

Before discussing the various prognostic factors, it is essential to define the different types of survival and response to therapy. The criteria for these are given in Table 10-7.[73–77] In the modern era of therapy, cure of many pediatric malignancies has become attainable. Disease-free survival for 2 years in children with solid tumors and for 5 years in children with leukemia are considered as evidence of "cure." Normal physical and mental health and rehabilitation are also important in defining "biologic" cure. It should be noted that malignancy can recur longer than 5 years after therapy is completed.

Effect of Age on Prognosis

It has been observed that certain pediatric tumors, such as sacrococcygeal teratoma, yolk sac carcinoma of testis, and neuroblastoma, have a benign or relatively less malignant behavior when they occur in the young infant as compared with an older child. On the other hand, as indicated above with the

TABLE 10-7 Criteria for Types of Response to Therapy and Types of Survival in Children with Malignancies

Type of response or survival	Criteria
Complete response (CR) (solid tumors)	Complete disappearance of all signs of disease based on clinical and imaging evidence
Partial response (PR) (solid tumors)	At least 50% reduction in the sum of the products of maximum perpendicular diameters of all measured lesions
Complete response (CR) in non-Hodgkin's lymphoma (NHL)	Disappearance of symptoms and signs of NHL
No response	Persistent disease
Progressive disease	Progression of disease, appearance of new lesions, or enlargement of existing lesions
Progression-free survival	Survival without relapse, progressive disease
Remission in acute lymphoblastic leukemia	Absence of leukemic cells on conventional examination of blood samples, <5% blast cells in bone marrow with evidence of recovering hematopoiesis, <5 mononuclear cells/ml in CSF
Event free survival in childhood acute lymphoblastic leukemia (also called failure-free survival or time to first event)	First occurrence of major events representing initial treatment failure (i.e., lack of response or death in the induction period), relapse at any site following remission, death in remission without preceding relapse or second malignancy
Disease-free survival (for solid tumors)	The time from starting treatment after judging disease-free by surgery to first failure (i.e., relapse or death)

Source: References 73–77.

availability of effective therapy, young age is not a statistically significant prognostic indicator of Wilms' tumor. The precise mechanism related to the phenomenon of better prognosis of tumors occurring in infants is not known. The primary and secondary embryonal inducers and organizers may exert a repressive influence on the pediatric tumors arising from embryonal cells. The repressive influence may lead to lysis, arrest of growth, and induction of differentiation.[14,78]

Oncogenes in Pediatric Tumors

About 20 different viral oncogenes have been isolated from viruses (Table 10-8).[79] There are a number of pediatric tumors in which oncogene expression has been detected or predicted (Table 10-9).[80] Oncogene overexpression or amplification may be of value in further characterizing certain rare pediatric tumors and also in predicting survival. Thus amplification and overexpression

TABLE 10-8 Retroviral Oncogenes[a]

Retrovirus	Oncogene
Abelson murine leukemia virus (mouse)	abl
Avian erythroblastosis virus (chicken)	erb A, erb B
E26 (chicken)	ets
Chicken sarcoma virus, feline sarcoma virus (cat)	fes, fps
Feline sarcoma virus (cat), chicken sarcoma virus	fgr, yes
Feline sarcoma virus (cat)	fms
Murine sarcoma virus (mouse)	fos
Murine sarcoma virus (mouse)	mos
Avian myeloblastosis virus (chicken), E26	myb
Myelocytomatosis-29 virus, Mill-Hill-2 virus, CMII/OK10 virus (chicken)	myc
Mill-Hill-2 virus (chicken), murine sarcoma virus (mouse)	raf
Harvey murine sarcoma virus (rat)	H-ras
Murine sarcoma virus (mouse)	bas
Kirsten murine sarcoma virus (mouse)	K-ras
Reticuloendothelial virus (turkey)	rel
VR2 (chicken)	ros
Simian sarcoma virus (Woolly monkey), feline sarcoma virus (cat)	sis
SKV770 (chicken)	ski
Rous sarcoma virus (chicken)	src

[a]Each viral oncogene (v-onc) has cell analogue, i.e., the c-onc.

of c-myc oncogene rather N-myc appears to characterize peripheral primitive neuroectodermal tumor (PNET) and can be of potential use in distinguishing PNET from neuroblastoma.[81] Amplification of the oncogene N-myc in neuroblastomas is associated with poor prognosis. Therefore, knowledge of oncogene abnormalities in a tumor is important in diagnosis, prognosis, and understanding the pathogenesis of tumors in children.

The discussion of oncogenes must begin with the RNA tumor viruses. All RNA tumor viruses are retroviruses (RV). In addition to Rous sarcoma virus[82] causing sarcomas in chickens, numerous other RV have been shown to cause

TABLE 10-9 Oncogene Expression in Tumors in Children

Type of tumor	Oncogene[a]
Rhabdomyosarcoma	src, H/K-ras, c-myb, rel
Ewing's sarcoma	src
Neuroblastoma	H/K-ras, c-myb
PNET[b]	ets-1, c-myc
Leukemia	src, H/K-ras, c-myb, abl
Lymphoma	c-myb, c-myc
Osteosarcoma	src
Glioblastoma	sis

[a]See Table 10-8 for the viral origin of the oncogenes.
[b](Peripheral) primitive neuroectodermal tumor
Source: Adapted from reference 80.

cancer in animals (e.g., murine leukemia, murine mammary tumors).[79] However, in humans, a rare type of leukemia (adult T-cell leukemia/lymphoma) has been the only tumor associated with RV.[83] The genome of RV consists of single-stranded RNA that codes for three major genes. Gag and env genes code for structural proteins, while pol codes for an RNA-dependent DNA polymerase called *reverse transcriptase* (RT). A double-stranded DNA copy of the RNA template is required for the replication of RV, which is accomplished via RT.[84] In addition to the three major genes, the animal RV that are associated with cancer contain sequences in their genome that are responsible for transformation of the host cell. These genes are called viral oncogenes (v-onc). In 1978 Spector et al discovered that normal cellular DNA in the human genome included genes that were highly homologous to the v-oncs.[85] These genes were called *cellular oncogenes* or *protooncogenes* (c-onc). Some investigators use the term *oncogene* to indicate activated protooncogenes. Protooncogenes have been shown to be present in normal cells of almost all vertebrates and even in Drosophila. The presence of protooncogenes in the normal cells of animals of such wide distribution indicates a fundamental role for them in growth, development, and differentiation. Expression of protooncogenes is normally tightly regulated in human cells. The products of these genes are critical proteins involved in the control of normal growth and differentiation of a cell.

It has been suggested that v-oncs were originally derived from genes in eukaryotic cells. It has been shown that although there is high homology between c-onc and v-onc, the latter are in fact aberrant forms of their normal corresponding c-onc counterparts. The oncogenes identified in tumor cells are also aberrant forms of the normal cellular protooncogene and act as transforming genes. About 50 transforming oncogenes have been recognized in human tumors. Changes that activate normal protooncogenes to become transforming oncogenes could occur at the DNA, RNA, or protein level. An oncogene can be defined as a gene that codes for a protein that in certain circumstances may lead to transformation of a normal cell into a malignant neoplastic cell. Carcinogenesis is a multistep process that requires the acquisition of several oncogene abnormalities within a cell before complete neoplastic transformation occurs.

Isolation of Oncogenes

The oncogenes are isolated by the following procedure: (1) extraction of DNA from a cell culture of the tumor or the tumor tissue itself, (2) cutting of DNA into small fragments (30–50 kbp) by restriction endonucleases, (3) separation of fragments according to size by electrophoresis, (4) transfection (uptake of a foreign DNA by mammalian cells resulting in the acquisition of new genes) of mouse fibroblast cultures by transferring each DNA fragment separately, (5) transformation of the fibroblast culture that is transfected by DNA fragment containing the oncogene, (6) preparation of c-DNA probe from the DNA fragment containing the oncogene, (7) labeling of the probe by radioisotope for subsequent detection of the oncogene by radioautography, and (8) isolation of oncogene in pure form (Figure 10-13).[86]

Translation Products and Function of Oncogenes

The translation products of many oncogenes are relatively small peptides that participate in the regulation of mitosis by various mechanisms acting as

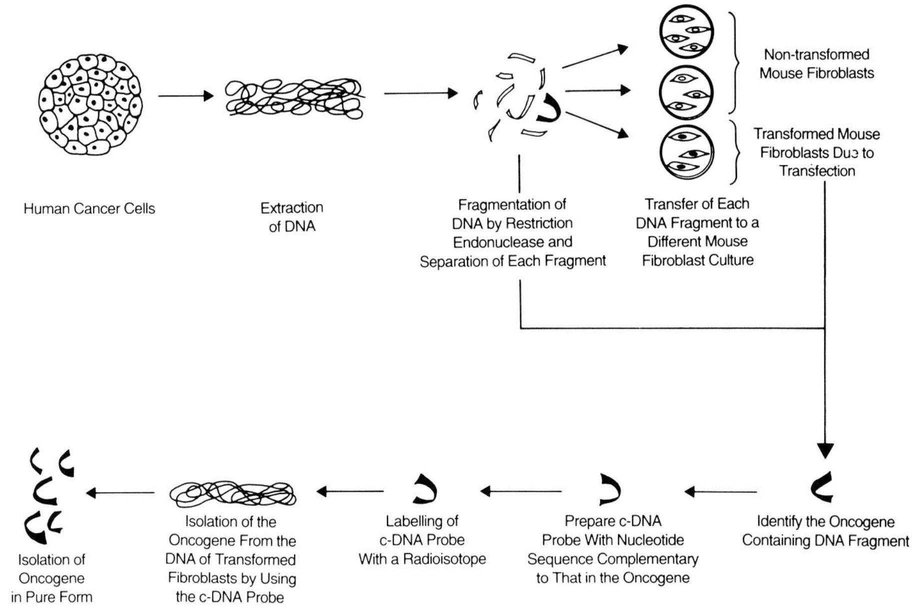

FIGURE 10-13. Diagrammatic representation of steps involved in the isolation of an oncogene (adapted from reference 86).

growth factors or at the inner side of the plasma membrane, in the cytoplasm or the nucleus. Cell multiplication is mediated by growth factors that bind to specific receptors on the cell surface. These external signals given by the growth factors are relayed by the receptors to membrane-associated cytoplasmic proteins that function as signal transducers. This information is further relayed to cytoplasmic or nuclear elements by second messenger proteins that are modified by the signal transducers. The receptor molecule may also modify the second messenger proteins directly. The gene expression is regulated by nuclear proteins resulting in synthesis of protein products that respond to the initial external signal appropriately. The oncogene products can be divided into four groups on the basis of their known or presumed function in the regulation of mitosis. A fifth group consists of products with unknown or uncertain function.[86,87] The groups are as follows:

1. *Growth factors*. Example: The cellular homolog c-sis, of the transforming gene, v-sis, of the simian sarcoma virus (SSV) has been shown to encode the platelet-derived growth factor (PDGF). PDGF released from platelets at the site of injury is a potent mitogen for the fibroblasts and smooth muscle cells. Cell lines transformed with SSV secrete a PDGF-like growth factor.

2. Growth factor receptors. Example: The receptor molecules on the external aspect of the cell membrane have an internal cytoplasmic tail that serves to transduce the stimulus to second messenger proteins. Most of the growth receptors are tyrosine kinases. The human neu oncogene which is now called c-erb B-2 or HER-2 neu encodes a protein which is 50% homologous with the

epidermal growth factor (EGF) receptor. The activated c-erb B-2 oncogene and its normal cellular homologue differ from each other only by a single amino acid substitution in the transmembrane portion of the protein.

3. *Signal transducers.* These proteins located along the inner aspect of the cell membrane transduce to the intracellular biochemical pathways the external stimuli received by cell surface components. Example: The gene product of c-src, which was the first protooncogene to be identified in the human genome, is a tyrosine-specific protein kinase that acts as a signal transducer when anchored to the inner surface of the membrane.

4. *Nuclear oncoproteins.* The external signals lead to activation of many second messenger proteins the identities of which are not known. The second messengers transmit the information of the external signals to the nucleus leading to activation of specific genes in the nucleus. It is possible that nucleoproteins encoded by oncogenes may be involved in the transmission of information from the second messengers to the nucleus. The activation of the specific genes constitutes the appropriate cellular response to the external signal. Example: N-myc gene product is a nuclear phosphoprotein that probably plays a role in regulating transcription of genes associated with proliferation. It is a basic helix-loop-helix (HLH)/leucine zipper protein that appears to form a heterodimer with another HLH protein called *Max.*[88] This heterodimer binds to a particular DNA recognition sequence CACGTG presumably of regulatory region of other genes involved in cell proliferation and activates transcription, whereas Max homodimers may repress this transcriptional activation.[88,89] The aforementioned heterodimers have been identified in human neuroblastoma cell lines.[90]

The functions of the oncogene products can be summarized as follows: (1) provide external stimulus to mitosis by secretion of growth factors (e.g., PDGF-like growth factor secreted by cell lines transformed with SSV, containing the cellular homologue of v-sis oncogene), (2) transduction of effect of exogenous growth factor by the growth factor receptors or activation of growth factor receptors at the plasma membrane (e.g., the EGF receptor-like product encoded by the cellular homologue of the Avian erythroblastosis virus oncogene v-erb B), (3) transduction of external signal to intracellular biochemical pathways (e.g., the tyrosine specific protein kinase encoded by c-src), and (4) DNA binding to activate specific genes (e.g., N-myc gene product and HLH protein Max binding to genes involved in cell proliferation).

Oncogenes and Neoplastic Transformation of Cells

Viral oncogenes were first identified in animal tumors and were determined to play a major role in the etiology of these tumors. Hence the designation *oncogene.* Now it has become apparent that the cellular homolog of the viral oncogenes are normal constituents of the genome and encode for proteins that play a vital role in the normal control of mitosis. Gordon[86] has suggested that the correct designation for these genes would be "mitogenes." In their natural state the oncogenes are relatively quiescent and control mitosis in an orderly manner. The result of disruption of regulation of oncogenes is disorderly cell division and differentiation, which are the hallmarks of cellular transformation. The following processes can result in abnormal deregulation of the oncogenes:[86]

1. The oncogene may be disordered by a point mutation. Point mutation may change a normal functioning gene product into a transforming peptide.
2. Oncogenes may be activated by altered chromosomal structure. For example, at its normal locus on the long arm of chromosome 8, the expression of c-myc gene is tightly regulated. As a result of 8;14 translocation in Burkitt's lymphoma, the c-myc gene is brought to 14*q*32 within the region of the gene for heavy-chain immunoglobulin, IgH. In its new location, the c-myc oncogene is brought under the regulatory elements of the transcriptionally active IgH gene. Therefore, c-myc oncogene is activated, resulting in marked increase in its product—a DNA-binding protein. The excessive binding of a DNA regulator of mitosis may be the mechanism by which the translocated and activated c-myc transforms normal cells to malignant ones.
3. Loss of regular sequences within the gene results in deregulation of the sequences responsible for coding of the gene product. When c-myc is translocated (as in Burkitt's lymphoma), it loses its regulator sequence in exon 1. This leads to overproduction of DNA binding protein encoded by the intact sequences within the gene.
4. Neoplastic cells frequently contain extra chromosomal material called *double minutes* (DM). There may also be large homogeneously staining regions (HSR) in some of the chromosomes of neoplastic cells. DNA probes for N-myc oncogene have been shown to bind to the DM and HSR in a human neuroblastoma cell line and HSRs contain multiple copies of part of the sequence of N-myc.[91] Excessive amount of the protein product is present in the cells that contain amplified copies of N-myc.[91] Amplification of N-myc is seen in advanced stages of neuroblastoma, thus correlating with poorer prognosis.[92] Amplification of N-myc gene may be associated with altered expression, resulting in abnormal protein product or normal protein product in abnormal amounts or synthesis of product at inappropriate times in the cell cycle.[93]
5. Interaction of oncogenes with exogenous agents may also initiate processes that deregulate the oncogenes. Infection of B lymphocytes by Epstein-Barr virus, a double-stranded DNA virus, results in their immortalization; i.e., these lymphocytes can grow continuously in tissue culture. The mechanism responsible for this immortalization of B lymphocytes probably involves an interation of EBV genome-coded protein with critical cellular proteins or genes. Burkitt's lymphoma arises from the immortalized lymphocytes when the *t*(8;14) and c-myc oncogene activation is superimposed on these immortalized lymphocytes.
6. Degree of methylation of the nucleotides is also related to the activity of the gene. Undermethylation is associated with heightened gene activity. Oncogenes could be activated by demethylation of its DNA by external agents.

Tumor Suppressor Genes

The presence of tumor suppressor genes (TSGs) or antioncogenes or emerogenes (from the Greek word meaning "to tame") was predicted by reversal of tumerigeneity in the hybrid cells resulting from fusion of normal cells with malignant cells in culture demonstrated in the 1960s and 1970s.[94] TSGs encode for proteins that are negative regulators of cell growth or differentiation. Normal expression of TSGs inhibits transformation. In contrast to oncogenes that act in a dominant manner (i.e., one abnormal allele is capable of causing malignant transformation), loss of both alleles of TSG is required for neoplatic transformation. Deletion of whole chromosomes or their fragments or mutation in the TSG itself results in inactivation of that TSG allele. Initially, mutation involving one allele of TSG makes it nonfunctional (heterozygous state). Complete inactivation of that TSG occurs with the loss of remaining normal allele as a result of chromosome nondisjunction, or recombination between affected and unaffected chromosomes during mitosis (loss of heterozygosity) (LOH).[95] Besides these mechanisms of inactivation at the DNA level, inactivation of TSG may also be accomplished by neutralization of its protein product by the binding of dominant oncoproteins.[87]

Retinoblastoma is the best example of pediatric tumor in which loss of a TSG, Rb on chromosome 13*q*14 has been demonstrated.[96–98] Structural rearrangement or mutations of the gene itself can lead to alterations and inactivation of Rb with synthesis of abnormal gene products coded by Rb.[97,98] Besides retinoblastoma, inactivation of Rb has been demonstrated also in osteogenic sarcoma, soft tissue sarcoma, and breast carcinoma. Inactivation of TSGs is suspected to involve the development of other pediatric tumors such as Wilms' tumor, embryonal rhabdomyosarcoma, hepatoblastoma, and neuroblastoma.[99–101] Another TSG that was initially designated as an oncogene is *p*53. Inherited mutations of *p*53 TSG are involved in the Li-Fraumeni syndrome (a rare familial syndrome characterized by high incidence of premenopausal breast carcinoma, childhood sarcomas, and other malignancies such as brain tumors and leukemias).[102] In a recent study, germ line mutations in *p*53 TSG were demonstrated in children and young adults who did not have family history of Li-Fraumeni syndrome but developed a second malignant neoplasm following therapy of the first one during childhood or at young age.[103] The first tumors were neuroblastoma, liposarcoma, soft tissue sarcoma, and non-Hodgkin's lymphoma. The second tumors were breast carcinoma, osteogenic sarcoma, gastric carcinoma, and colon carcinoma. Acquired mutations in *p*53 TSG are found in carcinomas of the colon, breast, and lung.

OTHER PROGNOSTIC MARKERS IN PEDIATRIC TUMORS

Besides histologic features, age, and oncogene amplification, other prognostic markers have also been described in pediatric tumors. These include serum lactate dehydrogenase (LDH),[104–106] serum ferritin,[107] DNA index,[20,108,109] and structural chromosomal abnormalities.[110]

Serum Markers of Prognosis

Elevated serum LDH, which is a nonspecific marker of poor prognosis in many different types of malignancies, reflects a large tumor burden and release of the enzyme from the tumor cells. In neuroblastoma and in Burkitt's lymphoma high serum LDH level (≥1000 or 1500 IU/liter) is associated with advanced stages and poor prognosis.[104–106] Serum ferritin levels of <75 ng/ml, 75–142 ng/ml, and >142 ng/ml (measured by radioimmunoassay) correlated respectively with better, intermediate, and poor prognosis in children with neuroblastoma.[107] Structural abnormalities of chromosome 1 (deletions and translocations of short arm with breakpoint at 1*p*32) are associated with poor prognosis in neuroblastoma.[110]

DNA Index

DNA index (DI) is a numerical value that expresses the amount of DNA content of tumor cells as compared with that of normal cells. Chicken and trout erythrocytes are used as internal controls and normal human peripheral lymphocytes as external controls to identify the normal human diploid G_0/G_1 portion. Thus DI of 1.57 for a tumor indicates that the aneuploid population of tumor cells has DNA content 1.57 times that of normal cells. DI has been shown to be of significant prognostic value in acute lymphoblastic leukemia (ALL),[20] medulloblastoma,[109] and neuroblastoma.[108] Thus in children with ALL, those with a DI of >1.16 showed significantly better response to therapy as compared with those whose leukemic cells had diploid DI or DI of 1.01–1.15.[20] In medulloblastoma aneuploidy is predictive of better outcome.[109] In contrast to aneuploid pediatric solid tumors, aneuploid solid tumors in adults such as carcinomas of breast or ovary are associated with advanced disease and worse survival.[111,112] In neuroblastoma DI of 1 is associated with worse survival.[108]

Of the various nonmorphologic prognostic markers described in this section, DI is the most important from the point of view of surgical pathologist, who is involved in sending a sample from the tumor for ploidy analysis and in some institutions actual determination of the DI by flow or image cytometry. It is essential to make certain that the sample represents viable tumor tissue and that an adequate amount of tumor tissue is sent. In a cellular tumor, a position measuring 0.3–0.5 cm^3 is usually sufficient to yield $0.5–1 \times 10^6$ tumor cells.[113] The sample does not have to be sterile. It should be removed from the fresh tumor as soon as possible after resection and placed in RPMI or other suitable transport medium and stored at 4°C until it is processed or sent at room temperature to the centralized laboratory of the national study group by overnight courier service. Tumor tissue frozen at −70°C and paraffin-embedded tumor tissue can also be used for determination of DI.

Cell Cycle and Ploidy Status

Knowledge of cell cycle is essential in the understanding of DI. The phases in the cell cycle are represented diagrammatically in Figure 10-14. After completing mitosis (M phase), the cell enters the presynthetic G_1 phase of cell growth. In G_1 phase the nucleus has a 2*N* or diploid amount of DNA (23 chromosome pairs). The cells with diploid DNA content that are not cycling are considered as being in G_0 or resting phase. The cycling cells that are considered as being G_1 phase begin to replicate their DNA content. After completion of DNA replication the cells have 4N amount of DNA. This phase of cell cycle is called "G_2." The minimum cell cycle transit time is about 5–10 hours for mammalian cells. Cell cycle can become delayed in the early G_1 phase. The cycling cells that are between G_1 and G_2 phases have a DNA amount varying between 2*N* and 4*N*. The phase between G_1 and G_2 is called "S phase." Proliferation in a population of

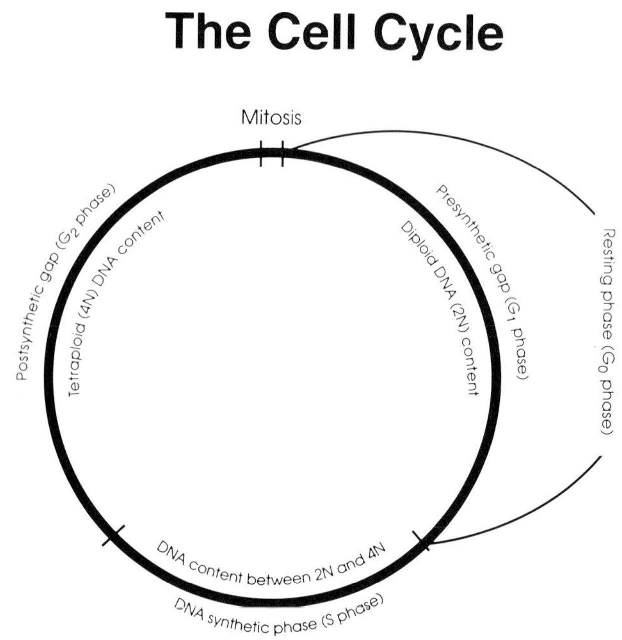

FIGURE 10-14. Diagrammatic representation of the various phases of the cell cycle and DNA content in each phase.

cells proceeds asynchronously. Therefore at any given time, cells can be found in all phases of cell cycle. The flow cytometric DNA analysis does not distinguish between G_2 and M nuclei (since they both have 4*N* amount of DNA). Therefore the term $G_2 + M$ is used. The amount of DNA within a nucleus is determined by flow cytometry by using fluorescence dyes (e.g., propidium iodide). The fluorescence intensity given by each stained nucleus is proportional to its DNA content. A histogram of the tumor cell population being analyzed is generated by collecting data on DNA content of a large number of nuclei. DNA histogram of central primitive neuroectodermal tumor of the brain in a 7-year-old boy is illustrated in Figure 10-15.

Another important measurement done by flow cytometry is the estimation of S-phase fraction (SPF). Other terms analogous to SPF are proliferative activity, proliferative capacity, proliferative potential, proliferative index, cell kinetics, and S-phase portion. SPF generally reflects the static measurement of cells with an S-phase amount of DNA, i.e., 2N–4N DNA. Proliferative index (PI), which reflects the ratio of proliferative compartment as compared with all compartments × 100, is calculated by the following formula:[114]

$$PI = \frac{100\,(S + G_2 + M)}{G_0G_1 + S + G_2 + M}$$

Most investigators have concentrated on the DNA content (ploidy) as a prognostic marker of malignancies. However, there is some evidence that high S-phase fraction may be predictive of a worse prognosis in certain malignancies (e.g., malignant lymphoma and Wilms' tumor).[115,116]

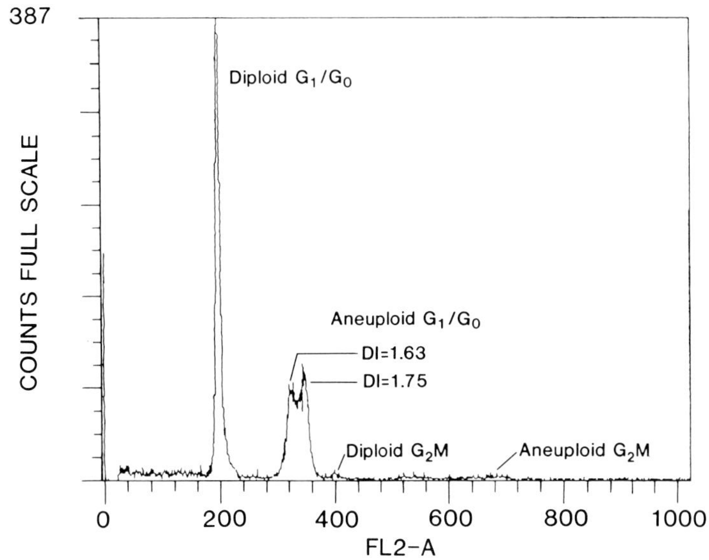

FIGURE 10-15. Histogram of a central primitive neuroectodermal tumor in a 7-year-old child showing three peaks. The first peak at channel number 200 is the diploid peak. The two subsequent closely placed peaks are indicative of aneuploid tumor cell populations with DI of 1.63 and 1.75 at channel numbers 326 and 350, respectively. Small peaks of diploid and aneuploid cells in G_2M phase are also present. (Courtesy of Dr. Greg Gagnon)

It should be noted that flow cytometric analysis does not pick up the individual chromosomal structural abnormalities in a diploid tumor cell population. It is not sensitive enough to pick up increased DNA content associated with oncogene amplification. It has been realized that flow cytometric analysis is likely to contain a significant margin of error. Reproducibility of data from one laboratory to another may not be satisfactory. The nature and preparation of the sample and analysis of histogram are major determinants of quality and consistency of results. Histologic evaluation of 5-μm-diameter sections from the sample analyzed by flow cytometry or of the cytospin should be performed by a surgical pathologist to ascertain that the sample is representative of the tumor under consideration and contains preferably at least 30% tumor cells. The proportion of lymphocytes and stromal cells and extent of necrosis and hemorrhage also should be noted in this evaluation. The suspension should contain single cells with minimal debris. Appropriate internal and external controls should be taken. Thus flow cytometric analysis requires stringent quality control.

Correlation between Different Nonmorphologic Prognostic Markers and between Morphologic and Nonmorphologic Prognostic Markers

A few reports in the literature have shown these correlations in Wilms' tumor and neuroblastoma. These are discussed in detail in Chapter 13, but briefly, anaplastic Wilms' tumor (containing foci of tumor cells with markedly hyperchromatic and enlarged nuclei and multipolar mitotic figures) are associated with hyperdiploidy with a DI of 1.7–3.2.[117] There is correlation between two nonmorphologic markers of poor prognosis of neuroblastoma, viz., N-myc gene amplification and DI of 1.[118] Correlation between high histologic grade, N-myc gene amplification, DI of 1, and high serum LDH values has also been shown in neuroblastomas.[119]

PRINCIPLES OF CHEMOTHERAPY

Although, as described in the introductory section of this chapter, the modern era of chemotherapy of malignancies was pioneered by a pediatric pathologist, present-day pediatric pathologists are not involved directly in the therapy of a child with a malignancy. The role of the pathologist in this area is indirect in terms of providing the accurate prognostic pathologic categorization (i.e., FH vs. UFH) or accurate diagnosis of a pathologic entity that requires specific therapeutic approach (e.g., clear cell sarcoma and malignant rhabdoid tumor of the kidney). The pediatric pathologist is involved in assessing certain types of drug toxicity seen in children with malignancies. Therefore, it is helpful to have a basic background of the principles and types of drugs used in chemotherapy.

The considerations of cell cycle described above in the section on flow cytometric analysis and of structure and organization of the tumor to be described presently are of vital importance in relation to discussion of chemotherapy. From the structural and organizational point of view, the tumor can be divided into the following fractions:[120] proliferative fraction (PF), differentiated fraction (DF), G_0 fraction (GF), and nonproliferative fraction (NPF). There is also cell loss from the primary tumor due to necrosis, apoptosis, exfoliation from skin, gastrointestinal and genitourinary tracts, exfoliation into several cavities, and metastasis. Necrosis in tumors is related to hypoxia due to hypovascularity or avascularity and direct killing of tumor cells by cell mediated immune response. The tumor growth is almost totally dependent on the tumor's ability to generate adequate blood supply by the phenomenon of neovascularization (tumor angiogenesis).[121] Presence of hypoxic cells has been demonstrated in solid tumors in experimental animals. Viable cells are usually within approximately 150 μm of a capillary.[122] Area of necrosis is seen beyond this distance. Proliferating tumor cells are found adjacent to the capillary. The cells between proliferating cells and area of necrosis are arrested in cell cycle because of insufficient nutrients. These cells constitute the NPF of the tumor.

The PF of the tumor represents the concentrated focus of attack in therapy. The hypoxic and nutritionally deprived cells of the NPF are inadequately penetrated by chemotherapeutic agents and are relatively radiation resistant because of hypoperfusion. The NPF and G_0 are the principal obstacles in the therapeutic goal of total eradication of tumor cell population. The cells of the DF (e.g., mature ganglion cells of a ganglioneuroblastoma) that are presumably the end-stage cells are not taken into consideration from therapeutic point-of-view.

Types of Chemotherapeutic Agents

Chemotherapeutic agents can be classified on the basis of their effect on the proliferating cell. Thus there are phase-specific and cycle-specific drugs. The former exert their cytotoxic effect in a specific phase of cell cycle, usually the S phase. Drugs interfering with DNA synthesis such as vincristine, and 6-mercaptopurine belong to this group. The cycle-specific drugs are cytotoxic to cells in all phases of the cell cycle. The chemotherapeutic agents are also classified according to their pharmacologic and chemical properties (Table 10-10). The sites of action of these agents include DNA synthesis, synthesis of RNA from DNA, and synthesis of proteins from messenger RNA. The modes of action of various chemotherapeutic drugs are summarized in Table 10-10.

Drug Toxicity

Antineoplastic agents acting on proliferating cells of the tumor also affect the proliferating cells in the normal tissues such as bone marrow, gastrointestinal

TABLE 10-10 Types of Drugs Used in Chemotherapy

Drug type	Examples	Mode of action
Alkylating agents	Cyclophosphamide, ifosfamide, cisplatin, melphalan, carmustine, dacarbazine, etc.	Alkylation of cellular macromolecules with damage to DNA template and DNA synthesis
Antimetabolites	Methotrexate, 6-mercaptopurine, 5-fluorouracil, cytarabine (cytosine arabinoside)	Binding to enzymes involved in the synthesis of DNA because of structural resemblance to normal metabolites, inhibition of synthesis of DNA, or synthesis of defective DNA
Antitumor antibiotics	Adriamycin, daunomycin, bleomycin, dactinomycin	Insertion into and binding to DNA helix, interfering with DNA replication, transcription and repair; free-radical formation with oxidative damage to macromolecules; formation of single-strand breaks in DNA, effects on cell membrane
Plant alkaloids	Vincristine, vinblastine, etoposide (VP-16), teneposide (VM-26)	DNA strand breaks, binding to tubulin with disruption of microtubular system and inhibition of mitotic spindle formation
Steroids	Prednisone, prednisolone, dexamethasone	Lympholysis
Miscellaneous	L-Asparaginase	Depletion of L-asparagine within leukemic cells with inhibition of protein synthesis

epithelial cells, and cells of the hair follicle. These agents have a low therapeutic index (ratio of toxic dose to therapeutic dose). Hence various toxic reactions are seen in children being treated for malignant disease. All antineoplastic drugs with the possible exception of bleomycin are immunosuppressive. Hence infectious complications are also seen in these children.

Clinically, hepatic, renal, cardiac, and neurologic dysfunction, nausea, vomiting, and alopecia are seen not infrequently in children who are given aggressive chemotherapy. In most instances, these are transient and reversible with appropriate supportive measures and/or withdrawal of the drugs. Hypersensitivity reactions ranging from urticaria to laryngeal edema, bronchospasm, and anaphylaxis are also seen in children given chemotherapy for malignant disease. Pathologic lesions are demonstrable if a biopsy is done or at autopsy if the patient dies.[63] The lesion may be so severe (e.g., fibrosis of urinary bladder due to cyclophosphamide toxicity) that it may require surgical resection.[123] The various types of toxic lesions and the drugs producing them are given in Table 10-11.[123–132] As pathologists we are likely to get bone marrow samples, liver biopsy, endomyocardial biopsy (Figure 10-16), lung biopsy, and for pulmonary infections bronchoalveolar lavage from those children who develop toxic reactions and infections following chemotherapy. Lesions related to toxicity and various infections are also seen at autopsy in fatal cases of pediatric malignancies.

In certain cases of advanced malignant disease refractory to conventional therapy, "experimental" drugs may be used as the last resort. The patient may respond to such therapy or may die despite the additional therapy. The pediatric oncologist would be interested in determining the extent of response to the new therapy in terms of reduction in the viable tumor in the local relapse or metastatic disease at autopsy. Careful gross examination to determine the extent of hemorrhage and necrosis in the tumor mass and appropriate number of sections from representative areas for histologic examination would enable the pediatric pathologist to answer these questions.

RADIATION THERAPY

In children with malignancies radiation therapy is used alone or in combination with chemotherapy. It may be associated with certain types of toxic reactions. Acute radiation effects are noted particularly in proliferating tissues such as skin, mucous membranes, gonads, and bone marrow, but most tissues show lesions of variable severity. Late effects in many of the tissues and organs are secondary to chronic radiation injury to arterioles and capillaries characterized by segmental sclerosis and luminal narrowing. The radiation effects are well described in the standard textbooks on pediatric oncology and general pathology and monographs on pediatric oncology.[132–135]

Bone marrow, lymph nodes, and gonads are highly radiosensitive. Lung, hair follicles and mucosal epithelium of gastrointestinal tract and other sites, show intermediate sensitivity to radiation. Vascular endothelium and epithelium of urinary bladder, kidney, breast, and pancreas, cartilage, bone, brain, muscle, and peripheral nerves show low to medium radiosensitivity. The

TABLE 10-11 Pathologic Lesions Related Toxicity of Chemotherapeutic Agents

Type of lesion	Drugs producing the lesion
Myelosuppression	Procarbazine, methotrexate, 5-fluorouracil, vinblastine, mechlorethamine, cyclophosphamide, ifosfamide melphalan, carmustine, lomustine, decarbazine, etoposide
Hepatic fibrosis	Methotrexate (chronic low dose regimen)
Interstitial pneumonia	Bleomycin, methotrexate, melphalan, carmustine, procarbazine, sesmustine, etc.
Diffuse alveolar damage	Bleomycin, cyclophosphamide, vinblastine, carmustine, lomustine, methotrexate, etc.
Obliterative bronchiolitis	Lomustine
Bronchiolitis obliterans—organizing pneumonia	Bleomycin, cyclophosphamide, methotrexate, etc.
Eosinophilic pneumonia	Bleomycin
Pulmonary venoocclusive disease	Bleomycin, carmustine
Pulmonary hemorrhage	Cyclophosphamide
Pulmonary edema	Methotrexate
Renal atrophy	Sesmutine, lomustine (cumulative dose of 1500 mg/m^2)
Encephalopathy	Mechlorethamine
Sclerosing thrombophlebitis	Mechlorethamine
Ulceration, fibrosis, and telangiectasia of urinary bladder	Cyclophosphamide, ifosfamide
Renal tubular necrosis predominantly of distal tubules and collecting ducts	Cisplatin
Peripheral neuropathy	Cisplatin, vincristine, etoposide
Hepatic venoocclusive disease	Dacarbazine (DTIC)
Hepatic vein thrombosis	Dacarbazine (DTIC)
Oral ulcers and stomatitis	Dactinomycin, methotrexate, etoposide, adriamycin, etc.
Gastrointestinal mucosal necrosis	Cytarabine
Loss of Purkinje cells and gliosis of cerebellum	Cytarabine
Dermatitis (erythema, desquamation, induration, pigmentation)	5- Fluorouracil, bleomycin, methotrexate, etc.
Cardiomyopathy (myofibrillar loss, vacuolar degeneration, interstitial fibrosis by light and electron microscopy)	Adriamycin (cumulative dose of >600 mg/m^2) and daunomycin (>559 ng/m^2)
Skin ulceration and soft tissue damage due to extravasation	Adriamycin, daunomycin, vincristine, etc.
Aseptic necrosis of bone	Corticosteroids

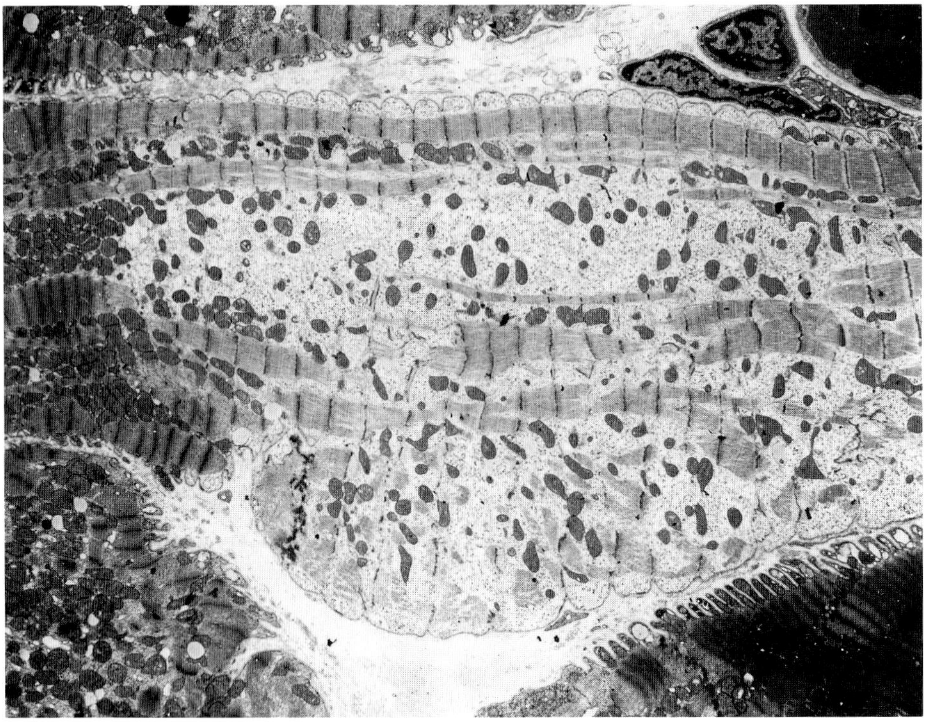

FIGURE 10-16. Electron micrograph of endomyocardial biopsy in a child with adriamycin cardiomyopathy. Note the loss of myofibrils (uranyl acetate and lead citrate, ×17,000).

lesions related to radiation toxicity that are listed in Table 10-12 are rarely biopsied. Surgical correction or resection may be required in some of the chronic cicatricizing lesions. These lesions should be carefully looked for in autopsies on fatal cases of pediatric malignancies. A serious late sequela of both chemotherapy and radiation therapy of pediatric malignancies, viz., development of a second primary malignancy, is described in a separate section below.

BONE MARROW TRANSPLANTATION

In recent years bone marrow transplantation (BMT) has been shown to be of benefit in the therapy of leukemias in children. BMT has also been employed in some of the children with NHL and neuroblastoma in whom conventional chemotherapy and radiation therapy had failed. Graft-versus-host disease (GVHD) is the main obstacle in the success of BMT. GVHD can be acute and chronic. Pediatric pathologists will be called on to confirm the diagnosis of GVHD in the biopsy specimens from skin, gastrointestinal tract, liver, lymphoreticular system, etc. Both acute and chronic lesions are present in the different tissues. Cytotoxic drugs and radiation that may be used in the pretransplantation preparatory period may produce similar lesions. Details of clinical history and

TABLE 10-12 Lesions Related to Radiation Injury

Tissue or organ	Lesions
Skin	Acute and chronic radiodermatitis
Bone marrow	Myelosuppression
Lymph nodes	Lymphocytic depletion, atrophy
Gonads	Necrosis of germ cells, atrophy, and fibrosis
Lung	Acute radiation pneumonitis, pulmonary edema, interstitial fibrosis
Gastrointestinal tract	Ulceration, hemorrhage, mucosal atrophy, submucosal fibrosis, stricture (e.g., of rectum)
Brain and spinal cord	Infarction, necrosis
Heart	Pericarditis with effusion, constrictive pericarditis, myocardial fibrosis
Blood vessels	Endothelial and medial necrosis, collagenous hyaline thickening with luminal narrowing
Urinary bladder	Acute (hemorrhagic) cystitis, contracture
Breast	Lack of development
Kidney	Acute and chronic radiation nephritis, atrophy
Liver	Acute and chronic radiation hepatitis, portal fibrosis (children more susceptible than adults, nutritional status influences extent of injury)
Growing cartilage and bone	Growth arrest, dwarfing, deformity
Mature cartilage and bone	Necrosis, fracture, sclerosis
Eye	Retinopathy, corneal ulceration, cataract
Peripheral nerves	Neuritis
Ureters	Stricture
Endocrine glands	Hypofunction of thyroid, adrenals, pituitary
Muscle	Atrophy

other modes of therapy the child may have received should be taken into consideration before the biopsy findings are interpreted. A number of articles and a monograph describing systematically the findings of biopsies of various organs in GVHD following BMT are available.[136–139] The basic diagnostic feature in skin, liver, intestine, labial, and oral mucosa, salivary and lacrimal gland ducts, and conjunctiva is individual cell death with formation of eosinophilic bodies involving the epithelial cells in these organs (in the liver the bile duct epithelium is the main target cell). The characteristic findings in various biopsies are summarized here: (1) *skin*—basal vacuolar degeneration and individual cell necrosis of keratinocytes with formation of eosinophilic bodies (after day 20), lymphocytic satellitosis around the necrotic cells, basal cell vacuolar degeneration; (2) *liver*—degeneration of bile duct epithelium, portal triaditis, lobular inflammatory infiltrate, hepatocyte degeneration, and necrosis; (3) *intestine* (particularly rectum)—necrosis of individual cells lining the crypts, mononuclear cell infiltration, crypt abscess; (4) *labial and oral mucosa*—individual cell necrosis of squamous epithelial cells, vacuolar degeneration of basal cells with mononuclear infiltration; and (5) *salivary or lacrimal gland ducts*—ductal epithelial cell necrosis, periductal mononuclear infiltrate.[139]

SPONTANEOUS REGRESSION

Spontaneous regression has been defined as "partial or complete disappearance of a malignant tumor in the absence of all therapy or following therapy considered inadequate to exert significant influence on neoplastic disease."[140] Among the pediatric tumors, neuroblastoma is known to show spontaneous regression.[141–143] Spontaneous regression can occur in solitary tumors as well as disseminated (stage D-S) disease. Hormonal and immunologic factors and cytodifferentiation with maturation have been implicated as the mechanisms in spontaneous regression. In neuroblastomas cytodifferentation with maturation appears to be the primary mechanism.[144] Both cellular and humoral cytotoxicity against neuroblastoma cells is present in children with neuroblastoma,[145] and it is possible that immunologic factors also play a role in the spontaneous regression. The frequent presence of lymphocytic infiltrates in ganglioneuroma and ganglioneuromatous component of ganglioneuroblastoma is of interest from this point of view.

SECOND PRIMARY MALIGNANCIES

Since about 50% of the children with newly diagnosed malignancy will be alive at 5 years from diagnosis, and a fairly large proportion of these are likely to survive to adulthood, the problem of second malignancy has assumed greater importance in recent years. Of the various pediatric malignancies, Wilms' tumor, Hodgkin's disease, and retinoblastoma are associated with the best prognosis. Therefore, children with these malignancies are most likely to develop second malignancy. The risk of development of second malignancy in a child with one malignancy is 10 times that seen in age-matched population controls.[146] Patients treated with kilovoltage radiotherapy or alkylating agents and those with immunodeficiency syndrome are at particularly high risk. Up to 12% of the children will develop a second malignancy within 20 years of the diagnosis of the first malignancy. Osteosarcoma and chondrosarcoma were the most frequent second malignancies in the retrospective study reported by Meadows et al.[147] Leukemias, tumors of central nervous system, soft tissue sarcomas, and carcinomas (of skin, breast, colon, etc.) are also encountered. In a recent series of acute lymphoblastic leukemia, CNS tumors were particularly more common as second malignancies.[148] The interval between diagnosis of first and second malignancy varies from less than a month to over 40 years with a peak incidence between 5 and 15 years after the diagnosis of first malignancy.

Radiation therapy and chemotherapy (particularly with alkylating agents, nitrosoureas, procarbazine, and cisplatin) have been implicated in the pathogenesis of second malignancy. It is possible that genetic factors also play a role. Thus children who develop a malignancy may have inherent increased susceptibility to development of second malignancy. The recent demonstration of germline mutations in the TSG *p53* in a group of children and young adults who developed second malignancy is of great interest in this respect.[103] The possibility of second malignancy necessitates regular periodic monitoring of patients who had a successfully treated childhood malignancy.[149]

TABLE 10-13 Late Nonneoplastic Sequelae of Therapy of Pediatric Malignancies

Tissue or Organ	Sequela(e)
Bone	Short stature, uneven growth, avascular necrosis
Muscle or soft tissue	Scoliosis, fibrosis
Eye	Cataract, retinopathy
Central nervous system	Atrophy, calcification, neuropsychologic deficit
Kidneys	Atrophy
Genitourinary tract	Contracture
Gonads	Sterility
Gastrointestinal tract	Stricture, malabsorption
Heart	Cardiomyopathy
Pericardium	Constrictive pericarditis
Lung	Interstitial fibrosis
Liver	Hepatic fibrosis (?cirrhosis)

NONNEOPLASTIC SEQUELAE OF THERAPY

The late effects of drug and radiation toxicity (listed in Table 10-11 and 10-12) can leave permanent imprints and result in structural deformities and/or impairment of function. These sequelae are listed in Table 10-13.[150] The pediatric pathologist does not have to deal with these directly but should be aware of these sequelae in autopsy cases of pediatric malignancies.

REFERENCES

1. Farber S, Diamond LK, Mercer RD, et al: Temporary remissions in acute leukemia in children produced by folic acid antagonist, 4-aminopteroyl-glutamic acid (aminopterin). *N Engl J Med* 238:787–793, 1948.
2. Farger S, Cutler EC, Hawkins JW, et al: Action of pteroyl glutamic conjugates on man. *Science* 106:619–621, 1947.
3. Farber S, D'Angio G, Evans A, et al: Clinical studies of actinomycin D with special reference to Wilm's tumor in children. *Ann NY Acad Sci* 89:421–424, 1960.
4. Miller RW, McKay FW: Decline in US childhood cancer mortality. *JAMA* 251:1567–1570, 1984.
5. Young JL, Ries LG, Silverberg E, et al: Cancer incidence, survival and mortality for children younger than 15 years. *Cancer* 58:598–602, 1986.
6. Wolff JA: History of pediatric oncology. *Pediatr Hematol Oncol* 8:89–91, 1991.
7. Hammond GD, Bleyer WA, Hartmann JR, et al: The team approach to the management of pediatric cancer. *Cancer* 41:29–35, 1978.
8. Young JL, Miller RW: Incidence of malignant tumors in children. *J Pediatr* 86:254–258, 1975.
9. Jussawalla DJ, Yeole BB, Natekar NV: Cancer in children in Greater Bombay (1964–1972): Comparative study. *Indian J Cancer* 86:254–258, 1975.
10. McWhirter WR, Stiller CA, Lennox EL: Carcinomas in childhood. A registry-based study of incidence and survival. *Cancer* 63:2242–2246, 1989.

11. Ikeda H, Okumura H, Nagashima K, et al: The management of prenatally diagnosed sacrococcygeal teratoma. *Pediatr Surg Inter* 5:192–194, 1990.
12. Fraumeni JF Jr, Miller RW: Cancer deaths in the newborn. *Am J Dis Child* 117:186–189, 1969.
13. Crom DB, Wilimas JA, Green AA, et al: Malignancy in the neonate. *Med Pediatr Oncol* 17:101–104, 1989.
14. Bolande RP: Models and concepts derived from human teratogenesis and oncogenesis in early life. *J Histochem Cytochem* 32:878–884, 1984.
15. Miller RW: Relation between cancer and congenital defects in man. *N Engl J Med* 275:87–93, 1966.
16. Breslow NE, Beckwith JB: Epidemiological features of Wilms' tumor: Results of the National Wilms' Tumor Study. *J Natl Cancer Inst* 68:429–436, 1982.
17. Sandberg AA, Turc-Carel C: The cytogenetics of solid tumors. Relation to diagnosis, classification and pathology. *Cancer* 59:387–395, 1987.
18. Trask BJ: Fluorescence in situ hybridization: Applications in cytogenetics and gene mapping. *Trends Genet* 7:149–154, 1991.
19. Douglass EC, Valentine M, Etcubanas E, et al: A specific chromosomal abnormality in rhabdomyosarcoma. *Cytogenet Cell Genet* 45:148–155, 1987.
20. Look AT, Roberson PK, Williams DL, et al: Prognostic importance of blast cell DNA content in childhood acute lymphoblastic leukemia. *Blood* 65:1079–1085, 1985.
21. Douglass EC, Green AA, Hayes FA, et al: Chromosome 1 abnormalities. A common feature of pediatric solid tumors. *JNCl* 75:51–54, 1985.
22. Brodeur GM: Genetic and cytogenetic aspects of Wilms' tumor. In Pochedly C, Baum ES (eds): *Wilms' tumor: Clinical and biological manifestations*, Chapter 9, pp 125–146. New York, Elsevier, 1984.
23. Melnick S, Cole P, Anderson D, et al: Rates and risks of diethylstilbestrol-related clear cell adenocarcinoma of the vagina and cervix: An update. *N Engl J Med* 316:514–516, 1987.
24. Sedlis A, Robboy SJ: Diseases of the vagina. In *Blaustein's pathology of the female genital tract*, 3rd ed, Kurman RJ (ed): Chapter 4, pp 98–140. Springer-Verlag, New York, 1987.
25. O'Brien PC, Noller KI, Robboy SJ, et al: Vaginal epithelial changes in young women enrolled in the National Cooperative Diethylstilbestrol Adenosis (DESAD) project. *Obstet Gynecol* 53:300–308, 1979.
26. Sherman S, Roizen N: Fetal hydantoin syndrome and neuroblastoma. *Lancet* 2:517, 1976.
27. Kersey JH, Spector BD, Good RA: Cancer in children with primary immunodeficiency diseases. *J Pediatr* 84:263–264, 1974.
28. Frizzera G, Rosai J, Dehner LP: Lymphoreticular disorders in primary immunodeficiencies: New findings based on an up-to-date histologic classification of 35 cases. *Cancer* 46:692–699, 1980.
29. Frizzera G, Hanto DW, Gail-Peczalska KJ, et al: Polymorphic diffuse B-cell hyperplasia and lymphomas in renal transplant recipients. *Cancer Res* 41:4262–4279, 1981.
30. Penn I: Cancers following cyclosporine therapy. *Transplantation* 43:33–35, 1987.
31. Purtilo DT: Immune deficiency, Epstein-Barr virus and lymphoproliferative disorders. In Purtilo DT (ed): *Immunodeficiency and cancer: Epstein Barr virus and lymphoproliferative malignancies*. New York, Plenum Medical Book Co, 1984.
32. Hanto DW, Gail-Peczalska KJ, Frizzera G, et al: Epstein-Barr virus (EBV) induced polyclonal and monoclonal lymphoproliferative disease occuring after renal transplantation. *Ann Surg* 198:356–369, 1983.
33. Andiman WA, Eastman R, Martin K, et al: Opportunistic lymphoproliferation

associated with Epstein-Barr viral DNA in infants and children with AIDS. *Lancet* 1:1390–1393, 1985.
34. Weinberg KI, Parkman R: Interface between immunodeficiency and pediatric cancer. In Pizzo PA, Poplack DG (eds): *Principles and practice of pediatric oncology*, Chapter 4, pp 65–79. Philadelphia, Lippincott, 1989.
35. Starzl TE, Nalesnick MA, Porter KA, et al: Reversibility of lymphomas and lymphoproliferative lesions developing under cyclosporine-steroid therapy. *Lancet* 1:583–587, 1984.
36. McLoughlin LC, Nord KS, Joshi W, et al: Disseminated leiomyosarcoma in a child with AIDS. *Cancer* 67:2618–2621, 1991.
37. Lee E, Dickman PS, Jaffe R, et al: Post-transplant spindle cell tumor (PTST): An entity associated with Epstein-Barr virus. *Mod Pathol* 6:127A, 1993.
38. Timmons CF, Richards S, Katz WS: Hepatic leiomyosarcoma of donor genotype in a liver transplant recipient. *Mod Pathol* 6:9P, 1993.
39. Fernbach DJ, Vietti TJ: General aspects of childhood cancer. Chapter 1. In Fernbach DJ, Vietti TJ (eds): *Clinical pediatric oncology*, 4th ed, pp 1–10. St Louis, Mosby Year Book, 1991.
40. Murphy SB, Cohn SL, Craft AW, et al: Do children benefit from screening for neuroblastoma? Consensus statement from the American Cancer Society Workshop on Neuroblastoma Screening. *Lancet* 337:344–345, 1991.
41. Beckwith JB: Wilms' tumor and other renal tumors of childhood: A selective review from the National Wilms' Tumor Study Pathology Center. *Hum Pathol* 14:481–492, 1983.
42. Miettinen M, Rapola J: Immunohistochemical spectrum of rhabdomyosarcoma and rhabdomyosarcoma-like tumors: Expression of cytokeratin and the 68-kD neurofilament protein. *Am J Surg Pathol* 13:120–132, 1989.
43. Murphy JJ, Blair GK, Fraser GC, et al: Rhabdomyosarcoma arising within congenital pulmonary cysts: Report of three cases. *J Pediatr Surg* 27:1364–1367, 1992.
44. Valderrama E, Sabja G, Shende A: Pulmonary blastoma. A report of two cases in children. *Am J Surg Pathol* 2:415–417, 1978.
45. Joshi VV, Cantor AB, Altshuler G, et al: Recommendations for modification of terminology of neuroblastic tumors and prognostic significance of Shimada classification. *Cancer* 69:2183–2196, 1992.
46. Haas JE, Muczynski KA, Krailo A, et al: Histopathology and prognosis in childhood hepatoblastoma and hepatocarcinoma. *Cancer* 64:1082–1095, 1989.
47. Dehner LP: Gonadal and extragonadal germ cell neoplasia of childhood. *Hum Pathol* 14:493–511, 1983.
48. Joshi VV, Kaur P, Ryan B, et al: Mucoid anaplastic hepatoblastoma. *Cancer* 54:2035–2039, 1984.
49. Zuppan CW, Beckwith JB, Luckey DW: Anaplasia in unilateral Wilms' tumor. *Hum Pathol* 19:1199–1209, 1988.
50. Cozzutto C, Carbone A: Pleomorphic (anaplastic) neuroblastoma. *Arch Pathol Lab Med* 112:621–625, 1988.
51. Kodet R, Newton WA, Hamoudi AB, et al: Childhood rhabdomyosarcoma with anaplastic (pleomorphic) features. A report of the intergroup rhabdomyosarcoma study. *Am J Surg Pathol* 17:443–453, 1993.
52. Dehner LP: Anaplasia in solid malignant tumors of childhood. *Arch Pathol Lab Med* 113:11–12, 1989.
53. Heppner GH: Tumor heterogeneity. *Cancer Res* 44:2259–2265, 1984.
54. Foulds L: The experimental study of tumor progression: A review. *Cancer Res* 14:327–339, 1954.
55. Foulds L: *Neoplastic development*. New York, Academic Press, 1975.

56. Horn RC, Enterline HT: Rhabdomyosarcoma: A clinicopathological study and classification of 39 cases. *Cancer* 11:181–199, 1958.
57. Joshi VV, Frei JV: Gross and microscopic changes in the lymphoreticular system during genesis of malignant lymphoma induced by a single injection of methylnitrosourea in adult mice. *J Natl Cancer Inst* 44:379–394, 1970.
58. Walker NI, Harmon VB, Gobe GC, et al: Patterns of cell death. *Meth Achiev Exp Pathol* 13:18–54, 1988.
59. Shimada H, Chatten J, Newton WH, et al: Histopathologic prognostic factors in neuroblastic tumors: Definition of subtypes of ganglioneuroblastoma and an age-linked classification of neuroblastomas. *J Natl Cancer Inst* 73:405–416, 1984.
60. Dehner LP: Favorable vs unfavorable histologic appearance: The lesion of pathologic grading of solid malignant neoplasms in children. *Arch Pathol Lab Med* 116:817–819, 1992.
61. Beckwith JB, Palmer NF: Histopathology and prognosis of Wilms' tumor: Results of the National Wilms' Tumor Study. *Cancer* 41:1937–1948, 1978.
62. Joshi VV, Cantor AB, Altshuler G, et al: Age-linked prognostic categorization based on a new histologic grading system of neuroblastomas: A clinicopathologic study of 211 cases from the Pediatric Oncology Group. *Cancer* 69:2197–2211, 1992.
63. Viadana E, Bross IDJ, Pickren JW: An autopsy study of the metastatic patterns of human leukemias. *Oncology* 35:87–96, 1985.
64. Nigro JF, Gresik MV, Fernback DJ: Value or postmortem examination in pediatric populations with leukemia. *J Pediatr* 116:350–354, 1990.
65. Mahoney DH Jr, Fernbach DJ: Occult ovarian leukemia in childhood acute lymphoblastic leukemia. *N Engl J Med* 306:993, 1982.
66. Joshi VV, Kauffman S, Oleske JM, et al: Polyclonal polymorphic B cell lymphoproliferative disorder with prominent pulmonary involvement in children with AIDS. *Cancer* 59:1455–1462, 1987.
67. Mueller BV, Butler KM, Higham MC, et al: Smooth muscle tumors in children with HIV infection. *Pediatrics* 90:460–463, 1992.
68. Dahm B: The autopsy in pediatrics (editorial). *Am J Dis Child* 140:335, 1986.
69. Hays DM: General principles of surgery. In Pizzo PA, Poplack DG (eds): *Principles and practice of pediatric oncology*. Chapter 10, pp 207–232. Philadelphia, Lippincott, 1989.
70. Hays DM, Fryer CJ, Pringle KC, et al: An evaluation of abdominal staging procedures performed in pediatric patients with advanced Hodgkin's disease: A report from the Children's Cancer Study Group. *J Pediatr Surg* 27:1175–1180, 1992.
71. Urba WJ, Longo DL: Hodgkin's disease. *N Engl J Med* 326:678–687, 1992.
72. D'Angio GJ, Evans A, Breslow N, et al: The treatment of Wilms' tumor. Results of the second National Wilms' Tumor Study. *Cancer* 47:2302–2311, 1982.
73. Mauer HM, Gehan EA, Beltangady M, et al: The intergroup Rhabdomyosarcoma Study—II. *Cancer* 71:1904–1922, 1993.
74. Murphy SB, Hustu HO: A randomized trial of combined modality therapy of childhood non-Hodgkin's lymphoma. *Cancer* 45:630–637, 1980.
75. Mastrangelo R, Poplack D, Bleyer A, et al: Report and recommendations of the Rome workshop concerning poor prognosis acute lymphoblastic leukemia in children: Biologic basis for staging, stratification and treatment. *Med Pediatr Oncol* 14:191–194, 1986.
76. Miller AB, Hoogstraten B, Staguet M, et al: Reporting results of cancer treatment. *Cancer* 47:207–214, 1981.
77. Murphy SB: Non-Hodgkin's lymphomas of childhood: An analysis of the histology, staging and response to treatment of 338 cases at a single institution. *J Clin Oncol* 7:186–193, 1989.

78. Bolande RP: Benignity of neonatal tumors and concept of cancer regression in early life. *Am J Dis Child* 122:12–14, 1971.
79. Bishop JM: Viral oncogenes. Cell 42:23–38, 1985.
80. Israel MA: Molecular and cellular biology of pediatric malignancies. In Pizzo PA, Poplack DG (eds): *Principles and practice of pediatric oncology*, Chapter 3, pp 39–64. Philadelphia, Lippincott, 1989.
81. Yeger H, Mor O, Pawlin G, et al: Importance of pheotypic and molecular characterization for identification of a neuroepithelioma tumor cell line, NUB-20. *Cancer Res* 50:2794–2802, 1990.
82. Rous P: Transmission of a malignant new growth by means of a cell-free filtrate. *JAMA* 56:198, 1911.
83. Yoshida M, Miyoshi I, Hinuma Y: Isolation and characterization of retrovirus from cell lines of human adult T-cell leukemia and its implication in the disease. *Proc Natl Acad Sci USA* 79:2031–2035, 1982.
84. Varmus HE: Reverse transcriptase rides again. *Nature* 314:583–584, 1985.
85. Spector DH, Varmus HE, Bishop JM: Nucleotide sequences related to the transforming gene of avian sarcoma virus and present in DNA of uninfected vertebrates. *Proc Natl Acad Sci USA* 75:4102–4106, 1978.
86. Gordon H: Oncogenes. *Mayo Clin Proc* 60:697–713, 1985.
87. Carroll WI, Schwartz AL: Molecular oncology. In Fernback DJ, Vietti TJ (eds): *Clinical pediatric oncology*, 49th ed, pp 29–68. St Louis, Mosby Year Book, 1991.
88. Blackwood EM, Eisenman RN: Max: A helix-loop zipper protein that forms a sequence-specific DNA-binding complex with Myc. *Science* 251:1211–1217, 1991.
89. Makela TP, Koskinen PJ, Vastrik I, et al: Alternative forms of Max as enhancers or suppressors of Myc-Ras co-transformation. *Science* 256:373–377, 1992.
90. Wenzel A, Cziepluch C, Hamann U, et al: The N-myc oncprotein is associated in vivo with the phosphoprotein Max (p20/22) in human neuroblastoma cells. *EMBO J* 10:3703–3712, 1991.
91. Schwab M, Alitalo K, Klempnauer KH, et al: Amplified DNA with limited homology to myc cellular oncogene is shared by human neroblastoma cell lines and a neuroblastoma tumor. *Nature* 305:245–248, 1983.
92. Brodeur GM, Seeger RC, Schwab M, et al: Amplification of n-myc in untreated human neuroblastomas correlates with advanced disease stage. *Science* 224:1121–1124, 1984.
93. Michitsch RW, Montgomery KT, Melera PW: Expression of the amplified domain in human neuroblastoma cells. *Mol Cell Biol* 4:2370–2380, 1984.
94. Stanbridge EJ: Genetic analysis of human malignancy using somatic cell hybrids and monochromosome transfer. *Cancer Surv* 7:317–324, 1988.
95. Brodeur GM: The involvement of oncogenes and suppressor genes in human neoplasia. *Adv Pediatr* 34:1–44, 1987.
96. Murphree AL, Benedict WF: Retinoblastoma: Clues to human oncogenesis. *Science* 223:1028–1033, 1984.
97. Friend SH, Bernards R, Rogelj S, et al: A human DNA segment with properties of the gene that predisposes to retinoblastoma and osteosarcoma. *Nature* 323:643–646, 1986.
98. Fung Y-K, Murphree AL, Tang A, et al: Structural evidence for the authenticity of the human retinoblastoma gene. *Science* 236:1657–1661, 1987.
99. Fong CT, Morita M, Griffith RC, et al: Analysis of human neuroblastomas for loss of heterozygosity for chromosome 1. *Proc Am Soc Can Res* 28:52, 1987.
100. Koufos A, Hansen MF, Lampkin BC, et al: Loss of alleles at loci as human chromosome 11 during genesis of Wilms' tumor. *Nature* 309:170–172, 1984.

101. Koufos A, Hansen MF, Copeland NG, et al: Loss of heterozygosity in three embryonal tumors suggests a common pathogenetic mechanism. *Nature* 316:330–334, 1985.
102. Li FP, Fraumeni JF: Prospective study of a family cancer syndrome. *JAMA* 247:2692–2694, 1982.
103. Malkin D, Jolly KW, Barbier N, et al: Germline mutations of the *p53* tumor-suppressor gene in children and young adults with second malignant neoplasms. *N Engl J Med* 326:1309–1315, 1992.
104. Shuster JJ, McWilliams NB, Castleberry RP, et al: Serum lactate dehydrogenase in childhood neuroblastoma: A Pediatric Oncology Group Recursive Partitioning Study. *Am J Clin Oncol* 15:295–303, 1992.
105. Magrath IT, Lee YJ, Anderson T, et al: Prognostic factors in Burkitt's lymphoma: Importance of total tumor burden. *Cancer* 45:1507–1515, 1980.
106. Csako G, Magrath IT, Elin R: Serum total and isoenzyme lactate dehydrogenase activity in American Burkitt's lymphoma. *Am J Clin Pathol* 78:712–717, 1982.
107. Hann HW, Evans AE, Siegel SE, et al: Prognostic importance of serum ferritin in patients with Stages III and IV neuroblastoma: The Children's Cancer Study Group experience. *Cancer Res* 45:2843–2848, 1985.
108. Look AT, Hayes FA, Nitschke R, et al: Cellular DNA content as a predictor of response to chemotherapy in infants with unresectable neuroblastoma. *N Engl J Med* 311:231–235, 1984.
109. Tomita T, Yasue M, Engelhand HT, et al: Flow cytometric DNA analysis of medulloblastoma: Prognostic implication of aneuploidy. *Cancer* 61:744–749, 1988.
110. Christiansen H, Lampert F: Tumor karyotype discriminates between good and bad prognostic outcome in neuroblastoma. *Brit J Cancer* 57:121–126, 1988.
111. Cornelisse CJ, Van de Velde CJH, Caspers RJC, et al: Ploidy and survival in breast cancer patients. *Cytometry* 8:225–235, 1987.
112. Friedlander ML, Hedley DW, Taylor IW, et al: Influence of cellular DNA content on survival in advanced ovarian cancer. *Cancer Res* 44:397–400, 1984.
113. Dressler LG, Bartow SA: DNA flow cytometry in solid tumors: Practical aspects and clinical applications. *Semin Diagn Pathol* 6:55–82, 1989.
114. Haag D, Goerttler K, Tschahargane C: The proliferative index (PI) of human breast cancer as obtained by flow cytometry. *Pathol Res Pract* 178:315–322, 1984.
115. Cavalli C, Danova M, Gobbi PG, et al: Ploidy and proliferative activity measurements by flow cytometry in non-Hodgkin's lymphomas. Do spectulative aspects prevail over clinical ones? *Eur J Cancer Clin Oncol* 25:1755–1763, 1989.
116. Kumar S, Marsden HB, Cowan RA, et al: Prognostic relevance of DNA content in childhood renal tumors. *Brit J Cancer* 59:291–295, 1989.
117. Douglass EC, Look AT, Weber B, et al: Hyperdiploidy and chromosomal rearrangements define the anaplastic variants of Wilms' tumor. *J Clin Oncol* 4:975–981, 1986.
118. Look AT, Hayes FA, Shuster JJ, et al: Clinical relevance of tumor cell ploidy and N-myc gene amplification in childhood neuroblastomas: A Pediatric Oncology Group Study. *J Clin Oncol* 9:581–591, 1991.
119. Joshi VV, Cantor AB, Brodeur GM, et al: Correlation between morphologic and other prognostic markers of neuroblastoma: A study of histologic grade, DNA index, N-myc gene copy number and lactic dehydrogenase in patients in the Pediatric Oncology Group. *Cancer* 71:3173–3191, 1993.
120. Steel GG: *Growth kinetics of tumors.* Bristol, Oxford Clarendon Press, 1977.
121. Folkman J: How is blood vessel growth regulated in normal and neoplastic tissue? *Cancer Res* 46:467–473, 1986.
122. Pardee AP: Principles of cancer biology: Biochemistry and cell biology. In DeVita VT, Hellman S, Rosenberg SA (eds): *Cancer: Principles and practice of oncology.* Philadelphia, Lippincott, 1985.

123. Johnson WW, Meadows DC: Urinary bladder fibrosis and telangiectasia associated with long-term cyclophosphamide therapy. *N Engl J Med* 284:290–294, 1971.
124. Stillwell TJ, Benson RC, Burgert EO: Cyclophosphamide induced hemorrhagic cystitis in Ewing's sarcoma. *J Clin Oncol* 6:76–82, 1988.
125. Bleyer WA: Cancer chemotherapy in infants and children. *Pediatr Clin N Am* 32:557–574, 1985.
126. Luna M, Bedrossian C, Lichtiger B, et al: Interstitial pneumonitis associated with bleomycin therapy. *Am J Clin Pathol* 58:501–510, 1972.
127. Myers JL: Pathology of drug induced lung disease. In Katzenstein AA, Askin FB (eds): *Surgical pathology of nonneoplastic lung disease*, Chapter 4, pp 97–127. Philadelphia, Saunders, 1990.
128. Bolis FM, Holcenberg JS, Poplack DG: General principles of chemotherapy. In Pizzo PA, Poplack DG (eds): *Principles and practice of pediatric oncology*, Chapter 9, pp 165–205. Philadelphia, Lippincott, 1989.
129. Gonzalez-Vitale JC, Hays DM, Cvitkovic E, et al: The renal pathology in clinical trials of cis-platinum (II) diammine dichloride. *Cancer* 39:1362–1371, 1977.
130. Paschke R, Heine M: Pathophysiological aspects of dacarbazine-induced human liver damage. *Hepatogastroenterology* 32:273–275, 1985.
131. Billingham ME, Mason JW, Bristow MK, et al: Anthracycline cardiomyopathy monitored by morphologic changes. *Cancer Treat Rep* 62:865–872, 1978.
132. Arya S, Gilbert EF, Wiedrich TA: Complications of treatment of neoplasia in childhood, including second malignancies. In Finegold M (ed): *Pathology of neoplasia in children and adolescents*, Chapter 17, pp 433–464. Philadelphia, Saunders, 1986.
133. Cotran RS, Kumar V, Robbins SL: Environmental pathology. In *Robbins' pathologic basis of disease*, Chapter 9, pp 469–514. Philadelphia, Saunders, 1989.
134. Anderson RE: Radiation injury. In Kissane JM (ed): *Anderson's pathology*, 9th ed, Chapter 5, pp 247–288. St Louis, Mosby, 1990.
135. Mandell LR, Wharam MD: Radiotherapy. In Fernbach DJ, Vietti TJ (eds): *Clinical pediatric oncology*, 4th ed, pp 155–172. St Louis, Mosby Year Book, 1991.
136. Sale GE, Shulman HM: *The pathology of bone marrow transplantation*. New York, Masson Publishing, 1984.
137. Wick MR, Moore SB, Gastineau DA, et al: Immunologic, clinical, and pathologic aspects of human graft versus hot disease. *Mayo Clin Proc* 58:603–612, 1983.
138. Slavin RE, Santos GW: The graft versus host reaction in man after bone marrow transplantation: Pathology, pathogenesis, clinical features and implication. *Clin Immunol Immunopathol*. 1:472–498, 1973.
139. Sale GE: Bone marrow and thymic transplantation. In *Pathology of organ transplantation*, Chapter 9, pp 229–260. Boston, Butterworth, 1990.
140. Everson TC, Cole WH: *Spontaneous regression of cancer*. Philadelphia, Saunders, 1966.
141. Evans AE, Gerson J, Schnaufer L: Spontaneous regression of neuroblastoma. *Natl Cancer Inst Monogr* 44:49–54, 1976.
142. Cole WH: Spontaneous regression of cancer and importance of finding its cause. *Natl Cancer Inst Monogr* 44:5–9, 1976.
143. Cushing H, Wolbach SB: Transformation of malignant paravertebral sympathicoblastoma into benign ganglioneuroma. *Am J Pathol* 3:203–216, 1927.
144. Bolande RP: Spontaneous regression and cytodifferentiation of cancer in early life: The oncogenic grade period. *Surv Synth Pathol Res* 4:296–311, 1985.
145. Hellstrom IE, Hellstrom KE, Pierce GE, et al: Demonstration of cell bound and humoral immunity against neuroblastoma cells. *Proc Natl Acad Sec USA* 60:1231–1238, 1968.

146. Mike V, Meadows AT, D'Angio GJ: Incidence of second malignant neoplasms in children: Results of an international study. *Lancet* 2:1326–1331, 1982.
147. Meadows AT, D'Angio GJ, Mike V, et al: Patterns of second malignant neoplasms in children. *Cancer* 40:1903–1911, 1977.
148. Neglia JP, Meadows AT, Robison LL, et al: Second neoplasms after acute lymphoblastic leukemia in childhood. *N Engl J Med* 325:1330–1336, 1991.
149. Kingston JE: Second primary tumors. *Arch Dis Child* 60:695–697, 1985.
150. Carter MC, Thompson EI, Simone JV: The survivors of childhood solid tumors. *Ped Clin N Am* 38:505–526, 1991.

11 CLASSIFICATION AND GRADING OF TERATOMAS IN CHILDREN

INTRODUCTION

Teratomas occur in gonads and in various extragonadal sites and in various pediatric age groups, including fetuses, neonates, infants, children, and adolescents. I have seen partially cystic and partially solid teratoma of the mediastinum causing intrauterine death due to cardiac compression in two antepartum stillborn fetuses. Prenatal ultrasonographic examination has resulted in the recognition of sacrococcygeal teratomas (SCT) in the fetus. Twenty such cases were reported up to 1990.[1] The sites of 526 teratomas reported in children by various authors include sacrococcygeal region (42%), ovary (24%), testis (9%), mediastinum (7%), central nervous system (6%), head and neck (5%), retroperitoneum (4%), and miscellaneous (~3%).[2] The exact incidence is not known, but these tumors may constitute about 10% of all "serious" pediatric solid tumors[3] and about 3% of malignancies in children.[4] Teratomas of certain sites have sex predilection. For example, gastric teratomas occur in boys and SCT in girls. Teratomas are the second commonest tumors in newborn period and the most frequent gonadal tumors in children.

Behavior of teratomas is related to degree of maturity and presence of the following malignant germ-cell components: germinoma (G) composed of "germ cells," embryonal carcinoma (EC) composed of undifferentiated "embryonal" cells, choriocarcinoma (CCA) composed of cytotrophoblastic and syncytiotrophoblastic cells, and yolk sac carcinoma (YSC) composed of cells and patterns (e.g., endodermal sinuses) indicative of yolk sac differentiation. Various methods of pathologic grading of ovarian teratomas containing immature elements have been described. For reproducibility and comparability, when applied to teratomas arising in other sites, relative lack of complexity of the criteria used for grading is essential. Accuracy of grading is important for making the decision regarding the necessity of additional therapy besides surgical resection. The main emphasis of this chapter is to review (1) the grading systems originally described for ovarian immature teratomas and their applicability to immature teratomas of extraovarian sites and (2) the significance of glial "implants" seen in the peritoneum and lymph nodes in the cases of ovarian immature teratomas.

DEFINITION

Willis defined teratoma as a true tumor or neoplasm composed of multiple tissues of kinds foreign to the part in which it arises.[5] Ganzales-Crussi gives the following definition: Teratomas are neoplasms that originate in pluripotent cells and that are composed of wide diversity of tissues foreign to the organ or anatomic site in which they arise.[6] Willis[5] emphasized that teratoma is not a quiescent malformation. Neither definition specifies the number of germlayers (ecto-, mono- and endoderm) that are represented in a teratoma. Willis believes that the demonstration of representation of all three germ layers depends on the thoroughness of sampling for histologic examination. However, "monodermal" teratomas composed exclusively or predominantly of one type of tissue or derivatives of only one germ layer foreign to the site are recognized in the ovary and other organs. Carcinoid, struma ovarii (normal thyroid tissue or thyroid adenoma being the predominant or sole component of the teratoma), benign cystic teratoma composed of purely neurogenic tissue and malignant neuroectodermal tumor of the ovary, and hepatocellular adenoma of placenta serve as examples of these "monodermal" teratomas.[7–9] It must be emphasized, however, that extensive sampling of the tumor is essential before the diagnosis of monodermal teratoma is made. The term "ovarian dermoid cyst" also connotes that it is a monodermal teratoma. In fact, these tumors are composed of a variety of tissues (ectodermal, mesodermal, and endodermal). Therefore, the term, mature cystic teratoma is preferable. A pure YSC or CCA of any site may be considered as a monodermal malignant teratoma. When the tumor is composed exclusively of germ cells, the term "seminoma," "dysgerminoma," or "germinoma" is used to designate tumors arising in the testis, ovary, and extragonadal sites, respectively.

Although orderly arrangement of the three germ layers is not evident in all the areas of teratoma, and the histologic patterns of the different tissues in the teratomas are characteristically described as chaotic, a certain degree of organization and replication of normal "organ" structure is evident in the mature tumors. Thus organized and differentiated tissues such as cerebellum, with orderly arrangement of the granular layer and Purkinje cells, gastric mucosa in apposition to smooth muscle bundles, choroid plexus in an ependyma-lined cavity and bronchus with respiratory epithelium and cartilage are not infrequently found in the mature teratomas. Thus in the case reported by Woodfield et al[10] all portions of the gastrointestinal tract were demonstrated on histologic examination of a mature ovarian teratoma.

GROSS FEATURES AND PROCESSING OF GROSS SPECIMEN

The specimen should be carefully examined for completeness of resection. In SCT the coccyx must be specifically identified, photographed and sent through for histologic examination. Capsular tears and adhesions are not uncommon in immature ovarian teratomas. For example, Robboy and Scully[11] found one or the other of these abnormalities in 11 of 12 cases in their series. Therefore, in all teratomas the capsule should be examined for presence of tear, invasion by tumor, or adhesion to surrounding structures and portions of omentum. Adhesion to a portion of omentum may be overlooked or considered as "nonspecific" connective tissue component of the capsule itself. Ideally, the surgeons should identify the site of omental adhesion for the pathologist, but in

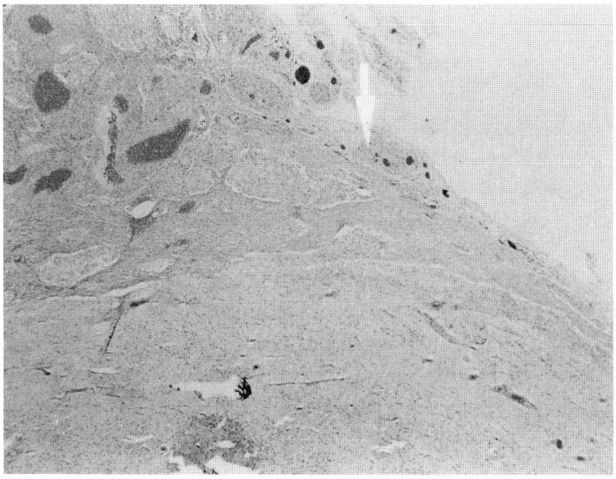

FIGURE 11-1. Extension of glial tissue through the capsule of an immature ovarian teratoma. A small glial nodule is seen on the surface of the capsule (arrow). The omentum is adherent to the capsule left to the arrow. (H&E, ×100.)

practice it may not be done. The pathologist should therefore examine the capsule carefully. The histologic sections taken through such adhesions may reveal extension of glial tissue through the capsule (Figures 11-1, 11-2).

Gross description should clearly mention whether the tumor is totally solid, totally cystic, or partially cystic and solid (Figures 11-3, 11-4). Grossly identifi-

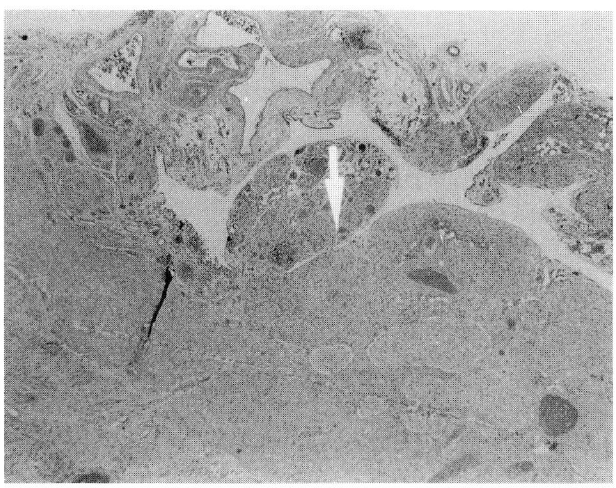

FIGURE 11-2. Extension of glial tissue through the capsule at the site of omental adhesion to an immature ovarian teratoma. The arrow points to a glial implant on the surface of the capsule. The top portion of the figure shows fibrofatty tissue of the adherent omentum. Glial implants are present also in the adherent omentum. (H&E, ×250.)

able structures such as teeth, hair shaft, or sebaceous material may be present (Figure 11-5). In a predominantly cystic teratoma, solid areas should be looked for. Serial slicing ("bread-loafing") of the gross specimen can be done with better results after overnight or several hours of formalin fixation. Fleshy-appearing areas, foci of hemorrhage and/or necrosis, or solid areas in a predominantly cystic tumor and capsule should be extensively sampled. In an almost exclusively cystic tumor multiple strips should be taken from the septa of the cysts in individual cassettes so that large amount of tissue from the septa can be examined in the individual slides. One section for each centimeter of the longest dimension of the tumor or 10 sections, whichever is larger, is the usual recommended guideline for histologic sampling.[6] Dehner[12] recommends that up to 15 sections should be studied from a teratoma. If immature tissues are found on microscopic examination, it may be advisable to go back to the specimen to take more sections. The importance of adequate sampling of teratomas within practical limits mentioned above cannot be overemphasized. It is possible that the case of mature teratomas with raised α-fetoprotein (AFP) levels or with subsequent metastasis represent inadequately sampled teratomas that have a "malignant" component originally. All the lymph node and peritoneal implants sampled by the surgeon should be submitted for histologic examination.

HISTOLOGIC CLASSIFICATION

Teratomas are classified according to the maturity and presence or absence of germ-cell elements mentioned in the introduction. There are three broad categories: (1) mature, (2) immature, and (3) malignant teratomas.

Mature Teratomas

Mature teratomas contain only mature tissues in all the extensive samples taken for histology. These tumors are often predominantly cystic. In ovarian teratomas, skin and its adnexa are the frequent components. However, other

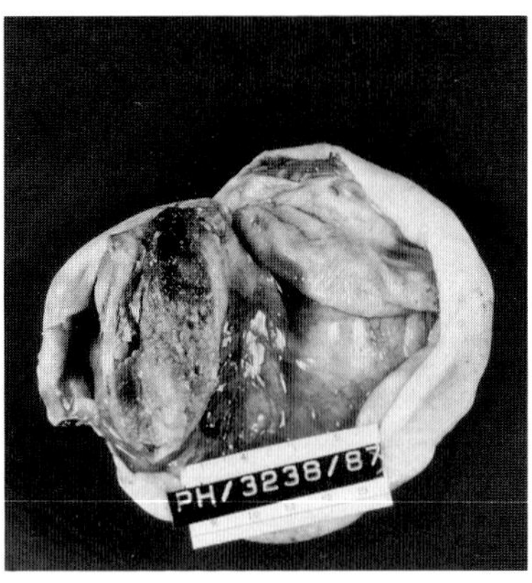

FIGURE 11-3. Cystic teratoma of ovary with a tuft of black hair and sebaceous material within the cyst cavity.

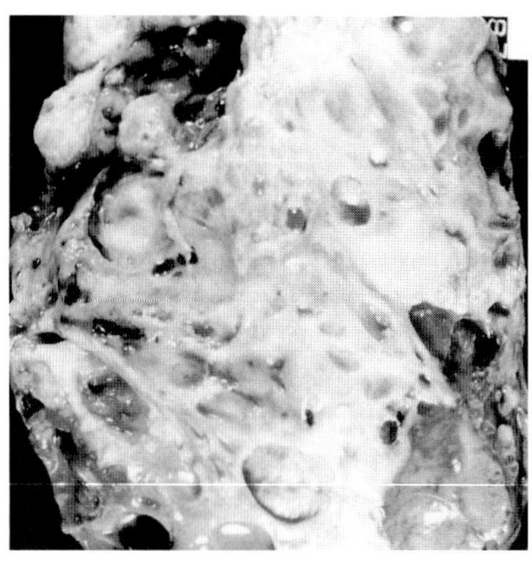

FIGURE 11-4. Partly cystic and partly solid teratoma of mediastinum.

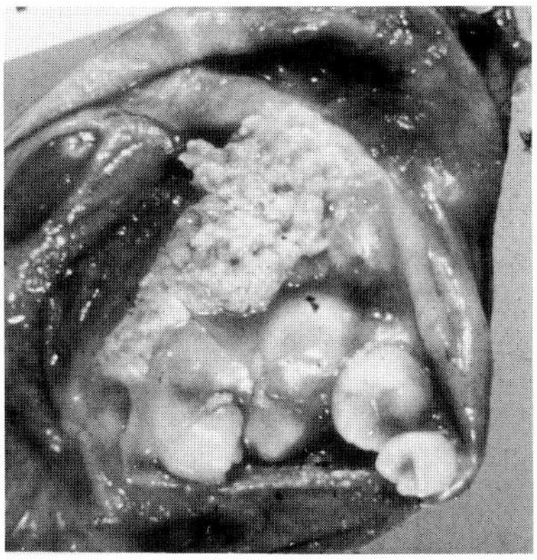

FIGURE 11-5. Sebaceous material and teeth in a teratoma of the ovary.

elements such as glial tissue, fat, fibrous tissue, cartilage, and bone are always detected when adequate numbers of sections are taken from the minor solid component of the tumor. Foci of mature tissues showing organization with formation of structures mentioned above are not uncommon in mature teratomas.

Fetus in the fetu (FIF) should be distinguished from mature teratomas. FIF, which is considered to belong to the spectrum of twinning, is a rare condition. Only 37 cases were reported up to 1988.[13] It represents a monozygotic malformed twin included within the body of its cotwin. FIF contains a vertebral column that forms an axis around which variable combinations of rudimentary or well-formed organs and limbs are arranged.[14] The presence of vertebral column is demonstrated by radiographic and pathologic examination.

Malignant Teratomas

Malignant teratomas contain germ cell, yolk sac or trophoblastic components mentioned above exclusively or in combination with mature and/or immature tissues. The criteria for various types of malignant teratomas given below are adapted from those recommended by the Pediatric Oncology Group.[15]

Dysgerminoma

This tumor is composed of large, round, oval, or polygonal cells with abundant clear cytoplasm and large round nuclei with prominent nucleoli. The cells are arranged in nests separated by septa of fibrous tissue. Lymphocytic infiltrate with or without granulomas is present within the fibrous septa. Foci of necrosis are seen. Isolated syncytial giant cells resembling syncytiotrophoblast may be present. The tumor cells are positive for the immunoperoxidase stain for placental alkaline phosphatase.

Embryonal Carcinoma

The following features are seen:

1. The tumor is composed of sheets of large epithelial-like cells with round, oval, or irregularly outlined nuclei containing one or more nucleoli and

having a coarse nuclear membrane. There may be considerable pleomorphism. The cells have abundant cytoplasm.

2. A tubulopapillary arrangement of tumor cells may be seen focally, but it is not associated with intracytoplasmic or extracellular hyaline globules of the type seen in YSC (see below). Necrotic tumor cells may resemble hyaline globules, but their location in assocation with dying or necrotic cells distinguishes them from true hyaline globules.
3. A few embryoid bodies may be present. The embryoid bodies are organoid structures resembling perfect or imperfect embryos of about 2 weeks' gestation. They are composed of "embryonic disks" containing ectoderm and endoderm and of cavities on either side resembling amniotic cavity, yolk sac, and extraembryonic coelom with extraembryonic mesenchyme.[16]
4. The stroma may be loose and edematous or fibrous. Occasionally it is quite cellular.
5. When the tumor is composed exclusively or predominantly of embryoid bodies, a diagnosis of polyembryoma is made.

Embryonal carcinoma is sometimes subclassified into infantile and adult type.[12] The adult type has the features described above, whereas the infantile type is in fact the YSC described below. Adult type of EC is rare in children. This subclassification is confusing and should be avoided. The tumors should be designated as EC or YSC depending on the histologic features.

Choriocarcinoma

The tumor is composed of syncytiotrophoblast (ST) and cytotrophoblast (CT). ST is a large cell with multiple hyperchromatic nuclei and moderate to abundant eosinophilic cytoplasm. Vacuoles may be present in the cytoplasm. CT is present in compact nests of medium-sized, relatively uniform cells with clear cytoplasm, distinct cell margins, and a vesicular nucleus. Both ST and CT must be present for the diagnosis of choriocarcinoma. (Individual ST without accompanying CT can be seen in other malignant germ-cell tumors.) ST can be further identified by immunoperoxidase stain for β_1 human chorionic gonadotrophin (hCG).

Yolk Sac Carcinoma

These tumors are composed of small cells with variable-sized nuclei in which prominent nucleoli may be present. The tumor cells are arranged in one or more of the following patterns in various combinations:[17] (1) loose network of cystic spaces lined by flat mesothelioid cells, (2) endodermal sinus structures (Schiller–Duval bodies or glomeruloid bodies) composed of central small blood vessel surrounded by a mantle of epithelial cells, (3) honeycomb pattern with meshwork of microcysts, (4) labyrinthine structure consisting of communicating cavities and spaces, (5) regularly arranged cystic structures lined by flat cells with protruding nuclei, (6) polyvesicular vitelline pattern consisting of isolated "yolk sac" vesicles, (7) compact aggregates of embryonal cells, and (8) myxoid stroma resembling the extraembryonic mesoderm. In some foci the tumor cells show hyaline, eosinophilic intracytoplasmic (or extracellular) globules that are PAS-positive after diastase digestion and on immunoperoxidase stain for AFP. Foci of hematopoiesis may be present.

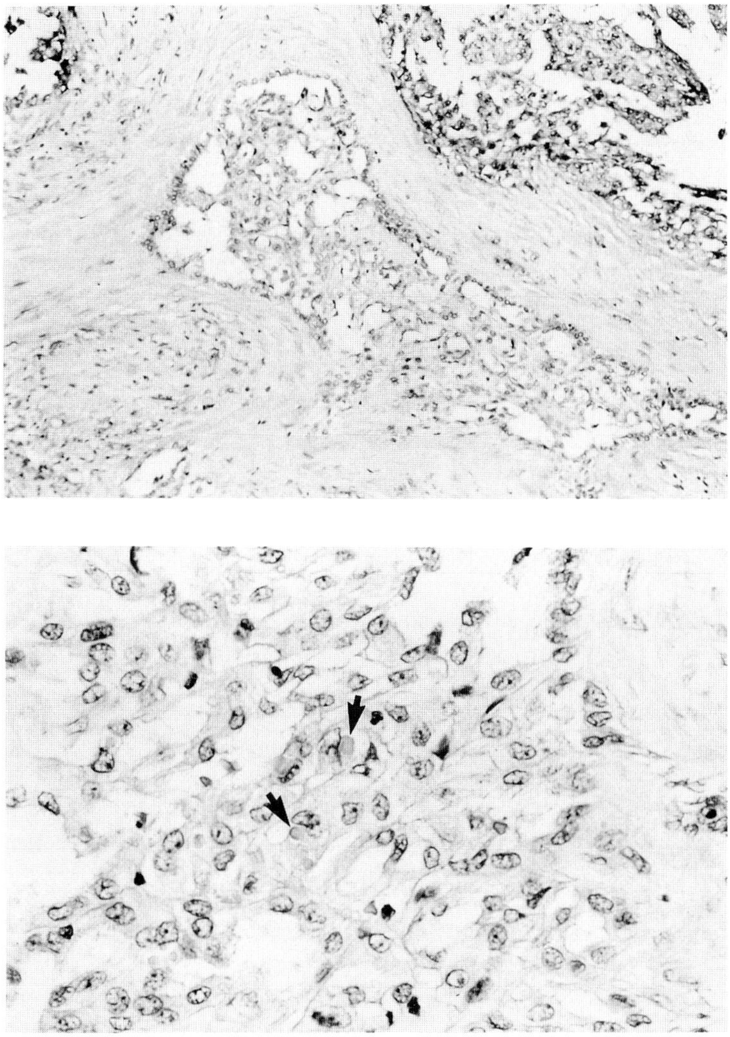

A

B

FIGURE 11-6. (A) Note the epithelial hyperplasia of rete testis in a case of embryonal carcinoma of the testis (top right-hand corner) (H&E, ×100); (B) hyaline globules (arrows) in the hyperplastic epithelial cells of the rete testis (H&E, ×400). (Courtesy of Dr. James L. Finley.)

Epithelial hyperplasia of the rete testis (EHRT) with presence of eosinophilic hyaline globules simulates YSC.[18] EHRT is seen in association with invasive testicular tumors of both germ-cell and non-germ-cell origin. The epithelial hyperplasia develops in reaction to an invasive testicular neoplasm (Figure 11-6). The hyaline globules, which give a negative or equivocal result with the immunoperoxidase stain for AFP, probably represent proteins that are absorbed and retained by the hyperplastic epithelial cells from the human rete testis (Figure 11-6). It is of great practical importance to accurately diagnose EHRT and not make a diagnosis of mixed germ-cell tumor because of features simulating YSC.

Teratomas with Mixed Histologic Pattern

The malignant teratomas defined above usually occur in pure form in children. However, admixture of EC and YSC or CCA and immature non-germ-cell elements may occur in rare instances. The occurrence of ST in germinomas (particularly of the testis) can also be considered as an example of admixture of different germ-cell elements. Such combinations are more frequently observed in adults than in children.

Teratomas with non-germ-cell malignant component such as malignant neuroectodermal tumor,[8] sarcomas of various types,[19,20] carcinomas,[21–23] or lymphoma[24] found in the original tumor or in a subsequent recurrence is designated as a (mature or immature) teratoma with malignant non-germ-cell elements.

Immature Teratoma

Immature teratomas contain incompletely differentiated tissues of various types, in varying proportion and varying grades of immaturity. Neuroectodermal and mesenchymal tissues are the most frequent among the immature elements. Microscopic foci of yolk sac carcinoma may be present in a tumor that otherwise has the features of immature teratoma. Such foci may be overlooked unless all the slides of the adequately sampled tumor are carefully reviewed. Hawkins et al[25,26] have described three cases of immature SCT (and three cases of mature SCT) removed at birth in which recurrences developed. The recurrent tumor in each case contained YSC. Retrospective review of the slides of tumors revealed microscopic foci of YSC that were originally overlooked.[25,26] These foci of YSC were found within the nests of immature mesenchymal elements. Foci of immature mesenchymal elements should also be carefully reviewed to exclude the possibility of sarcomatous foci such as leiomyosarcoma, angiosarcoma, rhabdomyosarcoma, and liposarcoma.[19,20] Presence of any malignant germ-cell or non-germ-cell component negates the diagnosis of immature teratoma. Such tumors should be labelled as malignant teratomas or teratomas with non-germ-cell malignant element(s) as the case may be. These guidelines for making a diagnosis of malignancy may be applied when areas with features resembling neuroblastoma or nephroblastoma are predominant.

Morphologic Criteria for Incompletely Differentiated Tissues

These criteria are not standardized. In general, increased cellularity of tissue with relatively smaller amount of matrix, large size of nuclei, small amount of cytoplasm, basophilia of cytoplasm, and hyperchromasia of nuclei are the features indicative of immaturity (Figures 11-7–11-9). Mitotic figures may be present. Atypical features associated with malignancy such as atypical mitotic figures and marked pleomorphism are not present.

Immaturity is also seen in the structural organization. For example, immature cerebellar tissue shows an external granular layer that is not present in mature cerebellar tissue (Figure 11-10). Neuroepithelial tubules or medullary canals lined by ependymal cells and glial tissue with increased cellularity are seen in immature neuroectodermal tissue (Figures 11-11–11-13). Nephrogenic tissue contains groups of blastemal cells, immature tubules and glomeruli (Figure 11-14). Immature lung tissue has also been described. The concept of immaturity of some of the tissues may not be applicable to the teratomas seen in

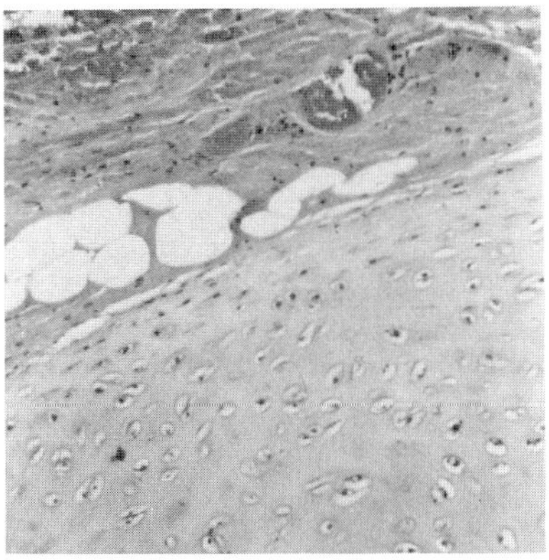

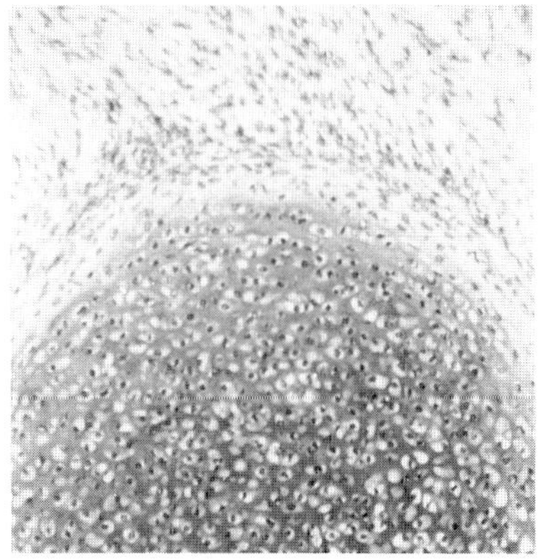

FIGURE 11-7. (A) Normocellular mature cartilage with slight basophilia of the moderate amount of matrix in a mature teratoma; note also the surrounding mature fibrofatty tissue (H&E, ×100). (B) Increased cellularity with decreased amount and increased basophilia of the matrix of an immature cartilage in an immature teratoma; note also the surrounding immature mesenchyma (H&E, ×100).

newborn and young infants since some of the tissues generally are not mature at this age. Thus the presence of an external granular layer in the cerebellar tissue in a teratoma in a premature infant, although indicative of immaturity, is of appropriate maturity for the age of the patient.

Criteria for Grading of Immature Teratomas

When immature tissues are detected in a teratoma, the next step is to grade the teratoma on the basis of amount of immature tissues. Various methods for

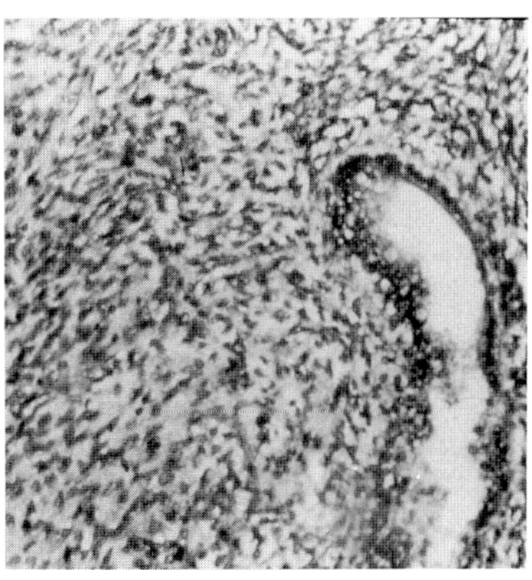

FIGURE 11-8. Immature mesenchyme surrounding an immature tubular structure; note the moderately dense cellularity and nuclear hyperchromasia of the mesenchyme (H&E, ×100).

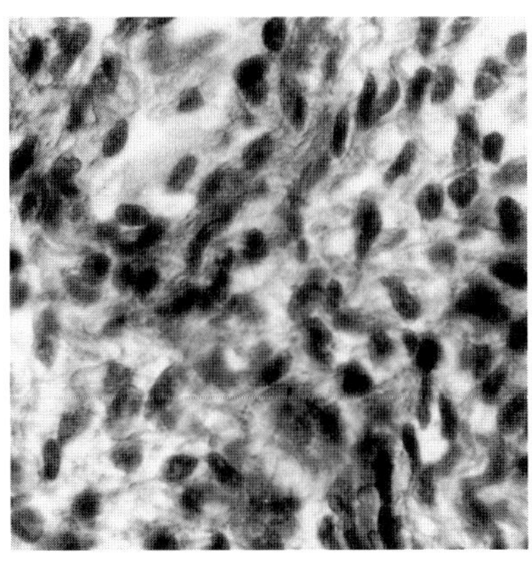

FIGURE 11-9. Large hyperchromatic nuclei of immature mesenchyme (H&E, ×250).

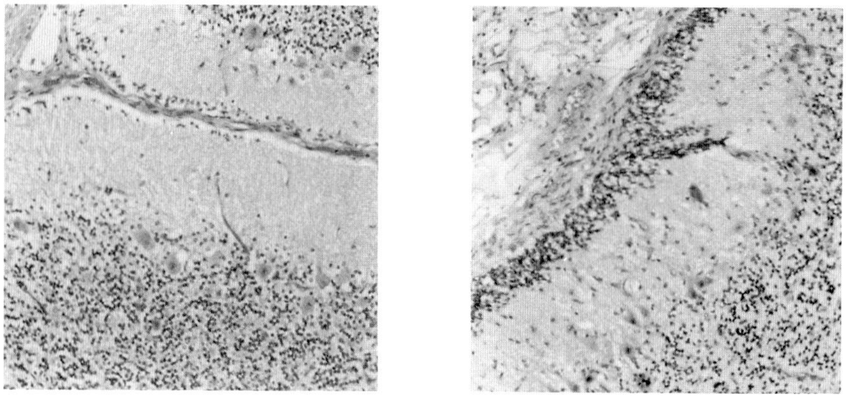

FIGURE 11-10. (A) Mature cerebellar tissue characterized by the inner granular layer and well-differentiated Purkinje cells in a mature sacrococcygeal teratoma; note the absence of external granular layer (H&E, ×100). (B) Immature cerebellar tissue characterized by the presence of external granular layer and immature Purkinje cells (H&E, ×100).

assessing the amount of immature tissues have been described (Table 11-1).[6,11,27] These grading systems have been used primarily for ovarian teratomas. It is not clear whether these systems can be extrapolated to immature teratomas occurring in other sites (see below). However, Pediatric Oncology Group protocols have recommended the grading system of Norris et al[27] for both ovarian and extraovarian immature tertomas. In general the criteria for grading include semiquantitative assessment of the amount of immature tissue in the various histologic sections of the tumor (Table 11-1). Mitotic activity is used as a criterion only by Robboy and Scully.[11] It is important to note that amount and

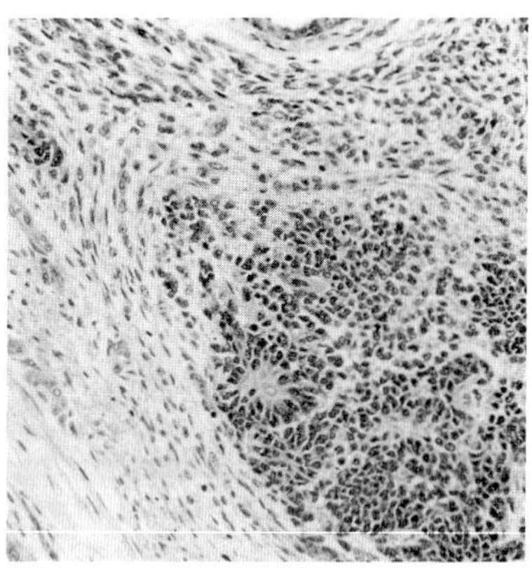

FIGURE 11-11. Immature neuroectodermal tissue with neuroepithelial tubules surrounded by immature neuroglial tissue (H&E, ×100).

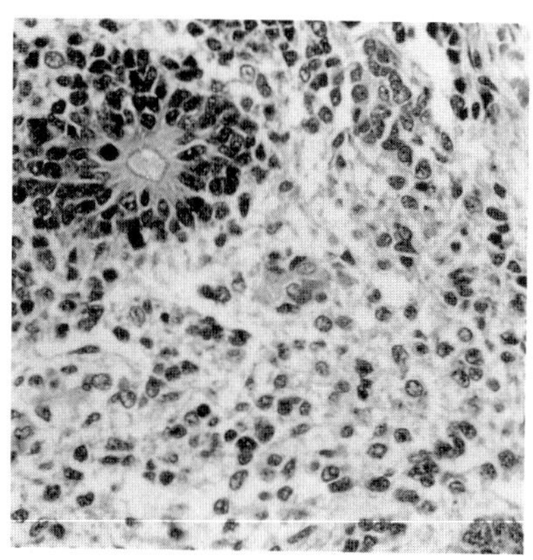

FIGURE 11-12. Immature neuroglial tissue and neuroepithelial tubule (H&E, ×250).

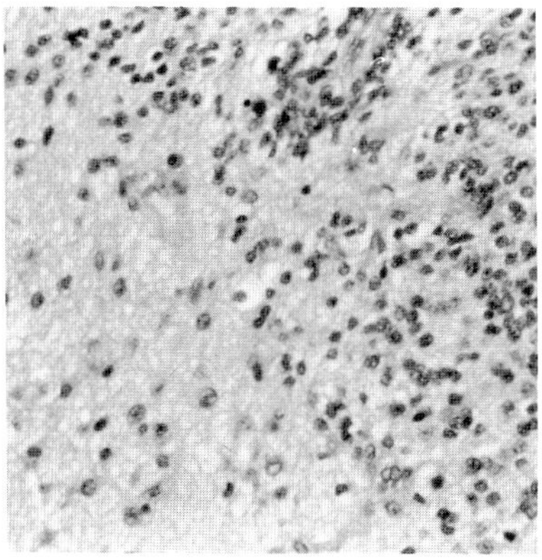

FIGURE 11-13. Mature neuroglial tissue with adjacent immature neuroglial tissue (H&E, ×250).

not degree of immaturity of the immature tissues is included in the grading system of primary tumors. However, for grading of the glial implants in the peritoneum or glial tissue in the lymph nodes the degree of cellularity, i.e., degree of immaturity of the glial tissue and mitotic activity, are taken into consideration. The amount of immature glial tissue in the implants cannot be assessed since (1) only a few of the numerous implants may be submitted by the surgeon for histologic examination, although it is recommended that the surgeon sample the peritoneal glial implants in cases of ovarian teratomas as extensively as is feasible; and (2) each implant is usually small and shows uniform maturity or degree of immaturity as the case may be. The criteria for grading these implants are essentially the degree of cellularity and extent of mitotic activity.

Critical review of the original articles and the photographs shows that histologic criteria of immaturity are not described and illustrated adequately.

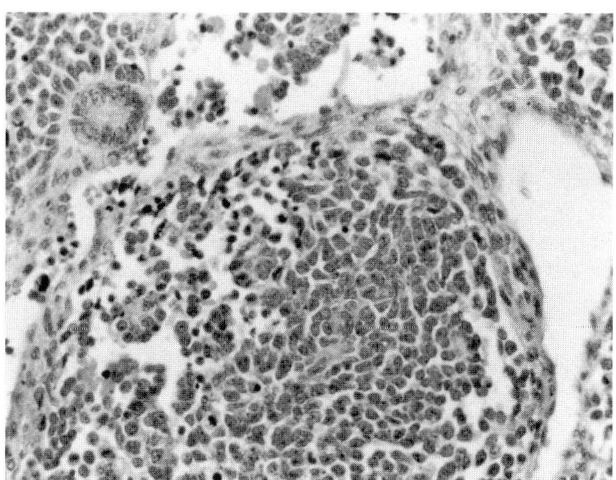

FIGURE 11-14. Nephrogenic tissue with blastemal cells; note an immature tubule (H&E, ×250).

TABLE 11-1 Grading System for Ovarian Teratomas Recommended by Various Authors

Robboy and Scully (reference 11)	
Grade 0	All tissues mature, no mitotic activity
Grade 1	Minor foci of abnormally cellular or embryonal tissue mixed with mature elements; rare mitoses
Grade 2	Moderate quantities of embryonal tissue mixed with mature elements; moderate mitotic activity
Grade 3	Large quantities of embryonal tissue present
Gonzalez-Crussi[a] (reference 6)	
Grade 0	All well-differentiated tissues
Grade 1	<10% of sampled tumor contains incompletely differentiated tissues
Grade 2	10–50% of sampled tumor contains immature tissues
Grade 3	>50% of sampled tumor contains undifferentiated tissue of uncertain metastatic potential
Norris et al (reference 27)	
Grade 0[b]	All mature tissues and absent or rare mitotic activity
Grade 1	Some immaturity[c] and neuroepithelium[d] absent or limited to a rare 40x field and no more than one such focus per slide
Grade 2	Greater immaturity than in grade 1 and neuroepithelium limited to 2 to 3 40x fields per slide
Grade 3	Greater immaturity than in grade 2 and neuroepithelium in >4 40x fields per slide

[a] The author considers grade 0 and grade 1 teratomas as mature and grade 2 and grade 3 teratomas as immature teratomas.

[b] These are mature teratomas.

[c] It appears that authors are referring to immaturity in nonneural tissues.

[d] This term is equivalent to primitive neuroectoderm. From their illustrations it appears that neuroepithelial tubules are included in their definition of neuroepithelium. Note that the semiquantitative criteria apply only to neuroepithelium. But these could be used for other immature tissues such as metanephric blastema, immature mesenchyme and primitive neuroectoderm without neuroepithelial tubules.

What is also missing from these descriptions are the guidelines and standardization for the selection of areas of the tumor for histologic sampling based on gross features. Moreover, all the authors imply that the same criteria are used for grading the primary tumor and glial implants. However, primitive neuroectoderm with neuroepithelial tubules (Table 11-1) is usually not seen in the implants and as indicated above the amount of immature glial tissue cannot be estimated from the sections available for histologic examination. Although none of the authors state so, in fact the criteria for grading the implants are based on the degree of cellularity and/or mitotic activity.

In my own practice, I have put particular emphasis on extensive histologic sampling of the areas with the following types of features on gross examination: (1) fleshy appearance, (2) soft "encephaloid" appearance, (3) firm "mesenchy-

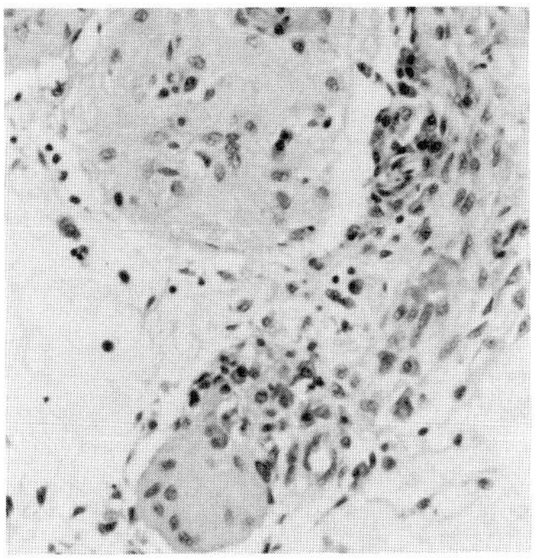

FIGURE 11-15. Grade 0 glial implants composed of mature glia; note scattered lymphocytes around and within the implants (H&E, ×250).

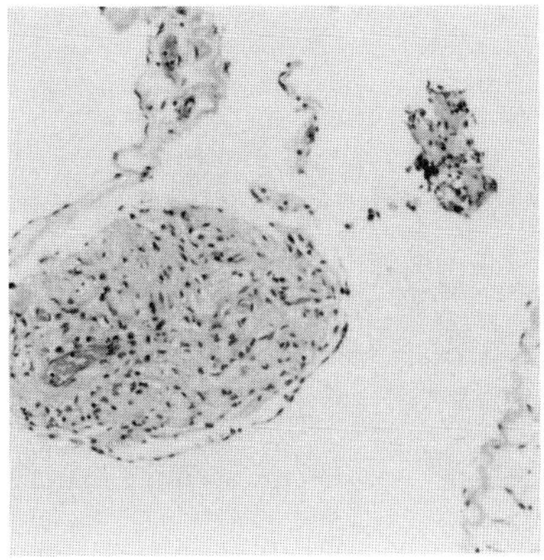

FIGURE 11-16. Grade 1 glial implant showing increased cellularity (H&E, ×100).

mal" areas, and (4) borderline of what appear to be hemorrhagic and/or necrotic foci with the surrounding viable areas. If adequate number of blocks for histologic examination are not taken from the areas of a teratoma with these types of features seen on gross examination, the grading may not accurately reflect the degree of immaturity and the malignant germ-cell or non-germ-cell components may not be sampled.

The criteria for grading of glial implants are as follows:

Grade 0. mature glia showing normal cellularity (Figure 11-15)

Grade 1. glia showing slightly greater cellularity than normal mature glial tissue and/or rare mitoses in the entire implant of small size or per high field in larger implants (Figures 11-16, 11-17)

Grade 2. glial implant showing moderate cellularity and/or occasional mitoses (Figure 11-18)

Grade 3. glial implant showing marked cellularity (Figure 11-19)

Occasionally lymphocytic infiltrates may be present in the glial implants, giving an impression of increased cellularity and of higher than the actual grade (Figures 11-20, 11-21). Such lymphocytic "infiltrates" may also be present in glial areas of the primary tumor, giving an impression of immaturity. The lymphocytic nature of the cells can be confirmed by immunoperoxidase stain for leukocyte common antigen (LCA) (Figures 11-22, 11-23).

BIOLOGIC BEHAVIOR OF TERATOMAS

Mature Teratomas

Mature teratomas are benign. It is, however, possible that in a teratoma diagnosed as "mature," immature or malignant elements may be present in those

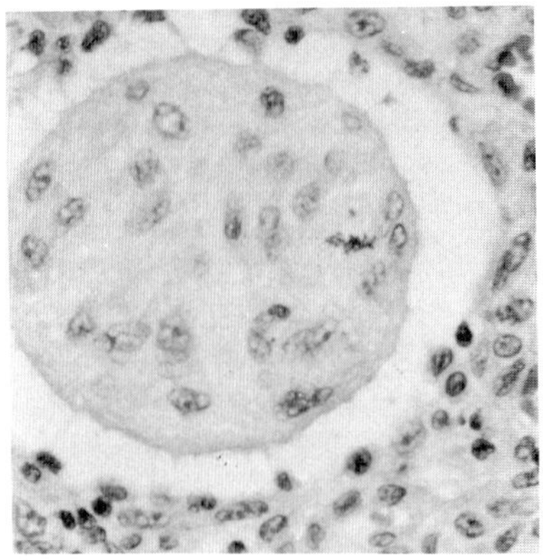

FIGURE 11-17. A small grade 1 glial implant showing a mitotic figure (H&E, ×400).

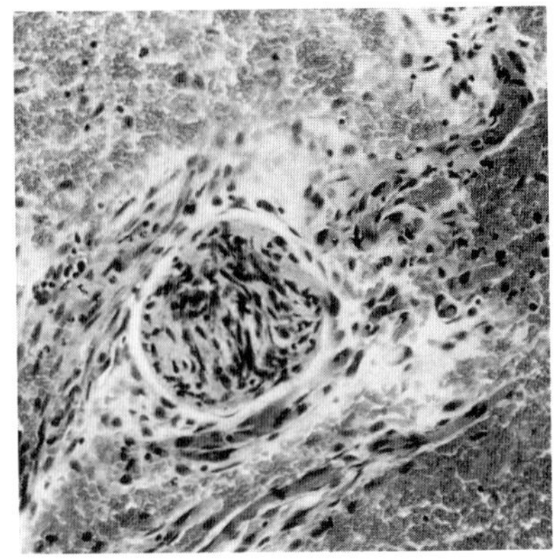

FIGURE 11-18. Grade 2 glial implant with moderate cellularity (H&E, ×100).

parts of the tumor not included in the samples taken for histologic examination. As described above in a tumor diagnosed originally as mature or immature neonatal SCT, local recurrence as YSC can occur.[25,26] In rare instances:

1. Metastases from a mature teratoma may show only mature tissues.[28]
2. Local recurrence consisting of mature tissue may occur as a result of incomplete resection.
3. A focus of malignant tumor such as squamous cell carcinoma[29] or predominant neuroblastoma-like areas[30] may be present in an otherwise mature cystic teratoma. These tumors should be designated as teratoma with a malignant non-germ-cell component. The youngest patient with squamous cell carcinoma in an otherwise "mature" cystic ovarian teratoma in the series reported by Hirakawa et al[29] was 32 years old and the patient with neuroblastoma in an otherwise "mature" cystic ovarian teratoma was 18 years old.[30]
4. Peritoneal implants of mature glial tissue (grade 0) (gliomatosis peritonei) can occur in very large predominantly solid or partly cystic mature teratoma of the ovary.

Gliomatosis peritoneai is considered to be benign in almost all cases (see section on peritoneal implants of glial tissue below). Lipogranulomas of regional lymph nodes in the absence of any metastasis may be seen in mature (grade 0) teratoma of testis.[31] It is possible that leakage of lipid from sebaceous material into the stroma of the tumor is followed by its drainage via lymphatics. The lipid thus deposited in the lymph node incites a foreign-body-type giant cell reaction. Deaths occurring in mature teratomas may be due to surgery-related complications or non-tumor-related factors. For example, a premature newborn infant with mature SCT may die of idiopathic respiratory distress syndrome or other perinatal disorders.

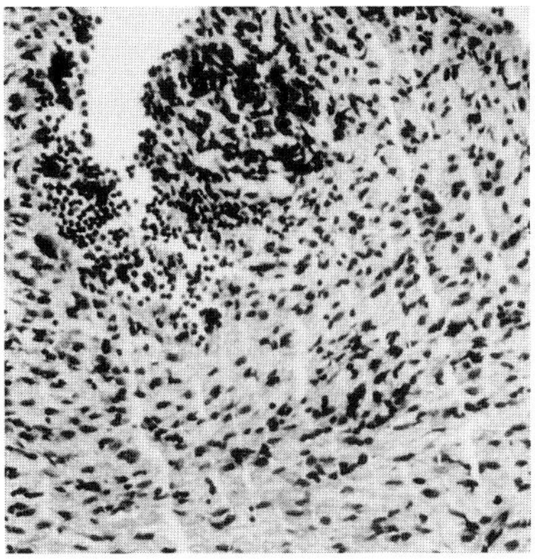

FIGURE 11-19. Grade 3 glial implant with marked cellularity (H&E, ×100).

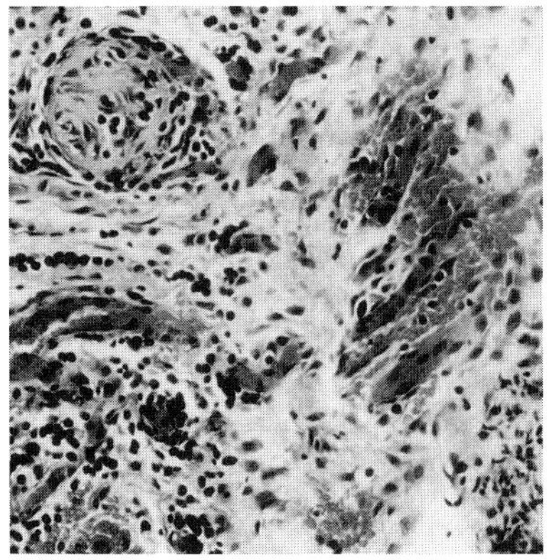

FIGURE 11-20. Grade 1 glial implant with lymphocytic infiltrate within and around it giving the implant an appearance of increased cellularity (H&E, ×100).

Malignant Teratomas

Malignant teratomas as the name indicates behave in a malignant fashion. EC, CCA, and YSC show more aggressive behavior than G. YSC of the testis in children younger than 2 years of age is thought to have better prognosis than in older children. However, analysis of recent data collected by the Section on Urology of American Academy of Pediatrics suggests that no such difference exists in the two age groups.[32] Most of the children with YSC of testis in the series reported by Kaplan et al presented with stage I disease (160 of 181 cases), and the median age in that series was 17 months.[32] It has been argued that the mortality

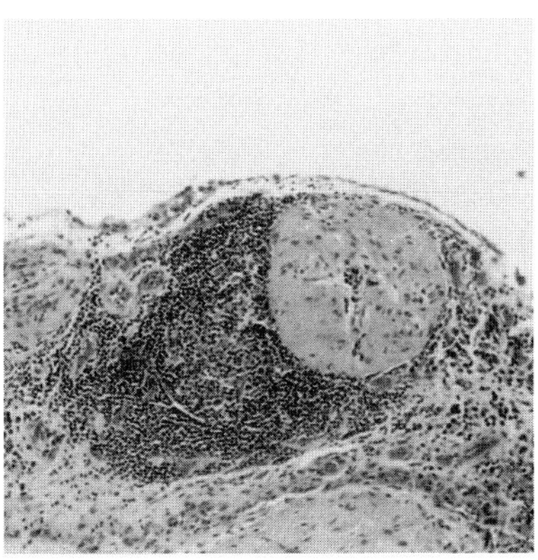

FIGURE 11-21. Grades 0 and 1 glial implants (on the right and left, respectively) with a dense lymphocytic infiltrate around them (H&E, ×40).

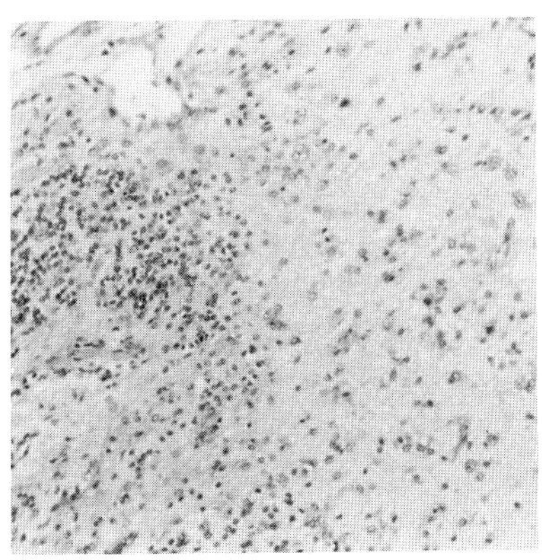

FIGURE 11-22. Mature glial tissue in a teratoma showing a focus of increased cellularity due to lymphocytic infiltration (H&E, ×100).

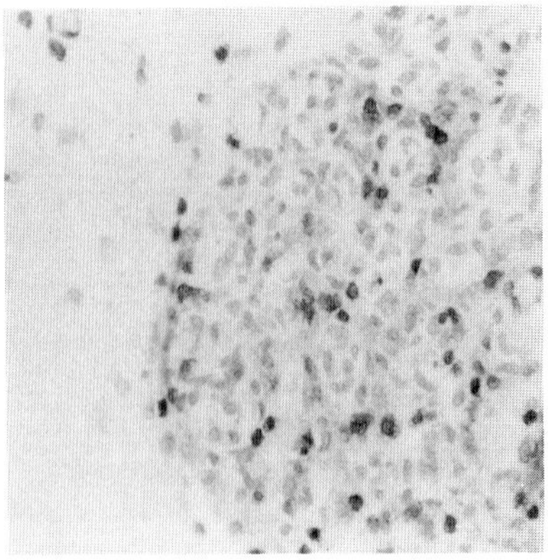

FIGURE 11-23. Immunoperoxidase stain for leukocyte common antigen showing positive reaction in the lymphocytes (H&E, ×250).

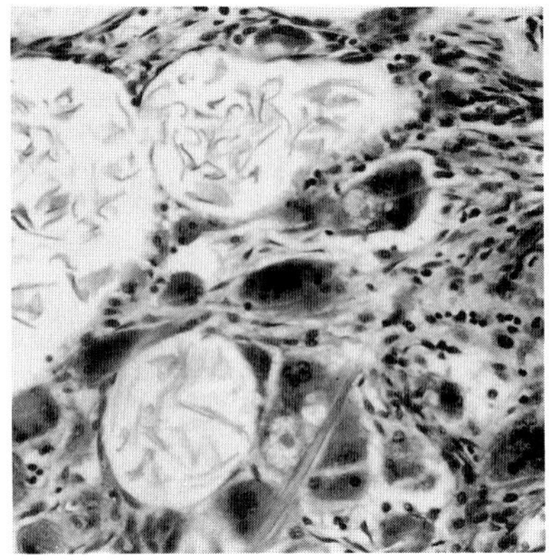

FIGURE 11-24. Peritoneal "implant" composed of keratin flakes surrounded by foreign-body-type giant cell reaction (H&E, ×400).

is correlated with the stage of the disease rather than age of the patient. However, it is possible that YSC of testis occurring in children <2 years of age is biologically different and inherently less aggressive than YSC of testis in older individuals. Therefore in most cases it remains restricted to stage I. It is of interest to note that in a preliminary report Perlman et al[33] have shown in YSC of testis (and other sites) in infants, the absence of chromosomal abnormality *i*(12*p*), which is present in most adult germ-cell tumors.

One of the notable features of metastases detected after chemotherapy in some of the cases of malignant teratomas is the presence of mature elements on histologic examination.[34] It has been suggested that the metastases composed of mature elements are remnants persisting following the eradication of the malignant elements that are responsive to chemotherapy. An alternative explanation is the possible maturation of the immature malignant elements as a result of chemotherapy.

Biochemical Markers of Malignant Teratomas

Malignant teratomas, (EC, YSC, and CCA) are associated with two biochemical markers, AFP and hCG. EC is associated with both AFP and hCG; YSC, with AFP; and CCA, with hCG. There is generally good correlation between elevated serum levels and demonstration of the marker(s) in the tumor tissue by immunoperoxidase stain.[35] These markers are useful for diagnosis, assessing the completeness of resection of the tumor and in follow-up of the patients for recurrence.

In mature and immature teratomas (i.e., teratomas without the malignant germ-cell components such as EC, YSC, or CCA), AFP and hCG cannot be demonstrated by immunoperoxidase stain and serum levels of AFP and HCG are normal. However, in rare cases of mature and immature teratoma serum AFP levels may be slightly elevated.[36,37] In such instances AFP may be demonstrable in the tubular structures lined by GI-type epithelium and in fetal liver tissue in mature and immature teratomas.[38] AFP, which probably behaves as fetal albumin and has the same structure and osmotic and carrier functions as albumin, is synthesized by fetal liver cells, by yolk sac, and in trace amounts by the fetal gastrointestinal tract.[39] In a recent report Nogales et al[40] have described two cases of solid immature ovarian teratomas with focal cystic change occurring in two girls (9 and 10 years of age) in whom there were moderate elevations of AFP (case 1, 500 ng/ml; case 2, 730, normal 0–15) and of hCG (case 1, 30 mU/ml; case 2, positive pregnancy test, normal, 0–10 mU/ml). On histologic examination, there was no neuroectodermal component. The tumors consisted of tissues of endodermal and mesenchymal derivation. Thus columnar cell lined cysts, embryonic lung tissue, esophagus and intestine, primitive mesoblast, cartilage, smooth muscle, and foci of hematopoiesis were present. Large syncytial cells were seen in the embryonic intestinal structures. The immunoperoxidase stain for AFP was positive in the epithelial lining of many of the aforementioned structures. The large syncytial cells mentioned above were positive for hCG. These cases reinforce the point that AFP synthesis can occur in endodermally-derived epithelium. It should be noted that the elevations of AFP in these cases of immature teratoma were only moderate in contrast to values of $\geqslant$100,000 ng/ml in YSC (and $\geqslant$500,000 ng/ml in hepatoblastoma).

AFP levels are moderately raised also in neonatal hepatitis, biliary atresia, cirrhosis, and inflammatory bowel disease. Malignant teratoma (or hepatoblastoma), which generally produces very high levels of serum AFP levels, can be easily distinguished from the nonmalignant conditions mentioned above. Nevertheless, elevated serum AFP levels in a case diagnosed histologically as a mature or immature teratoma should prompt an intensive search for YSC component by careful reexamination of the histology slides and by taking additional sections from the remaining gross specimen. Besides AFP, carcinoembryonic antigen has also been demonstrated in the well-differentiated columnar and squamous epithelium, pancreatic ducts and neuroepithelium in some cases of mature and immature sacrococcygeal teratomas.[38]

Immature Teratomas

Behavior of immature teratomas is unpredictable and can vary from benign, borderline (local recurrence) to malignant (metastasis). In cases of incompletely resected immature teratomas there are three possibilities: (1) immature tissues may mature, (b) the tissue may show enhanced proliferation with recurrence, or (3) the tissue may undergo malignant transformation with metastasis.[6]

The relationship between histologic grade and behavior has been studied primarily in ovarian teratomas. Neuroectodermal tissue is among the commonest immature tissues in immature teratomas. These areas resemble neuroblastoma but do not show malignant behavior in most instances. Only rare cases of metastatic neuroblastoma have been reported.[30,41] However, Dehner[42] cautions that presence of neuroepithelial tubules (or primitive mesenchyme) (Figures 11-8, 11-9, 11-11, 11-12) in an SCT even in a neonate should alert the pathologist (and the clinician) to the possibility of unpredictable behavior of such a tumor. Immature mesenchymal, nephrogenic, and lung tissue has also been described in immature teratomas.[43,44] Presence of metanephric blastemal tissue resembling Wilms' tumor in an SCT has been considered as evidence of malignancy, although metastasis was not present.[45] In the case reported by Ward and

Dehner,[45] the SCT in a 3-year-old girl was composed predominantly of nephroblastomatous tissue. Gonzalez-Crussi et al[43] have described metanephric blastemal foci in SCT without evidence of metastasis. Besides these reports of nephroblastomatous or metanephrogenic blastemal tissue in SCT, occurrence of similar tissue has also been described in rare cases of retroperitoneal, mediastinal, and ovarian teratomas.[46–48] Nogales et al[48] suggested that Wilms' tumor may arise from such metanephrogenic blastemal foci. Although occasional small foci of nephrogenic and other embryonic tissues may not be necessarily associated with malignant behavior, Gonzalez-Crussi cautions against complacency when large or abundant amounts of such nongerminal immature tissue (i.e., excluding YSC, EC, and CCA) are present.[6]

Peritoneal Implants of Glial Tissue

Peritoneal (and omental) implants composed of glial tissue are found in up to one-third of cases of immature ovarian teratoma.[37] These implants occur probably as a result of tears and defects in the capsule.[11] These defects may be present de novo or may occur as a result of biopsy procedure or break in the capsule at the time of surgery. In some cases in the sections taken from the appropriate site, glial tissue can be demonstrated to extend through the capsule to the peritoneum (Figures 11-1, 11-2).[11] These implants are graded histologically as described above. When all the glial implants in a case are mature, i.e., histologic grade 0, the term "gliomatosis peritonei" (GP) is used. Truong et al[37] reviewed 32 cases of GP including two of their own. The primary ovarian teratoma may be of any grade. Thus in the 29 of the 32 cases reviewed by Truong et al[37] the grades of the primary tumor were as follows: grade 0 (2 cases), grade 1 (15 cases), grade 2 (7 cases), and grade 3 (5 cases). It should be noted that the tumors producing GP tend to be very large in size ($\leqslant$35 cm and $\leqslant$4000 g) and predominantly or partly solid. GP may also occur in mature (grade 0) ovarian teratomas. Despite such spread to the peritoneum, 29 of these 32 patients survived from 6 months to 38 years in the cases reviewed by Truong et al.[37] In two of the three patients who died, GP was replaced by teratomatous and malignant glial tissue at autopsy. In addition to glial implants, implants composed of keratin flakes and squamous epithelial cells surrounded by foreign-body-type giant cell reaction (Figure 11-24) and of teratomatous elements may also occur on the peritoneum in association with capsular tears or defects of immature ovarian teratomas. The former implants are probably due to implantation of the squamous elements through the rupture or tears in the capsule. The teratomatous implants composed of admixture of various types of tissues such as skin adnexa, mucous glands, and cartilage are usually few in number and tend to be of a large size in contrast to the multiple small white glial implants measuring a few millimeters.[37,49–51] Presence of mature (grade 0) glial implants, i.e., GP, is considered to be benign, requiring no additional therapy in virtually all cases. The teratomatous implants may imply poor outcome, and consideration may have to be given to additional therapy.

Nodal Gliomatosis

In rare cases of immature teratoma of the ovary, microscopic nodules of glial tissue may be found in the omental, mesenteric or para-aortic lymph nodes.[11,52,53] In two of the three cases showing nodal metastasis the glial tissue was mature, i.e., histologic grade 0.[52,53] In the third case, the glial tissue was given grade 1 because of the presence of a single mitosis.[11] The glial tissue is seen in the subcapsular sinus (Figure 11-25) or in a deeper portion of the lymph node. When the glial tissue in the lymph nodes is mature, the term "nodal gliomatosis" is used. The location of the glial tissue within the subcapsular sinus and deeper part of the lymph node indicates that the process represents "metastasis" occurring via lymphatics. Therefore the term nodal "implants" used by Perrone et al[53] is not appropriate. The primary ovarian tumors were grade 1 in two of these cases. In the third case it is stated to be mature solid grade 0 teratoma. Despite the presence of glial tissue in the lymph nodes, two of the three patients in whom follow-up data are given were alive and well 5 years after surgery. One case of grade 1 ovarian teratoma with nodal involvement seen in personal experience (Figure 11-25) also has survived for 3 years after surgery. No additional chemotherapy is indicated in these cases.

Prognosis in Immature Teratomas

Available data suggest that grade of immature ovarian teratomas is a determinant of their behavior, although more data in larger series of cases of immature teratomas of ovaries and other sites are needed to provide the risk estimates.[11,27,43]

Norris et al[27] have presented detailed data in 58 cases of immature ovarian teratomas. In their series:

1. The age range was 14 months to 40 years with median age of 19 years. Of the 58 patients, 19 were less than 15 years and 17 were between 15 and 20 years of age. Thus this is a tumor predominantly of childhood and adolescence.
2. Age of the patient, size of the tumor, stage, and histologic grade of the primary tumor and grade of metastases appeared to be related to prognosis.
3. Detailed statistical analyses after adjusting for various prognostic factors and data regarding statistical significance have not been provided but following trends in prognostic significance of the aforementioned factors were noted. The survival in patients younger than 13 years tended to be better. Teratomas measuring <10 cm were associated with 100% survival. In contrast, 67 and 54% patients with teratomas measuring 10–19.9 cm and ≥20 cm, respectively, were living and well. The survival in stage I patients was 74%, in

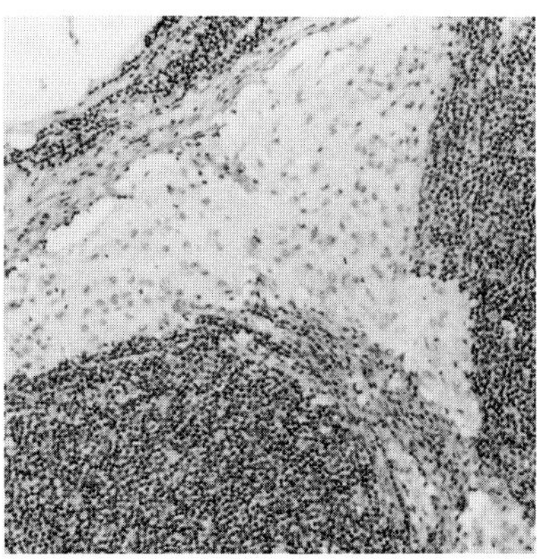

FIGURE 11-25. Nodal gliomatosis characterized by mature grade 0 glial tissue in the subcapsular sinus of an omental lymph node (H&E, ×250).

TABLE 11-2 Staging of Ovarian Tumors

Stage I	Tumor limited to one or both ovaries; capsule intact; absence of malignant cells in peritoneal fluid
Stage II	Tumor within or beyond the ovarian capsule with local pelvic extension; absence of malignant cells in peritoneal fluid and no metastasis in retroperitoneal lymph nodes
Stage III	Metastasis to retroperitoneal nodes, presence of malignant cells in the peritoneal fluid, or abdominal extension
Stage IV	Extraabdominal dissemination

Adapted from reference 54.

contrast to 38% survival in stages II and III patients. (The criteria for staging of ovarian, testicular and extragonadal teratomas are given in Tables 11-2, 11-3, and 11-4, respectively.[54]) The survival rates in patients with grades 1, 2, and 3 of the primary tumors were 82, 63, and 30% respectively and in patients with grades 0, 1, and 2 of the metastases were 83, 40, and 50% respectively. The authors state that although the size and stage of the tumors were related to survival, the grade of the primary tumor was the major determinant of extraovarian spread and the grade of metastases shows the best correlation with subsequent course.

In a more recent series of 41 cases of immature ovarian teratomas from M. D. Anderson Hospital and Tumor Institute,[55] the tumors were graded histologically according to the criteria of Norris et al.[27] Metastases were present in the peritoneum, lymph node, omentum, intestine, diaphragm, uterus, liver capsule, and fallopian tube in some cases. The data regarding relationship of metastases to histologic grade are not given. The differences in progression-free survival (PFS) in the various stages were not statistically significant. The PFS rates in patients with grades 1, 2, and 3 neoplasms were 75, 55, and 31%, respectively. However, none of these differences was statistically significant. Interestingly AFP was elevated in 31% of patients. In six patients there was a mature cystic teratoma in the contralateral ovary. The authors recommended the following guidelines for therapy: (1) grade 1 stage I patients—surgical resection alone; (2) all other tumors—surgical resection followed by combination chemotherapy.

A second-look laparotomy done in immature teratoma may show implants of only mature glial tissue. It has been suggested this may represent maturation of previously immature implants due to chemotherapy (chemotherapeutic retro-

TABLE 11-3 Grouping of Testicular Tumors in Children

Group I	Tumor restricted to the testis, AFP levels normal within 1 month after orchiectomy; chest radiograph and retroperitoneal imaging normal
Group IIA	Same as group I, but retroperitoneal lymph node dissection reveals unsuspected metastases in the nodes
Group IIB	Retroperitoneal metastasis revealed by imaging studies, AFP levels persistently high
Group III	Demonstrable metastases beyond the retroperitoneum

Adapted from reference 54.

conversion) or necrosis and disappearance of immature elements due to chemotherapy with persistence of the mature elements which are unresponsive to chemotherapy.[55,56]

Application of Histologic Grading System Used in Immature Ovarian Teratomas to Other Sites

As indicated above, the histologic grading systems described in Table 11-1 have been primarily developed and tested in the cases of immature ovarian teratomas. Dehner[12] states that "application of a similar histologic grading system to the SCT, however, has yielded only equivocal result." No data with respect to this statement are given. Gonzales-Crussi et al[43] applied to the SCT the grading system used for the ovarian tumors by Norris et al.[27] In their series of 40 cases of SCT there were 18 cases of immature teratomas (grade 1, 3 cases; grade 2, 5 cases; and grade 3, 10 cases). Numerous recurrences and metastases were seen in the patients with grades 2 and 3 SCTs. However, it should be noted that they considered SCT with foci of YSC as grade 3 immature teratoma. According to current recommendation these tumors are considered as malignant teratoma with YSC component. Valdiserri and Yunis[57] also applied to SCT the criteria for grading used by Norris et al[27] for ovarian teratomas. In their series of 68 cases, 8 were immature teratomas (grade 2, 2 cases; grade 3, 6 cases). Four of these patients had no recurrence after a follow-up of 4–13 years (average, 7.5 years). There were two postoperative deaths. One death which was unrelated to immature teratoma occurred at 3 years after surgery. One patient was lost to follow-up. Carter et al[44] reviewed the reported cases of immature mediastinal teratomas in children and added two new cases. One of the cases described by these authors was a grade 2 immature teratoma, while the second one was grade 1 apparently according to the criteria applied to immature ovarian teratomas by Norris et al.[27] Both patients in whom the diagnosis was made in the neonatal period or infancy were alive and well and 6 years after surgery. In one of these patients only a partial resection of the mediastinal teratoma was possible because of close apposition to the great arteries. These authors also reviewed 13 cases of immature mediastinal teratoma in children who were 15 years old or younger. Sufficient data was not available in these cases for assessment of the histologic grade. However, all the 13 cases had survived at the last follow-up varying from 1 to 3 years after surgery. The Pediatric Oncology Group recommends that the grading system described by Norris et al[27] for ovarian teratomas be used for teratomas of other sites. The data using the grading system for sites other than ovary in the Pediatric Oncology Group cases has not been published as yet.

Terminology and Follow-up of Immature Teratomas

There is considerable confusion regarding the terminology of immature teratomas. Grade 2 and grade 3 immature teratomas have been and are still designated outright as malignant teratomas.[27,58] Although immature tissues are potentially malignant, labeling all immature teratomas as "malignant" is not indicated. Age of the patient and site and stage of the teratoma are also related to the biologic behavior of immature teratomas. In the pathology report the diagnostic term "immature teratoma" should be used, and it should be qualified by specific reference to histologic grade of the primary tumor, completeness of resection, capsular penetration, and grade of implants whenever applicable. The recurrence in immature teratomas may be related to incomplete resection or to a malignant germ-cell component that may have been missed despite extensive sampling. AFP and hCG levels in the serum should be determined preoperatively and a regular follow-up of the patient by monitoring by noninvasive imaging techniques is advisable. If a teratoma that consists mostly or focally of immature tissues but has a small malignant germ-cell component (such as YSC), the designation malignant teratoma (with the appropriate germ-cell component) should be used. Immature teratomas of grade 3 should be designated as such and the outright use of the designation malignant immature teratoma is not indicated. Presence of metanephric blastemal or immature "neuroblastoma-like" neuroectodermal tissue should be assessed semiquantitatively in terms "small," "moderate," or "abundant amounts." The amounts of such tissue should be specifically stated in the description. The possibility of aggressive behavior particularly in cases with abundant amount of such tissues should be brought to the attention of the clinician and the association of high grade in immature teratomas with relatively poor outcome should also be indicated in a comment.

SUMMARY

Teratomas are divided into mature, immature, and malignant types. Extensive sampling is essential to detect immature and malignant elements in teratomas and for confirming or determining the stage of the tumor. A definitive diagnosis of mature or immature teratoma in an incisional biopsy of a large teratoma cannot be made because "malignant" elements may be present in the remaining tumor mass. Data regarding survival and management of immature teratomas are not conclusive at this stage. But in view of the available data, older children with high-grade and/or high-stage immature teratomas are probable candidates for chemotherapy. The pathologist should therefore take an adequate number of sections for determining the grade of immature teratomas. The surgeon should give an adequate number of peritoneal glial implants for histologic examination in the cases of ovarian immature teratomas since the grade of the implants is an important determinant of survival. In the pathology report "mature" and "immature" may be used as diagnostic terms rather than "benign" and "malignant" to designate teratomas with mature and immature elements, respectively. Teratomas containing germ-cell elements focally or exclusively are malignant. A comment regarding potential for malignant behavior, particularly in high-grade immature teratomas, may be included in the report. Immature teratomas, if excised, completely may behave in a benign manner. The age, stage, and location of teratomas are also related to behavior. Immature tissues in ovarian vs. sacrococcygeal vs. mediastinal teratomas and in neonates vs. young children vs. individuals older than 15 years of age may not have the same significance in terms of behavior. Thus immature tissues in a SCT in a newborn infant may not raise the same degree of concern as those in an ovarian teratoma in a 15-year-old girl. The following guidelines for therapy of immature teratomas have been recommended:[54] stage I, grade 1 immature teratomas can be treated by surgery alone. Older children with higher-stage

TABLE 11-4 Staging for Extragonadal Tumors

Stage I	Tumor limited to one organ or structure with complete resection at initial surgical operation using a single incision
Stage II	Tumor extending to structures adjacent to the primary tumor but completely resected at the time of the initial operation
	Tumors requiring more than one incision for removal but without tumor spillage during operation
Stage III	Tumors with microscopic residual following operation, due to spillage or presence of tumor at resection margins
	Tumors incompletely resected at surgery
Stage IV	Disseminated disease

Adapted from reference 54.

disease and perhaps with higher-grade disease should receive chemotherapy. The guidelines for staging are given in Tables 11-2–11-4. Ovarian teratomas with grade 0 peritoneal implants probably require no treatment other than excision of the ovarian tumor.

REFERENCES

1. Ikeda H, Okumura H, Nagashima K, et al: The management of prenatally diagnosed sacrococcygeal teratoma. *Pediatr Surg Int* 5:192–194, 1990.
2. Dehner LP: Gonadal and extragonadal germ cell neoplasia of childhood. *Hum Pathol* 14:493–511, 1983.
3. Marsden HB, Steward JK: Tumors in children. In *Problems of children's tumors in Britain*, Springer-Verlag, New York, 1968, Chap 1, pp 1–12.
4. Young JL Jr, Miller RW: Incidence of malignant tumors in U.S. children. *J Pediatr* 86:254–258, 1975.
5. Willis RA: The teratoma. In *Pathology of tumors*, 4th ed. Butterworths, London, 1967, Chap 61, pp 959–1003.
6. Gonzales-Crussi F: Extragonadal teratomas: Fascicle 18 in second series of Atlas of tumor pathology, Armed Forces Institute of Pathology, Washington, DC, 1984.
7. Spaun E, Rix P: Benign cystic monodermal teratoma of neurogenic type. *Int J Gynecol Pathol* 9:283–290, 1990.
8. Aquirre P, Scully RE: Malignant neuroectodermal tumor of ovary, a distinctive form of monodermal teratoma: Report of five cases. *Am J Surg Pathol* 6:283–292, 1982.
9. Chen KTK, MA CK, Kussel SH: Hepatocellular adenoma of the placenta. *Am J Surg Pathol* 10:436–440, 1986.
10. Woodfield B, Katz DA, Cantrell CJ, et al: A benign cystic teratoma with gastrointestinal tract development. *Am J Clin Pathol* 83:236–240, 1985.
11. Robboy SJ, Scully RE: Ovarian teratoma with glial implants on the peritoneum: An analysis of 12 cases. *Hum Pathol* 1:643–653, 1970.
12. Dehner LP: Gonadal and extragonadal germ cell neoplasms—teratomas in childhood. In *Pathology of neoplasia in children and adolescents* (Finegold M, Ed). Saunders, Philadelphia, pp 282–312, 1986.
13. Sutherland SF, Singh S: Fetus in fetu. *Pediatr Surg Int* 3:368–372, 1988.
14. Willis RA: *The borderline of embryology and pathology*, 1st ed). Butterworths, London, 1958, pp 147, 641.

15. Hawkins E: Personal communication, 1993.
16. Nakashima N, Murakami S, Fukatsu T, et al: Characteristics of embryoid body in human gonadal germ cell tumors. *Hum Pathol* 19:1144–1154, 1988.
17. Teilum G: *Special tumors of the ovary and testis and related extragonadal lesions. Comparative pathology and histological identification*, 2nd ed. Copenhagen, Musksgaard, 1976, pp 33–47.
18. Ulbright TM, Gersell DJ: Rete testis hyperplasia with hyaline globule formation. A lesion simulating yolk sac tumor. *Am J Surg Pathol* 15:66–74, 1991.
19. Ulbright TM, Loehrer PJ, Roth LM, et al: The development of non-germ cell malignancies within germ cell tumors: A clinicopathologic study of 11 cases. *Cancer* 54:1824–1833, 1984.
20. Manivel C, Wick MR, Abenoza P, et al: The occurrence of sarcomatous components in primary mediastinal germ cell tumors. *Am J Surg Pathol* 10:711–717, 1986.
21. Ulbright TM, Boheen MP, Roth LM, et al: The differentiation of carcinomas of teratomatous origin from embryonal carcinoma: A light and electron microscopic study. *Cancer* 57:257–263, 1986.
22. Genadry R, Parmley T, Woodruff JD: Secondary malignancies in benign cystic teratomas. *Gynecol Oncol* 8:246–251, 1979.
23. Chumas JC, Scully RE: Sebaceous tumors in ovarian dermoid cysts. *Int J Gynecol Pathol* 10:356–363, 1991.
24. Sefier DB, Weiss LM, Kempson RL: Malignant lymphoma arising within thyroid tissue in a mature cystic teratoma. *Cancer* 58:2459–2461, 1986.
25. Hawkins E, Isaacs H, Cushing B, et al: Occult malignancy in neonatal sacrococcygeal teratomas. *Mod Pathol* 5:5P, 1992 (abstract).
26. Hawkins EP, Finegold MJ, Hawkins HK, et al: Nongerminomatous malignant germ cell tumors in children. A review of 89 cases from the Pediatric Oncology Group, 1971–1984. *Cancer* 58:2579–2584, 1986.
27. Norris HJ, Zirkin HJ, Benson WL: Immature (malignant) teratoma of the ovary. A clinical and pathologic study of 58 cases. *Cancer* 37:2359–2372, 1976.
28. Kusuda L, Leidich RB, Das S: Mature teratoma of the testis metastasizing as mature teratoma. *J Urol* 135:1020–1022, 1986.
29. Hirakawa T, Tsuneyoshi M, Enjoji M: Squamous cell carcinoma arising in mature cystic teratoma of the ovary: Clinicopathologic and topographic analysis. *Am J Surg Pathol* 13:397–405, 1989.
30. Reid H, Van Derm Walt JD, Fox H: Neuroblastoma arising in a mature cystic teratoma of the ovary. *J Clin Pathol* 36:68–73, 1983.
31. Epstein HD, Schitt SJ, Brodsky G: Lipogranulomas in lymph nodes (letter to the editor). *Arch Pathol Lab Med* 110:467–468, 1986.
32. Kaplan GW, Cromie WC, Kelais PP, et al: Prepubertal yolk sac testicular tumors: report of the testicular tumor registry. *J Urol* 140:1109–1112, 1988.
33. Perlman EJ, Henneberry J, Hawkins E, et al: Cytogenetic and ploidy analysis of endodermal sinus tumors (EST) in infants. *Mod Pathol* 6:7P, 1993 (abstract).
34. Logothetis CJ, Samuels ML, Trindada A, et al: The growing teratoma syndrome. *Cancer* 50:1629–1635, 1982.
35. Kurman RJ, Scardino Pt, McIntire KR, et al: Cellular localization of alpha-fetoprotein and human chorionic gonadotropin in germ cell tumors of the testis using indirect immunoperoxidase technique. A new approach to classification utilizing tumor markers. *Cancer* 40:2136–2151, 1977.
36. Nogales FF, Favara BE, Major FJ, et al: Immature teratoma of the ovary with a neural component ("solid" teratoma). *Hum Pathol* 7:625–642, 1976.
37. Truong LD, Jurro S, McGarran MK: Gliomatosis peritonei: Report of two cases and review of literature. *Am J Surg Pathol* 6:443–449, 1982.

38. Kuhjda FP, Taxy JB: Oncofetal antigens in sacrococcygeal teratomas. *Arch Pathol Lab Med* 107:239–242, 1983.
39. Gitlin D, Boesman M: Sites of serum alpha-fetoprotein synthesis in human and in the rat. *J Clin Invest* 46:1010–1016, 1967.
40. Nogales FF, Avila IR, Concha A, et al: Immature endodermal teratoma of the ovary: Embryologic correlations and immunohistochemistry. *Hum Pathol* 24:364–370, 1993.
41. Block M, Gilbert M, Davis C: Metastatic neuroblastoma arising in an ovarian teratoma with long-term survival: Case report and review of the literature. *Cancer* 54:590–595, 1984.
42. Dehner LP: Pediatric surgical pathology. In *Soft tissue, peritoneum and retroperitoneum*, 2nd ed. Williams & Wilkins, Baltimore, 1987, Chap 14, pp 869–938.
43. Gonzales-Crussi F, Winkler RF, Mirkin DL: Sacrococcygeal teratomas in infants and children. Relationship of histology and prognosis in 40 cases. *Arch Path Lab Med* 102:420–425, 1978.
44. Carter D, Bibro MC, Touloukian RJ: Benign clinical behavior of immature mediastinal teratoma in infancy and childhood: Report of two cases and review of the literature. *Cancer* 49:398–402, 1982.
45. Ward SP, Dehner LP: Sacrococcygeal teratoma with nephroblastoma (Wilms' tumor): A variant of extragonadal teratoma in childhood. *Cancer* 33:1355–1363, 1974.
46. Carney JA: Wilms' tumor and renal cell carcinoma in retroperitoneal teratoma. *Cancer* 35:1179–1183, 1975.
47. Willis RA: The structure of teratomata. *J Pathol Bacteriol* 40:1–36, 1935.
48. Nogales FF, Ortega I, Rivera F, et al: Metanephrogenic tissue in immature ovarian teratoma. *Am J Surg Pathol* 4:297–299, 1980.
49. Thurlbeck WM, Scully RE: Solid teratoma of the ovary. *Cancer* 13:804–811, 1960.
50. Nogucki TT, Lonser ER: Unusual teratoma of the ovary with implantation in the abdominal cavity. *Am J Obstet Gynecol* 82:381–385, 1961.
51. deGraaf J, van der Harten JJ: Alpha-fetoprotein in ovarian teratomas with glial implants on the peritoneum. *Eur J Obstet Gynecol Reprod Biol* 10:335–341, 1980.
52. El Shafie M, FurayRW, Chablani LV: Ovarian teratoma with peritoneal and lymph node metastases of glial tissue: A benign condition. *J Surg Oncol* 27:18–22, 1984.
53. Perrone T, Steiner M, Dehner LP: Nodal gliomatosis and alpha-fetoprotein production: Two unusual facets of grade 1 ovarian teratoma. *Arch Pathol Lab Med* 110:975–977, 1986.
54. Ablin A, Isaacs H: Germ cell tumors. In *Principles and practice of pediatric oncology* (Pizzo PA, Poplack DG, Eds). Lippincott, Philadelphia, 1989, pp 713–732.
55. Gershenson DM, Junco GD, Silva EG, et al: Immature teratoma of ovary. *Obstet Gynecol* 68:624–629, 1986.
56. Disaia PG, Saltz A, Kagan AR, et al: Chemotherapeutic retroconversion of immature teratoma of the ovary. *Obstet Gynecol* 49:346–350, 1977.
57. Valdiserri RD, Yunis EJ: Sacrococcygeal teratomas: A review of 68 cases. *Cancer* 48:217–221, 1981.
58. Wollner N, Gharimi F, Wachtel A, et al: Germ cell tumors in children: Gonadal and extragonadal. *Med Pediatric Oncol* 19:228–239, 1991.

12 SMALL ROUND CELL TUMORS AND RELATED LESIONS IN CHILDREN

INTRODUCTION

The small round cell tumors (SRCTs) conventionally include neuroblastoma (NB) (which may be considered as the prototype), rhabdomyosarcoma (RMS), Ewing's sarcoma (ES), and malignant lymphoma [non-Hodgkin's lymphoma (NHL)].[1–5] Peripheral primitive neuroectodermal tumor (PNET), which includes peripheral neuroepithelioma, Askin tumor, and certain cases designated as Ewing's sarcoma of soft tissue also belong to the conventional spectrum of SRCTs.[6] Certain other tumors such as small cell osteogenic sarcoma,[7] undifferentiated "anaplastic" small round cell hepatoblastoma,[8] germ-cell tumors, cellular hemangioma, malignant schwannoma, granulocytic sarcoma, blastemal Wilms' tumor,[9] extracranial metastasis of PNET of brain, and metastasis or extraocular extension of retinoblastoma, have to be included in the differential diagnosis for the sake of completeness. Only the SRCT in the conventional spectrum will be considered in detail in this chapter. Undifferentiated malignancies in childhood reviewed by Plotsky et al,[10] intraabdominal small cell desmoplastic tumors with divergent differentiation described by Gonzales-Crussi et al,[11] and other tumors will be described briefly. All these common and rare SRCTs and related tumors are listed in Table 12-1.

Although these tumors are designated as SRCTs, the tumors may not always contain small cells. Thus there are large cell NHLs, cells of ES are as large as histiocytes, and there is a large cell variant of ES. The cells of RMS are also large (Figures 12-1, 12-2). The cells may not necessarily be round. Thus, in embryonal RMS many of the tumor cells are fusiform in shape and in its spindle cell variant most of the cells are spindle-shaped (Figures 12-2, 12-3). Cells with irregulr outline are present in certain types of large cell NHLs. The nuclei may be convoluted (e.g., lymphoblastic NHL) (Figure 12-4) or cleaved (e.g., large cell NHL). The cells are blue in the sense that they have large hyperchromatic nuclei and indiscernible or a thin rim of cytoplasm (Figure 12-5), although some of the tumors may have cells with vesicular nuclei (e.g., ES of soft tissues or large cell NHL) and moderate amounts of cytoplasm (Figure 12-1).

INCIDENCE

SRCTs are common tumors in childhood since NB, RMS, and NHL are among the commonest malignancies in children. The tumors belonging to

TABLE 12-1 Small Round Cell (SRCT) and Related Tumors

Conventional spectrum
Neurobalstoma (prototype): undifferentiated and poorly differentiated types
Peripheral primitive neuroectodermal tumors (PNET), including peripheral neuroepithelioma, Askin tumor, neural type of Ewing's sarcoma, and "peripheral neuroblastoma"
Ewing's sarcoma of bone and soft tissues
Rhabdomyosarcoma: embryonal and alveolar (classical and solid) types
Malignant lymphoma: lymphoblastic, small cell noncleaved and large cell types
Other tumors to be considered in the differential diagnosis of SRCT
Undifferentiated small cell hepatoblastoma (primary or metastasis), blastemal
Wilms' tumor (primary or metastasis)
Small cell osteosarcoma, malignant schwannoma, cellular hemangioma
Retionoblastoma (extraocular extension or metastasis), extracranial metastasis of PNET of brain
Granulocytic sarcoma
Germ cell trumors (embryonal carcinoma, yolk sac tumors)
Small cell desmoplastic tumors with divergent differentiation of abdomen
"Undifferentiated"[a] malignancies in children
Anaplastic carcinoma
Malignant histiocytosis
Carcinoma (pancreas, nasopharynx)
Granulosa cell tumor
Malignant mesothelioma
Hemangiopericytoma
Inflammatory psuedotumor

[a]Initially diagnosed as "undifferentiated" with definitive diagnosis made following subsequent ancillary study: Plotsky C: *Am J Hematol Oncol* 12:141, 1990.

SRCTs have the following overall incidence of all childhood cancers:[2] NB (8% or 9.6 per million children per year), RMS (4% or 5.3 million^{-1} year^{-1}), ES (1% or 1.7 million^{-1} year^{-1}), and NHL (6% or 7.4 million^{-1} year^{-1}). The incidence of PNET is not known, but Marina et al[6] found 26 cases of PNET in contrast to 169 cases ES and 406 cases of NB between 1962 and 1987 at St. Jude Children's Research Hospital. SRCTs have been described in all pediatric age groups, but some of these are particularly more common in the second decade.[5] The child most likely to present a diagnostic problem is usually an older child or an adolescent with an SRCT.[5] SRCTs do not present a diagnostic problem in all cases. For example, differentiating NB, typical Burkitt's lymphoma, embryonal RMS with readily recognizable rhabdomyoblasts, etc. can be readily diagnosed. The diagnosis will be evident in most instances after taking into consideration all the morphologic features revealed by various methods of study. In rare instances, clinical, routine histologic, ultrastructural, and immunohistochemical features may not reveal the correct diagnosis. In such cases, one or more of the features such as biochemical data (e.g., urinary catecholamines in NB), cytogenetic abnormalities (e.g., in NB and PNET), oncogene overexpression (N-myc vs. c-myc in NB vs. PNET), enzyme patterns (e.g., in NB and PNET), or specific gene expression (e.g., in RMS) may have to be taken into consideration for diagnosis.

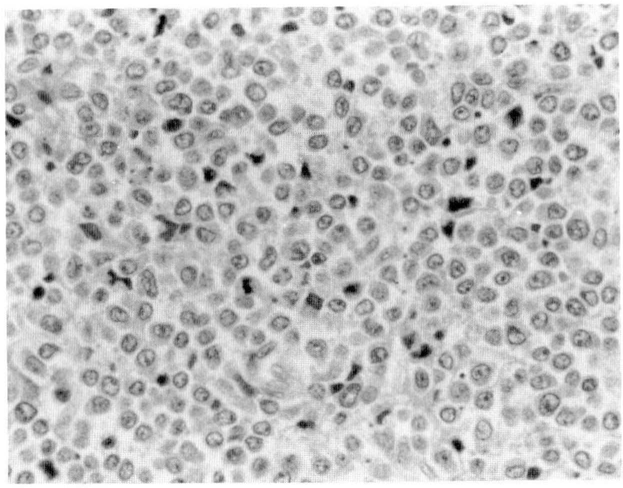

FIGURE 12-1. Large cell lymphoma composed of cells which have nuclei larger than the nuclei of histiocytes; note the vesicular appearance of the nuclei, prominent peripherally located nucleoli, and moderate amount of cytoplasm (H&E, ×400).

CHARACTERISTICS OF CONVENTIONAL SRCTS

The following characteristics are described below and summarized in Tables 12-2–12-14: clinical features; primary sites; metastatic sites; and histologic, ultrastructural, immunohistologic, and other features.

Neuroblastoma (NB)

NB is the most common extracranial solid tumor of childhood, accounting for 50% of malignancies in infants. The median age is about 2 years with a slight

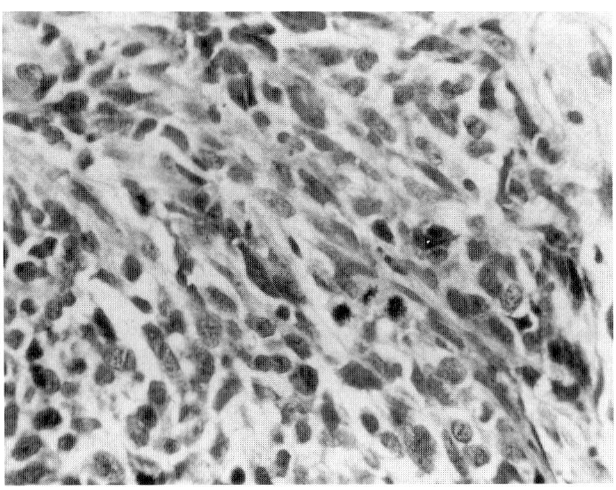

FIGURE 12-2. Admixture of fusiform to spindle-shaped cells and large round cells in embryonal RMS (H&E, ×400).

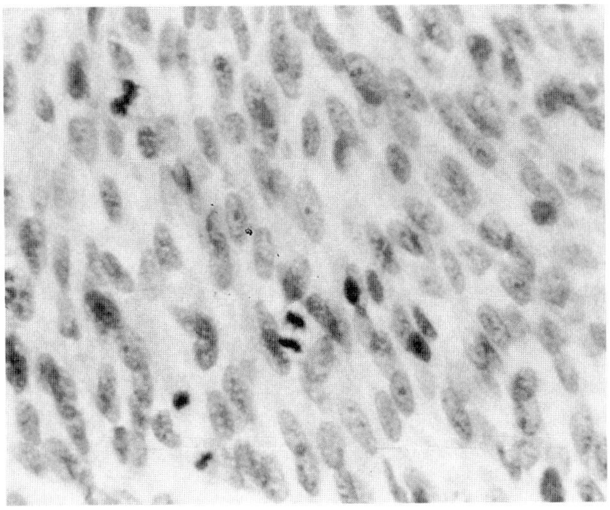

FIGURE 12-3. Spindle cells in embryonal RMS; there is high mitotic activity (H&E, ×400).

preponderance of males.[12] The incidence is 7.0 per million per year in black children and 9.6 in white children. NB is rare in certain areas of Africa. Familial cases of NB have been described. Increased frequency of NB has been observed in patients with neurofibromatosis, Beckwith–Wiedmann syndrome, but no specific congenital anomalies are associated with NB.

Clinical Features

Abdominal mass, which often crosses the midline, is the major finding in abdominal NBs. About 50% of infants and 70% of older children present with

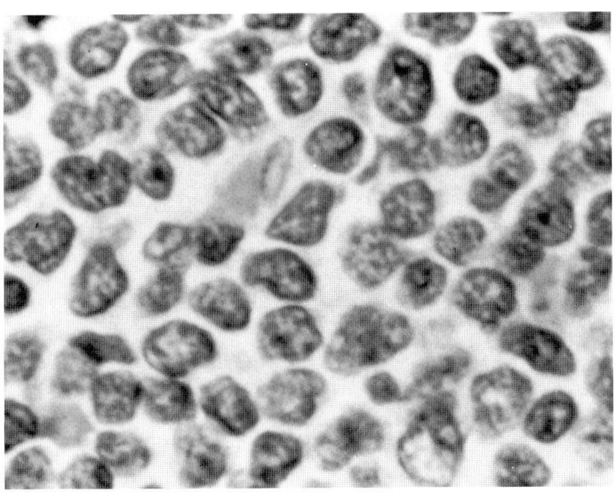

FIGURE 12-4. Convoluted nuclei of lymphoblastic non-Hodgkin's lymphoma (H&E, ×1000).

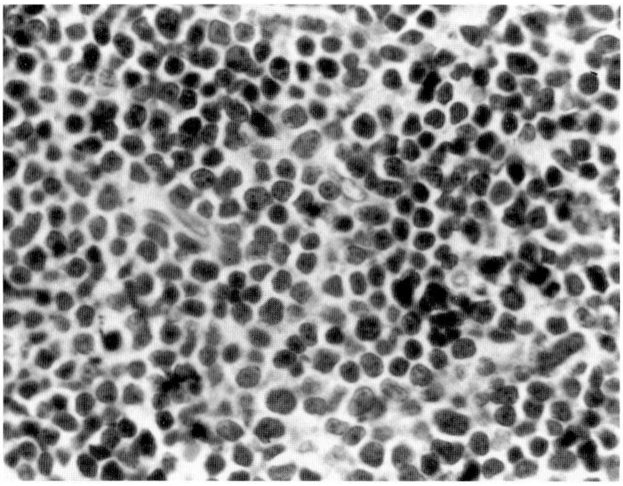

FIGURE 12-5. Small round cell tumor. Note the hyperchromatic round nuclei and indiscernible cytoplasm. There is lack of cohesion between tumor cells. (H&E, ×100.)

metastasis. About 70% of patients are <5 years, and 90% are <10 years.[13] Enlarged lymph nodes, skin nodules, hepatomegaly, and bone pain are the presenting features associated with metastasis (or multifocal involvement) of NB.

Primary Sites

Adrenal and sympathetic ganglia (thoracic, abdominal, cervical), pelvis, and retroperitoneum[12] are the primary sites (adrenals, 40%; paraspinal abdomen, 25%; paraspinal thorax, 15%; neck, 5%; pelvis, 5%). Kidney is a rare primary site.

Metastatic Sites

Lymph nodes, bone marrow, liver, bone, and skin are the well known sites. Rare sites include skeletal muscle, brain, and testes (Joshi: Unpublished data 1992).

Histologic Features

The various nomenclatures and prognostic categories of neuroblastic tumors based on morphologic features are summarized in Table 12-10 to Table 12-14. The histologic findings are summarized below. NBs with one or more of the features such as moderate to abundant neuropil, with or without Homer Wright rosette formation, differentiating neuroblasts, and ganglion cells can be readily diagnosed on routine histology (Figures 12-6–12-8). Rosettes are present in about 45% of cases.[14] The undifferentiated NBs or poorly differentiated NBs with little neuropil and ≤5% of differentiating neuroblasts are difficult or impossible to diagnose on routine histology (Figure 12-9). Arrangement into nests surrounded by fibrovascular septa, rosettes, calcification, and karyorrhectic tumor cells are characteristic but not diagnostic features of NB (Figure 12-10).[14–16] In rare instances, the following unusual features may be seen in NBs: spindle-shaped or fusiform or large anaplastic neuroblasts with moderate amount of eosinophilic

TABLE 12-2 Primary Sites of SRCT[a]

SRCT	Primary sites	Comments
NB	Adrenal medulla and sympathetic ganglia (abdomen, pelvis, thorax, neck)	Abdomen (adrenals) the commonest site; kidney is a rare primary site
PNET	Abdomen, thorax (chest wall and mediastinum), pelvis, extremities (peripheral nerves and ? soft tissue)	Sympathetic ganglia and adrenals are usually not a primary site; however, in Marina's series two cases apparently arose in the adrenals (reference 6)
OE	Bones of lower extremities (44%), humerus and ilium (21%) most frequent sites; axial skeleton, hands and feet less common	Osseous Ewing's sarcoma can extend to the soft tissue
EOE	Paravertebral and intercostal regions and lower extremities commonest; retroperitoneum, pelvis, hips less common	Soft tissue extension of an osseous Ewing's sarcoma can occur
Rhabdomyosarcoma	Genitourinary (21%), extremities (20%), cranioparameningeal region (14%), other head and neck except orbit (13%), and orbit (10%)	Obstruction of urinary tract, cranial nerve palsy, etc. may be seen clinically; primary site may be occult in rare cases
Non-Hodgkin's lymphoma	Abdomen, mediastinum, head and neck equal distribution, extranodal in majority; multiple sites at presentation in the majority	Unusual sites include liver, spleen, brain, gastrointestinal tract, bone, skin, thyroid, etc.; in children with AIDS primary site is commonly brain

[a] Abbreviations: SRCT—small round cell tumors; NB—neuroblastoma; PNET—peripheral primitive neuroectodermal tumor; OE—osseous Ewing's sarcoma; EOE—extraosseous Ewing's sarcoma.

cytoplasm, rhabdoid–pseudorhabdoid change in neuroblasts, pseudoalveolar, papillary-like and "starry sky" patterns in some areas, and microcystic change due to degenerative changes (Figures 12-11–12-13).[17] Some of the characteristic features mentioned above are also seen in other SRCTs (e.g., rosettes in PNET). In undifferentiated NB, the routine histologic features will be suggestive but not

TABLE 12-3 Metastatic Patterns of SRCT[a]

SRCT	Metastatic pattern	Comments
NB	Lymph nodes (61%), bone marrow (54%), bone (48%), lung (5%). Also metastasizes to skin, liver	Unusual sites include skeletal muscle of extremities, brain and testes (Joshi VV: Unpublished data)
PNET	Lung (31%), lymph nodes (31%), bone and bone marrow (12% each)	Local extension more frequently seen than in NB
Ewing's sarcoma of bone	Lung (43%), bone (37%), bone marrow (10%), lymph nodes (16%)	Local extension in 18%
Rhabdomyosarcoma	Lung, lymph nodes, bone, bone marrow, CNS and liver are the known sites (lymph nodes infrequent, lung relatively more frequent)	Bone marrow involvement may occur at presentation in stage IV patients (primary site may be occult in some of these cases)
Non-Hodgkin's lymphoma	Generalized disease in majority of cases	Skin, bone marrow and CNS involvement may occur; unusual sites include lung and brain; multiple lymph node group involvement and hepatosplenomegaly are common

[a] Abbreviations: SRCT—small round cell tumor; NB—neuroblastoma; PNET—peripheral primitive neuroectodermal tumor.

diagnostic; therefore, in such instances knowledge of primary or metastatic site, immunohistologic and ultrastructural features (see below), and data regarding catecholamines would be considered in making a definitive diagnosis of undifferentiated NB in some cases. A poorly differentiated NB may show a single isolated ganglion cell or rare scattered ganglion cells, which would be helpful in making a definitive diagnosis (Figure 12-14). The prognostic categorization on the basis of histologic features is discussed in the chapter on neuroblastic tumors.

Ultrastructural Features

Dense-core neurosecretory granules (50–200 n*M*) generally of uniform size and located at the periphery of the cytoplasm and in the cell processes mimicking neuritic processes are the diagnostic ultrastructural features (Figure 12-15). Neurotubules are also present in the neuritic processes. These ultrastructural features are poorly developed in the undifferentiated NB. Thus, the dense-core granules may be few in number and atypical in terms of size, variation in size, and location and the neurotubules may be disorganized.[2] The neurosecretory granules should be distinguished from the lysosomal granules (LG), which are located in the perinuclear Golgi region and are pleomorphic. LG

TABLE 12-4 Histologic Features in SRCT[a]

Histologic feature	SRCTs showing the feature	Comments
Large round cells	ES, large cell NHL, RMS	The cells are as large as histiocytes
Large round cells having bright eosinophilic fibrillary cytoplasm with or without cross striations (rhabdomyoblast) or strap-shaped cells with cross striations	Rhabdomyosarcoma	Cross striations can be accentuated by trichrome or PTAH stains; immunohistochemical staining helpful to prove rhabdomyoblastic nature although not required by IRS; normal degenerating skeletal muscle cells in other SRCTs that infiltrate surrounding muscle should be distinguished from rhabdomyoblasts
Cells with vesicular nuclei, small neucleoli and slight to moderate amount of cytoplasm	Neuroblastoma	These cells are intermediate between neuroblasts and ganglion cells
Monotonous round cells having amphophilic and pyroninophilic cytoplasm with lipid vacuoles	NHL, small cell noncleaved type (Burkitt's subtype)	Stain for fat and methyl green-pyronine stain can be performed on imprints of the tumor; the cells lack cohesion; however, cohesive pattern may be seen in rare cases
Fusiform or spindle-shaped cells	Embryonal RMS	The spindle-shaped cells may be present exclusively (spindle cell variant of embryonal RMS) or admixed with a few round tumor cells; neuroblastoma may show focal spindle cell pattern
Nuclear pleomorphism	NHL, small cell noncleaved type (non-Burkitt's subtype)	The distinction between Burkitt's and non-Burkitt's types of small cell noncleaved NHL is not clinically significant
Convoluted nuclei of monotonous "round" cells	NHL, lymphoblastic type	Variable number (rare to majority) show convolutions, PAS stain accentuates convolutions
Vesicular nuclei with prominent nucleoli in apposition to nuclear membrane	NHL, large cell cleaved or noncleaved type	
Vesicular nuclei with prominent centrally located nucleoli	NHL, large cell, immunoblastic type	

TABLE 12-4 Continued

Histologic feature	SRCTs showing the feature	Comments
Clear cytoplasm containing glycogen (PAS with or without diastase)	ES	Glycogen prominent in peripheral portion of tumor; abundant (4+) glycogen seen only in 26% cases of ES; glycogen absent in 23% cases; glycogen present in rhabdomyosarcomas and even in some neuroblastomas and NHL (particularly lymphoblastic and large cells types)
Pyroninophilic cytoplasm	Burkitt's lymphoma, immunoblastic lymphoma	The stain may be done on imprints
Mitotic karyorrhectic cells (MKC)	NB, PNET, ES, blastemal WT, NHL	Most characteristic of NB, various morphologic outlines of MKCs (cresentic, PMN-like, lymphocyte-like, punctate, complex)
Lymphoglandular bodies	NHL	These are better seen in cytologic preparations but careful examination of histologic section may reveal these structures; lymphoglandular bodies are seen in both reactive and neoplastic lymphoid lesions
Neuropil	NB	Fibrin strands, collagenous stroma may be mistaken for fibrillar background, PNET may show pale eosinophilic fibrillar cores in the rosettes when present
Homer Wright rosettes	NB, PNET	Best developed in NB, present in about 45% NB
Nests surrounded by fibrovacular septa	NB	Best developed and most common in NB, fibrovascular septa in NB may show nodular proliferation or hyalinization; focal nesting pattern in ES, PNET
Alveolar pattern	Alveolar rhabdomyosarcoma	Pseudoalveolar pattern may be rarely seen in NB; alveolar pattern in RMS may be present only in deeper portion of the tumor or may be totally absent (solid variant of alveolar RMS)

TABLE 12-4 Continued

Histologic feature	SRCTs showing the feature	Comments
Starry sky pattern	Most characteristically seen in Burkitt's NHL, but also seen in other NHLs	Size of nuclei of tumor cells smaller, same size and larger than the tingible body macrophages in lymphoblastic, Burkitt's, and large cell NHLs, respectively; starry sky may be seen focally in NB and blastemal Wilms' tumor in rare cases
Polypoid configuration and cambium layer	Botryoid rhabdomyosarcoma	Cambium layer necessary for diagnosis
Myxoid areas	Embryonal rhabdomyosarcoma	
Filigree pattern (biphasic pattern of light and dark cells)	ES	This pattern is related to degenerative changes in some of the cells or alternating arrangement of darkly staining tumor cells with lighter-staining fibrovascular septa; this pattern is to be distinguished from pseudofiligree pattern due to compression in the peripheral infiltrating portion of tumor; pseudofiligree pattern may be seen in other SCRTs
Diffuse pattern	ES, NHL, RMS	Lobular pattern may be seen focally; in NHL the tumor cells are noncohesive
Calcification	NB	Calcification is seen in germ cell tumors but rarely in others

Abbreviations: SRCT—small round cell tumors; NB—neuroblastoma; ES—Ewing's sarcoma; PNET—peripheral primitive neuroectodermal tumor; NHL—non-Hodgkin's lymphoma; RMS—rhabdomyosarcoma.

TABLE 12-5 Cytologic Features of Common Types of Non-Hodgkin's Lymphomas in Children

		Nucleus					
Type	Cell size	Shape	Nucleolus	Chromatin	Amount	Staining	Remarks
Lymphoblastic	Medium (12–14 μm)	Convoluted or round	Rare, inconspicuous	Delicate, stippled in convoluted; dust-like in nonconvoluted	Scanty ill-defined cell borders	Basophilic	Mitosis +, starry sky pattern may be seen (tumor cell nuclei < macrophage nuclei), variable pyroninophilia, admixture of prolymphocytes (coarse chromatin)
Small cell, noncleaved (Burkitt's subtype)	Uniform (10–25 μm)	Round	2–5 prominent basophilic	Coarse	Scanty to moderate	Amphophilic	Monotonous pattern, cytoplasmic fat vacuoles, pyroninophilia, starry sky pattern frequent (tumor cell nuclei = macrophage nuclei), mitoses +
Small cell, noncleaved (non-Burkitt's subtype)	Variable (>lymphocyte, <histiocytic)	Variable (but noncleaved)	Single prominent eosinophilic	Coarse	Scanty	Pale to amphophilic	Pleomorphism + mitosis + starry sky pattern may be seen (tumor cell nuclei = macrophage nuclei)

TABLE 12-5 Continued

Type	Cell size	Nucleus			Amount	Staining	Remarks
		Shape	Nucleolus	Chromatin			
Large cell	Large	Round or indented (cleaved or noncleaved)	Prominent (central in large cell cleaved or noncleaved subtype and peripheral in immunoblastic subtype)	Vesicular	Moderate	Pale eosinophilic to basophilic	Heterogenous groups, starry sky pattern may be seen (tumor cell nuclei >macrophage nuclei), aggressive behavior

TABLE 12-6 Immunohistological Features of SRCTs

Tumor type	Immunohistologic marker[a] NSE	LCA	MSA	VIM
Neuroblastoma	+	−	−	−
PNET	+	−	−	+
Ewing's sarcoma	±	−	−	+
Rhabdomyoma	−	+	−	±
Non-Hodgkin's lymphoma	±	−	+	+

[a]Abbreviations: NSE—neuron-specific enolase; LCA—leukocyte common antigen; MSA—muscle-specific antigen; VIM—vimentin.

can be present in all SRCTs and may be misinterpreted as neurosecretory granules. Thus the granules are identified as neurosecretory only when typical features and typical location are present. Undifferentiated NB may have LG and atypical or no neurosecretory granules.

Immunohistology

NBs are characteristically positive for neuron-specific enolase (NSE). NSE stains positively even when NBs lack specific neural features on light and electron microscopy.[2] However, NSE can be focally positive in nonneural tumors; e.g., weak NSE positivity may be observed in rhabdomyosarcoma.[18] NB is also positive for synaptophysin, although the reaction is variable in the poorly differentiated and undifferentiated NBs.[1] Immunoperoxidase stain using HSAN 1.2 monoclonal antibody recognizes neuroblastoma-associated antigen. This antibody is not available commercially. GD-2 and Leu-7 (a marker for natural-killer cells) are positive.[19] HLA is negative. Negative reaction is noted for vimentin and cytokeratin.[1] S-100 stain demonstrates Schwann cells along the fibrovascular septa in some cases of NB. Chromogranin and neurofilament triplet protein are variably positive.[1,22] Synaptophysin, chromogranin and NFP are not usually helpful in undifferentiated and poorly differentiated NB.

NSE is an isoenzyme of glycolytic enzyme enolase. This isoenzyme (gamma) is specific for neurons and neuroendocrine cells. Another isoenzyme (beta) is found in muscle. Nonneuronal (alpha) enolase (NNE) is found in many adult tissues, including muscle and liver. NSE obtained from commercial laboratories stains positively for almost all NB, but high concentrations of antiserum have to be used.[23] Cross reactivity with RMS was observed in rare instances by Tsokos et al[23] when commercial NSE antiserum was used. Of 20 RMS studied by Mierau et al,[18] 5 showed NSE positivity. (They had used NSE from a research laboratory.) Some degree of cross reactivity was observed by Tsokos et al[23] when B5-fixed NHLs were stained with NSE. Faint staining of tumor cells and stromal elements was observed in such instances.[23] Rare squamous and adenocarcinomas of lung and carcinoma of breast may be positive for NSE.[24] This staining pattern may be related to cross reactivity of NNE with NSE, nonspecific staining due to a high concentration of antiserum that may have to be used, and synthesis by tumor cells of enzymes that are not normally present in progenitor cell lines.[24] It is advisable to use monoclonal NSE antibody.

TABLE 12-7 Diagnostic Criteria for Small Round Cell Tumors of the Conventional Spectrum

Tumor type	Routine histology	Immunohistochemistry	Electron microscopy	Comment
Neuroblastoma	Small or large round cells, nesting pattern, fibrillar background with or without Homer Wright rosettes, cells intermediate between neuroblasts and ganglion cells, and/or typical or atypical ganglion cells may be present	Positive for neuron-specific enolase; other neural markers may also be present	Neuritic processes with neurotubules and neuroendocrine granules	Although NSE stain and electron microscopy are not essential for enrollment in the national cancer study protocols; for the diagnosis of undifferentiated neuroblastomas, and in cases with normal or unavailable catecholamine values, NSE stain and/or electron microscopy are essential
Ewing's sarcom (ES)	Primitive monomorphous tumor cells with delicate nuclear membrane, faintly stippled chromatin, inconspicuous nucleoli, clear scanty cytoplasm; diffuse pattern	One of the following neural markers may be positive: S-100, leu 7, NFP and NSE; MIC2 is positive in majority	Small round cells with relatively sparse organelles or intermediate filaments in the cytoplasm	Rosettes are absent in ES as currently defined by most investigators; demonstration of large amounts of glycogen by light and/or electron microscopy is helpful in the diagnosis; atypical ES with lobular pattern and large cell ES are also recognized

TABLE 12-7 Continued

Tumor type	Routine histology	Immunohistochemistry	Electron microscopy	Comment
Peripheral primitive neuroectodermal tumor (PNET)	Small round cells showing arrangement in rosettes, at least in a few foci	Two or more of the following neural markers (S-100, Leu 7, NFP, NSE)	Occasional cell processes with a few neuroendocrine granules	There is an overlap between ES and PNET; if a definitive diagnosis of one or the other entity cannot be made by using these criteria, the term "ES/PNET group tumor" or "ES group tumor" is used.
Rhabdomyosarcoma (RMS) embryonal, conventional variant	Fusiform or spindle-shaped cells admixed with round cells, myxoid stroma, variable number of rhabdomyoblasts (large round or strap-shaped cells with or without demonstrable cross striations on H&E or trichrome stain)	One or more of the following markers: desmin, myoglobin or muscle-specific actin are positive	Alternating thick and thin filaments *or* Z band material *or* Indian file arrangement of ribosomes along thick filaments	Rhabdomyoblastic nature of the neoplasm is ascertained by immunocytochemistry and/or electron microscopy
RMS, embryonal, spindle cell variant	Composed predominantly or almost exclusively of spindle-shaped cells; round rhabdo-myoblasts are rarely present; storiform pattern or leiomyosarcoma-like pattern is present	Same as above	Same as above	Occurs predominantly in paratesticular location; has better prognosis than conventional embryonal RMS

TABLE 12-7 Continued

Tumor type	Routine histology	Immunohistochemistry	Electron microscopy	Comment
RMS, botryoid	Same features as in conventional embryonal RMS; in addition, the variant has polypoid configuration with presence of subepithelial condensation of round and spindle-shaped tumor cells ("cambium" layer)	Same as conventional embryonal RMS	Same as conventional embryonal RMS. Prognosis is intermediate between embryonal RMS and alveolar RMS	Occurs predominantly in genitourinary tract and other subepithelial locations; has the best prognosis of the different variants of RMS; cambium layer is essential for diagnosis
RMS, alveolar, conventional variant	Round densely packed tumor cells showing alveolar pattern characterized by one or more peripheral layers of tumor cells closely applied to the fibrous trabeculae and central tumor cells showing detachment; "rare to occasional rhabdomyoblasts" present in the "alveoli"	Same as other variants of RMS	Same as other variants of RMS	Presence of rhabdomyoblasts must be confirmed by methods described above for embryonal RMS; alveolar pattern must be present in 50–70% of the tumor according to different investigators; alveolar pattern which may be present in the deeper portion of the tumor may be missed by a relatively superficial incisional or needle biopsy; this variant has the worst prognosis of all the different basic types of RMS

TABLE 12-7 Continued

Tumor type	Routine histology	Immunohistochemistry	Electron microscopy	Comment
RMS, alveolar, solid variant	Cytologically similar to the alveolar RMS, conventional variant; alveolar pattern is absent; dense collagenous bands without formation of alveolar pattern are present	Same as other variants or RMS	Same as other variants of RMS	There is no difference in the prognosis between solid and conventional variants of alveolar RMS; the diagnosis of solid variant is made by cytologic features different from those of embryonal or pleomorphic type of RMS
RMS, pleomorphic type	Cellular tumor composed of large elongated or strap-shaped cells; multinucleation and presence of moderate to abundant eosinophilic cytoplasm are frequently seen in the tumor cells	Same as other variants of RMS	Same as other variants of RMS	This is the rarest basic type of RMS. Most of the cases diagnosed as pleomorphic RMS in the past probably represent malignant fibrous histiocytoma of pleomorphic type; pleomorphic cells may also be found in other variants of RMS (see text for details)

TABLE 12-7 Continued

Tumor type	Routine histology	Immunohistochemistry	Electron microscopy	Comment
Non-Hodgkin's lymphoma (NHL)	Composed of round or variably shaped cells (depending upon the type of NHL) showing noncohesive diffuse pattern with effacement of lymph node architecture (follicular NHL are rare in children); effacement of lymph node architecture may be focal	Leukocyte common antigen demonstrated by immunohistochemistry or by flow cytometry distinguishes NHL from other SRCTs	Absence of cell junctions is a characteristic ultrastructural feature of NHL	Specific cell markers are described in the text; extranodal NHL are more common in children than in adults

TABLE 12-8 Approach to Diagnosis of SCRTs of a Biopsy or a Resected Specimen

Patterns of tumor cells. The following patterns are seen in various SRCTs: diffuse, lobular (nesting) with fibrovascular septa, filigree, pseudofiligree, cambium layer, myxoid pattern, rosettes (see Tables 12-4 and 12-7 for details).

Cellular features. The following features are seen in various SRCTs: monotonous round cells, convoluted nuclei, "large" cells, pleomorphism, prominent central or peripheral nucleoli, PAS-positive cytoplasm, pyroninophilic cytoplasm, lipid vacuoles in the cytoplasm (use imprints for details of cytologic features and also for special stains such as methyl green pyronin or stain for fat) (see Tables 12-4 and 12-5 for details)

Differentiating cells. Rhabdomyoblasts, cells intermediate between neuroblasts and ganglion cells, rare ganglion cells (see Table 12-7 for details)

Immunoperoxidase stains. A battery of stains may be needed (NSE, vimentin, LCA and muscle-specific antigen are the most important one) (see Table 12-6 and text for each SRCT for details)

Electron microscopy. If the diagnosis is not clear at this point, electron microscopy might be helpful (see text for details)

Other features. If the diagnosis is not clear at this point, cytogenetics and other biochemical and biologic features of the tumor may be helpful (see text for details)

Clinical features. Site of primary tumor or of metastasis and age might be supportive of one or more of the possible diagnoses

Other Features

Extracellular matrix proteins have been studied in NB cell lines.[25] Purely stromal proteins (fibronectin; collagen types I, II, and III) are not synthesized by NB. Only basal lamina associated proteins (laminin and collagen type IV) have

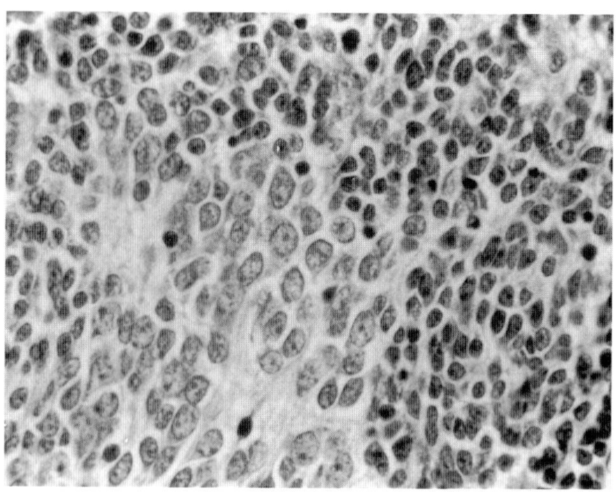

FIGURE 12-6. Neuroblastoma showing cells intermediate between neuroblasts and ganglion cells; note vesicular appearance of nuclei, presence of nucleoli, enlargement of size, and development of discernible cytoplasm in the intermediate cells (H&E, ×400).

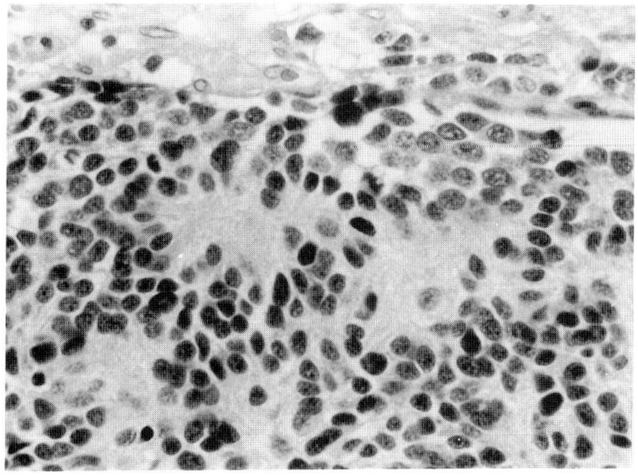

FIGURE 12-7. Neuroblastoma showing Homer Wright rosettes characterized by somewhat circular arrangement of tumor cells around a tangle of neuropil (H&E, ×400).

been identified.[19,25] Immunohistochemical stain is available to demonstrate type IV collagen.

Cells of NB contain one or multiple copies of N-myc gene. Multiple copies of N-myc gene are found in clinically aggressive NBs.[20,21] There is correlation between N-myc gene (DNA) amplification and expression of N-myc RNA.[19] Expression of c-myc is not found in NBs. Chromosomal abnormalities are detected in about 80% of NBs.[12,26] Deletions and translocations of the short arm of chromosome 1 with the most frequent breakpoint at 1p32 were found in 15 of

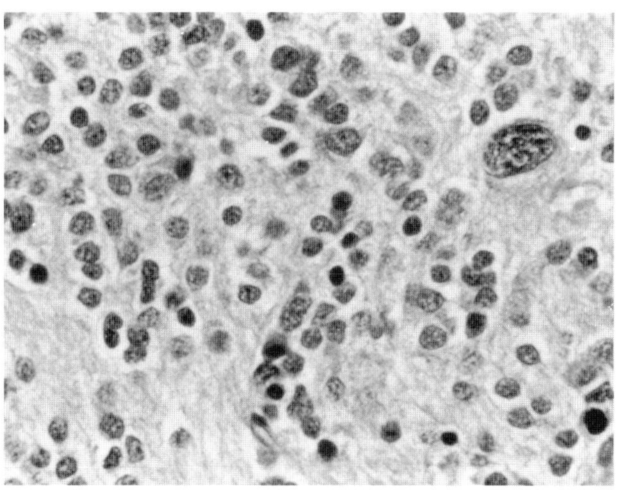

FIGURE 12-8. Neuroblastoma showing neuropil in the background. Note the uninucleated tumor giant cell. There is no rosette formation. (H&E, ×400.)

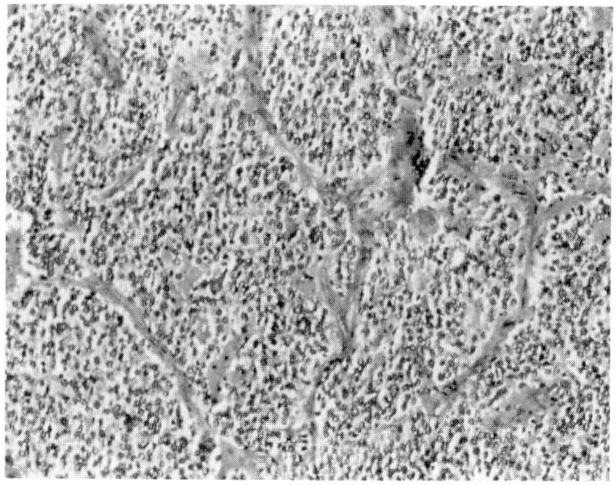

FIGURE 12-9. Undifferentiated neuroblastoma showing nesting pattern with fibrovascular septa (H&E, ×100).

18 patients with stage IV disease and 2 of 3 patients with stage III, but in none of 7 patients with stage I, II, or IV-S disease.[26] These 7 patients had hyperdiploid tumor karyotype (triploid range). Double minutes (DMs) and homogeneously staining regions (HMRs) were found in 12 of 21 stages III and IV patients. N-myc gene amplification (30 to 60 copies) was detected in 3 of 8 stages III and IV patients in whom the determination was made; these patients also showed DMs/HMRs.[26–28] There are high levels of N-myc protein in aggressive NBs.[29,30] N-myc gene is not specific for NB. One copy of the gene is present in other SRCTs (PNET, ES, RMS, and NHL). With the exception of rare cases of RMS,[31]

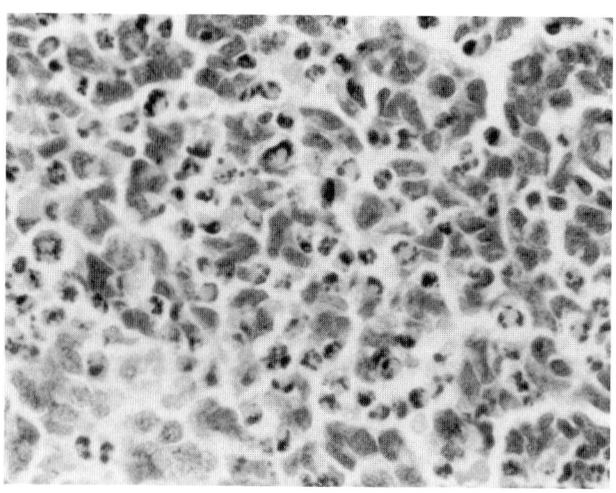

FIGURE 12-10. "Mitotic karyorrhectic" cells in neuroblastoma H&E, ×400).

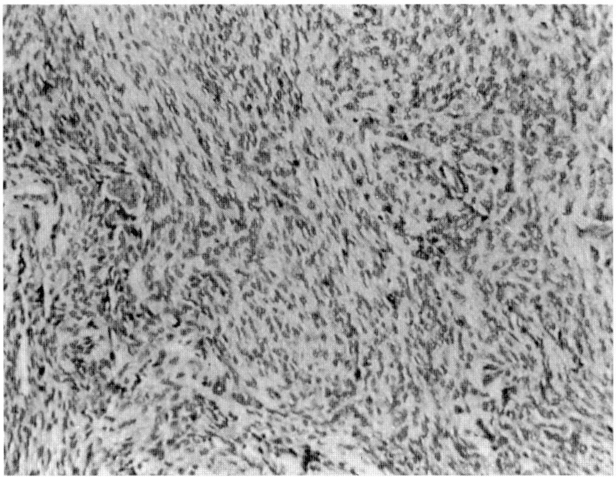

FIGURE 12-11. Neuroblastoma showing foci of spindle-shaped neuroblasts arranged in vague bundles (H&E, ×100).

retinoblastoma, astrocytoma and small cell carcinoma of lung,[32] N-myc gene amplification is not found in SRCT, other than NB. Thus N-myc gene amplification is highly characteristic of NB among the SRCTs under consideration in this discussion. NB associated N-myc gene is normally found in chromosome 2, but it appears to be translocated to the short arm of chromosome 1 and amplified in advanced neuroblastoma.[19] In NBs found on VMA mass screening abnormalities of chromosome 1, DMs or HMRs were not found.[28] Triploidy was noted in almost all the cases. All these patients were free of tumor at 4–32 months.

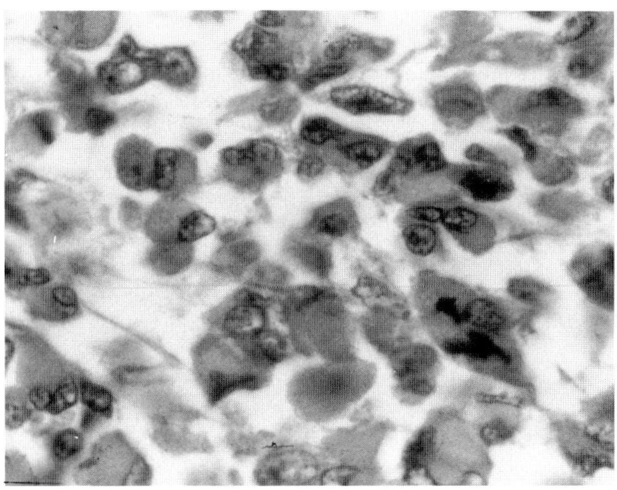

FIGURE 12-12. Neuroblastoma showing pseudorhabdoid change characterized by eccentric nucleus and abundant dense eosinophilic cytoplasm; the nuclei do not have prominent nucleoli (H&E, ×400).

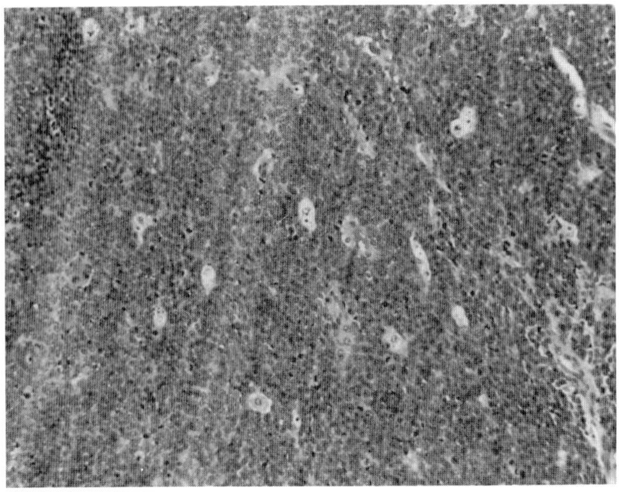

FIGURE 12-13. Undifferentiated neuroblastoma showing starry sky pattern (H&E, ×100).

The survival probabilities of patients with and without 1p abnormality were 10 and 90%, respectively. Thus chromosomal abnormality was related to prognosis.[26] Abnormality of chromosome 17 has also been described.[12] It may be pointed out that abnormalities of chromosome 1 (trisomy of 1q and breakpoints of 1p) have been detected in other pediatric tumors (Wilms' tumor, ES, PNET, RMS, and hepatoblastoma).[27]

Biochemical investigations have revealed mixed adrenergic and cholinergic enzyme profile consisting of dopamine beta hydroxylase and choline acetyl-

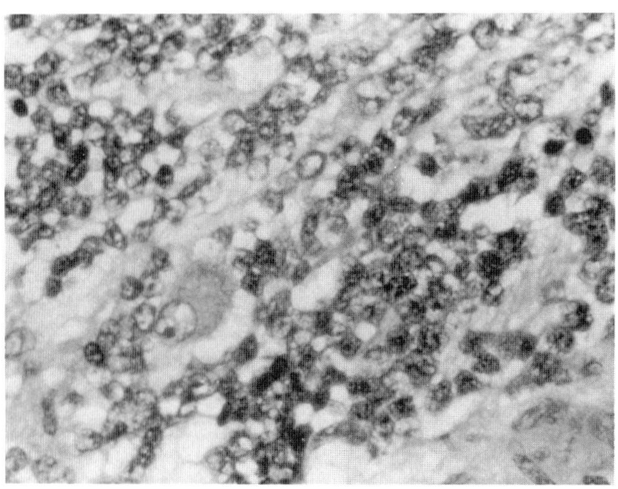

FIGURE 12-14. Poorly differentiated neuroblastoma showing a single isolated ganglion cell (H&E, ×400).

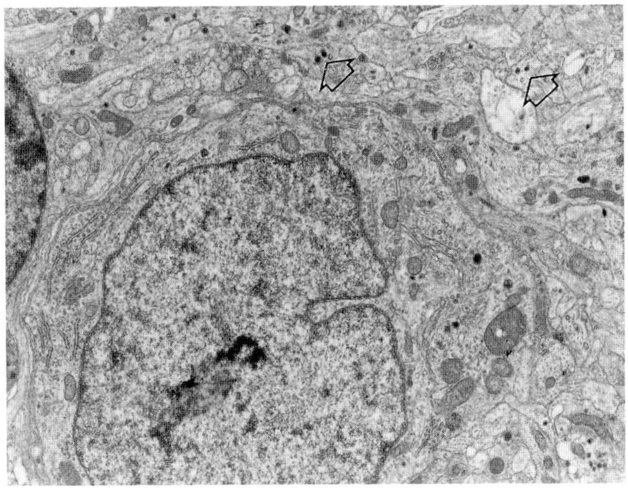

FIGURE 12-15. Electron micrograph of neuroblastoma cells showing neuritic processes containing neuroendocrine granules (arrows). Neurotubules (not well visualized at this magnification) were also present in these neuritic processes (×6100). (Courtesy of Dr. Gary Mierau.

transferase.[19,33] Catecholamine synthesis and secretion is a characteristic and diagnostic feature of NB. HVA (homovanillic acid) and VMA (vanillylmandelic acid) levels are elevated in serum and urine. The levels are generally determined in urine. In the more undifferentiated tumors, HVA levels are higher than VMA (HVA is a precursor of VMA). The vast majority of NBs secrete catecholamines; at least some of the tumors that were described as nonsecretors may in fact have been PNETs. Tissue culture of NB reveals characteristic neurite formation.

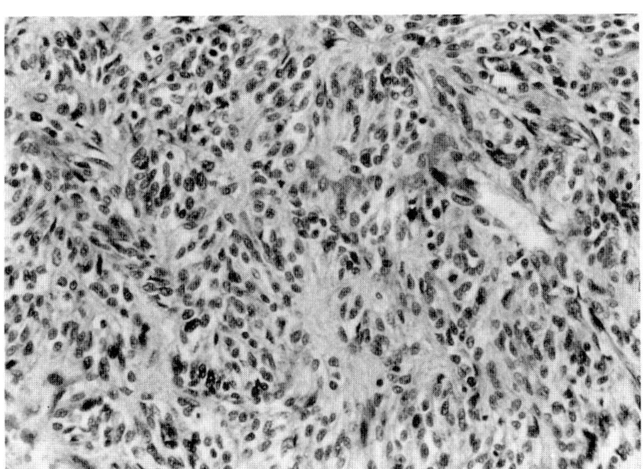

FIGURE 12-16. Peripheral primitive neuroectodermal tumor showing rosettes (H&E, ×400).

Peripheral Primitive Neuroectodermal Tumor (PNET)

The term "PNET" is used to include a variety of tumors: malignant small cell tumor of thoracopulmonary region (Askin tumor), extraskeletal Ewing's sarcoma (ES), peripheral neuroepithelioma, and peripheral neuroblastoma. Neural differentiation has been described in ES.[34] Many cases of skeletal ES probably belong in the spectrum of PNET. However, conventionally only extraosseous Ewing's sarcoma is included in PNETs. The term "neuroepithelium" indicates cells of the neuroectoderm. The term "neuroepithelioma" was first used by Stout.[35] Most authors prefer the term "PNET" and reserve the term "neuroepithelioma" for tumors showing glandular features. Central PNETs are seen in the brain.

Clinical Features

The median age in the series of Marina et al[6] was 14 years (range 2–19 years). Most of the patients had stage III or IV disease at presentation. PNET can also occur in adolescents and adults. PNET is extremely rare in black children.[36]

Primary Sites

Chest wall, trunk, retroperitoneum, pelvis, and extremities are the primary sites.[6,36] In some instances, the peripheral nerves in the extremities can be the primary site.[9] Adrenal was considered as the primary site in a few cases reported by Marina et al.[6]

Sites of Metastasis

PNETs are more aggressive locally (50% of the cases) and also have metastatic potential. In the series of 26 cases from St. Jude Children's Research Hospital,[6] 31% metastasized to the lungs, 12% to bone, 12% to bone marrow, and 31% to lymph nodes. In contrast NB in a series of 406 cases from the same institution showed the following metastatic pattern: 54% to bone marrow, 48% to bone, 61% to lymph nodes, and only 5% to the lungs. ES of bone (169 cases) metastasized to lungs (43%), bone (37%), bone marrow (10%), and lymph nodes (16%). Local extension was seen in 16% of NB, 18% of ES, and 50% of PNE.

Histologic Features[36,37]

In some cases of PNET, the histologic features are similar to those of ES,[9] in others the features are "neural." PNET is composed of small round cells arranged generally in a diffuse pattern. Nesting pattern with presence of fibrovascular septa may be present focally. The cells are monotonous primitive cells with scant cytoplasm. The nuclei have features similar to those of ES (oval uniform nuclei with inconspicuous nucleoli and indistinct cell borders). Homer Wright pseudorosettes with pale eosinophilic cores and less frequently, perivascular pseudorosettes or true Flexner-type rosettes with central lumen can be demonstrated in some cases. Careful search is required since these rosettes may be poorly defined and only focally present (Figure 12-16). Light and dark cells of the type seen in ES may be evident. Glycogen can be demonstrated by PAS stain with and without diastase in some of the tumors. Ganglion cells are rarely, if ever, found.[36] However, Marina et al[6] state that maturation of round tumor cells into ganglion cells was present in two cases and a ganglioneuroblastomatous focus with neurofibrillary stroma was seen in one case. In the majority of cases the aforementioned features of neural differentiation are inconspicuous and a definitive diagnosis of PNET is often not possible on the basis of routine histologic features (see discussion of relationship between PNET and ES below).

Occasional nests of epithelial-like cells, numerous mitoses, foci of necrosis with calcification, and cartilaginous and osseous metaplasia have been described in some cases by Hashimoto et al.[38] Resemblance of many cases to ES has been described by Marina et al[6] and Schmidt et al.[37] Myoid and melanocytic cells are identifiable in a minority of PNET.[39] Binucleate cells were present in some cases described by Llombart-Bosch et al,[40] but they did not find ganglion cells or multinucleated giant cells in any of the cases. Fibrillar background was noted by these authors.[40] Tubular structures were noted in one case by Schmidt et al.[37]

Ultrastructural Features

Dense core granules (120–150 n*M*) were noted in 11 of 14 cases in which specimens were processed in the series reported by Marina et al.[6] Intertwining cell processes are seen in most of the tumors. Microtubules may be present. Cytoplasmic glycogen can be demonstrated in a few cases.[37] Small desmosome-like junctions may be present.[37] In one of the cases studied by Marina et al[6] in which NSE stain was negative and there was no glycogen or rosette formation, short cytoplasmic processes without dense core granules were noted. Some of the ultrastructural features are illustrated in Figure 12-17.

Immunohistochemical Features

Most of PNETs are positive for NSE.[6] Positive staining for Leu-7 is also seen in some cases.[9] All of the 19 cases in the series reported by Marina et al[6] in which immunohistochemical staining was done were negative for desmin and muscle-specific actin except for two cases in which focal positivity was seen. Vimentin, NFP, and GFAP are other markers present in some of the cases of PNET.[4] HLA is positive in PNET, while HSAN 1.2, GD_2, and Leu-7 are weak to negative or variably positive.[19] Cytokeratin is positive in many cases.[39] In the cases studied by Llombart-Bosch et al,[40] NSE, chromogranin, Leu-7, and β_{2-} microglobulin were positive, whereas synaptophysin, GFAP, NFP, and S-100 were negative. However, Schmidt, et al[37] found positive staining for S-100, NFP, and GFAP in occasional cases in their series of 17 cases. In a study of 40 cases of PNET the following immunohistological staining pattern was noted: NSE (40/40), vimentin (31/33), β_2 microglobulin (33/36), synaptophysin (16/20), S-100 protein (27/40), NFP (12/20), keratin (4/18), chromogranin (0/30), desmin (0/40), and amylase sensitive PAS positivity (17/40).[41] They suggested that a diagnosis of PNET may be made when NSE and β_2 microglobulin are positive preferably with positive synaptophysin and supportive EM. In a recent article Parham et al have described two cases of PNET that were positive for desmin by immunohistology and Western blot.[42] A cell surface glycoprotein designated as HBA71 or p30/ 32^{MIC2} (abbreviated as MIC2) has been identified in PNET and ES (see section on ES below).

Other Features

PNETs do not secrete catecholamines, although exceptions may occur.[36] The enzyme profile consists of choline acetyltransferase. Cytogenetic studies

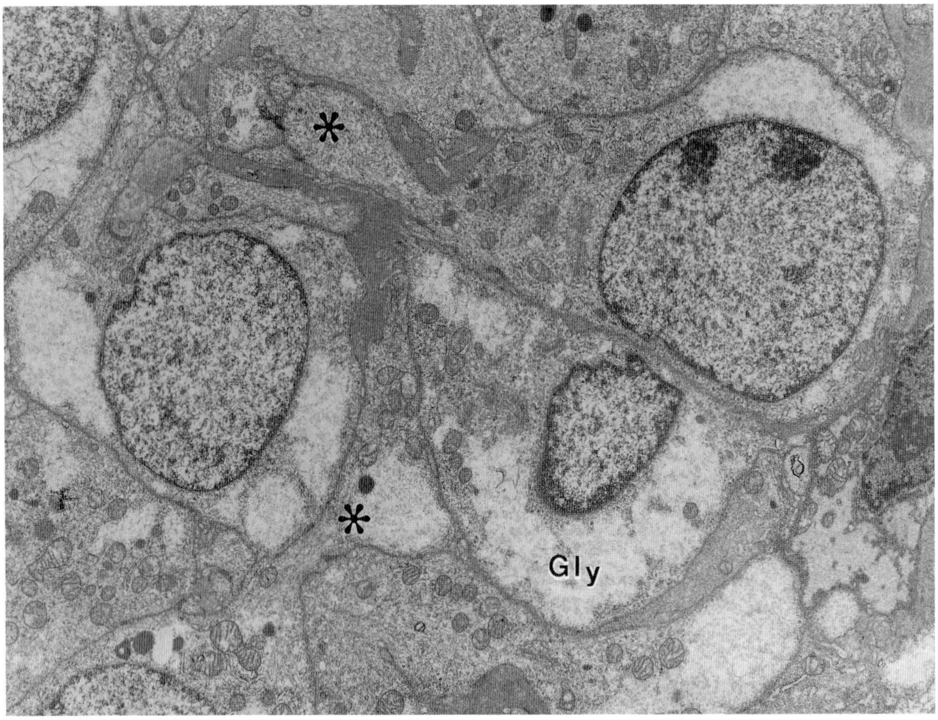

FIGURE 12-17. Electron micrograph of peripheral primitive neuroectodermal tumor cells. The cells share features of classical Ewing's sarcoma cells, including large glycogen deposits (Gly), but additionally display cytoplasmic processes (×3600). (Courtesy of Dr. Gary Mierau.)

have shown reciprocal translocation (11;22) (q24;q12). In some cases, supernumerary chromosome 8 has been demonstrated.[36] (Both these cytogenetic abnormalities are also present in ES.) There is overexpression of c-myc gene with high levels of c-myc protein.[36] (The c-myc gene is on chromosome 8.) A single copy of N-myc gene is present in PNET, but there is no gene expression.[19]

Ewing's Sarcoma

Ewing's sarcoma (ES) was originally described as a primary tumor of bone by Ewing in 1921.[43] ES of bone not infrequently extends into the soft tissues; but ES also occurs as a primary neoplasm of soft tissue.[44] It is referred to as "ES of soft tissues" or "extraosseous Ewing's sarcoma" (EOE). Both osseous Ewing's sarcoma (OE) and EOE have similar histologic features. These tumors were considered as primitive tumors of mesenchymal origin because of complete lack of specific features (except for presence of glycogen in 75–80% of cases) and absence of any specific markers such as NSE, desmin, cytokeratin, or factor VIII.[44] However, in recent years, some investigators have favored a neuroectodermal origin on the basis of certain histologic features (rosettes), immunohistochemical staining, ultrastructural features, and tissue culture.[34,35] There may thus be two subtypes of ES, the classical subtype and the neural subtype (see below). The latter is included under the broad category of PNET. In this regard, it is of interest to note that Willis considered ES as examples of metastatic NB in most cases.[46] In this discussion, ES will be considered as one entity, and the various neural features seen in some of the cases will be described. The term ES will be used to designate both OE and EOE.

Clinical Features

In the series of EOE reported by Angerwall and Enzinger[47] the median age was 20 years (range 20 months to 63 years with 70% of patients between 10 and 20 years of age and slight male predominance). This age distribution corresponds to that for OE.[48] However, it should be noted that OE can occur in children <3 years of age. Maygarden et al recently reviewed 19 cases of OE seen in this age group representing 2.6% of all patients registered with the Intergroup Ewing's Sarcoma Study.[49] There was predominance of girls in this age group (15 girls vs. 4 boys), and the survival rate of 56% for this age group was comparable to that in older children. The authors emphasized that OE needs to be considered the differential diagnosis of SRCTs even in infants and young children. For unknown reasons, both OE and EOE are rare in black children.[50] Catecholamine determinations are normal.[51] OE has been observed to occur in siblings and in association with multiple congenital anomalies, particularly of urogenital tract.[51] Recently ES of left fibula has been reported in 6.1-year-old boy with vertically transmitted HIV infection.[53]

Primary Sites

Principal sites of involvement of EOE are paravertebral and intercostal regions and lower extremities. Uncommon sites include soft tissues of pelvic and hip regions, retroperitoneum, and upper extremities. The tumor presents as a rapidly growing deeply located mass 5–10 cm in longest dimension.[44] In the intergroup ES study, the principal sites of OE were femur, fibula and tibia (41%), humerus (11%), and ilium (12.5%); axial skeleton, ribs, hands, feet, tail, and calvarium were less frequent sites.[54]

Metastatic Sites

Principal sites of metastasis in 169 cases of OE from St. Jude were lung (43%), bone (37%), bone marrow (10%), and lymph nodes (16%); local extension occurred in about 18% of cases.[6] In different series, about 14–50% patients have evidence of metastasis at the time of diagnosis.[51]

Histologic Features

Histologic features of OE and EOE are similar.[44,51,54,55] The statement that ES essentially consists of structureless array of small hyperchromatic blue cells represents an oversimplification.[54] The cells of ES are as large as histiocytes (which are not ordinarily regarded as small cells). The cells have round nuclei with delicate nuclear membrane, faintly stippled chromatin, inconspicuous nucleoli, clear scanty cytoplasm, and indistinct cell outline (Figure 12-18). A large cell variant of both OE and EOE has been described. In this variant the cells are larger than the conventional type of ES and show more variation in sizes and shapes, and the nuclei often have conspicuous nucleoli.[55,56] There are no differences in the clinical behavior of the conventional and large cell ES. The

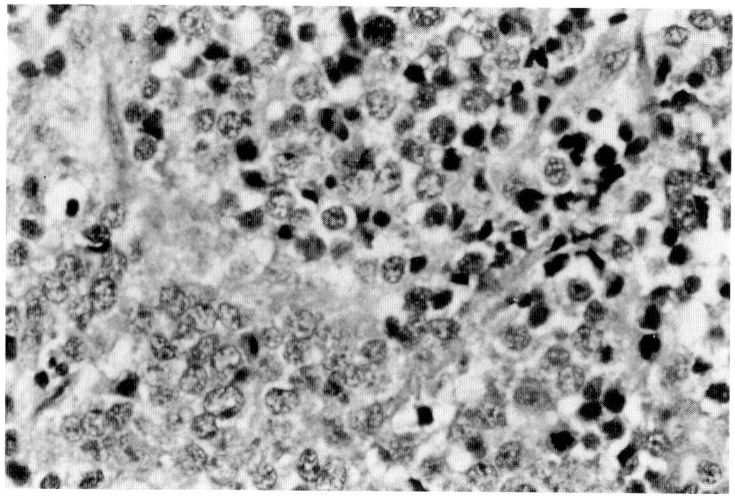

FIGURE 12-18. Soft tissue Ewing's sarcoma composed of cells with round nuclei, delicate nuclear membrane, stippled chromatin, inconspicuous nucleoli, scant clear cytoplasm, and indistinct outline. Note absence of rosettes and a few darkly staining degenerating tumor cells. (H&E, ×400.)

most common pattern noted is a diffuse pattern; however, a lobular (nesting) pattern may also be seen with presence of fibrovascular septa. The tumor is richly vascular. A filigree pattern (also referred to as "biphasic pattern of light and dark cells") results from foci of dark-staining degenerating tumor cells (Figure 12-18).[44] A similar pattern also results from alternating arrangement of tumor cells with lighter-staining fibrovascular septa (Figure 12-19).[54] A pseudofiligree pattern may be seen in the compressed peripheral portion of the tumor due to presence of darkly staining tumor cells infiltrating the pale-staining collagenous fibrous tissue of the surrounding area. Similar pseudofiligree pattern may be seen in peripheral portions of other SRCTs (Figure 12-20).

The cytoplasm of the cells is clear and contains glycogen. The amount of glycogen varies from tumor to tumor and in different portions of the same tumor.[44] The peripheral portions of tumor tend to contain more glycogen. Complete absence of glycogen is rare in EOE, according to Enzinger and Weiss.[44] However, Kissane et al[54] found absence of glycogen in 23% of 268 cases of OE. (Glycogen was 1 to 2 + in 39% and 3 to 4 + in 26% of their cases of EOE.) Glycogen is demonstrated by PAS stain with and without diastase. None of the authors comment about improvement in the demonstration of glycogen in ES by alcohol fixation. The mere presence of glycogen on light or electron microscopy is not a reliable feature for diagnosis of ES. As a general rule, a very large amount of glycogen supports a diagnosis of ES, but such a large amount of glycogen (i.e. 4+) is seen in only about 12% of cases.[54] Variable amounts of cytoplasmic glycogen are present in all SRCTs, including NBs and NHLs.[2] About 50% NB seen at NCI by Triche et al[2] showed readily demonstrable glycogen. Mierau et al[18] found glycogen in 10% of cases of lymphomas in children. Ganglion cell

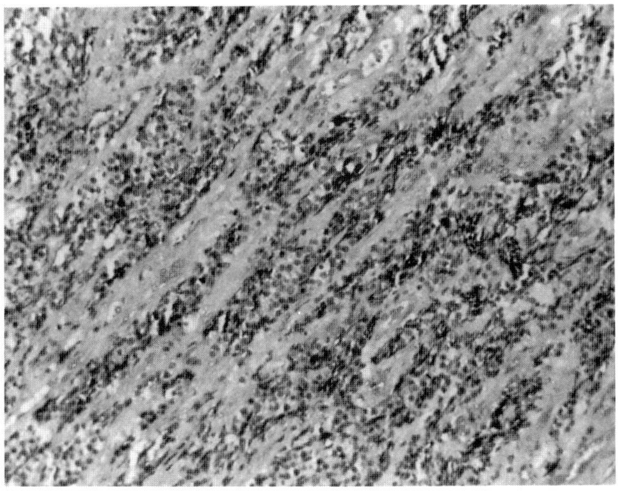

FIGURE 12-19. Light and dark pattern in Ewing's sarcoma due to darker staining tumor cells alternating with light staining fibrovascular septa (H&E, ×250).

differentiation is not seen in the neural types of ES. However, Jaffe et al[34] noted the tendency of a few cells at the periphery of the lobules of tumor cells toward ganglion cell differentiation as evidenced by routine morphologic features and NSE staining.

Shimada et al[45] studied 74 cases of EOE from the Intergroup Rhabdomyosarcoma Study (IRS). They found rosettes in 18 (24%) and 1 to 2+ glycogen in 36

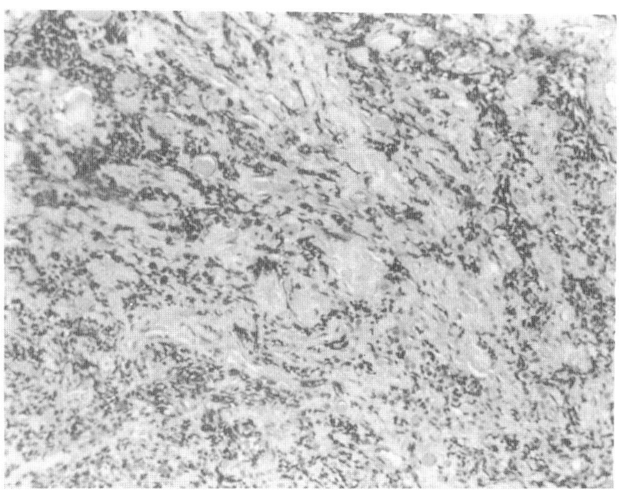

FIGURE 12-20. Pseudofiligree pattern in the peripheral infiltrative portion of a neuroblastoma; note the compressed darkly staining tumor cells and pale-staining collagenous fibrous tissue (H&E, ×100).

(48%) cases. Glycogen was considered as equivocal to absent in 13 (17%) cases. Jaffe et al[34] described four cases of small round cell tumors of bone occurring in children and having clinical and radiologic features of ES. They found poorly formed to well-defined focal rosettes and lobular (nesting) pattern in all of them. Glycogen was sparse in imprints and sections. Mitotic activity is variable. Coagulative necrosis is commonly noted, but these foci rarely show calcification unlike those in NB. These rosette containing ES-like tumors will be considered as PNET by the criteria recommended at present (see below, sections on relationship between PNET and ES and current criteria for their diagnosis).

Ultrastructural Features

The ultrastructural features of OE and EOE are similar.[44] Although the cells of ES do not have specific ultrastructural features, electron microscopy is usually helpful in the diagnosis.[18] Large amounts of glycogen with focal cytoplasmic distribution are demonstrable in most examples even in cases with negative PAS stain (Figure 12-21). Cell junctions are a second helpful feature when present (60–70% of cases). The cell junctions may take various forms (tight junctions to desmosomes). The cytoplasm contains few organelles (a few mitochondria, poorly developed Golgi, inconspicuous RER). Few ribosomes are seen. Occasionally cytoplasmic filaments may be present.[57] External lamina and Weibel Palade bodies are absent. Neural features have been recently described in electron-microscopic studies of some cases of both OE and EOE.[34,45,58] These consist of processes containing microtubles. Rare to few neurosecretory granules (150–200 nM), sometimes with atypical features were seen in the cytoplasm and/or cytoplasmic processes[34,45] (see the section on relationship between PNET and ES below).

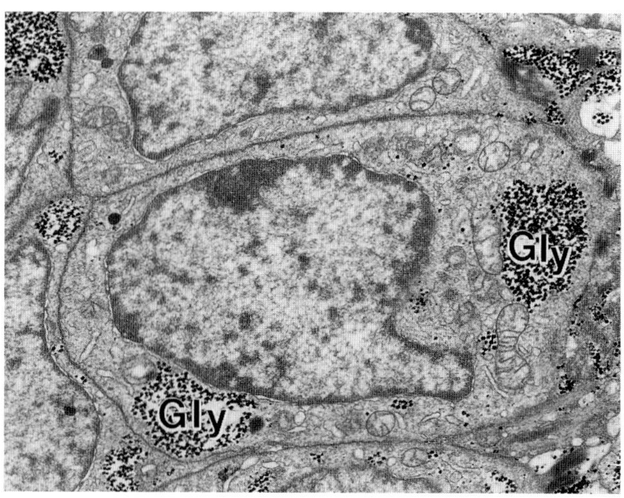

FIGURE 12-21. Electron micrograph of Ewing's sarcoma cells, which characteristically display large focally distributed accumulations of multiparticulate glycogen (Gly) and poorly developed cell junctions (×8200). (Courtesy of Dr. Gary Mierau.)

Immunohistochemical Features

According to the experience of most authors,[44,59,60] both OE and EOE stain positively for vimentin and negatively for S-100 protein, neurofilaments, GFAP, desmin, myoglobin, factor VIII, *Ulex europaeus* I lectin, and cytokeratin. However, recent reports indicate presence in some cases of OE and EOE of neural markers such as NSE and S-100.[34,45] The NSE-positive cells (cytoplasmic positivity only) were found in groups, whereas the S-100-positive cells (both nuclear and cytoplasmic positivity) were scattered.[45] Moll et al[61] have demonstrated variable positivity with simple epithelium cytokeratin by immunofluorescence technique in both OE and EOE.

A cell surface glycoprotein HBA71 antigen or p30/32^{MIC2} has been identified in ES and PNET by using immunoperoxidase method on frozen and paraffin sections.[62,63] Fellinger et al found MIC2 positivity in 41 of 43 ES.[62] Of these, 21 were positive for NSE and 20 for vimentin. Fellinger et al in another study have reported positive HBA71 staining in 9 of 11 PNET.[63] NB, melanoma, small cell osteosarcoma, esthesioneuroblastoma, malignant ectomesenchymoma, desmoplastic SRCT, and medulloblastoma were negative for MIC2. This appears to be a unique antigen for ES and PNET. However, it should be noted that stain for MIC2 antigen may be focally positive in a few cases of RMS and large cell NHL and strongly positive in some cases of lymphoblastic NHL.[64] Another marker that has been investigated in ES/PNET and other SRCTs is the neural cell adhesion molecule (NCAM), which is a surface antigen contributing to cell adhesion and pattern formation during development of chicken neurons.[65] ES/PNET was surprisingly NCAM negative, whereas NB was positive. It may be noted that NHL is NCAM-negative while embryonal RMS is positive.[65]

Other Features

ES cell lines have been studied for synthesis of matrix proteins.[25] ES synthesized both stromal (fibronectin, collagen types I and III) and pericellular proteins (laminin and type IV collagen). This is consistent with the presumed pleuripotential stem cell origin of ES. The matrix protein synthesis of neural type ES has not been studied. Cytogenetic studies on ES have shown most commonly reciprocal translocation between chromosomes 11 and 22 [t(11;22)(q23;q11)].[66] Other chromosomal abnormalities included trisomy of 1q and deletion of 3p and 6q. The authors did not specify whether the cases were OE or EOE (however these were most likely OE). It is of interest to note that t(11;22) has also been noted in PNET. Tissue culture of OE and ES has been studied by Jaffe et al[34] and Triche et al.[2] Jaffe et al[34] found short branching processes in long-term cultures. Electron microscopy of these processes showed filaments and microtubules. ES appeared "fibroblastic" in the tissue cultures studies done by Triche et al.[2]

Relationship between PNET and ES

There are similarities in the clinical, histologic, immunohistological, ultrastructural, and cytogenetic characteristics of PNET and ES. Therefore it has been suggested that PNET and ES may be histogenetically related[67] and may constitute a spectrum in which typical undifferentiated ES lies at one end and PNET with clear evidence of neural differentiation at the other.[68] The histogenesis of

PNET and ES is not known. Cells of neural crest, primordial germ cells and uncommitted mesenchymal cells have been implicated as the cells of origin.[67] Fellinger et al[63] searched for HBA71-positive cells in normal fetal tissues without any success. On the basis of histologic features such as rosettes, immunohistologic neural markers, such as NSE, and NFP, ultrastructural evidence of neural differentiation and neural-type differentiation in tissue culture neural crest origin is favored by many investigators.

Criteria for Diagnosis of PNET and ES

Because of the overlap in the pathologic (and other) features of PNET and ES, it has proved to be difficult to develop diagnostic pathologic criteria for each type of tumor. Marina et al[6] have suggested that at least two and preferably three of the following criteria should be present for diagnosis of PNET: (1) rosettes (Homer Wright or Flexner type), (2) origin in peripheral nerve, (3) positive staining with NSE or Leu-7, (4) neural differentiation by EM (granules and microtubules), (5) t(11;22)(q24;q12), (6) detectable protooncogene expression (N-myc, c-myc, c-ets-1), and (7) activity of neurotransmitter biosynthetic enzymes (tyrosine hydroxylase, dopamine-β hydroxylase, and choline esterase). It appears to us that two criteria are not sufficient since many cases of NB will satisfy criteria 1, 3, 4, 6, and 7. The criteria regarding neurotransmitter enzymes (i.e., both adrenergic and cholinergic enzymes being present) and the expression of N-myc are at variance with the features of PNET given by Triche.[19] Cavazzana et al[41] suggested that the diagnosis of PNET is warranted when the tumor consists of primitive round cell tumor showing lobular pattern, rosettes, NSE, and β_2 microglobulin positivity and ultrastructural features of primitive neuritic extensions and dense-core granules in the cellular processes or cytoplasm. β_2 microglobulin is usually intensely positive in PNET. It is only focally positive in ganglion cells of differentiating NB and stage IV-S NB.

Schmidt, et al[69] used the following criteria for PNET and ES in the past: (1) *PNET*—at least one positive immunohistologic neural marker (NSE, S-100, Leu-7, GFAP, NFP) and/or presence of rosettes in an otherwise primitive SRCT; and (2) *ES*—lack of neural differentiation and of reticulin fibers between tumor cells and presence of PAS-positive granules (of glycogen) in an undifferentiated SRCT. They revised these criteria as follow: (1) *PNET*—presence of rosettes and/or expression of at least two neural markers (NSE, S-100, NFP, Leu-7, GFAP); and (2) *ES*—absence of rosettes and expression of no or only one neural marker in a tumor consisting of primitive monomorphic cells. Most investigators currently use these revised criteria recommended by Schmidt et al.[69] In addition, ultrastructure features of neural differentiation are also accepted for the diagnosis of PNET. Hijazi et al[70] have given the following criteria:

1. PNET
   a. True rosettes by light microscopy (LM) or
   b. Two or more of neural markers (NSE, S-100, Leu 7, NFP) by immunohistology (IMH), or
   c. Dense-core granules in the cell process by electron microscopy (EM)
2. ES:
   a. Primitive monomorphic tumor cells by LM and

b. Absence of neural markers by IMH and
c. Small cells lacking a fair number of organelles by EM.

These authors also recognize an atypical variant of ES by the following criteria: (1) lobular architecture and/or cellular pleomorphism, prominent nucleoli, more than 2 mitoses/10 hpf, absence of true rosettes by LM, (2) one neural marker by IMH, (3) moderate number of cell organelles, and cell processes lacking dense-core granules by EM.

The need for distinction between PNET and ES is stressed because of the worse prognosis in PNET as compared with that in ES.[9,69,71] However, large prospective multicenter studies of possible prognostic differences between PNET and ES have not yet been done. In a preliminary report, Hjazi et al[70] found no differences in survival in patients with ES (8 cases) and PNET (26 cases) after using the same therapeutic protocol for patients with both types of tumor. Despite the attempts to define the criteria for PNET and ES, it is not possible to make a specific diagnosis in some cases because of either insufficient material, insufficient morphologic studies, or marked overlap of pathologic features. In such cases, the designation ES group tumor or Ewing's sarcoma/PNET group tumor has been used. The importance of making an attempt to distinguish between ES and PNET lies in the different chemotherapy protocols used currently for these tumors (Table 12-9) and possible differences in prognosis.

Rhabdomyosarcoma

Rhabdomyosarcoma (RMS) is the most common soft tissue malignancy in patients under 21 years of age, accounting for 50% of cases.[72] The term RMS is used to describe a tumor that shows at least some evidence of differentiation toward striated muscle. A diagnosis of RMS is rendered conventionally by demonstration of light-microscopic evidence of differentiation on H&E and special stains. Rhabdomyoblast is a large round or oval cell with abundant eosinophilic cytoplasm containing fibrillar material concentrically arranged around the nucleus. These cells rarely show cross striations in the fibrillar material. The other cell type is a fusiform, spindle-shaped, tadpole- or racquet-shaped cell. These cells have eosinophilic cytoplasm containing fibrillar material with cross striations. The cross striations are often better marked in a trichrome or PTAH stain.[44] In current practice of surgical pathology, the evidence for such differentiation is sought by electron microscopy and/or

TABLE 12-9 Chemotherapeutic Drugs Used in the Treatment of SRCTs

Tumor	Drugs
Neuroblastoma	Cisplatin (C), VP-16, cytoxan (CX), adriamycin (A)
Primitive neuroectodermal tumor	Vincristine (V), actinomycin (AC), ifosfamide (I), VP-16, CX, platinum
Ewing's sarcoma	V, AC, I, VP-16, CX
Rhabdomyosarcoma	V, dactinomycin, CX, VP-16, C
Non-Hodgkin's lymphoma	CX, A, V, prednisone, methotrexate

immunohistochemistry for a definitive diagnosis of RMS. Various antibodies against muscle proteins such as desmin, muscle-specific actin, and myoglobin are used for immunoperoxidase stains.

The criteria for diagnosis of RMS used by Intergroup Rhabdomyosarcoma Study (IRS) include demonstration of rhabdomyoblastic differentiation by routine histologic methods. The minimum histologic criteria for rhabdomyoblastic differentiation is presence of large round cells with bright eosinophilic cytoplasm and eccentric nucleus. Cross striations may or may not be present. (By definition fibrillar material with cross striations in the cytoplasm should be present but in practice cross striations are difficult to demonstrate). The histologic classification of RMS used by IRS in the United States[73] and International (European) Society of Pediatric Oncology (ISPO)[74] is based on the one suggested by Horn and Enterline in 1958.[75] Recently Toskos et al of the National Cancer Institute (NCI) group have described a new classification based on WHO classification of RMS to prognosis.[72] This classification is referred to as NCI classification.

IRS Classification[73]

Embryonal RMS

These tumors are composed mainly of fusiform to spindle-shaped cells, with admixture of a few round cells, and myxoid stroma (Figure 12-2). Scattered pleomorphic cells or clusters of pleomorphic cells may be seen in some cases[76] (see section on pleomorphic RMS below). Collagen bands separating groups of tumor cells may be present. There is little collagen between tumor cells. Variable numbers of "rhabdomyoblasts" (large round eosinophilic and broad strap shaped cells with or without demonstrable cross striation) are seen (Figures 12-22, 12-23). Cross striations could be demonstrated in only 24 of 65 or 37% of cases of embryonal RMS in the series reported by Bale et al.[77] Depending on the absence or presence of cells with identifiable skeletal muscle features (large eosinophilic round or strap-shaped cells), Bale et al[76] divide embryonal RMS into undifferentiated, poorly differentiated, and differentiated subtypes. In my opinion, such a subclassification of embryonal RMS is confusing and unacceptable since the minimum criterion for the diagnosis of RMS consists of presence of "rhabdomyoblasts." Some of the "undifferentiated" embryonal RMS may represent SRCT other than RMS.

Recently a spindle cell variant of embryonal RMS has been described by the investigators of IRS and German-Italian cooperative soft tissue sarcoma study.[78,79] The conventional embryonal RMS is composed mainly of spindle, tadpole or strap-shaped cells with an admixture of a few round cells (Figures 12-2, 12-22). The variant described by Cavazzana et al[78] and Leuschner et al[79] is composed predominantly of medium-sized spindle-shaped cells (Figure 12-3). Round "rhabdomyoblasts" or giant cells are rarely present. The diagnosis of RMS was established in these cases by immunohistology for muscle-specific actin (MSA), desmin, and/or myoglobin. Electron microscopy done in a small proportion of their cases showed ultrastructural features diagnostic of RMS (see below). Two patterns are recognized in this variant: (1) storiform pattern with tumor cells arranged in whorls and separated from each other by abundant collagen (these tumors are of relatively low cellularity) and (2) more elongated tumor cells

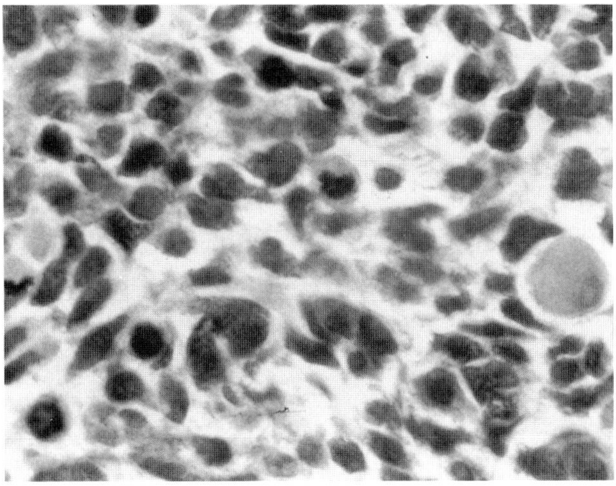

FIGURE 12-22. Embryonal rhabdomyosarcoma composed of fusiform cells and large round cells; note the rhabdomyoblast characterized by larger size, dense eosinophilic cytoplasm and a round faintly visible nucleus (H&E, ×400).

with eosinophilic cytoplasm, arranged in bundles with slight to moderate amount of collagen between tumor cells (these tumors resemble leiomyosarcoma). Paratesticular region is the predominant site of these tumors that have a significantly lower frequency of lymph node metastasis and better prognosis than conventional embryonal RMS occurring at this site (95.5% vs. 80% 5-year survival).[79] These tumors can also occur at other sites such as head and neck

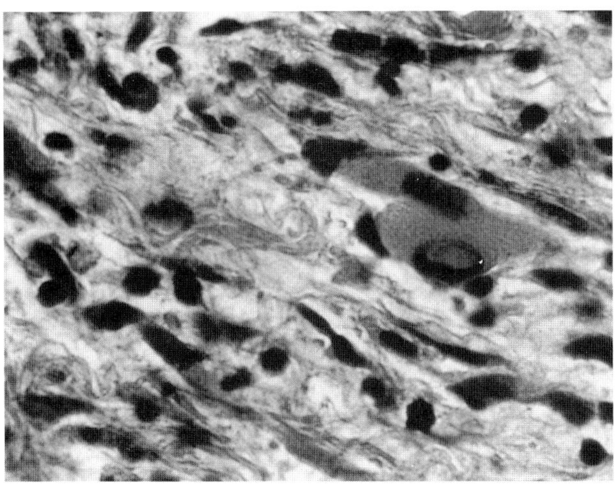

FIGURE 12-23. Embryonal rhabdomyosarcoma showing large elongated and strap-shaped rhabdomyoblasts with cross striations in the cytoplasm (H&E, ×400).

region, extremities, and orbit. It is not clear whether the tumors occurring at other sites are also associated with better prognosis.

Botryoid RMS

These are bulging submucosal polypoid tumors showing histologic features of embryonal type. In addition, there is a subepithelial "cambium" layer consisting of condensation of round or spindle shaped tumor cells (Figure 12-24). The cambium layer is an essential criterion for diagnosis.

Alveolar RMS

According to IRS I and II criteria, the tumor characteristically shows an alveolar pattern in at least 50% of the areas sampled for histology. Bale et al[77] require 70% or areas showing alveolar pattern. IRS-III is evaluating the prognostic significance of any evidence of alveolar pattern or even of cytology associated with alveolar pattern. The alveolar pattern may be present only in the deeper portion of the tumor. In such cases alveolar pattern is not evident if only a small superficial biopsy of the tumor is available (Figure 12-25). The tumor cells that are round (not spindle-shaped) are usually densely packed. Myxoid stroma is not seen. The alveoli are separated by connective tissue trabeculae of varying vascularity and delicacy (Figure 12-26). One or more layers of the cells are usually closely applied to the trabeculae, but in the central portion there are variable number of detached cells (Figure 12-27). Multinucleated giant cells and rhabdomyoblasts are present within the "alveoli." Pleomorphic tumor cells may be seen in rare cases.[76] Investigators from National Cancer Institute describe a solid variant of alveolar RMS in which there is no alveolar pattern but the cytologic features are those of alveolar RMS[72] (see below). (This variant of alveolar RMS will have to be considered in the differential diagnosis of SRCTs.

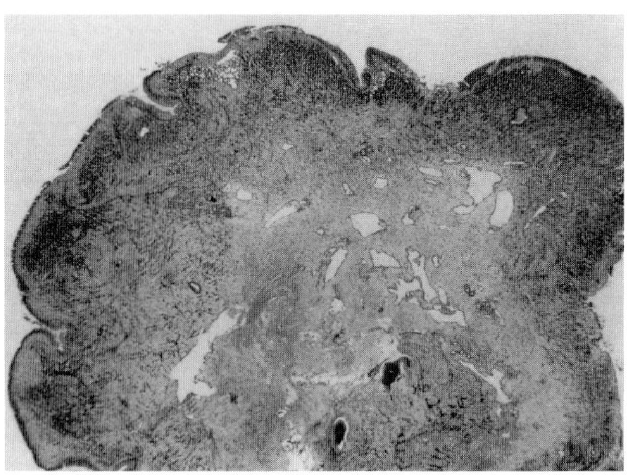

FIGURE 12-24. Sarcoma botryoides characterized by polypoid configuration and presence of condensed layers of tumor cells under the epithelium of the ethmoid sinus (H&E, ×40).

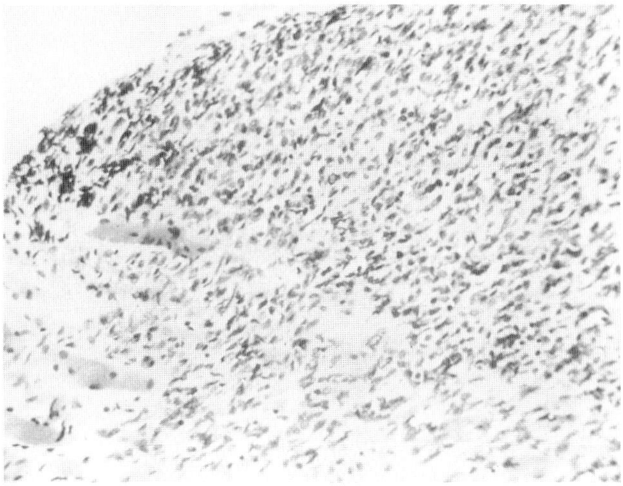

FIGURE 12-25. Superficial biopsy of a tumor which turned out to be an alveolar rhabdomyosarcoma. Note that tumor cells which are round or oval in shape are arranged in diffuse "solid" sheets and infiltrate the surrounding skeletal muscle. Alvelar pattern is absent. (H&E, ×400.)

Rhabdoid change characterized by eccentric nucleus, prominent nucleolus, abundant eosinophilic cytoplasm, and a cytoplasmic inclusion may be seen in some cases of embryonal RMS (and less commonly in alveolar RMS).[80] The cytoplasmic inclusions are positive for vimentin and desmin. There was no

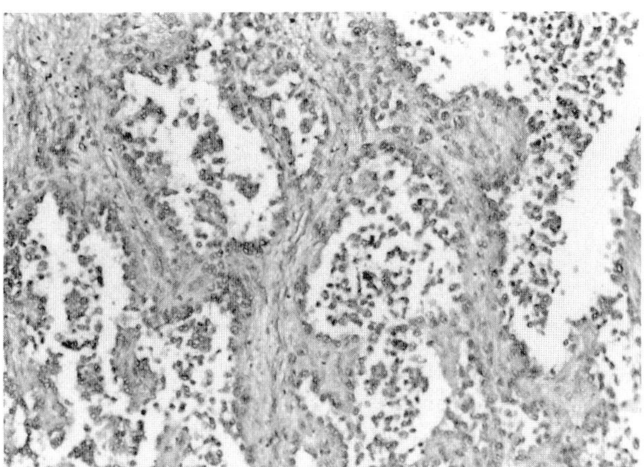

FIGURE 12-26. Alveolar rhabdomyosarcoma characterized by present of fibrovascular septa separating alveoli-like structures filled with tumor cells (H&E, ×100).

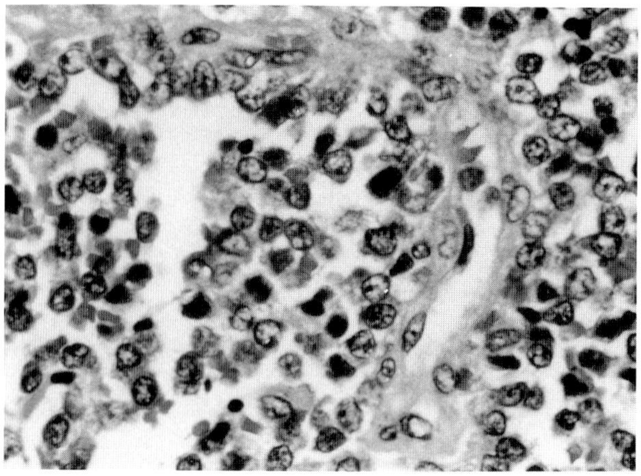

FIGURE 12-27. Alveolar rhabdomyosarcoma showing detached large round tumor cells in the lumen of the "alveolus" and a layer of similar cells closely applied to the fibrous trabecula (H&E, ×400).

statistically significant difference in survivals in patients with RMS showing rhabdoid change versus in those with nonrhabdoid RMS.

Pleomorphic RMS

This was considered at one time as the classical type of RMS.[75] However, it is rare in children and most of the cases described even in adults probably represent malignant fibrous histiocytoma. This type of RMS is characterized by cellularity and pleomorphism. The tumor shows large, broad, elongated, or strap-shaped cells, often with multiple nuclei and bright eosinophilic cytoplasm.[75] Pleomorphism (anaplasia) may also be seen in embryonal and alveolar RMS. Kodet et al in a recent review of about 3000 cases of RMS registered with IRS I, II, and III[76] found pleomorphism (anaplasia) in some cases of embryonal RMS and rare cases of alveolar RMS. Transition from typical nonpleomorphic embryonal RMS to pleomorphic embryonal RMS was noted in many of these cases. Therefore Kodet et al indicated that pleomorphic RMS as defined originally does not occur in children.[76]

RMS with Mixed Pattern

In 7% (90 of 1319 IRS cases) mixed patterns (embryonal, alveolar, pleomorphic) were noted.

Extraosseous Ewing's Sarcoma (EOE)

A number of cases submitted to IRS as RMS turned out to be EOE (tumor composed uniformly of small undifferentiated cells with immature nuclei and abundant cytoplasmic glycogen, indistinguishable from OE).

Small Round Cell Sarcoma, Type Undetermined (STI)

These are sarcomas composed of small round or spindle cells that could not be included in any of the subtypes due to lack of specific histologic features. This is also called "undifferentiated sarcoma." This probably corresponds to embryonal sarcoma in the classification used by the ISPO Pathology Panel[74] (see below).

Sarcoma, Not Classified (NOS)

A category of sarcoma, not classified (NOS), has also been included for those tumors that could not be classified as any of the preceding categories because of inadequacy of material.

Frequency and Prognostic Significance of Various Types

The frequency of various types in the IRS cases is as follows: embryonal (54%), botryoid (5%), alveolar (21%), pleomorphic (<1%), STI (8%), EOE (5%), and NOS (5%). The prognosis varied by histology: alveolar and STI had the worst; botryoid, the best; and embryonal and EOE, an intermediate prognosis.[73] The results of IRS-II showed that in nonmetastatic patients, the 5-year survival rate was 89% for botyroid RMS, 74% for embryonal RMS, 66% for alveolar RMS, and 61% for other types of RMS (undifferentiated, EOE, pleomorphic RMS, and RMS not otherwise specified) ($p < .001$). Comparable statistically significant differences were also noted for metastatic RMS.[80] Kodet et al[76] noted a statistically significant difference between the survival in patients with nonpleomorphic embryonal RMS (68%) and those with embryonal RMS showing clusters or sheets of pleomorphic (anaplastic) cells (46%). Scattered pleomorphic cells were not of any prognostic significance.

ISPO Classification

This classification[74] is basically similar to the IRS classification. There are more subtypes in each histologic type (loose, dense, poorly differentiated etc.). The ISPO classification recognizes embryonal sarcoma, which has histologic features similar to embryonal RMS except that rhabdomyoblasts are absent.

NCI Classification

The WHO classification divides RMS into botryoid, embryonal, alveolar, and pleomorphic types.[82] A mixed embryonal–alveolar subtype is also recognized. In the NCI classification two basic types of RMS, viz., embryonal and alveolar, are recognized.[83] The tumor cells of these two types have different cytologic features and patterns of arrangement. In embryonal RMS the tumor cells are spindle-shaped and show a diffuse loose pattern with myxoid areas. Botryoid RMS is a subtype of embryonal type with characteristic features described above in the IRS classification. The alveolar type is composed of round cells showing an alveolar arrangement. A solid alveolar subtype is recognized. This subtype is cytologically similar to alveolar type. Specifically, the cells are round with large round or irregular nuclei and coarse chromatin pattern. Alveolar pattern is absent. The tumor cells are densely packed without any collagen/reticulin between individual tumor cells. However, dense collagenous bands similar to those seen in alvelar RMS are seen commonly. These bands produce a focal lobular pattern. The third category of RMS in the NCI classification consists of the rare pleomorphic RMS. In addition, other rate tumors that cannot be categorized according to the aforementioned criteria are also seen. These tumors which show myoblastic or fibrosarcoma-like pattern are included in a heterogeneous group termed "other."

Statistical analysis of 159 cases of RMS classified according to these criteria showed prognostic value of the NCI classification even after stratification for age, site, and stage.[83] Specifically the embryonal RMS had better prognosis than alveolar RMS, which included both the conventional and solid variants. Therefore, embryonal RMS was labelled as "favorable histologic" type and alveolar RMS as "unfavorable histologic" type. The results of the prognostic significance of the NCI classification reported by Tsokos et al indicate the practical importance of recognition of a solid variant of alveolar RMS, which is associated with poor prognosis. Solid alveolar RMs may show alveolar pattern in the deeper parts of the tumor or in the metastasis.

Clinical Features

The presence of a visible and/or palpable mass and/or disturbance of body function by an unsuspected critically located mass are the two main clinical features—the details varying according to the primary site. Thus, for example, RMS of bladder and prostate would present with hematuria and/or urinary obstruction. The median age in the IRS-I series consisting of 686 patients was 7 years with 4% patients younger than 1 year, 38% patients younger than 5 years, and 63% patients 10 years or younger.[84] Congenital anomalies involving CNS, GU (genitourinary) system, and CVS occur with higher frequency than in normal children.[85]

Primary Sites

In the IRS-I study, the primary sites were as follows: GU tract 21%, extremities 20%, cranioparameningeal region (nasopharynx, mastoid, middle ears, orbit, sinuses, etc.) 14%, and other head and neck excluding orbit 13%. Besides the bladder, the prostate, vagina, uterus, and soft tissues of the pelvis or perineum may also be the primary sites. The common histologic types by primary sites are as follows: GU tumors—embryonal 71%, botryoid 20%; extremities—alveolar 50%; head and neck—embryonal 71%. Douglas et al[86] describe three patients of alveolar RMS with occult primary site. The diagnosis was made in these patients on the basis of bone marrow involvement.

Metastatic Sites

Lung, lymph nodes, bone marrow, bone, liver, and CNS are the known metastatic sites. Overall lymph node involvement is infrequent but does occur (e.g., in paratesticular tumors retroperitoneal LNs are involved in 30% of the cases). LN involvement also occurs in uterine and/or vaginal tumors and in tumors of the extremities. Lung is relatively more frequently involved than other sites.[72] Ruymann et al[85] reported bone marrow involvement in 29% of stage IV IRS-I patients at presentation. Douglas et al[86] described three cases of alveolar RMS in which there was such extensive involvement of the bone marrow by metastatic RMS, that initially a diagnosis of leukemia was made. The true nature of the neoplastic process was demonstrated by cytogenetic studies and follow-up of the patients (see below). However, as compared with NB, this type of presentation is seen less frequently in RMS. (In IRS-I stage IV was seen in 19% patients; in contrast, stage IV or D disease was seen in 63% of 237 POG cases of NB.[12,84]

Histologic Features

These have already been described in the introductory section and in the discussion of various pathologic classifications. RMS as a broad group are composed of cells of various shapes (round, tadpole, strap, and spindle cells). The points to be emphasized with respect to classification are as follow. Embryonal RMS has mainly fusiform to spindle shaped cells and myxoid areas. A spindle cell variant of embryonal RMS described above has also been recognized recently.[78,79] Alveolar RMS has predominantly round or pear-shaped cells. The solid variant of alveolar RMS (i.e., without alveolar pattern) described by the NCI group[83] contains round cells. This variant is designated as monomorphic RMS by Palmer et al.[88,89] The histologic feature that is required for diagnosis of RMS is the rhabdomyoblasts (large round cells or elongated cells with abundant bright red cytoplasm and hyperchromatic nucleus or nuclei). Cross striations may or may not be present. Embryonal sarcoma of ISPO classification and STI of IRS classification will have to be considered in the differential diagnosis of SRCTs.

Ultrastructural Features

Historically electron microscopy was the only alternative to routine and special stains in the diagnosis of RMS. With the advent of immunohistochemistry, it has assumed a complementary role. Most cases of RMS are more easily distinguished by light microscopy, including immunohistochemistry.[72] However, Mierau et al[18] are of the opinion that electron microscopy is more helpful in making a diagnosis of RMS than immunohistochemical stains, particularly when one is dealing with undifferentiated or poorly differentiated tumors as seen by light microscopy and with cases in which immunohistochemical stains may be equivocal. The essential ultrastructural criteria for rhabdomyoblastic nature of the cells are as follow: alternating thick and thin filaments in hexagonal array *or* Z band material *or* Indian file arrangement of ribosomes along thick filaments (Figure 12-28).[18] Less convincing but helpful criteria include monoparticulate glycogen, external lamina, and pinocytotic vesicles.[18]

Immunohistochemistry

Myoglobin, desmin, and MSA are the three stains that are helpful in RMS. The number of cells showing positivity with MSA may be higher than that of desmin positive cells in some of the tumors. On the basis of his experience, Parham states that myoglobin has higher specificity but poor sensitivity as compared with desmin and MSA.[91] The poor sensitivity of myoglobin particularly in primitive RMS may be related to relatively late synthesis of this protein during the muscle development.[92] Occasional cases may show NSE and S-100 positivity.[18,90] Cytokeratin and NFP have also been demonstrated in some cases of embryonal and alveolar RMS.[90] Myosin and myoglobin seem specific for skeletal muscle. Actin and desmin react with both smooth and striated muscle; however, skeletal muscle isotypes are apparently specific for striated muscle. It should be noted that cytoplasm of tumor cells and of histiocytes in tumors of

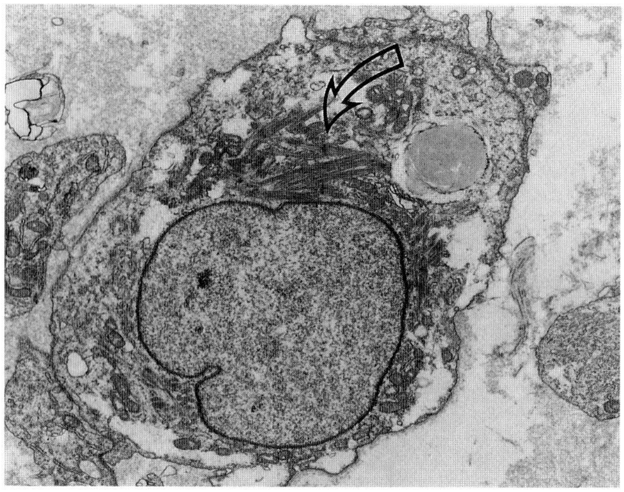

FIGURE 12-28. Electron micrograph of rhabdomyoblast showing presence of thick and thin filaments with Z bands (arrow)(×5500). (Courtesy of Dr. Gary Mierau.)

nonmuscular origin such as lymphoma, breast carcinoma, and melanoma infiltrating the skeletal muscle may show positive reaction in the immunoperoxidase stain for myoglobin.[93] The myoglobin may be transferred to the histiocytes by phagocytosis and to the tumor cells by passive diffusion of the protein in vivo or as a fixation artifact. I have seen one case of lymphoma infiltrating pelvic muscles that gave a positive result on immunoperoxidase stain for MSA. Enzymes such as creatine kinase subunit M (muscle type), or β-enolase can be demonstrated by immunohistochemistry or standard histochemistry on frozen sections.[94,95] Immunohistochemical stains are helpful in cases in which routine histology and electron microscopy may be negative.[72,90] However, Mierau et al[18] consider electron microscopy more helpful.

Other Features

Genetic studies have shown that muscle differentiation is under the control of a set of related regulatory genes including MyoD1, myogenin, myf-5, and myf-6.[96–98] Transfection of murine fibroblasts by a single gene MyoD1 results in their conversion to myoblasts. MyoD1 encodes a nuclear phosphoprotein (MyoD1 protein) whose expression is restricted to skeletal muscle in the mouse. Scrable et al[96] detected MyoD1 gene expression by demonstrating specific mRNA by Northern blotting of homogenized tumor tissue from RMS. These investigators also demonstrated that in embryonal RMS there is loss of heterozygosity for certain loci (D11S2y, CAT, PTH, etc.) on chromosome 11 whereas alveolar RMS retained the heterozygosity. Dias et al[97,98] have demonstrated MyoD1 protein in the nuclei of cells of RMS by immunofluorescence and immunohistochemical method on frozen sections of the tumor tissue. There was positive staining in all the specimens of RMS (including these in which desmin was negative), fetal muscle, and human RMS cell lines. The staining was confined to the nucleus. The punctate nature of MyoD1 destribution within the nucleus was confirmed by immunoelectromicroscopy. In addition, the staining was positive in two of the five specimens that were originally designated as sarcoma type undetermined according to the IRS classification and in two of three specimens designated as extraosseous Ewing's sarcoma diagnosed by the criteria used in IRS classification of RMS. Because of the positive results, these cases were categorized as RMS. NB, PNET, NHL, embryonal sarcoma of liver, malignant fibrous histiocytoma, malignant rhabdoid tumor, and osseous Ewing's sarcoma were negative for MyoD1.[97] MyoD1 protein thus appears to be a marker for RMS. It is of interest to note that strong MyoD1 protein expression has been demonstrated by immunofluorescence in a case of alveolar soft part sarcoma raising the possibility of skeletal muscle origin of that tumor.[99]

Shapiro et al[100] determined cellular DNA content (ploidy) of RMS in 37 patients with unresectable tumors. They found that patients with unresectable RMS having diploid DNA content have a significantly high risk of treatment failure. They also found that in the group with abnormal ploidy, hyperdiploidy (DNA index of 1.10–1.80), and tetraploidy (DNA index of 1.80–2.60) were strongly associated with embryonal and alveolar RMS, respectively. A specific translocation, t(2;13) (q35;q14) has been found to occur in alveolar RMS.[101] Alveolar RMS with this translocation tend to take a high aggressive course with shorter median survival. RMS can be xenografted into immune deprived inbred mice.[102]

MALIGNANT LYMPHOMAS (NON-HODGKIN'S LYMPHOMAS)

Malignancies in general are neoplastic proliferations of a localized tissue or organ. Non-Hodgkin's malignant lymphomas (NHL) in children are generalized at presentation in most cases. The systemic involvement mimics the pattern of circulation of normal lymphoid cells. The following differences have been noted between NHL in children and adults:[103] (1) higher frequency in boys (3 : 1, M : F in adults 1 : 1); (2) three histologic types according to National Cancer Institute working formulation of NHL[104] constitute the overwhelming majority of cases—lymphoblastic (mostly in supradiaphragmatic sites), small cell, noncleaved (Burkitt's and non-Burkitt's subtypes) (mostly in abdomen) and large cell lymphoma; (3) follicular lymphomas are extremely rare in children (50% of NHL in adults are of follicular type); (4) all NHL in children are high-grade; (5) extranodal sites are more common in children; (6) cure rate of NHL in children has doubled in the last decade; and (7) in children there is considerable overlap in clinical and pathologic features of acute lymphoblastic leukemia (ALL) and NHL. Many children with anterior mediastinal mass or massive lymphadenopathy, which are considered as characteristic features of NHL, have bone marrow involvement. The malignant T cells of lymphoblastic lymphoma and T cells of ALL are morphologically similar as are the cells of Burkitt's lymphoma and B-cell ALL. However, there may be immunophenotypic differences between T-cell ALL and T-cell lymphoblastic lymphoma. There is some evidence that T-cell ALL arises from early thymocyte stage whereas T-cell lymphoblastic lymphoma arises from intermediate or mature cell type.[105] In practice, the percentage of blast cells in the bone marrow is an arbitrary criterion used for distinguishing ALL from lymphoblastic lymphoma. The usual cutoff point used by investigators >25% blasts for the diagnosis of ALL.

Clinical Features

The age ranged from 7 months to 19 years in the series from St. Jude.[103] Only 16 of the 338 cases were under 3 years of age at diagnosis. The racial distribution in the series was 85% white and 15% nonwhite. In the Pediatric Oncology Group (POG) series,[106] nearly all patients with NHL had lymphoblastic and nonlymphoblastic (i.e., undifferentiated and large cell) NHL, respectively. NHL are the commonest malignancy in children with AIDS (see chapter 2 pathology of AIDS). NHL also occurs with high frequency in children with congenital immunodeficiency syndromes, including immune deficiency to Epstein–Barr virus (cross-linked lymphoproliferative syndrome).

Primary Sites

In the series from St. Jude Children's Research Hospital,[103] abdomen, mediastinum, and head and neck regions were involved almost equally. Majority of these tumors were extranodal. Only 6.5% of the cases presented with tumors in peripheral lymph nodes outside the neck. In general, supradiaphragmatic and infradiaphragmatic NHL are of lymphoblastic and small cell noncleaved types, respectively. The less common locations included bone, skin, epidural space, thyroid, liver, spleen, and gastrointestinal tract.[103,107–109] In children with AIDS brain is a common primary site.[110]

Involvement of Other Sites

The disease is generalized in majority of the cases. Skin, bone marrow, and CNS involvement can occur. Unusual sites of involvement include lung and brain.[105] Testicular and renal involvement has also been described.[111,112]

Histologic Features

Lymphoblastic (33%), small cell noncleaved (about 50%), and large cell (15%) types were the three main types of NHL in the Childrens Cancer Study Group series.[113] In the POG series of 227 cases, the figures were 47, 21, and 32%, respectively.[106] Virtually all NHL in children are of diffuse type. Follicular lymphomas are rare.[114] The cells of lymphomas are noncohesive and are arranged in diffuse sheets (Figure 12-1). Lobular or nesting pattern with fibrovascular septa is not seen. However, in rare cases the cells because of extremely compact arrangement may appear to be cohesive (Figure 12-29). Lymphoglandular bodies, which are fragments of cytoplasm, may be present, which are better demonstrated in the imprints (Figure 12-30). Starry sky pattern due to presence of tingible body macrophages is seen most commonly in small cell noncleaved NHL (Burkitt's type) but also occurs in the other two types. The comparison of the sizes of the lymphoma cells and the macrophages of the starry sky can be helpful in the differential diagnosis between different types of childhood NHL. Thus the nuclei of tumor cells are smaller than, of the same size as, and larger than the nuclei of starry sky macrophages in lymphoblastic. Burkitt's, and large cell NHL, respectively (Figures 12-29, 12-31).[113] There is disagreement among the hematopathologists regarding which dimensions of the tumor cells and the starry sky macrophages should be compared. According to Kjeldsberg et al,[113]

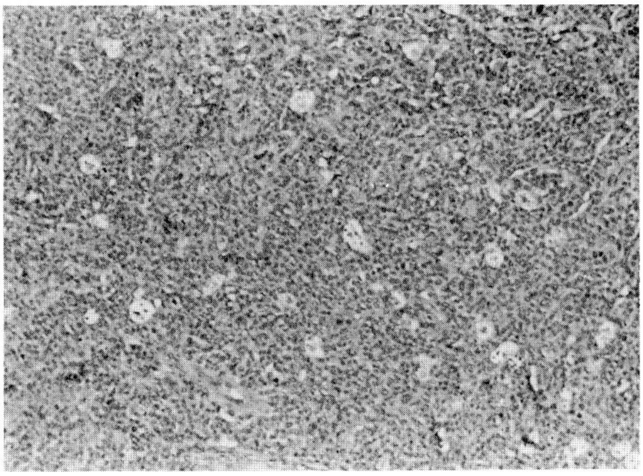

FIGURE 12-29. Lymphoblastic lymphoma showing arrangement of tumor cells in diffuse densely packed sheets giving an appearance of cohesiveness to the cells; note also the starry sky appearance with nuclei of tumor cells being smaller than those of the macrophages (arrows) (H&E, ×40).

nuclear sizes of the two types of cells are compared. Cossman,[115] on the other hand states that in Burkitt's NHL the diameter of the tumor cells is the same as the nuclei of the starry sky macrophages. Mitosis and karyorrhexis are prominent, particularly in Burkitt's NHL. The cytologic features for the different types are as follows:

1. *Lymphoblastic NHL.*[106] These lymphomas show monotonous cells with nuclei smaller than those of reactive histiocytes (but larger than small

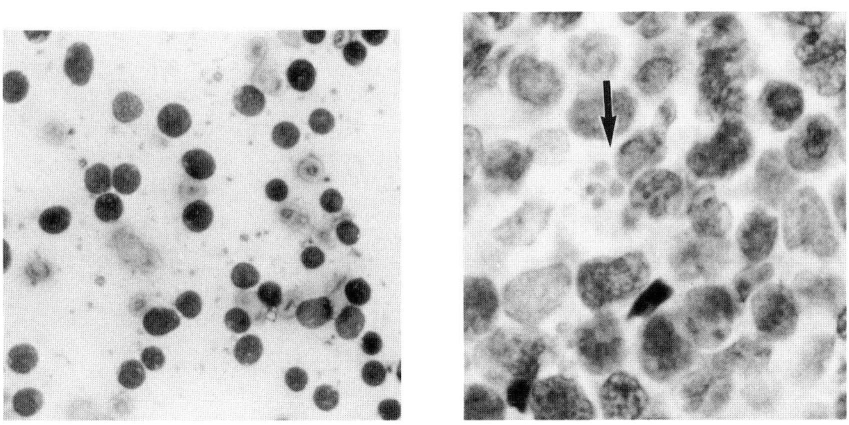

A B

FIGURE 12-30. (A) Lymphoglandular bodies in an imprint of non-Hodgkin's lymphoma (Diff-Quik, ×400); (B) histologic section of non-Hodgkin's lymphoglandular bodies (arrow) (H&E, ×1000).

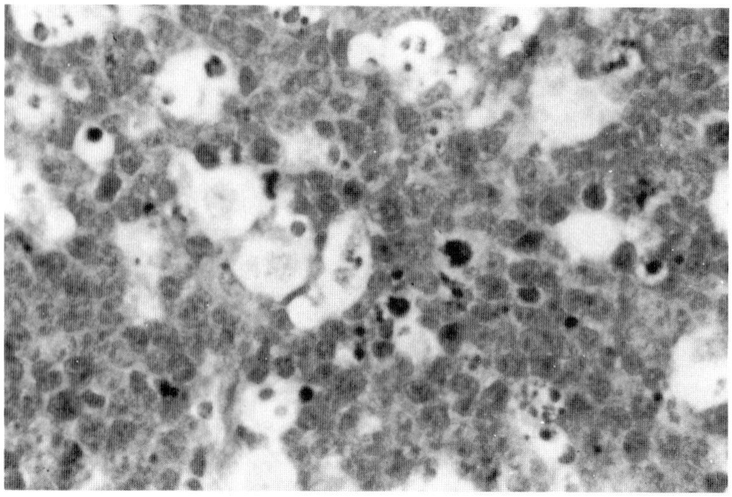

FIGURE 12-31. Burkitt's lymphoma showing starry sky pattern. Note that the nuclei of tumor cells are of the same size as those of the macrophages. The nuclear chromatin is unevenly distributed and one or more prominent nucleoli are present. Note the high mitotic activity in the tumor cells around the macrophages (H&E, ×400).

lymphocytes). The nuclei are round to avoid with variable number showing convolutions (none to majority). Convolutions can be best appreciated in a PAS stain. The nuclear chromatin is delicate, dusty, and dispersed. There are inconspicuous nucleoli. The cytoplasm is scanty. PAS stain is positive in some cases. Lymphoblastic NHL isnot morphologically distinguishable from ALL in the tissue sections or bone marrow aspirates. Griffith et al,[106] in a study of 106 POG cases, recognized three histologic subtypes: convoluted (83%), nonconvoluted (4%), and a large cell variant (11%). The last subtype had larger cells with one or two relatively prominent nucleoli. Nuclear convolutions were not as conspicuous as in the convoluted subtype. It was difficult to distinguish the large cell variant from undifferentiated and large cell NHLs. Reliance was placed on finely dispersed chromatin for the diagnosis of lymphoblastic NHL. Most of the lymphoblastic NHLs are supradiaphragmatic (primarily mediastinal) in location. However, large cell NHL can also occur in the mediastinum.[116]

2. *Small cell noncleaved NHL*[117]
   a. *Burkitt's type*. The histologic features of African and non-African Burkitt's are identical. The cells are monotonous, and have round to oval nuclei that are of the same size as the nuclei of reactive histiocytes. The nuclear chromatin is irregularly distributed and one or more usually prominent nucleoli are present (Figure 12-31). The cytoplasm is scanty to moderate, amphophilic, and pyroninophilic and has lipid vacuoles (Figure 12-32).
   b. *Non-Burkitt's type*. The cytologic features are the same as above but there is nuclear pleomorphism (greater variation in size and shape). The histologic distinction between Burkitt's and non-Burkitt's is sometimes difficult. There is no difference in prognosis between the two subtypes.

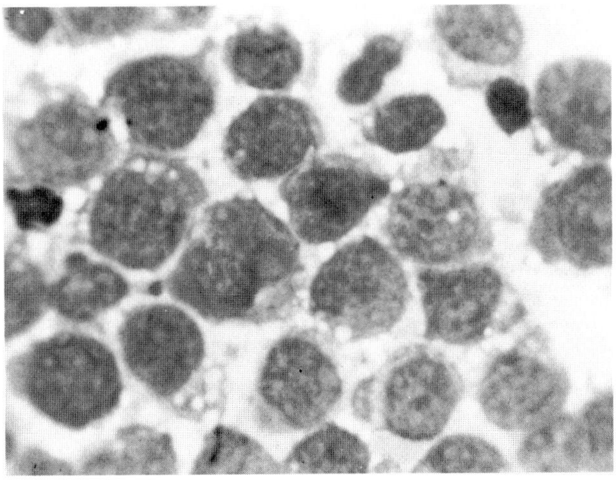

FIGURE 12-32. Imprint of Burkitt's lymphoma showing lipoid vacuoles in tumor cells (H&E, ×1000).

3. *Large cell lymphoma.*[118] These lymphomas have cells with nuclei that are larger than the nuclei of reactive histiocytes. They are divided by NCI working formulation[104] into cleaved and noncleaved [follicular center cell (FCC) (44%) (Figure 12-1) and immunoblastic subtype (56%).

The last subtype may have plasmacytoid, clear cell, or polymorphous features or may have epithelioid cell component. The cells of large cell cleaved and noncleaved NHL have round to oval vesicular nuclei with two or three prominent nucleoli often in apposition to the nuclear membrane. The narrow rim of cytoplasm is amphophilic and pyroninophilic. The immunoblastic lymphomas have one or several centrally located nucleoli and abundant cytoplasm which is basophilic or clear depending upon the subtype. The polymorphous variant is characterized by large atypical cells with irregular nuclei. Nathwani et al[118] concluded that the morphologic subclassification of large cell lymphomas currently has limited clinical prognostic significance in children. The cellular features of various types of NHLs are summarized in Table 12-5.

Ultrastructural Features

The cells of NHLs have nonspecific features, which, with experience, enable recognition of the nature of the cell. There are a few scattered mitochondia. Polyribosomes are present (Figure 12-33). Endoplasmic reticulum with serpentine outline may be present. Glycogen may be seen in the cytoplasm. In over one hundred cases examined by Mierau et al,[18] convincing cell junctions were not found in any of the cases. Nuclear convolution may be present in lymphoblastic NHL. Herrera et al[119] described neurosecretory-like granules in four cases of NHL in adults. Electron-dense granules may be overinterpreted if the criteria of neurosecretory granules are not stringently applied[2] (see section on NB above).

Immunohistochemistry

Leukocyte common antigen (LCA) distinguishes NHL from other SRCTs.[120] LCA may be negative in some cases (8 out of 40 in the series of Mierau et al[18]).

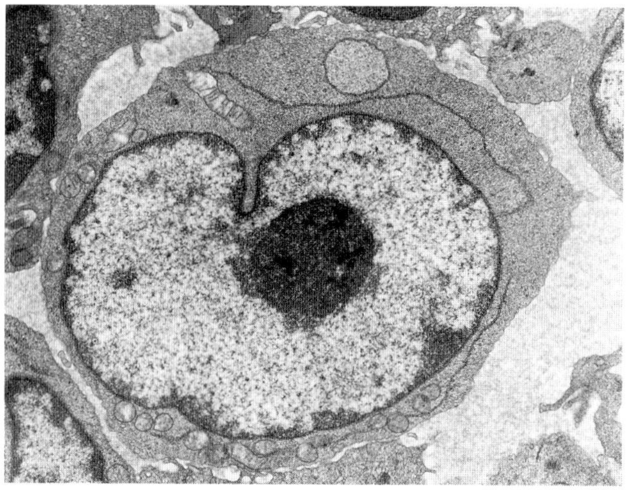

FIGURE 12-33. Electron micrograph of tumor cells of a large cell non-Hodgkin's lymphoma showing abundant polyribosomes in the cytoplasm, which is nearly devoid of other organelles (×7100). (Courtesy of Dr. Gary Mierau.)

Extreme caution is required in the interpretation of the results. Faint positivity may be difficult to interpret. Reactive lymphocytes present in certain SRCTs—particularly NBs may be abundant in some foci and will stain positively. Vimentin may be positive.[1] NSE, synaptophysin, cytokeratin, neurofilament protein, actin, and desmin are negative. Faint positive staining of tumor cells and stromal elements by NSE may be seen in B5-fixed NHLs.[23]

Segal et al[121] have recommended the panel of following three antibodies for immunophenotyping of NHL in paraffin sections: (1) L-26 identifying the CD20 antigen of normal and neoplastic B cells, (2) UCHL-1 identifying the CD45RO present on most T cells and T-cell NHL, and (3) Leu-22 identifying the CD43 antigen present on normal T cells and monocytes but not on normal B cells. Lineage assignments were identical for paraffin section immunohistology and immunophenotyping on fresh or frozen tumor tissue done by immunocytometry is 48 of the 50 cases. Despite the efficiency and overall reliability of immunophenotyping on paraffin sections, it is recommended that these determinations be done on fresh or frozen tissue to get more accurate results.[122] Obtaining fresh and frozen tumor tissue also enables the determination of gene rearrangements.[121] It has been shown that coexpression of CD43 (Leu-22) and CD20 (L-26) antigens correlates with malignant B-cell lymphoproliferation.[123]

Detailed immunophenotyping by using panels of monoclonal antibodies and clinicopathologic analysis of cases NHL have resulted in recognition of the following cases of uncommon types of NHL, which also occur in children and adolescents:

1. *Ki-1 NHL.* Ki-1 antibody, initially believed to be specific for Reed–Sternberg cells of Hodgkin's disease, has been shown to react with neoplastic cells of

certain large cell NHL of T-cell lineage. Initially, Ki-1 antibody could be used on frozen sections only. An antibody (BERH2) that can be used on paraffin section is available now. Ki-1 staining may be focal or diffuse. Schnitzer et al[124] reported three cases Ki-1 NHL in children. These lymphomas characteristically show large bizarre neoplastic cells. The lymph node involvement shows a sinusoidal pattern. Because of these features, Ki-1 NHL may be mistaken for malignant histiocytosis.

2. *T-cell-rich B-cell lymphomas.* In the series reported by Macon et al[125] two of the 19 patients were 18 years of age at the time of diagnosis.
3. *Peripheral/post thymic T-cell lymphomas.* In a series of 79 cases reported by Pinkus et al,[126] two patients were 17 years of age.
4. *Pre-B-cell NHL.* Most B cell NHL in children represent malignant counterpart of more mature B lymphocytes. NHL derived from B-cell precursors are extremely rare in children. Kamps et al[127] reported one pediatric case and reviewed eight pediatric cases reported in the literature. In their case, the antigens CD19, CD22, and CD24 of B-cell precursors were detected in frozen sections.

Thus the cell markers for various stages of T and B cells need to be determined for immunophenotyping of the NHL. Cell markers should also be determined by flow cytometry. As indicated above, on rare occasion there may be discrepancy between the two techniques. In addition to the antigens described above, the following markers are also recognized in various types of NHL: (1) terminal deoxynucleotidyl transferase (TdT), a DNA polymerase occurring in immature thymic lymphocytes, is present in the cells of lymphoblastic NHL[105] (imprints or frozen sections are required for its demonstration, and <90% of cases are positive); and (2) a few large cell lymphomas may be histiocytic in type. These are recognized by demonstration of lysozyme (muramidase), nonspecific esterase and by Cathepsin B.[123]

Other Features

Translocation between chromosomes 8 and 14 has been demonstrated in Burkitt's lymphoma. This involves the translocation of c-myc gene from chromosome 8 to the immunoglobulin heavy-chain locus on chromosome 14 [t(8;14)(q24;q32)].[95] Variant translocations, viz., t(2;8) (p12;q24) and t(8;22) (q24;q11), result in juxtaposition of c-myc gene with the loci for immunoglobulins [kappa (κ) light chains on chromosome 2 and lambda (λ) light chains on chromosome 22]. B cell lineage/monoclonality can be recognized by genotypic methods if rearrangement of heavy-chain and/or light-chain immunoglobulin is found. T-cell lineage–monoclonality can be recognized by demonstration of T-cell receptor B constant region (TCRB) gene rearrangements.

UNCOMMON TUMORS IN DIFFERENTIAL DIAGNOSIS OF SRCTS:

Intraabdominal Desmoplastic Small Round Cell Tumors with Divergent Differentiation

Gonzales-Crussi et al[11] reported three cases in which the tumors were attached to the peritoneum. The age varied from 6 to 8 years. The histologic pattern suggested metastatic "epithelial" tumor. But there was no evidence of primary neoplasm in the abdominal organs. Grossly the tumors presented well-circumscribed pseudoencapsulated and multilobulated or multinodular masses. In one case, there were metastases to the liver. Two children died at 6 and 8 years. The third patient was in good health 18 months after surgery. Histologically, there were discrete islands of compact, small epithelium-like cells encased in a fibrous stroma producing a nesting pattern. The vesicular nuclei had fine chromatin and one to three small nucleoli. There were abundant mitoses. In one case a tendency to formation of tubular lamina was noted. In addition to the nesting pattern, diffuse growth was also present. Focal deposits of eosinophilic hyalin material were noted intra- and extracellularly. Immunohistochemical studies revealed coexpression of epithelial (cytokeratin) and mesenchymal (desmin) markers. Neural markers gave variable results. NSE was faintly positive in one case. Synaptophysin was slightly to moderately positive in all cases. Chromogranin was strongly but focally positive in all cases. Ultrastructural examination showed the following features: (1) complex subcellular structure of cells characterized by prominent Golgi apparatus, occasional focal glycogen accumulation, numerous free ribosomes, and RER, etc.; (2) microvillous-like structures; (3) no basement lamina; (4) poorly developed cell junctions despite close cell–cell apposition; and (5) a few electron-dense inclusions that could *not* be identified as neurosecretory granules. Differential diagnosis includes extrarenal Wilms' tumor, conventional SRCTs, and germ-cell tumors. The histogenesis of the neoplasm remains undetermined.

Forty-six additional cases of intraabdominal desmoplastic SRCT have been described by Gerald et al.[128–130] The age range was 7–48 years with a mean of 20.8 years. The tumor is strikingly more common in males. It is characterized by multiple peritoneal nodules with direct invasion of organs (urinary bladder, intestine, or stomach). Two cases of thoracic (pleural) involvement alone were also seen.[130] Histologically there was nesting pattern and marked desmoplastic reaction containing myofibroblasts. Focal rhabdoid features were noted. Small acini were observed in the two cases reported by Variend et al.[131] Positive reaction for keratin, epithelial membrane antigen, neuron-specific enolase, and desmin was demonstrated by immunohistologic methods. Histogenesis of this tumor with divergent differentiation remains undetermined. Sawyer et al[132] have recently demonstrated a reciprocal translocation t(11;22) (p13;q12) in a case of intraabdominal desmoplastic SRCT. It should be noted that the translocation affected the breakpoint on chromosome 22 (q12), but it is different from that seen in ES and PNET [t(11;22) (q24;q12)]. It is possible that this tumor is more common than is generally realized. Since a diagnosis of atypical variant of one or other of the conventional SRCT, malignant mesothelioma, undifferentiated carcinoma, carcinoid tumor, and germ-cell tumor may have been made by pathologists before the characterization of this tumor.

Blastemal Wilms' Tumor

Occasionally Wilms' tumor may be predominantly or exclusively blastemal. Wilms' tumor can also occur at extrarenal sites in rare instances. Small biopsies from such cases may pose diagnostic difficulties. Histologic features such as absence of well-defined nesting pattern and presence of rare glomeruloid or tubular structures may be helpful. I have seen Homer Wright and Flexner rosettes in rare cases of blastemal Wilms' tumor (Figure 12-34). Blastemal cells of Wilms' tumor are positive for both cytokeratin and vimentin. Ultrastructural examination shows flocculent basement-membrane-like material, oligocilia, phagolysosomes, and microvilli. The details are described on the chapter on renal tumors in children.

A unique case of a small round cell tumor of fallopian tube in a 15-year-old girl was reported by Bendit et al.[133] Histologically, it was composed of small round cells with sparse eosinophilic cytoplasm. Numerous typical and atypical mitoses were present. The tumor cells were arranged in solid masses surrounded by fibrovascular stalks giving the appearance of pseudorosettes. Cords and pseudoacini were occasionally observed. The tumor cells were positive for vimentin and keratin and negative for EMA, GFAP, NSE, CEA, PAP, and chromogranin. The impression on histologic examination was neuroectodermal neoplasm or undifferentiated (blastemal) extrarenal Wilms' tumor. Electron microscopy revealed undifferentiated cells with basement-membrane-like material around some of them. No microfilaments, neurotubules, or neurosecretory granules were seen. These observations were considered as more consistent with Wilms' tumor. Molecular biologic studies revealed that the N-myc gene was overexpressed in the RNA extracted from the tumor. Analysis of DNA revealed a single copy of N-myc gene. Extensive overexpression of N-myc without gene amplification has been described in Wilms' tumor.[32] Therefore, the tumor was considered as most consistent with undifferentiated (blastemal) extrarenal Wilms' tumor.

Malignant Histiocytoma in Children

Cozzutto et al.[134] have reported four cases in children varying from 6 to 8 years. The tumors arose in the soft tissues of shoulder, supraclavicular, or knee region and one case in the soft palate. Another site includes thymus.[135] The tumor is composed of large pleomorphic epithelium-like cells with abundant

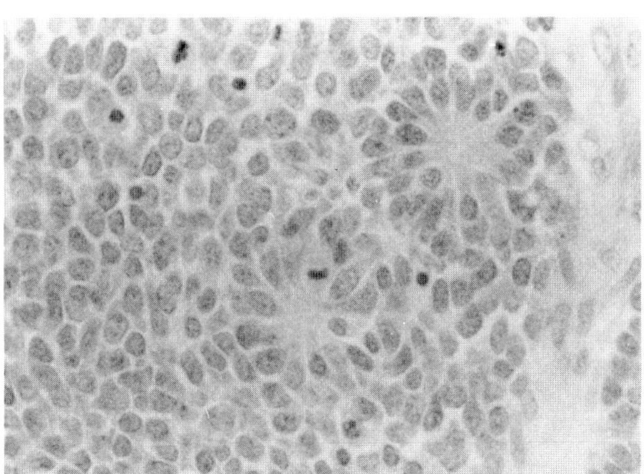

FIGURE 12-34. Blastemal Wilms' tumor showing Homer Wright rosettes (H&E, ×400).

cytoplasm. Lysozyme (muramidase) and α_1-antichymotrypsin can be demonstrated by immunoperoxidase technique.[135] SRCTs and extrarenal malignant rhabdoid tumor are to be considered in the differential diagnosis. In fact, the tumor designated as "malignant histiocytoma of the thymus" by Lemos and Hamoudi[136] probably represents extrarenal malignant rhabdoid tumor. Malignant histiocytoma is different from "polyhistiocytoma" described by Jacobsen.[137] The latter consists of small round cells resembling those seen in ES. These small round cells show focal mesenchymal differentiation with formation of cartilage, ostoid, bone, fibrovascular tissue, lipoid elements, etc. The youngest patient in the series reported by Jacobson[137] was 2.5 years old, and about one-third of the cases occurred in the second decade.

Inflammatory Pseudotumors in Children

Scott, et al[138] reported five cases in children 2–6 years of age. In four cases, the lesions arose in the abdomen (mesentery, pancreas, bladder, uterus) and in one at the typical site, viz., lung. The preoperative clinical diagnosis in all the cases was a malignant tumor (neuroblastoma, lymphoma, sarcoma). Histologically, the lesions consisted of localized proliferation of mononuclear cells (plasma cells, lymphocytes, eosinophils) and spindle-shaped mesenchymal cells or myofibroblasts. The lesions can be readily distinguished from SRCTs.

Undifferentiated Malignancy in Childhood

Plotsky et al[10] reviewed 20 cases seen at Children's Hospital of Pittsburgh from 1971 to 1987 in which a diagnosis of "malignant tumor," "undifferentiated malignancy," "undifferentiated carcinoma," or "anaplastic tumor or carcinoma" was made. The slides and electron micrographs, when available, were reviewed. Fresh sections cut from the blocks were used for immunohistochemistry (cytokeratin, desmin, vimentin, actin, LCA, EMA, AFP, α_1-antichymotrypsin, lysozyme, S-100, factor VIII, placental alkaline phosphatase, keratin, and NSE). The revised diagnoses included malignant extrarenal rhabdoid tumor, large cell NHL, RMS, PNET, inflammatory pseudotumor, malignant histiocytosis, pancreatic carcinoma, anaplastic carcinoma, nasopharyngeal carcinoma, congenital hemangiopericytoma, malignant mesothelioma, and granulosa cell tumor. In three cases, a new but still only tentative diagnosis was possible. This series shows the importance of immunohistochemistry in making a definitive diagnosis of undifferentiated tumors in children, although in a few cases only tentative diagnosis may be possible.

Small Cell Osteosarcoma

The diagnosis is made by demonstrating osteoid. Osteoid may be present in only a few small foci. A small biopsy may not contain a convincing focus of osteoid (Figure 12-35). Diagnosis of ES or NHL may be made in such cases.[139]

Retinoblastoma (Extraocular Extension or Metastasis)

The characteristic Flexner rosettes are present. Clinical history would be helpful in making diagnosis of metastasis.

Undifferentiated, "Small Round Cell" Hepatoblastoma

In rare cases hepatoblastoma may be composed of sheets of undifferentiated small round cells without any of the characteristic "hepatic" features being

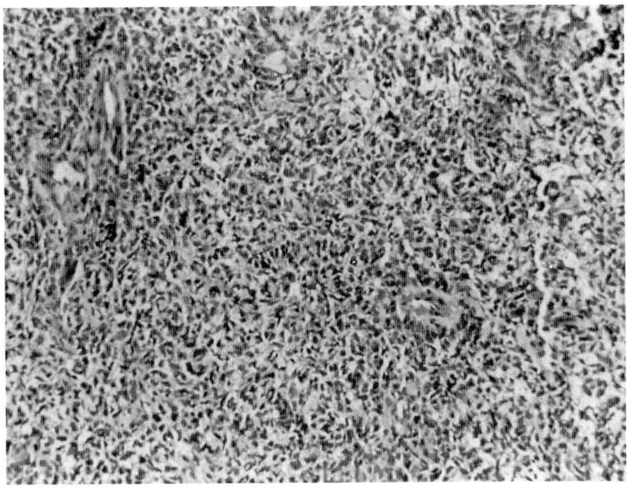

FIGURE 12-35. Small cell "undifferentiated" osteosarcoma. The biopsy specimen showed a small round cell tumor. No osteoid was seen in the biopsy specimen. However, in the resected specimen osteoid was present. (H&E, ×100.)

present (light and dark areas of embryonal and fetal hepatocytes, foci of hematopoiesis, arrangement in cords and trabeculae) (Figure 12-36). Abundant mucoid material was present. Immunoperoxidase stain for AFP was positive, and ultrastructurally bile canaliculi were identified in one of the cases.[8]

Granulocytic Sarcoma (Extramedullary Myeloid Tumor, Chloroma)

These tumors may precede the leukemic phase in occasional cases. Retroperitoneum, jaw, and orbit are among the sites of granulocytic sarcoma. Differ-

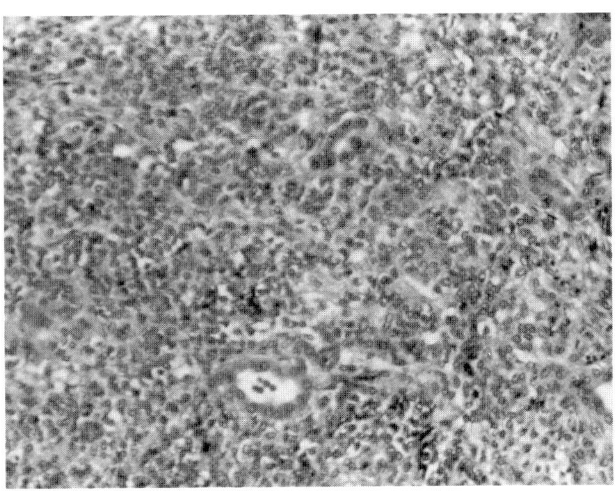

FIGURE 12-36. Small cell undifferentiated hepatoblastoma composed of sheets of darkly staining round cells; note entrapped bile ducts (H&E, ×250).

ential diagnosis in the orbital tumors includes embryonal RMS, NHL, and metastatic NB. Granulocytic sarcoma is characterized by sheets of large round cells. Cohesiveness is lacking. A careful search should be made for eosinophilic myelocytes. Chloroacetate esterase (Leder) strain is positive.[145] Myeloperoxidase and Sudan black will be positive in imprints of the biopsy.

Germ-Cell Tumors

Embryonal carcinoma, choriocarcinoma, and yolk sac tumors will show characteristic histologic features and positive staining for α fetoprotein (AFP) or human chorionic gonadotropin (HCG). Germ-cell tumors of seminoma type (germinoma) have large round cells with moderate cytoplasm. These tumors may have to be considered in the differential diagnosis, although in most instances the diagnosis can be readily made on the basis of characteristic histologic features (diffuse arrangement or arrangement into lobules, two types of cells, i.e., large round tumor cells and lymphocytes, granulomatous stromal reaction). Occasional "syncytiotrophoblastic" cells may be present) (Figure 12-37). AFP and HCG are negative in germinomas. Placental alkaline phosphatase (PAP) is positive.

Extracranial Metastasis of Central Primitive Neuroectodermal Tumor (PNET)

The previous history will be helpful in such cases. These metastases occur at variable time following surgery. Central PNET consists primarily of small round undifferentiated cells but may show foci of differentiation along astrocytic, ependymal, and neuronal lines. Medulloblastoma is considered as a type of central PNET. In one of the personally studied cases, metastasis to lung and liver were present in the biopsy specimens from a child who was previously operated on for central PNET. The lung metastasis showed pseudorhabdoid features.

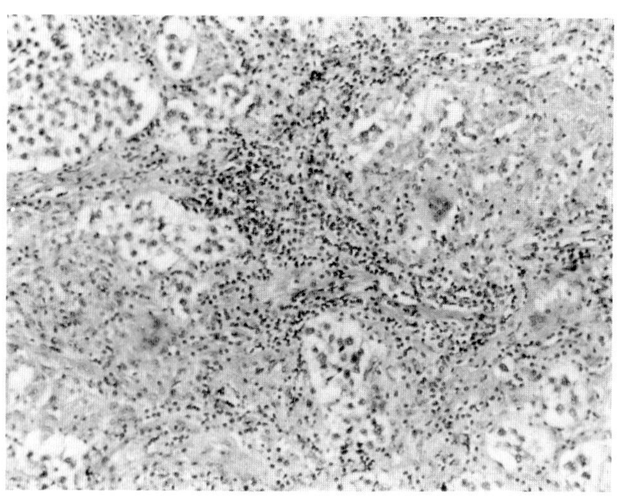

FIGURE 12-37. Germ cell tumor (dysgerminoma) showing large round tumor cells arranged into lobules, occasional syncytiotrophoblastic cells, and lymphocytic infiltration of the fibrous septa (H&E, ×250).

Extrarenal Malignant Rhabdoid Tumor (EMRT)

The malignant rhabdoid tumor of the kidney (MRTK) is a well recognized entitity.[140] Tumors with similar pathologic features and malignant behavior have also been reported to occur in both children and adults in extrarenal sites such as thymus, soft tissues, chest wall, liver, pelvis, etc.[136,139–143] The tumor cells of rhabdoid tumors are characterized by large eccentric nucleus, prominent nucleolus, abundant eosinophilic cytoplasm, and a cytoplasmic inclusion. The cytoplasm is composed of intermediate filaments on electron microscopy and stain for vimentin and keratin on immunoperoxidase stain. Thus the EMRT can be readily distinguished from SRCTs. However, some of the tumors that belong to the spectrum of SRCTs such as NB[17] and RMS[80] or other tumors that need to be considered in the differential diagnosis (e.g., intraabdominal small cell desmoplastic tumors with divergent differentiation or blastemal Wilms' tumor)[11,144] may show focal rhabdoid or pseudorhabdoid features. For making a diagnosis of rhabdoid tumors all the cytologic features described above should be present in the tumor cells. Presence of only abundant cytoplasm or cytoplasmic inclusion without the presence of prominent nucleoli or presence of only the latter without the former, described as "pseudorhabdoid" change,[144] should not be confused with rhabdoid change. The histogenesis of EMRT is not known. Histiocytic known. Histiocytic and neuroectodermal derivations have been suggested. The tumors are of a primitive nature, and many investigators favor neuroectodermal origin.

APPROACH TO DIAGNOSIS OF SRCT

Although in the vast majority of the cases of SRCT the diagnosis is evident or strongly suspected on the basis of routine histologic features, tumor specimen should be triaged as described below if adequate amount of tumor tissue is available. In cases in which the diagnosis is not evident using the routine methods, appropriately triaged portions of the specimen will then be available for demonstrating other diagnostic features.

Ideally, the diagnosis should be made on morphologic features alone, and this is possible in most SRCTs. However, the morphologic features showing overlap between different SRCT (e.g., rosettes) are to be considered in the clinical context (age of the patient, site of the tumor, etc.). Diagnostic morphologic features may not be present or fully developed in a given case. In such instances cytogenetic studies and molecular biologic studies will be helpful in arriving at the correct diagnosis. The 11;22 translocation seen in ES/PNET and the overexpression of N-myc of which a single copy is present in Wilms' tumor serve as examples of this situation and emphasize the importance of triaging of the specimen appropriately. The appproach to diagnosis of SRCTs is summarized in Table 12-8.

Triaging of the Specimen

The following types of specimen may be submitted for diagnosis: (1) FNA biopsy of primary or metastatic SRCT, (2) pleural or peritoneal fluid, (3) Trucut needle biopsy or incisional biopsy of primary or metastatic SRCT, and (4) incomplete or complete resection of primary or metastatic SRCT.

These specimens should be ideally triaged as follows:[5] (1) sterile fresh tissue for cytogenetics (and tissue culture), (2) glutaraldehyde-fixed tissue for electron microscopy, (3) nonsterile fresh tissue for cell marker studies of NHL and for DNA analysis by flow cytometry, (4) imprints for routine and special stains (such as oil red O or methyl green-pyronine) and for DNA analysis by image cytometry, (5) frozen tumor tissue for (a) frozen sections for immunohistologic studies (particularly in NHL), (b) biochemical and molecular biologic studies (enzymes, matrix proteins, RNA, oncogene, etc.), and (c) frozen tissue for tumor bank; (5) formalin-fixed tissue for routine histology; and (6) B-5 fixed tissue and tissue for plastic embedding in NHL. It is recommended that a minimum of 10 blocks be taken from the resected tumor for routine histology.

If only a small amount of tissue is present in the biopsy specimen, the triaging of the biopsy will have to be prioritized. Imprints should be made. Adequate tissue must be taken for routine histology. The formalin-fixed tissue can be used for immunohistochemistry in SRCTs, with reliable results in most instances including NHL and for DNA analysis by image cytometry. Since ultrastructural studies can be helpful in making a definitive diagnosis of certain types of SRCT (NB, RMS, etc.), tissue should always be taken for electron microscopy. Only minute amounts of tissue are required for electron microscopy. A small fresh portion of the biopsy may be saved for cell marker studies if sufficient amount of tissue is available. Tissue for studying other parameters may be taken depending on the type of tumor with high index of suspicion and facilities and research interests of the pathologists and other individuals in the institution.

Diagnosis of SRCT in an FNA Biopsy

In certain cases of SRCTs there may be an immediate need for instituting therapy because of acute signs and symptoms such as mediastinal compression or intestinal obstruction. In many of these cases the tumor may be unresectable, or an incisional biopsy may be contraindicated because of the general poor condition of the patient. (The latter situation is more likely to arise in developing countries). Under these circumstances an FNA biopsy done under ultrasound guidance is the only diagnostic method available. The National Pediatric Cancer Study Groups are now accepting such diagnoses for enrollment of the patients on the protocol.

The immediate review of the Diff-Quik-stained FNA smears provides clues regarding the probable diagnosis (nuclear molding, fibrillary background, cytoplasmic vacuoles, cytoplasmic tags, rosettes, lymphoglandular bodies, karyorrhectic cells, etc.) (Table 12-15).[146] Depending on the impression on this review, additional aspiration specimens can be triaged appropriately for immunoperoxidase stains, electron microscopy, and cytogenetics.[147,148] After final review of the Diff-Quik and Papanicolaou stains the definitive diagnosis may be evident. A cell block from the material remaining in the needle of the first aspirate and from an additional aspirate is desirable. Ancillary studies mentioned above will be helpful in confirming the impression or diagnosis made on this review.[149] Knowledge of primary or metastatic site of the SRCT as the case may be is also

TABLE 12-10 Comparison of Conventional, Shimada, and Modified Conventional Terminology of Neuroblastic Tumors[a]

Conventional terminology	Shimada terminology	Modified conventional terminology
Classical NB[b] (<5% differentiating neuroblasts)	NB, stroma-poor, undifferentiated	NB, undifferentiated and NB, poorly differentiated
GNB[c] (>5% mono and/or multinucleated ganglion cells with or without atypia)[d]	NB, stroma-poor, differentiating	NB, differentiating
Composite GNB (gross or microscopic nodules of NB in a ganglioneuromatous tissue)	NB, stroma-rich, well-differentiated; NB, stroma-rich, intermixed; and NB, stroma-rich, nodular	GNB, borderline[e]; GNB, intermixed[e]; and GNB, nodular
Ganglioneuroma[f]	Ganglioneuroma	Ganglioneuroma

Notes: a) See Tables 12-11 and 12-12 for criteria for various tumors defined by Shimada and modified conventional terminology respectively; b) NB—neuroblastoma; c) GNB—ganglioneuroblastoma; d) The conventional criteria for GNB are not standardized. Presence of ganglion cells is generally required. Presence of ganglioneuromatous areas is generally not considered as a criterion in conventional terminology. The definition given here is currently most widely used; e) Borderline or intermixed types of GNB may be designated as ganglioneuroma by some pathologists; f) Confusing terms such as "partially differentiated" and "immature ganglioneuroma" are sometimes used in conventional terminology. Such usage should be discouraged. Immature or partially differentiated ganglioneuroma is essentially a ganglioneuroblastoma.

TABLE 12-11 Terminology and Criteria of Neuroblastic Tumors According to Shimada Classification

Catetory	Criteria
NB[a], stroma-poor (SP)	Tumor that is poor in stromal elements, i.e., Schwannian elements (ganglioneuromatous component is absent). Two subtypes based on degree of differentiation are as follows: NB, SP, undifferentiated (<5% differentiating neuroblasts); NB, SP, differentiating (≥5% differentiating neuroblasts)
NB, stroma-rich (SR)	Tumor that is rich in stromal elements, i.e., predominant ganglioneuromatous component. Three subtypes based on distribution of SP elements within the predominant SR background are as follows: NB, SR nodular (one or more discrete, grossly visible nodules of stroma-poor neuroblastomatous tissue); NB, SR, intermixed (scattered nests of variably differentiated neuroblasts); and NB, SR, well-differentiated (a few randomly distributed immature neuroblastic cells)

a) NB—neuroblastoma.

TABLE 12-12 Recommended Terminology and Criteria for Neuroblastic Tumors

Tumor type	Criteria	Comment
Neuroblastoma (NB), undifferentiated, poorly differentiated, or differentiating*	Neuroblasts and neuropil constitute the predominant (>50%) or exclusive component of the tumor. A small minority of NBs contain small ganglioneuromatous focus or foci at the periphery or within the septa.	The three subtypes are recognized on the basis of proportion of differentiating neuroblasts (0, ≤5 and >5%, respectively). Shimada terminology for this tumor would be stroma-poor NB.
Ganglioneuroma (GN)	The tumor is composed exclusively of mature ganglion cells, neurites accompanied by Schwann cells, and fibrous tissue	Any degree of immaturity or atypia of ganglion cells or Schwann cells in a tumor that otherwise resembles GN, negates that diagnosis. Such tumors would be designated as borderline ganglioneuroblastomatous (see below). Adequate sampling is essential.
Ganglioneuroblastoma (GNB), nodular, intermixed, or borderline[a]	The tumor is composed of a predominant ganglioneuromatous component (>50%) and a small neuroblastomatous component.	The three subtypes are recognized on the basis of type of neuroblastomatous component (Shimada terminology for GNB would be stroma-rich NB). In almost all GNBs the GN component is far in excess of 50%. Nodular GNB has a single or few grossly demonstrable neuroblastomatous nodules; intermixed GNB has a few well-defined microscopic neuroblastomatous foci and borderline GNB has a few poorly defined neuroblastomatous foci (see comment with reference to GN above).

Table 12-12 Continued

Tumor type	Criteria	Comment
Transitional Neuroblastic Tumor	The tumor is composed of approximately equal proportions of neuroblastomatous and ganglioneuromatous components.	Presumptive tumor since no example was encountered in the review of cases.
Neuroblastoma, not otherwise specified (NOS)	Clusters of neuroblastic cells or foci of neuroblastoma are seen.	This diagnosis should be made when the features mentioned are seen in a bone marrow aspirate, bone marrow biopsy, FNA or incisional biopsy of primary or metastatic tumor or in a histologically inadequately sampled primary tumor resected before or after other mode(s) of therapy. (There is a remote possibility that the FNA or incisional biopsy may sample only the neuroblastomatous nodule of nodular GNB.)
Mixed neuroblastic tumor, not otherwise specified (NOS)	The tumor is composed of neuroblastomatous and ganglioneuromatous elements in unknown proportions.	The diagnosis should be made when the features mentioned are seen in an incisional or FNA biopsy of primary or metastatic tumor or in a histologically inadequately sampled primary tumor resected before or after other mode(s) of therapy.

[a]The subtyping of NB and GNB should be done only on histologically adequately sampled primary tumors resected before other mode(s) of therapy. Adequate histologic sampling is defined as one section for each centimeter of the longest dimension of the resected primary tumor.

TABLE 12-13 Prognostic Categorization of Neuroblastic Tumors According to Shimada Classification

Category	Favorable histology	Unfavorable histology
NB[a], stroma-rich[b] at any age	Well-differentiated[c] and intermixed subtypes	Nodular subtype
NB, stroma-poor at age <18 months	Any subtype with MKI[d] <200	Any subtype MKI >200
NB, stroma-poor at age 18 to 60 months	Differentiating subtype with MKI <100	Differentiating subtype with MKI >100 *or* undifferentiated subtype with any MKI
NB, stroma-poor, at age >60 months	None	All subtypes

Notes: a) NB—neuroblastoma; b) NB, stroma-rich category is designated as ganglioneuroblastoma in the modified conventional terminology; c) This subtype is designated as ganglioneuroblastoma of borderline subtype in modified conventional terminology; d) MKI—mitosis karyorrhexis index.

helpful in arriving at the correct interpretation, particularly in cases in which the diagnostic cytologic features may not be present. However, the precise primary site may not be known in a particular case, and it is the best policy to rely on whatever morphologic evidence one has for a particular interpretation. Electron microscopy of the FNA specimen would provide diagnostic clues in a case of retroperitoneal SRCT (e.g., oligocilia, microvilli, phagolysosomes, and basement-membrane-like flocculant material in blastemal Wilms' tumor and the typical ultrastructural features of NB described in the section on NB). It should be kept in mind that individual types of SRCTs can arise in and metastasize to unusual sites (e.g., NB of kidney and NB metastasis to the lung) (Tables 12-2, 12-3). In some instances the characteristic cytologic findings need to be considered in the clinical context. For example, a tumor arising in a black child or in a white infant showing mostly clusters of undifferentiated round cells with a few structures suggestive of rosettes is unlikely to be ES since ES is extremely rare in black children and ES usually is seen in older white children. Cytogenetic studies are helpful in distinguishing between NB and PNET and confirming the diagnosis of Burkitt's NHL.

TABLE 12-14 Histologic Grading of Neuroblastomas[a]

Grade	Criteria
1	Calcification *and* low mitotic rate[b]
2	Calcification or low mitotic rate
3	Absence of calcification and of low mitotic rate[c]

Notes: a) Shimada classification is used for prognostic categorization of ganglioneuroblastomas (Table 12-13); b) Low mitotic rate = ≤10/10 high power fields (hpf); c) Absence of low mitotic rate = presence of high mitotic rate (>10/10 hpf).

TABLE 12-15 Cytologic Differential Features of PNET and Other Small Round Cell Tumors of Childhood[a]

Cytologic features	PNET	NB	ES	BL	LL	RMS	WT
Nuclear molding	+	+	±	–	–	–	±
Nucleoli	–	–	–	+ (2–5)	–	±	–
Ganglion cells	–	±	–	–	–	–	–
Neuropil	–	+	–	–	–	–	–
Cytoplasmic vacuoles	+	–	+ (glycogen)	+ (lipid)	–	–	–
Cytoplasmic tags	±	±	–	–	–	+	–
Homer Wright rosettes	± Rare	+	± Rare	–	–	–	–
Tubules	–	–	–	–	–	–	+
Lymphoglandular bodies	–	–	–	+	+	–	–
Macrophages	±	±	–	+	±	–	–
Myxoid matrix	–	–	–	–	–	±	–
Fibrous matrix	–	–	–	–	–	–	+
Spindle-shaped cells	–	–	–	–	–	+	±
Tadpole or ribbon-shaped cells	–	–	–	–	–	+	±
Dense cytoplasm	–	–	–	–	–	+	±
Karyorrhectic cells	–	+	–	+	±	–	–

[a]Abbreviations: PNET—primitive neuroectodermal tumor; NB—neuroblastoma; ES—Ewing's sarcoma; BL—Burkitt's lymphoma; LL—lymphoblastic lymphoma; RMS—rhabdomyosarcoma; WT—Wilms' tumor; + = frequently present or prominent; ± = may be present (rare) or inconspicuous; + = absent.

Reprinted from Silverman et al: *Acta Cytol* 36:541, 1992.

Gross Features of SRCTs

Gross features can provide clues to the diagnosis. Foci of calcification are characteristically seen in NBs (Figure 12-38). Fish-flesh appearance is seen in NHLs. The embryonal RMS may show "myxoid" areas. The polypoid configuration is present in sarcoma botyroides. Dark-red to purple appearance of the external and cut surfaces is frequently present in NB because of hemorrhage probably related to surgical resection of the tumor. The hemorrhagic areas in rare instances may show cystic change.

Histologic Diagnosis of SRCT

The aforementioned comments pertaining to clinical considerations, primary and metastatic sites, and ancillary studies such as electron microscopy and cytogenetics also apply to the histologic diagnosis of SRCT on a biopsy or resection specimen. The triaging may have to be prioritized if only a needle biopsy or a small incisional biopsy is available. In some cases the crush artifact will further reduce the amount of diagnostic tissue available (Figure 12-39).

The diagnostic clues are provided by the features of individual tumor cells (nuclear shape, amount and staining quality of the cytoplasm, shape of the cell, etc.) and patterns (diffuse, nesting, lack of cohesiveness, etc.) (Tables 12-4, 12-7).

The details of nuclear and cytoplasmic features of the tumor cells are best seen in properly prepared and properly stained imprints of the cut surface of the

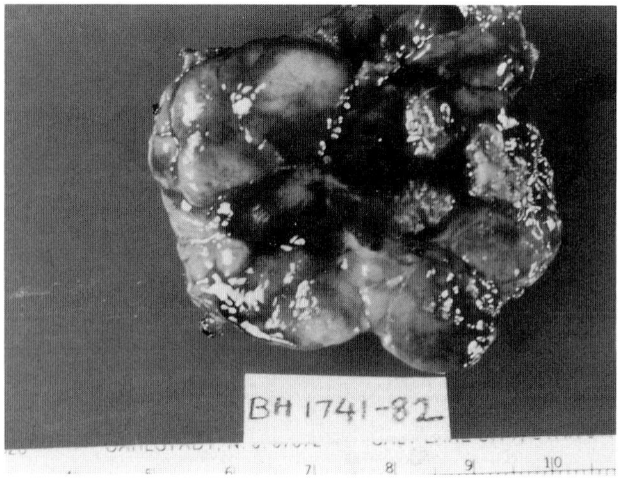

FIGURE 12-38. Gross photograph of neuroblastoma showing calcification (the whitish punctate areas shown by arrows).

tumor. Unusual or uncharacteristic features may be present in rare cases of SRCT; for example, cells of NHL may show cohesive pattern of starry sky pattern may be focally present in a NB.[17] Special attention should be paid to cytologic features that might be indicative of differentiation. For example, cells intermediate between neuroblasts and ganglion cells and rhabdomyoblasts would provide clues to the diagnosis. SRCTs infiltrating the muscle may produce secondary changes in the muscle cells that can be readily distinguished from features of neoplastic rhabdomyoblasts (Figure 12-40).

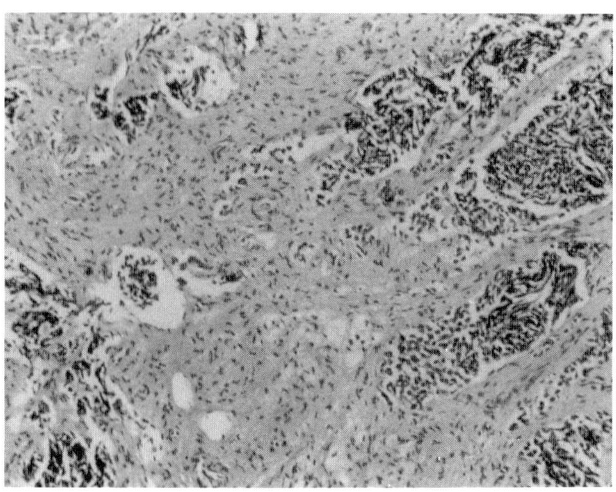

FIGURE 12-39. Small biopsy of a small round cell tumor showing crush artifact (H&E, ×40).

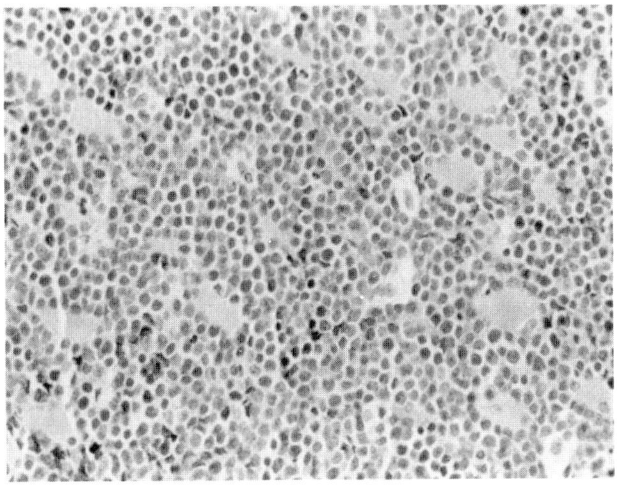

FIGURE 12-40. Lymphoblastic lymphoma infiltrating the pelvic muscle; note the entrapped muscle cells (H&E, ×250).

Special stains such as trichrome, reticulin, and PAS stains are often helpful in providing clues or confirming diagnosis. For example, the striations in rhabdomyoblasts may be better visible on a trichrome stain. The PAS with and without diastase is helpful in demonstrating the presence of glycogen in ES. Absence of reticulin is seen in ES. In the current era of immunoperoxidase stains, these simple special stains are often neglected.

Immunoperoxidase Stains in the Diagnosis of SRCT

These stains are widely applied in the current practice of surgical pathology. Although not required by the National Pediatric Cancer Study Groups, it is imperative that an attempt be made to confirm the histologic diagnosis of a particular type of SRCT by specific immunoperoxidase stain(s). NSE, LCA, muscle-specific actin (MSA), and vimentin could be used as the primary panel of immunohistological stains for diagnosis of SRCT. If the results of these are inconclusive, other "neural" markers (S-100, NFP, GFAP, Leu-7, etc.), muscle markers (myoglobin, desmin), and other markers (cytokeratin, β_2-microglobulin, MIC2) may be tested. In most instances results confirmatory of the histologic impression or diagnosis will be obtained. In cases with overlapping results, e.g., NSE and MSA being positive, or with totally negative results for all markers, other methods such as electron microscopy, cytogenetics, and molecular biologic studies may have to be used. If a diagnosis of NHL is made, the immunophenotyping is done by flow cytometry and/or by immunohistology on frozen or paraffin sections.

In the use and interpretation of the immunohistologic stains, the following aspects should be kept in mind:

1. Overfixation of tissue (for >72 hours in formalin) interferes with the quality of staining due to antigenic cross-linking.[150] Proteolytic enzymes such as

trypsin, pepsin, and pronase can be used for breaking the antigenic cross-linkage and to restore immunoreactivity.[151]
2. Monoclonal antibodies are preferred to polyclonal ones.
3. The concentration of antibody and enzyme complex components for getting a proper result may have to be worked out for the individual laboratory.
4. Commercially available kits should be obtained from reputable manufacturers. The type of tissue (frozen or fixed or either) for which the kit is suitable should be ascertained from the product representative.
5. Unexpected positive staining for a particular marker may be due to cross reactivity and therefore can be categorized as a false-positive reaction. This can happen with polyclonal antibodies. However, the unexpected positive result (e.g., cytokeratin in RMS, desmin in PNET) may be due to aberrant synthesis of a protein by the tumor, progenitor cells of which do not normally synthesize the protein.
6. Negative controls must be included in the immunostaining procedure.
7. Results of stain for certain markers may be more consistent in some laboratories than in other laboratories. For example, myoglobin may give more consistent results in one laboratory whereas MSA is preferred in another laboratory.
8. Specificity of a particular marker for a particular SRCT may not be absolute but may be related to quantitative differences in the level of expression and sensitivity of a particular technique. For example, Biggs et al[152] detected MIC2 expression by polymerase chain reaction on reversed transcribed mRNA in the cell lines derived from ES, PNET, NB, and RMS. The level of expression was markedly lower in RMS and NB than in ES and PNET. Immunohistologic stain for MIC2 on the cell lines showed focal staining in RMS and faint to absent staining in NB.
9. False-positive reaction may be obtained because of passive diffusion of proteins from surrounding or entrapped normal tissues to the tumor cells (Figures 12-40, 12-41).[93]

Immunohistology vs. Electron Microscopy

Electron microscopy (EM) as a method of diagnosis is being used less frequently since the advent of immunohistologic staining procedure. EM is also more expensive and time-consuming. However, EM can be helpful in cases in which immunohistology is inconvlusive. For example, in a case of PNET in whichNSE is negative, short cytoplasmic processes may be present on EM.[6] In certain cases of RMS, EM can be helpful when immunohistology is inconclusive.[18] EM is particularly helpful in the small FNA biopsy specimens of SRCT. It appears that in contrast to adult tumors, pediatric tumors and particularly SRCTs lend themselves better to specific ultrastructural diagnosis. Therefore, a small portion of the biopsy or resected tumor should always be fixed in glutaraldehyde. The decision regarding whether EM needs to be done can be taken after the results of routine histology and immunohistology are available. It should also be noted that in certain cases of NB and RMS with nondiagnostic EM features, immunohistology can give diagnostic results.[2,18]

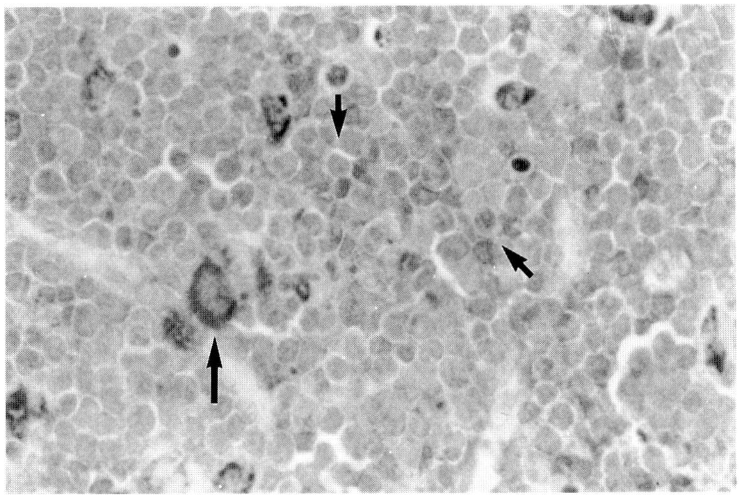

FIGURE 12-41. Immunoperoxidase stain for muscle-specific actin (MSA) showing positive staining in the muscle cells entrapped in an infiltrating lymphoblastic lymphoma (large arrow); note that a few of the tumor cells also show positive reaction (small arrows) (immunoperoxidase stain for muscle-specific actin, ×400).

Divergent Differentiation in SRCT

Evidence of divergent differentiation may be seen in SRCT. For example, myoid and epithelium-like cells, cartilage, and bone have been described in PNET[37,38] Divergent differentiation may be evident on immunohistologic staining; for example, cytokeratin, NSE, or NFP may be positive in certain cases of RMS.[90] However, positive staining for myoglobin seen in cases of non-RMS infiltrating the skeletal muscle is not due to divergent differentiation, but due to passive diffusion of protein into the tumor cells. True divergent differentiation characterized by presence of ganglion cells and rhabdomyoblasts is seen in ectomesenchymoma, which is a rare neuroectodermal tumor. Entrapped ganglion cells, neuritic processes, and skeletal muscle fibers in an infiltrating SRCT should not be misinterpreted as divergent differentiation.

Therapeutic Implications of the Pathologic Diagnosis of SRCT

There are specific protocols of chemotherapy and radiation therapy (alone or in combination) for specific types of SRCT. Table 12-9 (p. 391) lists the different drugs used in the treatment of specific SRCTs. These drugs are used in different dosages given at different intervals and for variable periods. Therefore, it is imperative that every attempt be made to render an accurate diagnosis of the SRCT in children.

Undiagnosed SRCTs and Related Lesions

In extremely rare instances, the precise diagnosis of the type of SRCT maynot be evident despite all the morphologic and cytogenetic studies done in that case.

It is imperative that such a case be sent to a consultant who will have more experience in dealing with undiagnosed SRTCs and the resources to do further immunocytochemical and molecular biologic studies. In any event, the consultant will be able to collect a sizable number of such cases that may have certain common previously unrecognized features. Thus a new entity in SRCTs or related lesions might emerge. Small cell desmoplastic tumors with divergent differentiation and extrarenal malignant rhabdoid tumor serve as examples of relatively recently characterized tumors.

REFERENCES

1. Dehner LP: A contemporary view of neoplasms in children: *Pediatr Clin N Am* 36:113–137, 1989.
1. Triche TJ, Askin FB: Neuroblastoma and the differential diagnosis of small-, round-, blue-cell tumors. *Hum Pathol* 14:569–595, 1983.
3. Variend S: Small cell tumors in childhood. A review. *J Pathol* 145:1–25, 1985.
4. Schmidt D, Harms D, Pilon VA: Small cell pediatric tumors: Histology, immunohistochemistry and electron microscopy. *Clin Lab Med* 7:63–89, 1986.
5. Triche TJ: Round cell tumors in childhood: The application of newer techniques to the differential diagnosis: *Pediatr Pathol* 7:279–322, 1982.
6. Marina NM, Etcubanas E, Parham DM, et al: Peripheral primitive neuroectodermal tumor (peripheral neuroepithelioma) in children. A review of the St. Jude experience and controversies in diagnosis and management. *Cancer* 64:1952–1960, 1989.
7. Spjut HJ, Ayala AG: Skeletal tumors in childhood and adolescence. In *Pathology of neoplasia in children and adolescents* (Finegold M, Ed. Saunders, Philadelphia, 1986, Chap 10, pp 256–281.
8. Joshi VV, Kaur P, Ryan B, et al: Mucoid anaplastic hepatoblastoma. *Cancer* 54:2035–2040, 1984.
9. Beckwith JB: Wilms' tumor and other renal tumors in children. *Hum Pathol* 14:481–492, 1983.
10. Plotsky C, Jaffe R, Curley J, et al: A retrospective review of undifferentiated malignancy in childhood. *Am J Pediatr Hematol Oncol* 12:141–146, 1990.
11. Gonzales-Crussi F, Crawford SE, Sun CCJ: Intraabdominal desmoplastic small-cell tumors with divergent differentiation. *Am J Surg Pathol* 14:633–642, 1990.
12. Hayes FA, Smith EI: Neuroblastoma. In *Principles and practice of pediatric oncology* (Pizzo PA, Poplack DG, Eds). Lippincott, Philadelphia, 1989, Chap 28, pp 607–622.
13. Wilson LMK, Draper GJ: Neuroblastoma, its natural history and prognosis: A study of 487 cases. *Br Med J* 3:301–307, 1974.
14. Joshi VV, Cantor AB, Altshuler G, et al: Age-linked prognostic categorization based on a new histologic grading system of neuroblastomas: A clinicopathologic study of 211 cases from the Pediatric Oncology Group. *Cancer* 69:2197–2211, 1992.
15. Joshi VV, Chatten J, Sather HN, et al: Evaluation of the Shimada classification in advanced neuroblastoma. *Mod Pathol* 4:139–147, 1991.
16. Joshi VV, Cantor AB, Altshuler G, et al: Recommendations for modification of terminology of neuroblastic tumors and prognostic significance of Shimada classification. *Cancer* 69:2183–2196, 1992.
17. Joshi VV, Silverman JF, Altshuler G, et al: Systematization of primary, histopathologic and fine-needle aspiration cytologic features and description of unusual histopathologic features of neuroblastic tumors. A report from the Pediatric Oncology Group. *Hum Pathol* (in press).

18. Mierau GW, Berry PJ, Orsini EN: Small round cell neoplasms: Can electron microscopy and immunohistochemical studies accurately classify them? *Ultrastr Pathol* 9:99–111, 1988.
19. Triche TJ: Neuroblastoma and other childhood neural tumors. A review. *Pediatr Pathol* 10:175–193, 1990.
20. Brodeur GM, Seeger RC, Schwab M, et al: Amplification of N-myc in untreated human neuroblastomas correlates with advanced disease stage. *Science* 224:1121–1124, 1984.
21. Seeger RC, Brodeur GM, Sather H, et al: Association of multiple copies of N-myc oncogene with rapid progression of neuroblastomas. *N Engl J Med* 313:1111–1116, 1985.
22. Chang TK, Chin-Yang L, Smithson WA: Immunocytochemical study of small round cell tumors in routinely processed specimens. *Pathol Lab Med* 113:1343–1348, 1989.
23. Tsokos M, Linnoila RI, Chandra RS, et al: Neuron-specific enolase in the diagnosis of neuroblastoma and other small round cell tumors in children. *Hum Pathol* 15:575–584, 1984.
24. Taylor CR: *Immunomicroscopy: A diagnostic tool for the surgical pathologist.* Saunders, Philadelphia, 1986, pp 169, 340.
25. Triche TJ, Silsby B, Scarpa S, et al: Extracellular matrix protein synthesis by childhood tumors. *Lab Invest* 48:14P, 1983.
26. Christiansen H, Lampert F: Tumor karyotype discriminates between good and bad prognostic outcome in neuroblastoma. *Br J Cancer* 57:121–126, 1988.
27. Douglass EC, Green AA, Hayes FA, et al: Chromosome 1 abnormalities: A common feature of pediatric solid tumors. *J Natl Cancer Inst* 75:51–54, 1985.
28. Hayashi Y, Inaba T, Hanada R, et al: Chromosome findings and prognosis in 15 patients with neuroblastoma found by VMA screening. *J Pediatr* 112:567–571, 1988.
29. Triche TJ, Cavazzana AO, Navarro CP, et al: N-myc protein expressions in small round cell tumors. *Adv Neurobl Res* 2:475–485, 1988.
30. Schwab M, Ellison J, Busch M, et al: Enhanced expression of the human gene N-myc consequent to amplification of DNA may contribute to malignant progression of neuroblastoma. *Proc Natl Acad Sci USA* 81:4940–4944, 1984.
31. Garson JA, Clayton J, McIntyre P, et al: N-myc oncogene amplification in rhabdomyosarcoma at release. *Lancet* 1:1496, 1986.
32. Nisen PD, Zimmerman K, Cotter S, et al: Enhanced expression of the N-myc gene in Wilms' tumors. *Cancer Res* 46:6217–6222, 1986.
33. Tsokos M, Scarpa S, Ross RA, et al: Differentiation of human neuroblastoma recapitulates neural crest development. Study of morphology, neurotransmitter enzymes and extracellular matrix proteins. *Am J Pathol* 128:484–496, 1987.
34. Jaffe R, Santamaria M, Yunis ES, et al: The neuroectodermal tumor of bone. *Am J Surg Pathol* 8:885–898, 1984.
35. Stout AP: A tumor of the ulnar nerve. *Proc NY Pathol Soc* 18:2–12, 1918.
36. Israel MA, Miser JS, Triche TJ, et al: Neuroepithelial tumors. In *Principles and practice of pediatric oncology* (Pizzo PA, Poplack DG, Eds). Lippincott, Philadelphia, 1989, Chap 29, pp 623–634.
37. Schmidt D, Harms D, Burdach S: Malignant peripheral neuroectodermal tumors of childhood and adolescence. *Virchows Arch (Pathol Anat)* 406:351–365, 1985.
38. Hashimoto H, Enjoji M, Nakajima T, et al: Malignant neuroepithelioma (peripheral neuroblastoma). A clinicopathologic study of 15 cases. *Am J Surg Pathol* 7:309–318, 1983.
39. Dehner LP: Primitive neuroectodermal tumors. ASCP Teleconference, June 15, 1990.

40. Llombart-Bosch A, Terrier-Lacombe MJ, Peydro-Olaya A, et al: Peripheral neuroectodermal sarcoma of soft tissue (peripheral neuroepithelioma): A pathologic study of ten cases with differential diagnosis regarding other small round cell sarcomas. *Hum Pathol* 20:273–280, 1989.
41. Cavazzana AO, Ninto V, Montesco M, et al: Peripheral neuroepithelioma. Morphologic and immunologic criteria for diagnosis. *Mod Pathol* 1:17A, 1988.
42. Parham DM, Dias P, Kelly DR, et al: Desmin positivity in primitive neuroectodermal tumors of childhood. *Am J Surg Pathol* 16:483–492, 1992.
43. Ewing J: Diffuse endothelioma of bone. *Proc NY Pathol Soc* 21:17, 1921.
44. Enzinger FM, Weiss SW: *Soft tissue tumors*, 2nd ed. Mosby, St. Louis, 1988, pp 951–958.
45. Shimada H, Newton WA, Soule EH, et al: Pathologic features of extraosseous Ewing's sarcoma: A report from the intergroup rhabdomyosarcoma study. *Hum Pathol* 19:442–453, 1988.
46. Willis RA: *Pathology of tumors*. Butterworths, London 1967, pp 702–703.
47. Angerwall L, Enzinger FM: Extraskeletal neoplasms resembling Ewing's sarcoma. *Cancer* 36:240, 1975.
48. Pritchard DJ, Daffin DC, Dauphine RT, et al: Ewing's sarcoma. *J Bone Joint Surg* 57A:10, 1974.
49. Maygarden SJ, Askin FB, Siegal GD, et al: Ewing's sarcoma of bone in infants and toddlers. A clinicopathologic report from Intergroup Ewing's Study. *Cancer* 71:2109–2118, 1993.
50. Fraumeni JF, Glass AG: Rarity of Ewing's sarcoma among US negro children. *Lancet* 1:366, 1979.
51. Miser JS, Triche TJ, Pritchard DJ, et al: Ewing's sarcoma and the nonrhabdomyosarcoma soft tissue sarcomas of childhood. In *Principles and practice of pediatric oncology* (Pizzo PA, Poplack DG, Eds). Lippincott, Philadelphia, 1989, pp 659–688.
52. McKeen EA, Hanson MR, Mulhivill J, et al: Birth defects in Ewing's sarcoma. *N Engl J Med* 309:1522, 1983.
53. Lyall EGH, Langdale-Brown B, Eden OB, et al: Ewing's sarcoma in a child with HIV (type 1) infection. *Med Pediatr Oncol* 21:127–131, 1993.
54. Kissane JM, Askin FB, Foulkes M, et al: Ewing's sarcoma of bone: Clinicopathologic aspects of 303 cases from the intergroup Ewing's sarcoma study. *Hum Pathol* 14:773–779, 1983.
55. Soule EH, Newton WA, Moon TE, et al: Extraskeletal Ewing's sarcoma. A preliminary review of 26 cases encountered in the intergroup rhabdomyosarcoma study. *Cancer* 42:259–264, 1978.
56. Nasimento AG, Unni KK, Cooper KL, et al: A clinicopathologic study of 20 cases of large cell (atypical) Ewing's sarcoma of bone. *Am J Surg Pathol* 4:29–36, 1980.
57. Erlandson RA: Ewing's sarcoma with intermediate filaments. *Ultrastr Pathol* 5:323–328, 1983.
58. Yunis EJ: Ewing's sarcoma and related small round cell neoplasms in children. *Am J Surg Pathol* 10:54–62, 1986.
59. Miettinen M, Lehto VP, Virtanen I: Histogenesis of Ewing's sarcoma. An evaluation of intermediate filaments and endothelial cell markers. *Virchows Arch B Cell Pathol* 41:277–284, 1982.
60. Navas-Palacios JJ, Aparicio-Duque R, Valdes MD: On the histogenesis of Ewing's sarcoma. An ultrastructural, immunohistochemical, and cytochemical study. *Cancer* 53:1882–1901, 1984.
61. Moll R, Lee I, Gould VE, et al: Immunochemical analysis of Ewing's tumors: *Am J Pathol* 127:288–304, 1987.
62. Fellinger EJ, Garin-Chesa P, Glasser DB, et al: Comparison of cell surface antigen

HBA71 (p30/32^{MIC2}), neuron-specific enolase, and vimentin in the immunohistochemical analysis of Ewing's sarcoma of bone. *Am J Surg Pathol* 16:746–755, 1992.
63. Fellinger EJ, Garin-Chesa P, Triche TJ, et al: Immunohistochemical analysis of Ewing's sarcoma cell surface antigen (p30/32^{MIC2}). *Am J Surg Pathol* 139:317–325, 1991.
64. Riopel MA, Dickman PS, Link M, et al: MIC2 analysis in pediatric lymphomas. *Mod Pathol* 6:128A, 1993 (abstract).
65. Garin-Chesa P, Fellinger EJ, Huvos AG, et al: Immunohistochemical analysis of neural cell adhesion molecules: Differential expression in small round cell tumors of childhood and adolescence. *Am J Pathol* 139:275–286, 1991.
66. Douglass EC, Valentine M, Green AA, et al: t(11,22) and other chromosomal rearrangements in Ewing's sarcoma. *J Natl Cancer Inst* 77:1211–1215, 1986.
67. Dehner LP: Primitive neuroectodermal tumor and Ewing's sarcoma. *Am J Surg Pathol* 17:1–13, 1993.
68. Editorial: Ewing's sarcoma and its congeners: An interim appraisal. *Lancet* 339:99–100, 1992.
69. Schmidt D, Herrmann C, Jurgens H, et al: Malignant peripheral neuroectodermal tumor and its necessary distinction from Ewing's sarcoma. *Cancer* 68:2251–2259, 1991.
70. Hijazi Y, Worthy E, Steinberg S, et al: Ewing's sarcoma (ES) vs. primitive neuroectodermal tumor (PNET)—Does histology play a role in prognosis? *Mod Pathol* 6:126A, 1993 (abstract).
71. Jurgens H, Exner U, Gadner H, et al: Multidisciplinary treatment of primary Ewing's sarcoma of bone: A 6 year experience of European co-operative trial. *Cancer* 61:23–32, 1988.
72. Raney RB, Hayes DM, Jeff M, et al: Rhabdomyosarcoma and the undifferentiated sarcomas: In *Principles and practice of pediatric oncology* (Pizzo PA, Poplack DG, Eds) Lippincott, Philadelphia, 1989, Chap 30, pp 635–658.
73. Newton WA, Soule EH, Hamondi AB, et al: Histopathology of childhood sarcomas, Intergroup Rhabdomyosarcoma Studies I and II: Clinicopathologic Correlation: *J Clin Oncol* 6:67–75, 1988.
74. Cailland JM, Gerard-Marchant R, Marsden HB, et al: Histopathologic classification of childhood rhabdomyosarcoma: A report from the International Society of Pediatric Oncology Pathology Panel. *Med Pediatr Oncol* 17:391–400, 1989.
75. Horn RC, Enterline HT: Rhabdomyosarcoma: A clinicopathologic study and classification of 39 cases: *Cancer* 11:181–199, 1958.
76. Kodet R, Newton WA, Hamoudi AB, et al: Childhood rhabdomyosarcoma with anaplastic (pleomorphic) features: A report of the Intergroup Rhabdomyosarcoma Study. *Am J Surg Pathol* 17:443–453, 1993.
77. Bale PM, Parsons RE, Stevens MM: Pathology and behavior of juvenile rhabdomyosarcoma. In *Pathology of neoplasia in childhood and adolescence* (Feingold M, Ed). Saunders, Philadelphia, 1986, pp 196–222.
78. Cavazzana AD, Schmidt D, Ninto V, et al: Spindle cell rhabdomyosarcoma: A prognostically favorable variant of rhabdomyosarcoma. *Am J Surg Pathol* 16:229–235, 1992.
79. Leuschner I, Newton WA, Schmidt D, et al: Spindle cell variants of embryonal rhabdomyosarcoma in the paratesticular region. *Am J Surg Pathol* 17:221–230, 1993.
80. Kodet R, Newton WA, Hamoudi AB, et al: Rhabdomyosarcomas with intermediate filament inclusions and features of rhabdoid tumors. Light microscopic and immunohistochemical study. *Am J Surg Pathol* 15:257–267, 1991.
81. Maurer HM, Gehan EA, Beltangady M, et al: The intergroup rhabdomyosarcoma study, II. *Cancer* 71:1904–1922, 1993.

82. Agamanolis DP, Dasu S, Krill CE: Tumors of skeletal muscle. *Hum Pathol* 17:778–795, 1986.
83. Tsokos M, Webber BL, Parham DM, et al: Rhabdomyosarcoma: A new classification scheme related to prognosis. *Arch Pathol* Lab Med 116:847–855, 1992.
84. Maurer HM, Beltangady M, Gehan EA, et al: The Intergroup Rhabdomyosarcoma Study—1. A final report. *Cancer* 61:209–220, 1988.
85. Ruymann FB, Maddux HR, Ragab A, et al: Congenital anomalies associated with rhabdomyosarcoma: An autopsy study of 115 cases. A report from the Intergroup Rhabdomyosarcoma Study Committee. *Med Pediatr Oncol* 16:33–39, 1988.
86. Douglas EC, Shapiro DN, Valentine M, et al: Alveolar rhabdomyosarcoma with the t(2;13): Cytogenetic findings and clinicopathologic correlations. *Med Pediatr Oncol* 21:83–87, 1993.
87. Ruymann FB, Newton WA, Ragab AH, et al: Bone marrow metastases at diagnosis in children and adolescents with rhabdomyosarcoma: A report from the Intergroup Rhabdomyosarcoma Study. *Cancer* 53:368–373, 1984.
88. Palmer N, Parsons RE, Stevens MM: Histopathology and prognosis in rhabdomyosarcoma (IRS-1): (Abstract C-660) *Proc Am Soc Clin Oncol* 1:120, 1982.
89. Palmer N, Foulkes M: Histopathology and prognosis in the second intergroup rhabdomyosarcoma study (IRS-II): *Proc Am Soc Clin Oncol* 2:229, 1983.
90. Miettinen M, Rapola J: Immunohistochemical spectrum of rhabdomyosarcomas and rhabdomyosarcoma-like tumors: Expression of cytokeratin and 68-kD neurofilament protein. *Am J Surg Pathol* 13:120–132, 1989.
91. Parham DM: Immunohistochemistry of childhood sarcomas: Old and new markers. *Mod Pathol* 6:133–137, 1993.
92. Carter RL, McCarthy KP, Machine LG, et al: Expression of desmin and myoglobin in rhabdomyosarcomas and in developing skeletal muscle. *Histopathology* 15:585–595, 1989.
93. Eusebi V, Bondi A, Rosai J, et al: Immunohistochemical localization of myoglobin in nonmuscular cells. *Am J Surg Pathol* 8:51–55, 1984.
94. DeJong SH, Van-Kessel-Van Vark M, Albus-Lutter Ch E, et al: Creatine kinase subunits M and B as markers in the diagnosis of poorly differentiated rhabdomyosarcomas in children. *Hum Pathol* 16:924–928, 1985.
95. Royds JA, Variend S, Timperley WR, et al: Comparison of beta enolase and myoglobulin as histological markers of rhabdomyosarcoma. *J Clin Pathol* 38:1258–1260, 1985.
96. Scrable H, Witte D, Shimada H, et al: Molecular differential pathology of rhabdomyosarcoma. *Genes Chromosom Cancer* 1:23–35, 1989.
97. Dias P, Parham DM, Shapiro DN, et al: Myogenic regulatory protein (MyoD1) expression in childhood solid tumors. Diagnostic utility in rhabdomyosarcoma. *Am J Pathol* 137:1283–1291, 1990.
98. Dias P, Parham DM, Shapiro DN, et al: Monoclonal antibodies to the myogenic regulatory protein MyoD1: Epitope mapping and diagnostic utility. *Cancer Res* 52:6431–6439, 1992.
99. Rosai J, Dias P, Parham DM, et al: MyoD1 protein expression in alveolar soft part sarcoma as confirmatory evidence of its skeletal muscle nature. *Am J Surg Pathol* 15:974–981, 1991.
100. Shapiro DN, Parham DM, Douglass EC, et al: Relationship of tumor-cell ploidy to histologic subtype and treatment outcome in children and adolescents with unresectable rhabdomyosarcoma. *J Clin Oncol* 9:159–166, 1991.
101. Douglass EC, Shapiro DN, Valentine M, et al: Alveolar rhabdomyosarcoma with the t(2;13): Cytogenetic findings and clinicopathologic correlations. *Med Pediatr Oncol* 21:83–87, 1993.

102. Houghton JA, Houghton PJ, Webber BL: Growth and characterization of childhood rhabdomyosarcomas as xenografts. *J Natl Cancer Inst* 68:437–443, 1982.
103. Murphy SB, Fairclough DL, Hutchison RE, et al: Non-Hodgkin's lymphomas of childhood: An analysis of histology, staging and response to treatment of 338 cases at a single institution. *J Clin Oncol* 7:186–193, 1989.
104. National Cancer Institute sponsored study of classifications of non-Hodgkin's lymphomas: Summary and description of a working formulation for clinical usage. The Non-Hodgkin's Lymphoma Pathologic Classification Project. *Cancer* 49:2112–2135, 1982.
105. Magrath IT: Malignant non-hodgkin's lymphomas: In *Principles and practice of pediatric oncology* (Pizzo PA, Poplack DG, Eds). Lippincott, Philadelphia, 1989, Chap 2, pp 415–456.
106. Griffith RC, Kelly DR, Nathwani BN, et al: A morphologic study of childhood lymphoma of lymphoblastic type: The Pediatric Oncology Group experience. *Cancer* 59:1126–1131, 1987.
107. Grumayer ER, Ladenstein RL, Alavc I, et al: B-cell differentiation pattern of cutaneous lymphomas in infancy and childhood. *Cancer* 61:303–308, 1988.
108. Miller ST, Wollmer N, Meyers PA, et al: Primary hepatic or hepatosplenic non-Hodgkin's lymphomas in children. *Cancer* 52:2285–2288, 1983.
109. Berry CL, Keeling JW: Gastrointestinal lymphoma in childhood. *J Clin Pathol* 23:459–463, 1970.
110. Epstein LG, DiCarlo FJ, Joshi VV, et al: Primary lymphoma of the central nervous sytem in children with AIDS. *Pediatrics* 82:355, 1988.
111. Haddy TB, Sandlund JT, Magrath IT: Testicular involvement in young patients with non-Hodgkin's lymphoma. *Am J Pediatr Hematol Oncol* 10:224–229, 1988.
112. Gilboa N, Lum GM, Urizar RE: Early renal involvement in acute lymphoblastic leukemia and nonHodgkin's lymphoma in children. *J Urol* 129:364–367, 1983.
113. Kjeldsberg CR, Wilson JF, Berard CW: Non-Hodgkin's lymphoma in children. *Hum Pathol* 14:612, 1983.
114. Pinto A, Hutchinson RE, Grant LH, et al: Follicular lymphomas in pediatric patients. *Mod Pathol* 3:308–313, 1990.
115. Cossman J: Diffuse aggressive non-Hodgkin's lymphomas. In *Surgical pathology of the lymph nodes and related organs* (Jaffe ES, Ed). Saunders, Philadelphia, 1985, Chap 8, pp 203–217.
116. Bunin NJ, Hvizdala E, Link M, et al: Mediastinal non-Hodgkin's lymphomas in children: A clinicopathologic study. *J Clin Oncol* 4:154–159, 1986.
117. Kelly DR, Nathwani BN, Griffith RC, et al: A morphologic study of childhood lymphoma of undifferentiated type: The Pediatric Oncology Group experience. *Cancer* 59:1132–1137, 1987.
118. Nathwani BN, Griffith RC, Kelly DR, et al: A morphologic study of childhood lymphoma of the diffuse "histiocytic" type: The Pediatric Oncology Group experience. *Cancer* 59:1138–1142, 1987.
119. Herrera GA, Crofts JL, Roberts CR: Neurosecretory granule-like structures in lymphomas. *Hum Pathol* 11:449–457, 1990.
120. Warnke RA, Gatter KC, Falini B, et al: Diagnosis of human lymphoma with monoclonal antileukocyte antibodies. N Engl J Med 309:1275–1281, 1983.
121. Segal GH, Stoler MH, Fishleder AJ, et al: Reliable and cost-effective paraffin section immunohistology of lymphoproliferative disorders. *Am J Surg Pathol* 15:1034–1041, 1991.
122. Andrade RE, Wick MR, Frizzera G, et al: Immunophenotyping of hematopoietic malignancies in paraffin sections. *Hum Pathol* 19:394–402, 1988.

123. Ngan BY, Picker LJ, Medieros LJ, et al: Immunophenotypic diagnosis of non-Hodgkin's lymphoma in paraffin sections: Coexpression of L60 (leu 22) and L26 antigens correlates with malignant histologic findings. *Am J Clin Pathol* 91:579–583, 1989.
124. Schnitzer B, Roth MS, Hyder DM, et al: Ki-1 lymphomas in children. *Cancer* 61:1213–1221, 1988.
125. Macon WR, Williams ME, Greer JP, et al: T cell rich B cell lymphomas. *Am J Surg Pathol* 16:351–363, 1992.
126. Pinkus GS, O'Hara CJ, Said JW: Peripheral/post-thymic T cell lymphomas: A spectrum of disease, clinical pathologic and immunologic features of 78 cases. *Cancer* 65:971–998, 1990.
127. Kamps WA, Poppema S: Pre-B cell non-Hodgkin's lymphoma in childhood. Report of a case and review of literature. *Am J Clin Pathol* 90:103–107, 1988.
128. Gerald WL, Rosai J: Desmoplastic small cell tumor with divergent differentiation. *Pediatr Pathol* 9:177–183, 1989.
129. Gerald WL, Miller HK, Battifora H, et al: Intra-abdominal desmoplastic small round cell tumor: Report of 19 cases of a distinctive type of high grade polyphenotypic malignancy affecting young individuals. *Am J Surg Pathol* 15:499–513, 1991.
130. Gerald WL, Rosai J: Desmoplastic small cell tumor. Further assessment of a distinctive primitive malignant tumor of unknown histogenesis. *Mod Pathol* 6:6A, 1993.
131. Variend S, Gerrard M, Norris PD, et al: Intraabdominal neuroectodermal tumor of childhood with divergent differentiation. *Histopathology* 18:45–51, 1991.
132. Sawyer JR, Tryka AF, Lewis JM: A novel reciprocal chromosome translocation t(11;22) (p13;q12) in an intraabdominal desmoplastic small round cell tumor. *Am J Surg Pathol* 16:411–416, 1992.
133. Bendit I, Johnston J, Valderrama E, et al: Molecular phenotype of a pediatric small round cell tumor. *Cancer* 66:1524–1528, 1990.
134. Cozzutto C, Bronzini E, Brandelloni R, et al: Malignant monomorphic histiocytoma in children. *Cancer* 48:2112–2120, 1981.
135. Dehner LP: *Pediatric surgical pathology*, 2nd ed. Williams & Wilkins, Baltimore, 1987, p 902.
136. Lemos LB, Hamoudi AB: Malignant thymic tumor in an infant (malignant histiocytoma). *Arch Pathol Lab Med* 102:84–89, 1978.
137. Jacobsen SA: Polyhistiocytoma. A malignant tumor of bone and extraskeletal tissues. *Cancer* 40:2116–2130, 1977.
138. Scott L, Blair G, Taylor G, et al: Inflammatory pseudotumors in children. *J Pediatr Surg* 23:755–758, 1988.
139. Ayala AG, Ro JY, Raymond AK, et al: Small cell osteosarcoma. A clinicopathologic study of 21 cases. *Cancer* 64:2162–2173, 1989.
140. Beckwith JB, Palmer NF: Histopathology and prognosis of Wilms' tumors: Results from the First National Wilms' Tumor Study. *Cancer* 41:1937–1948, 1978.
141. Parham DM, Jenkins JJ, Holt H, et al: Phenotypic diversity in pediatric rhabdoid tumors: A morphologic and immunohistochemical study. *Lab Invest* 56:58A, 1987 (abstract).
142. Sotelo-Avila C, Gonzalez-Crussi F, deMello D, et al: Renal and extrarenal rhabdoid tumors in children. A clinicopathologic study of 14 patients. *Sem Diagn Pathol* 3:151–163, 1986.
143. Niffeneger JH, Jakobiec FA, Shore JW, et al: Adult extrarenal rhabdoid tumor of the lacrimal gland. *Ophthalmology* 99:567–574, 1992.
144. Weeks DA, Beckwith JB, Mierau G, et al: Renal neoplasms mimicking rhabdoid

tumor of kidney: A report from the National Wilms' Tumor Study Pathology Center. *Am J Surg Pathol* 15:1042–1054, 1991.

145. Kant JA, Jaffe ES: The interpretation of nonlymphoid elements in lymph node biopsy specimens. In *Surgical pathology of the lymph nodes and related organs* (Jaffe E, Ed). Saunders, Philadelphia, 1985, pp. 412–437.
146. Silverman JF, Berns LA, Holbrook CT, et al: Fine-needle aspiration cytology of primitive neuroectodermal tumors. *Acta Cytol* 36:541–550, 1992.
147. Silverman JF, Finley JL, O'Brien KF, et al: Diagnostic accuracy and the role of immediate interpretation of fine-needle aspiration biopsy specimen from various sites. *Acta Cytol* 33:791–796, 1989.
148. Silverman JF, Frable WJ: The use of the Diff-Quik stain in the immediate interpretation of fine-needle aspiration biopsies. *Diagn Cytopathol* 6:366–369, 1990.
149. Silverman JF, Joshi VV: Fine-needle aspiration biopsy of small round tumors of childhood: Cytomorphologic features and the role of ancillary studies. *Diagn Cytopathol* (in press).
150. Culling CF, Reid PE, Sinnott NH: The effect of various fixatives and trypsin digestion upon the staining of routine paraffin-embedded sections by peroxidase-antiperoxidase and immunofluorescent techniques. *J Histochem Cytochem* 3:10–19, 1980.
151. Battifora H, Kopinski M: The influence of protease digestion and duration and fixation on immunostaining of keratins. *J Histochem Cytochem* 34:1095–1100, 1986.
152. Biggs C, Rowland J, Crabbe D, et al: MIC-2 expression in small round cell tumors of childhood. *Mod Pathol* 6:126A, 1993 (abstract).

13 PATHOLOGY OF RENAL TUMORS IN CHILDREN

INTRODUCTION

Renal tumors in children constitute about 8% of all pediatric malignancies and are the second most common category of solid tumors outside the central nervous system. There are over 450 cases of pediatric renal tumors occurring every year in the United States; the overwhelming majority of these are Wilms' tumors (WTs). Beckwith in his detailed systematic study of the pathology of renal tumors in children, carried out since the inception of the National Wilms' Tumor Study (NWTS) in 1969, has made fundamental contributions resulting in the recognition of anaplastic WT, characterization of new entities such as clear cell sarcoma of the kidney (CCSK) and malignant rhabdoid tumor of the kidney (MRTK), and systematization and understanding of the significance of nephrogenic rests (NRs) and nephroblastomatosis (NPB).[1–4] The pathology of Wilms' tumor and its variants and other principal renal tumors in childhood are described in this chapter.

HISTOGENESIS OF WILMS' AND OTHER RENAL TUMORS IN CHILDREN

For a discussion of the histogenesis of tumors and how it is determined, see Chapter 10 on Pathology of Tumors in Children—General Aspects. The reader is referred to the detailed descriptions and illustrations of complex events during the development of the kidney given by Ekblom,[5] Mierau et al,[6] and Gonzalez-Crussi and Franklin.[7] From the point of view of the histogenesis of nephroblastic tumors, there are two main components involved in the renal development: (1) nephrogenic mesenchyme (NM) which is derived from the lower part of the nephrogenic cord, and (2) inducted metanephric blastema–ureteric bud (MB–UB) complex (Figure 13-1). Metanephric blastema is derived from NM and UB from the lower end of the mesonephric duct. There is a very close and continuous interactive reciprocal inductive influence of MB and UB on each other, extending from 6 to 34 weeks. Two broad categories of nephroblastic tumors linked to these components are proposed: (1) tumors arising from (and recapitulating) the derivatives of NM, and (2) tumors arising from (and recapitulating) inducted MB-UB complex. In the first category, the mesenchymal tumors, namely, congenital mesoblastic nephroma (CMN), cellular variant of CMN (CCMN), and CCSK are included. In the second broader category, the remaining nephroblastic tumors, namely, neoplastic NR, NPB, nephrogenic adenofibroma (NAF), composite WT and renal cell carcinoma (RCC), some cases of RCC, cystic nephroma (CN), and cystic partially differentiated nephroblastoma (CPDN) are included. In this category the tumors may be divided into two subgroups: (a) tumors arising from and recapitulating derivatives of inducted MB, and (b) those arising from and recapitulating UB. It must be emphasized that some overlap between the two main categories may occur since in some cases the mesenchymal tumors may recapitulate derivatives of transitional MB (i.e., MB which is between the uninducted stage and the early stages of induction). Thus there may be neoplastic epithelial (tubular) elements in some cases of the mesenchymal tumors.

Controversy and uncertainty surround the histogenetic considerations of MRTK. Based on ultrastructural and immunohistochemical features, nephrogenic mesenchyme, neuroectodermal cells, pleuripotent parental cells, myogenous cells, histiocytes, and epithelial cells have been implicated in the histogenesis.[3,8–10] Primitive neuroectodermal origin or origin from nephrogenic mesenchyme involved in renal medullary development are the two most plausible theories. The evidence for histogenesis is not conclusive. Therefore, MRTK is categorized as tumor of undetermined histogenesis.

CLASSIFICATION OF RENAL TUMORS

Tumors of the kidney in children can be classified on a histogenetic, morphologic, or behavioral basis. Classification based on a combined histogenetic and morphologic approach is presented in Figure 13-1 and Table 13-1. It must be emphasized that this classification is based on presumed or known histogenesis. What is shown diagrammatically in Figure 13-1 and outlined in Table 13-1 represents a conceptual framework. More definitive evidence becoming available in the future may necessitate deletion from and additions to the scheme without altering the basic conceptual framework.

STAGING OF RENAL TUMORS IN CHILDREN

The guidelines were developed by NWTS primarily for WT but these also apply to other renal tumors such as CCSK and MRTK.[11,12] Staging criteria for RCC are summarized in the section on RCC. Accurate staging is of practical importance since the therapeutic protocols, particularly for WT, are stage-related. The criteria for the different stages are given in Table 13-2.

Gross and Histologic Examination of the Resected Specimens

Following are the specific objectives of pathologic examination of the specimen: (1) to render the precise pathologic diagnosis (WT, CCSK, etc.); (2) in the cases of WT, to determine whether the tumor belongs to favorable histology (FH) or unfavorable histology (UH) subgroups; (3) to confirm (or extend) the surgical staging; (4) to determine microsubstaging of cases of Stage I FH WT; (5)

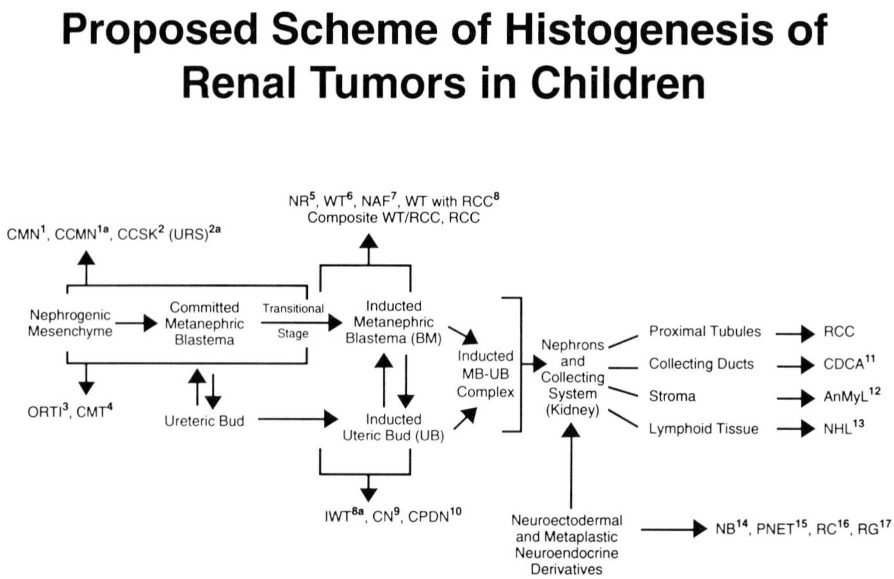

FIGURE 13-1. Diagrammatic representation of histogenesis of renal tumors of childhood. (1) CMN: congenital mesoblastic nephroma; (1a) CCMN: cellular variant of congenital mesoblastic nephroma; (2) CCSK: clear cell sarcoma of kidney; (2a) URS: Undifferentiated renal sarcoma; (3) ORTI: ossifying renal tumor of infancy; (4) CMT: cytodifferentiated mesenchymal tumor; (5) NR: nephrogenic rests; (6) WT: Wilms' tumor; (7) NAF: nephrogenic adenofibroma; (8) RCC: renal cell carcinoma; (8a) IWT: "intralobar" Wilms' tumor; (9) CN: cystic nephroma; (10) CPDN: cystic partially differentiated nephroblastoma; (11) CDCA: collecting duct carcinoma; (12) AnMyL: angiomyolipoma; (13) NHL: non-Hodgkin's lymphoma; (14) NB: neuroblastoma; (15) PNET: primitive neuroectodermal tumor; (16) RC: renal carcinoid; (17) RG: renal gastrinoma.

to determine whether the margins of surgical resection are free of tumor; and (6) to contribute adequate fresh tumor tissue for biologic studies undertaken by NWTS or other investigators and pathologic material for the NWTS pathology center. A thorough and systematic approach is required for meeting these objectives.[13,14] The details of gross examination and the technique of sampling for histologic examination are given in Table 13-3 and Figure 13-2. Careful examination of the external surface and margins of resection to detect any suspicious areas of invasion by tumor (Figure 13-3), prompt and proper collection of material for special studies (electron microscopy, flow cytometry, cytogenetics, molecular biologic studies for WT1 and other genes), and adequate histologic sampling are the most critical aspects of the gross examination. The histologic sections should be labeled so that one can determine what part of the resected specimen each section belongs to. The number of sections of the tumor is determined by the size of the tumor. The total number of sections should equal 1.5 times the mean of the three dimensions of the tumor (see Chapter 10 Pathology of Tumors in Children: General Aspects).

TABLE 13-1 Histogenetic[a] and Morphologic Classification of Renal Tumors in Children

I. Tumors arising from nephrogenic mesenchyme[b]
  1. Ossifying renal tumor of infancy
  2. Cytodifferentiated mesenchymal tumor (CMT)
  3. Classical congenital mesoblastic nephroma (CMN)
  4. Cellular or atypical variant of CMN (CCMN)
  5. Combined (classical and cellular) CMN
  6. Clear cell sarcoma of kidney (CCSK)
     (Focal or diffuse cystic change can occur in CMN, CCMN, and CCSK)

II. Tumors arising from inducted metanephric blastema–ureteric bud complex
  A. Tumors recaptiulating predominantly derivatives of inducted metanephric blastema
    1. Perilobar adenomatous nephrogenic rests (NRs)
    2. Nephrogenic adenofibroma (NAF)
    3. Perilobar nephroblastomatous NRs
    4. Nephroblastomatosis (NBM)
    5. Wilms' tumor (WR) ("perilobar" type)[c]
    6. WT showing foci of renal cell carcinoma (RCC)
    7. Composite WT and RCC
    8. Renal cell carcinoma (RCC)
  B. Tumors recapitulating predominantly inducted ureteric bud
    1. Intralobar adenomatous NRs
    2. Intralobar nephroblastomatous NRs
    3. WT ("intralobar" type)
    4. Cystic nephroma (CN)
    5. Cystic partially differentiated nephroblastoma (CPDN) conventional variant
       a. CPDN, papillonodular variant

III. Tumors arising from proximal tubules (originally derived from inducted metanephric blastema)
  1. Renal cell carcinoma (RCC)

IV. Tumors arising from collecting ducts (originally derived from inducted ureteric bud)
  1. Collecting duct carcinoma (CDCA)

V. Tumors arising from cells of juxtaglomerular apparatus
  1. Juxtaglomerular cell tumor

VI. Tumors of unknown histogenesis
  1. Malignant rhabdoid tumor of kidney (MRTK)

VII. Tumors arising from normally present, heterotopic or metaplastic neuroectodermal derivatives
  1. Neuroblastoma of kidney (NB)
  2. Primitive neuroectodermal tumor (PNET)
  3. Renal carcinoid (RC)
  4. Renal gastrinoma (RG)

VIII. Miscellaneous tumors
  1. Renal teratoma (RT)
  2. Benign and malignant mesenchymal tumors (angiomyolipoma, lymphangioma, rhabdomyosarcoma, leiomyosarcoma, unclassified sarcoma, etc.)
  3. Non-Hodgkin's lymphoma (NHL) (particularly Burkitt's type)

[a] Presumed or known histogenesis

[b] There may be some overlap, and tumors in this category may show derivatives of metanephric blastema which is between preinduction and early induction phase (transitional metanephric blastema)

TABLE 13-2 Criteria for Staging Malignant Renal Tumors in Children

Stage I.	Tumor limited to kidney with complete excision of tumor, intact renal capsule, and absence of: rupture of tumor before or during resection, residual tumor, extension of renal sinus infiltration beyond the renal hilus (outlined by the most medial extent of the renal parenchyma at the entrance to the sinus) or any extrarenal spread.
Stage II.	Extension of tumor beyond kidney (penetration of renal capsule and the perirenal soft tissue by tumor, renal sinus infiltration beyond the renal hilus, tumor thrombus in renal vein, biopsy including fine-needle aspiration with posterior approach,[a] local spillage during surgery confined to the flank), complete excision of tumor with no residual tumor and clear resection margins of the specimen.
Stage III.	Residual nonhematogenous tumor confined to abdomen characterized by any of the following: histologically proven metastasis to hilar, periaortic, or other distant abdominal lymph nodes; diffuse peritoneal contamination by tumor due to spillage of tumor beyond the flank before or during surgery or by penetration of peritoneal surface by tumor[a]; peritoneal implants of tumor; tumor at resection margin.
Stage IV.	Hematogenous metastasis (lung, bone, brain, liver).
Stage V.	Bilateral renal tumors (stage each side separately, e.g., right renal tumor, stage II; left renal tumor, stage I).

[a]Preoperative fine-needle aspiration biopsy (FNA) or intraoperative biopsy before nephrectomy will be considered as stage II or stage III depending upon the deemed extent of "spilling," i.e., whether it is confined to the local region (stage II) or whether there is peritoneal spillage (stage III). If anterior approach has been used for a biopsy (including FNA biopsy), the case may be considered as stage III.

PATHOLOGIC FEATURES OF RENAL TUMORS IN CHILDREN

The pathologic features of the principal tumors listed in Table 13-1 are described in this section. It should be emphasized that of all the pediatric renal tumors, WT is by far the commonest accounting for about 85% of the renal tumors in children. Many of the other tumors listed in Table 13-1, although relatively uncommon or rare are of importance because of the differences in their biologic behavior and the therapeutic approach.

Tumors Arising From or Recapitulating Derivatives of Nephrogenic Mesenchyme

Congenital Mesoblastic Nephroma (CMN)

Various diagnostic terms including spindle cell sarcoma, fibrosarcoma, leiomyoma, sarcoma, fibroma, leiomyomatous hamartoma, and fetal mesenchymal hamartoma had been used to designate this tumor until Bolande et al delineated it and gave it its current name.[15,16] In view of the subsequent recognition of the atypical or cellular variant of CMN with potential for aggressive behavior,[17] it is perhaps better to designate CMN merely as mesoblastic nephroma or as conventional or classical mesoblastic nephroma. But the term CMN is deeply entrenched and it appears that it will continue to be used. CMN accounts for about 2.8 to 5% of the renal neoplasms in childhood, i.e., about 12 to 20 cases are seen in the United States every year.

TABLE 13-3 Steps in the Gross Examination of Nephrectomy Specimen of Pediatric Renal Tumor

1. Weigh the specimen while still placed in the sterile container.
2. Examine the external surface for suspicious areas of invasion of renal capsule and perirenal fat by tumor (a bulge on the surface, adhesion between Gerota's fascia and renal capsule, area of roughening, etc.) (Figure 13-3).
3. Take histologic sections of the margin of resection of ureter and other hilar structures. Note whether a tumor thrombus is present at the resection margin of renal vein. If tumor is found at the margin of resection of the renal vein (Figure 13-3), the surgeon should be contacted to verify whether he indeed cut through the thrombus at the time of the operation. The apparent presence of tumor thrombus at the margin of renal vein may represent an artifact due to retraction of the vein after resection of the kidney.
4. Bivalve the specimen with sterile instruments, avoiding the area of concern on the external surface.
5. Take specimens for special studies (DNA analysis, cytogenetics, molecular biologic studies, electron microscopy, tumor bank). Make imprints from different portions of the tumor.
6. Photograph the external and cut surfaces of the entire specimen and the suspicious areas of the external surface.
7. Draw a diagram or take a Polaroid photograph of the external surface to show the location of the suspicious areas (Figure 13-2).
8. Ink the external surfaces of the two halves carefully.
9. Measure the specimen and the tumor. Note the gross characteristics of the tumor (single mass, multicentricity, location in the kidney, cystic change, etc.).
10. Remove lymph nodes, if any, from the hilus and send all of them for histologic examination.
11. Examine the renal sinus closely to note any tumor bulging or infiltrating into it. If there is renal sinus involvement, check whether it extends to the hilar plane.
12. Examine the surrounding uninvolved kidney for presence of grossly visible small (neoplastic nephrogenic rests) and large nodules (multinodular Wilms' tumor), cysts, or other abnormalities.
13. Make multiple incisions into the specimen, including incisions through the suspicious areas on the external surface, and examine the cut surface of these areas to note whether there is grossly visible infiltration of the perirenal fat or whether there is fusion of tumor capsule and renal capsule and further with the Gerota's fascia resulting in effacement of perirenal fat. Do *not* strip the capsule.
14. Fix the specimen in an adequate amount of formalin (5 to 10 times the size of the specimen) for several hours, make thinner slices of the tumor and the kidney or if the tumor appears to be multicystic, confirm that impression by serial bread-loafing of the tumor and ascertain that there are no solid mural tumor nodules.
15. Draw diagrams or take Polaroid photographs of the external and cut surfaces of the tumor to show the location of the tumor within the kidney and all notable features of the peripheral portions of the tumor (tumor and normal kidney interface, renal sinus, margin of resection of ureter, renal vein, etc.), hilar lymph nodes, and surrounding kidney.
16. Take sections from the suspicious area on the external surface, tumor and normal kidney interface, central portions of the tumor, renal sinus, hilar lymph node (if any), and the surrounding uninvolved kidney. Label each section and indicate on the diagrams or the Polaroid photographs the location of each section (Figure 13-2).

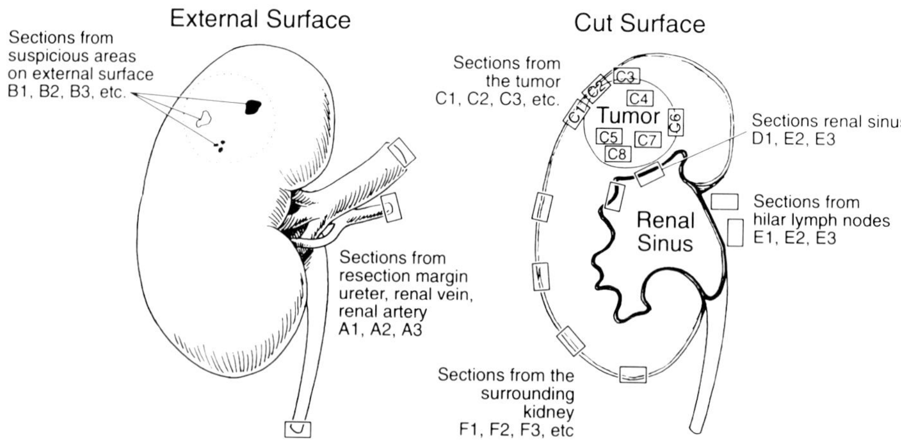

FIGURE 13-2. Diagram illustrating the histologic sampling and labeling of histologic sections of nephrectomy specimen.

Gross and Microscopic Features. In the 48 cases reviewed by Bolande,[16] the kidney was enlarged with an average weight of 138 g and measured 5–10 cm in the longest dimension. In the NWTS series,[18] the average weight was 290 g and extension of tumor into surrounding kidney, renal sinus, or perirenal fat was

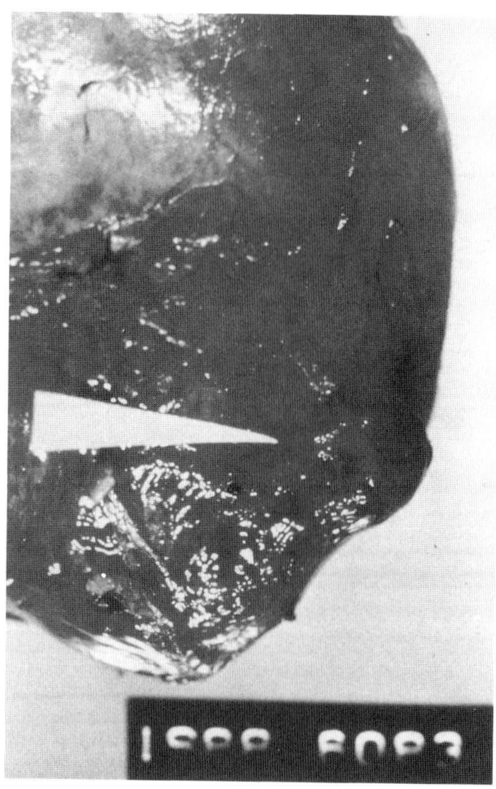

FIGURE 13-3A. Gross photograph of nephrectomy specimen showing a small bulge on the external surface (see Figure 13-33 for histologic features).

frequently noted. Extrarenal extension with involvement of colon or pancreas can occur in occasional cases. Renal vein invasion was present in one case in the NWTS series.[18] The histopathologic features of these NWTS cases were not described in the article and it is not clear whether any of the cases represented the cellular variant of CMN. The tumor is rubbery firm and gray-white to tan in color. On the cut surface it presents a characteristic trabeculated appearance reminiscent of uterine leiomyoma. A few cysts may be present. Rarely the entire tumor is multicystic due to dilatation of entrapped and possibly neoplastic tubular structures.[19] Areas of softening, necrosis, or hemorrhage are not seen in the classical CMN. Foci of calcification have been described by Fernbach et al.[20] On histologic examination no capsule can be demonstrated. The tumor is composed of spindle-shaped cells arranged in fascicles (Figure 13-4). These tumor cells are considered to be fibroblastic on the basis of histologic features seen by routine methods. Myxoid pattern may be focally present. CMN has characteristically low cellularity although occasional small areas or areas even up to 25% of the total tumor area examined microscopically may show increased cellularity.[16,21] The areas of normal and high cellularity merge abruptly (Figure 13-5A). Mitotic figures are rare. However, the more cellular areas may show somewhat prominent mitosis. There is often extension of tumor cells into the surrounding renal parenchyma due to an interdigitating growth pattern. The tumor may also extend to the renal hilus, the wall of renal pelvis and ureter and perirenal fat. Tubular and glomerular structures lined by cytologically normal

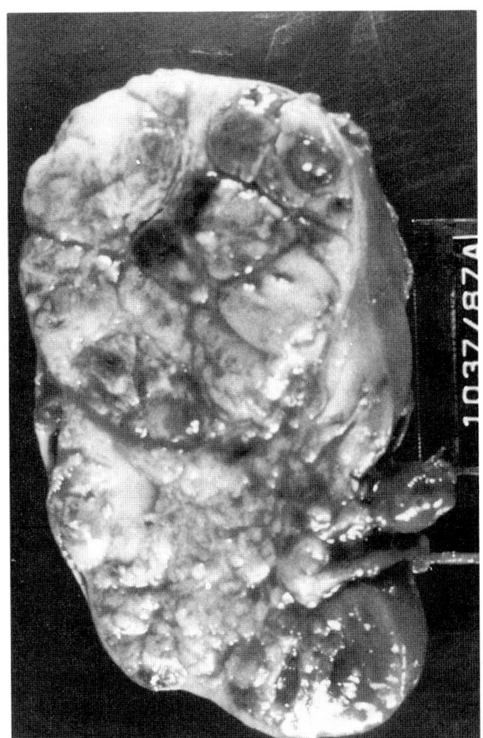

FIGURE 13-3B. Gross photograph of nephrectomy specimen showing marked renal vein distension (due to tumor thrombus which was seen in the section of the resection margin; not shown). Note the massive lobulated fleshy tumor replacing a large portion of the kidney and invading the renal sinus.

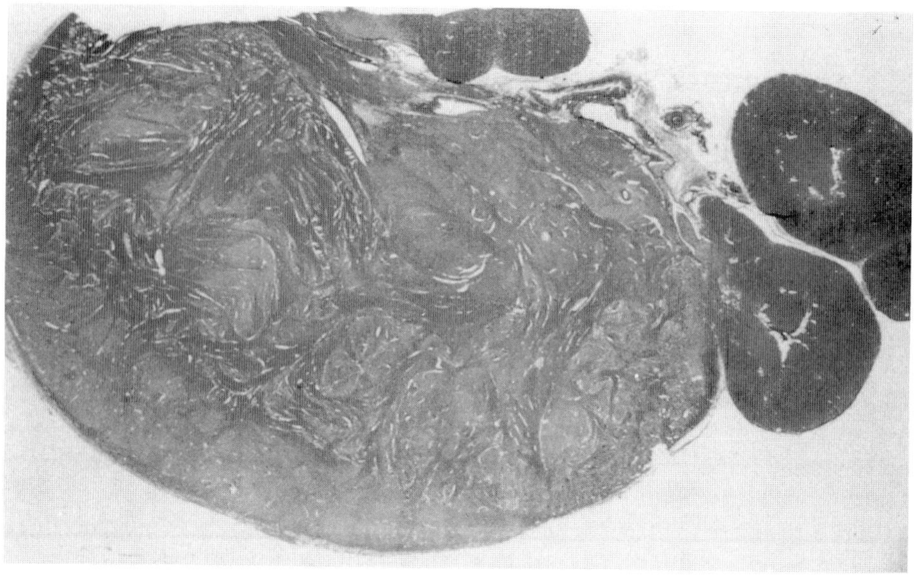

FIGURE 13-4A. Whole mount of congenital mesoblastic nephroma showing the trabecular appearance throughout the tumor. (Courtesy of Dr. John Fisher.)

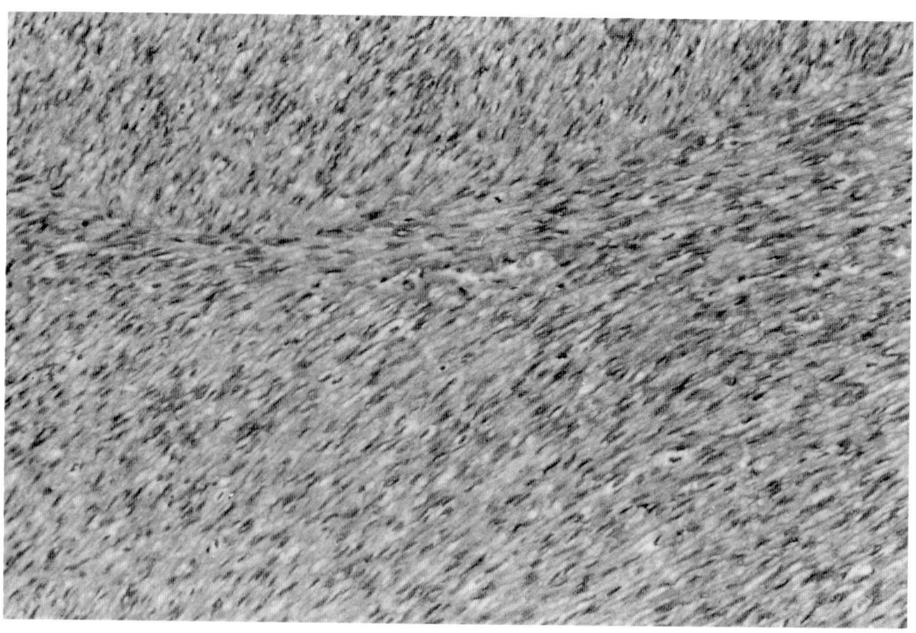

FIGURE 13-4B. Congenital mesoblastic nephroma composed of spindle-shaped cells arranged in fascicles (H&E, ×100).

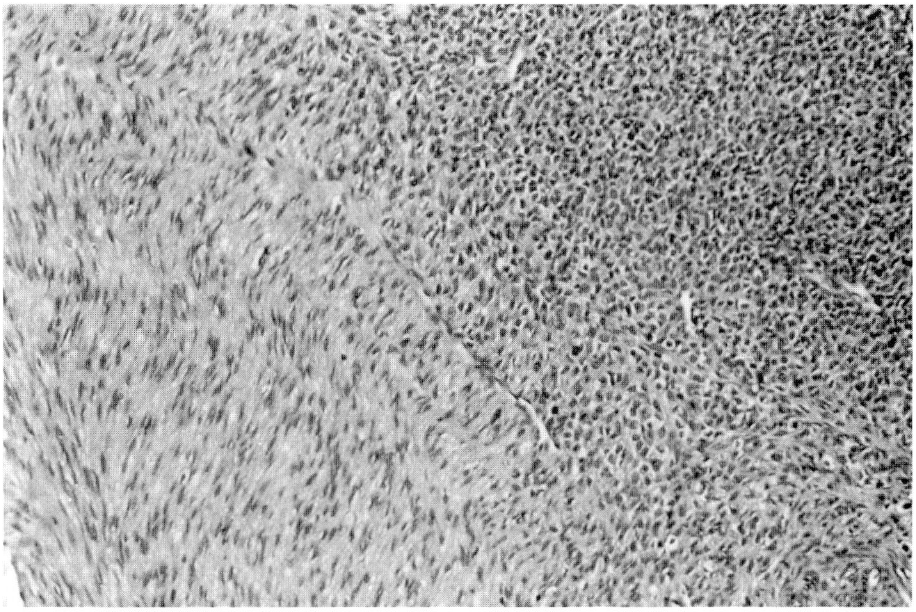

FIGURE 13-5A. Congenital mesoblastic nephroma showing a focus of high cellularity. The cellular area is composed of fusiform to oval compactly arranged cells. No fascicles are seen in the hypercellular area which merges abruptly with the normocellular area (H&E, ×100).

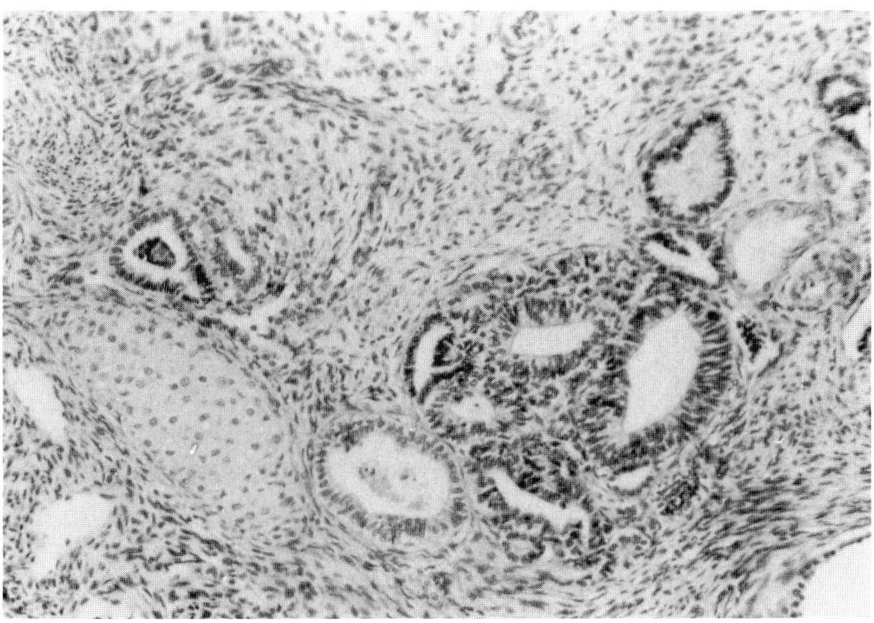

FIGURE 13-5B. A cluster of tubules lined by stratified epithelial cells with darkly staining nuclei in a congenital mesoblastic nephroma. Note the spicule of cartilage (H&E, ×100). (Courtesy of Dr. Robert P. Bolande.)

cells are often found at the periphery of the tumor. These constitute the entrapped structures belonging to the surrounding kidney. However, tubular and glomerular structures with irregular configuration lined by cells with hyperchromatic nuclei found in the deeper portion of the tumor probably represent neoplastic structures derived from the tumor (Figure 13-5B).[22] The other histologic features of CMN include presence of foci of hematopoiesis, spicules of cartilage, and prominent vascular structures exhibiting tortuosity and dilatation (Figure 13-5B). Squamous epithelium may be rarely seen.[23] Bolande[16] described and illustrated focal rhabdomyocytic differentiation occurring in some cases of CMN. However, it is generally believed that presence of rhabdomyocytic differentiation in a renal tumor negates the diagnosis of CMN. The cysts that may be present in CMN are lined by flattened to cuboidal epithelium. Taking sections from margins of resection of ureter, renal sinus, and any suspicious areas on the external surface is of great importance in the histological assessment of the nephrectomy specimen.

Immunohistochemical Features. Fibronectin and epithelial membrane antigen are absent while laminin is present in CMN.[24] Varying degree of staining for vimentin was noted in the tumor cells in a series of eight cases studied by Nadasdy et al.[25] Actin and desmin positivity was also seen in four and two of these cases respectively. Interestingly more nuclei showed staining for proliferating nuclear antigen (PCNA) in CCMN and in the cellular areas of classical CMN than in areas of low cellularity of CMN. In a series of 13 cases of CMN and CCMN, Pettinato et al demonstrated positive staining for vimentin, actin, and in some cases desmin. They concluded that the tumor cells are of myofibroblastic type.[26]

Ultrastructural Features. The ultrastructural features include focally dilated rough endoplasmic reticulum, bundles of thin filaments with dense bodies, external lamina and pinocytotic vesicles. These features, which were not consistently observed by all investigators, were focal or of variable degree of development. The tumor cells have been interpreted as fibroblasts or myofibroblasts.[6,26–28]

Cytologic Features. Diagnosis by fine-needle aspiration (FNA) biopsy has been described in two cases.[29,30] The smears showed isolated cells or small groups of spindle-shaped or tadpole-shaped cells with round to oval nuclei containing small nucleoli and fine chromatin pattern.[29] Coarse chromatin pattern and minimal nuclear atypia may also be present.[30]

Prognosis and Therapy. Before CMN was characterized as a distinct entity, it was frequently misdiagnosed as WT and chemotherapy and/or radiation therapy was given. Complications such as kyphoscoliosis and poor outcome due to adverse effects of therapy occurred in a few cases. Bolande and his colleagues noted the benign behavior of CMN and recommended nephrectomy alone as the therapy of choice.[15,16] This recommendation is being currently followed by pediatric oncologists. However, it should be noted that the tumor exhibits an interdigitating infiltrative pattern of growth. Therefore the surgeon should secure wide margins and the pathologist should ascertain that the margins are tumor free.[1] Thus, a more radical resection procedure is required for surgical treatment of CMN than for a stage I WT. Furthermore, rupture of the tumor during surgery may occur. It was noted in 10 out of 51 NWTS cases reported by Howell et al although as indicated above, it is not clear whether any of these cases represented cellular variant of CMN.[18] It is recommended that consideration should be given to additional therapy (chemotherapy and/or local radiation) in those cases in CMN in which the tumor is incompletely resected (e.g., presence of tumor at the margin of resection) or ruptured during surgery.[1]

Cellular or Atypical Variant of CMN

Typical cases of CMN exhibit low to moderate cellularity and the spindle-shaped tumor cells are arranged in fairly well demarcated fascicles. However, there may be some foci of hypercellularity in some cases of CMN (Figure 13-5). These foci do not exceed 25% of the tumor.[16,21] The cells in these hypercellular areas tend to be fusiform and the arrangement in the form of bundles is vague or absent. Variants of CMN in which there were large areas of hypercellularity or the entire tumor was hypercellular were recognized. Local recurrences of tumor and rarely metastasis were observed in some cases.[31,32] Joshi et al[17] reviewed the literature in 1986 and found 18 cases in which atypical morphologic features with or without atypical clinical behavior were noted. Sixty-two more cases including 20 from the International Society of Pediatric Oncology (Europe)[33] have been reported up to early 1993. However, the tumor is probably not as uncommon as these figures would imply, for Beckwith[1] mentions that 25 to 30% of NWTS cases of CMN show dense cellularity and high mitotic rate. However, it is not clear whether these features are focally or difusely present and whether these occur primarily in tumors in infants <3 months of age. Joshi et al[17] preferred the term "atypical mesoblastic nephroma" (AMN) to designate these tumors. The other term that has been used to designate these tumors is "cellular variant of CMN" (CCMN). The latter term, which has been widely used even after our suggestion of the term AMN, will be used in this chapter and is abbreviated CCMN.

Gross and Microscopic Features. A review of 18 cases reported until 1986 indicated that there are similarities and differences between CMN and CCMN.[17] The similarities include presence of a few areas of low CMN-like cellularity and spindle-shaped cells arranged in fascicles, foci of hematopoiesis, spicules of cartilage, and tubular and glomerular structures in CCMN. However, there are differences in other pathologic features of these two tumors (Table 13-4). It must be emphasized that all the atypical features listed in Table 13-4 may not be present in every case of CCMN. But at least one atypical gross feature (fleshy areas, focus/foci of hemorrhage and/or necrosis, involvement of surrounding structures other than connective tissues) and the two atypical microscopic features, viz. high cellularity and high mitotic index, are present in every case of CCMN (Figures 13-6 to 13-8). Cystic change due to dilatation of tubular structures or accumulation of mucoid material may be present. Foci of hematopoiesis and spicules of cartilage may be seen in CCMN. These and other features are illustrated in Figures 13-9 to 13-11 and summarized in Table 13-4. The importance of systematic examination of the margins of resection of ureter, the renal vessels, and the external surface of the resected specimen for presence of tumor cannot be overemphasized.

TABLE 13-4 Clinical, Gross, and Microscopic Differences Between Congenital Mesoblastic Nephroma (CMN) and Cellular Variant of Congenital Mesoblastic Nephroma (CCMN)

Feature	CMN	CCMN
Mean age	3.44 months	3.6 months
Age range	1 day to 9 years	1 day to 10 months
Size (range)	5 to 10 cm	3.2 to 21.5 cm
Weight (range)	35 to 450 g	47 to 1200 g
Cut surface	Firm, trabeculated appearance	Fleshy appearance, focus/foci of hemorrhage, and/or necrosis
Growth pattern	Infiltrative pattern with frequent involvement of perirenal and hilar connective tissue	Infiltrative pattern, adhesion to or invasion of surrounding structures (colon, pancreas, adrenal, spleen, diaphragm) may occur
Cellularity	Low (a few small cellular areas may be present)	High (few areas of low CMN-like cellularity may be present)
Tumor cell shape	Spindle-shaped	Fusiform to ovoid (foci of polygonal cells with clear cytoplasm may be present)
Arrangement of tumor cells	Well-defined fascicles	Vague fascicles or diffuse sheets
Mitotic activity	Low	Usually high (5–20/10 hpf [a] to as much as 5/hpf)
Gross cystic change	Rare	More common than in CMN
Microcystic change	Rare	More common (microcysts contain acid mucopolysaccharide[b])
Vascularity	Not prominent	Focally prominent
Staining for PCNA[c]	Low	High
DNA content	Diploid	Diploid or aneuploid
AgNOR count[d]	Low	High
Chromosomes	No abnormalities	Trisomy or tetrasomy for chromosome 11

[a] hpf: high-power field.
[b] Alcian blue–positive and PAS-negative acid mucopolysaccharide may be present also in the background of solid cellular areas.
[c] PCNA: proliferating cell nuclear antigen.
[d] AgNOR: silver-staining nucleolar organizing region.

Immunohistochemical Features. Positive staining for vimentin, actin, and α_1-antichymotrypsin has been reported in a variable proportion of cases.[25,26] Staining of a larger number of cells by PCNA in CCMN as compared with CMN has been mentioned above.

Ultrastructural Features. These have been studied in one case by Joshi et al[17] and in four cases by Pettinato et al.[26] Mierau et al have also described briefly

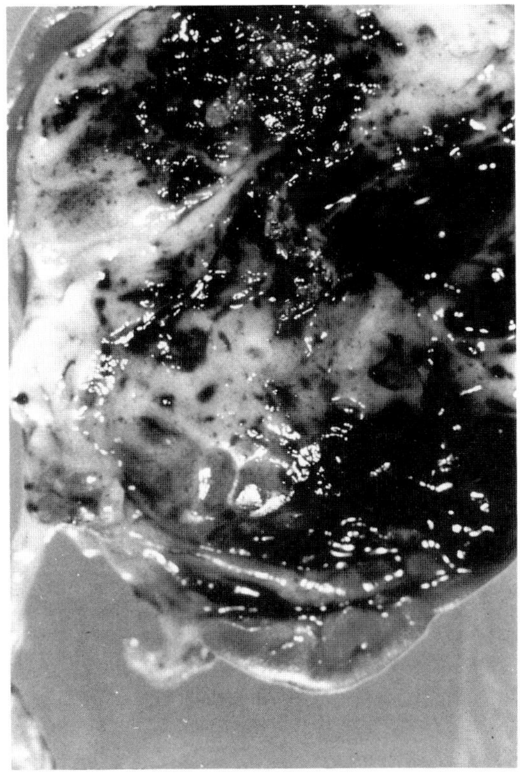

FIGURE 13-6. Gross photograph of cellular variant of congenital mesoblastic nephroma showing a fleshy appearance and large areas of hemorrhage and necrosis. Note extension to the renal pelvis. (Courtesy of Dr. John Fisher.)

the ultrastructural features of CCMN.[6] The round to oval tumor cells have large nuclei with prominent nucleoli. The cytoplasm contains dilated cisterns of rough endoplasmic reticulum (Figure 13-12). Poorly formed cell junctions may be present. External lamina and pinocytotic vesicles are absent. Rare collections of microfilaments with dense bodies have been described.

Differential Diagnosis. CCMN needs to be differentiated from monomorphous blastemal WT, CCSK, and MRTK. The compactly arranged oval or fusiform cells of CCMN may be mistaken for blastemal cells. The blastemal WT tends to show more dense cellularity. The blastemal cells are primitive cells arranged in masses circumscribed by thin fibrovascular strands. In CCMN, although a few areas of very dense cellularity may resemble the blastemal WT, the presence of fusiform cells arranged in vague bundles and a general mesenchymal appearance of the tumor cells and overall less dense cellularity as compared with blastemal WT are helpful in the diagnosis of CCMN. The arbitrary criterion that if the ratio of length to width of the nucleus is greater than 3 to 1, the cells should be considered mesenchymal, as described by Beckwith and Palmer,[2] may be useful in distinguishing the majority of the cells of CCMN from the blastemal cells of monophasic WT. Some overlap between CCMN and CCSK may be seen focally in some cases. Thus the epithelioid-appearing clear cells and focally prominent vascularity in CCMN may be confused with features of CCSK. However, CCSK shows a classical pattern characterized by arrange-

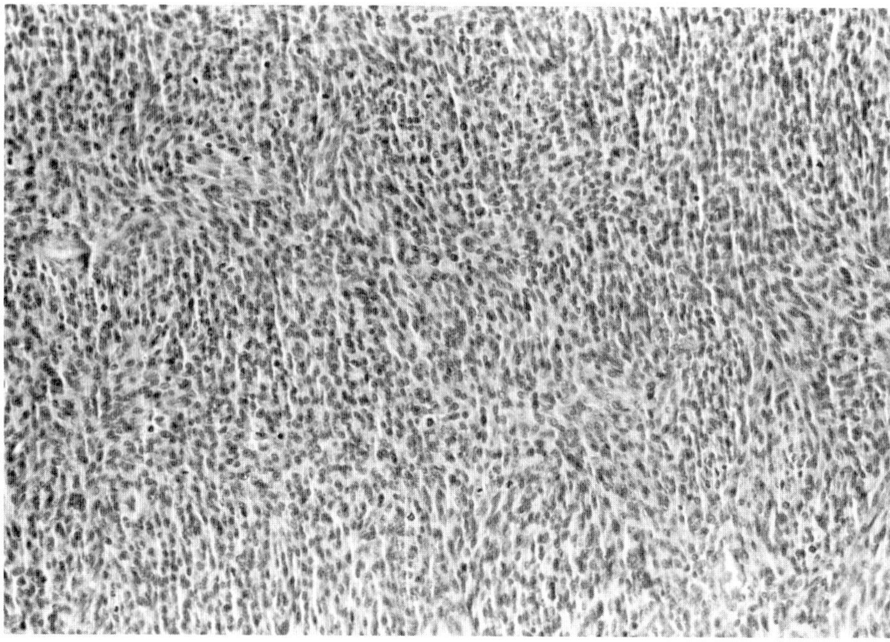

FIGURE 13-7. Cellular variant of congenital mesoblastic nephroma showing a highly cellular tumor composed of fusiform cells arranged diffusely and vague bundles (H&E, ×100). (Reprinted with permission from Joshi VV et al: *Arch Pathol Lab Med* 110:100–106, 1986.)

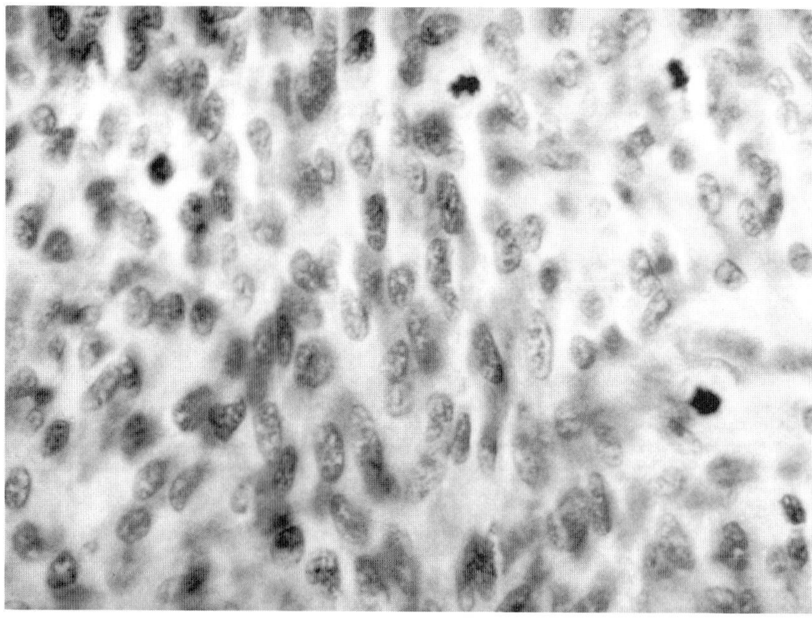

FIGURE 13-8. Cellular variant of congenital mesoblastic nephroma showing high mitotic activity in the oval to fusiform tumor cells (H&E, ×400).

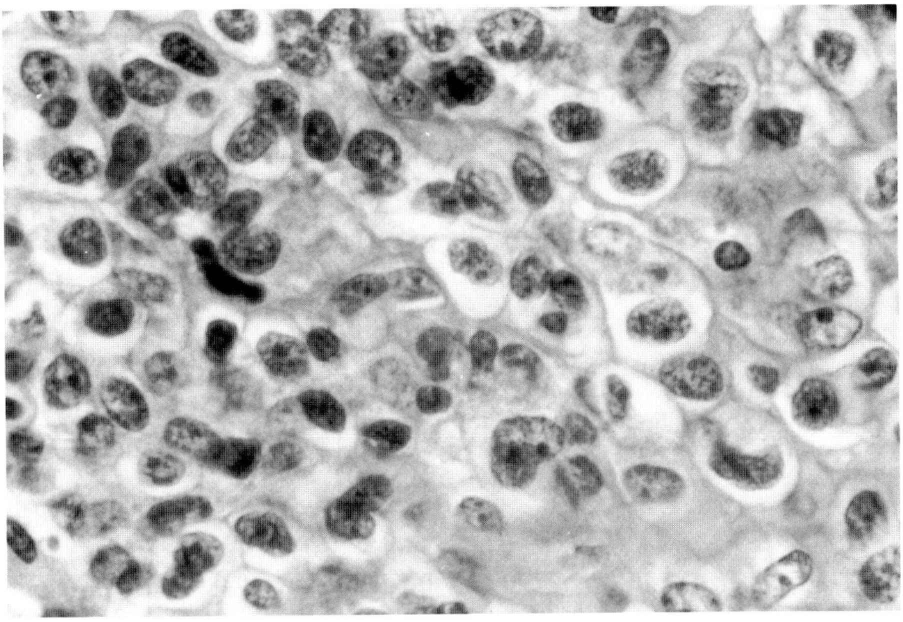

FIGURE 13-9. Cellular variant of congenital mesoblastic nephroma showing a focus of "epithelioid" cells (H&E, ×400). (Reprinted with permission from Joshi VV et al: *Arch Pathol Lab Med* 110:100–106, 1986.)

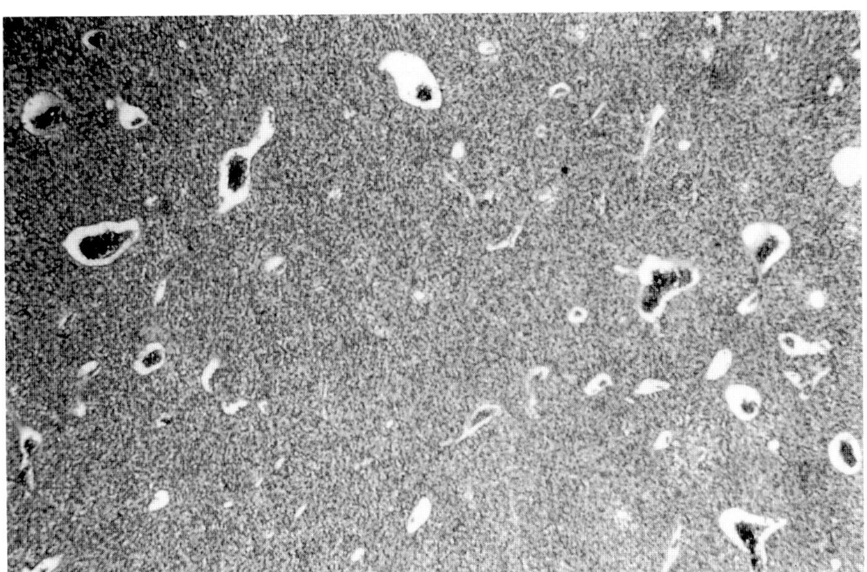

FIGURE 13-10. Cellular variant of congenital mesoblastic nephroma showing prominent dilated slightly tortuous blood vessels (H&E, ×25).

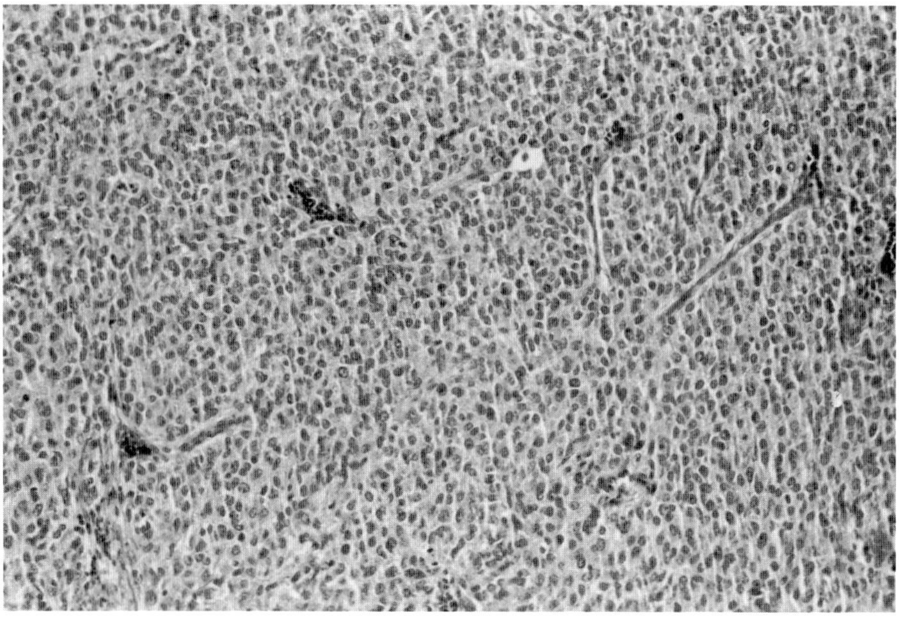

FIGURE 13-11. Cellular variant of congenital mesoblastic nephroma showing thin vascular channels in delicate septa. Note also minute foci of hematopoiesis (H&E, ×400). (Reprinted with permission from Joshi VV et al: *Arch Pathol Lab Med* 110:100–106, 1986.)

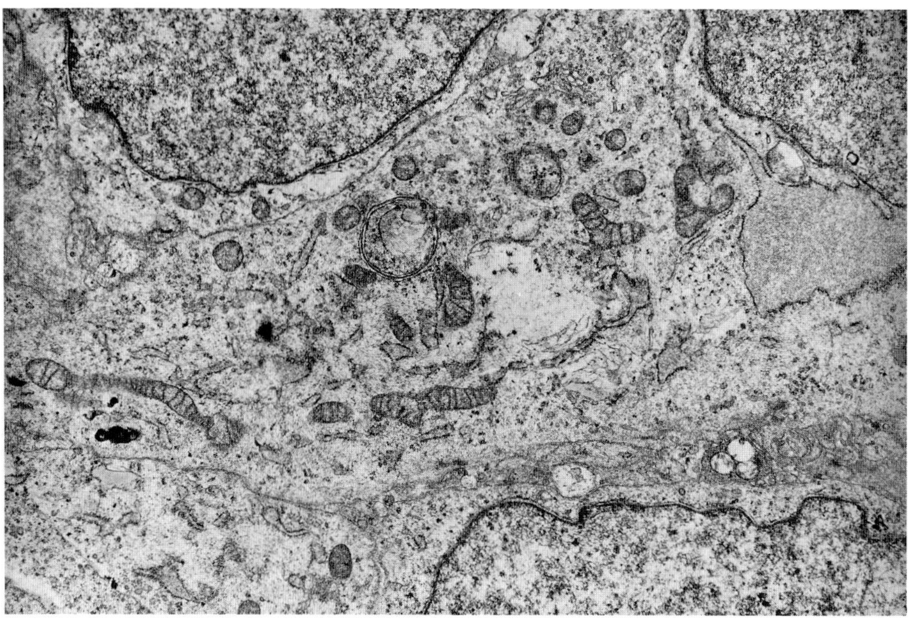

FIGURE 13-12. Electron micrograph of cellular variant of congenital mesoblastic nephroma showing dilated cisternae of rough endoplasmic reticulum containing granular electron-lucent material (uranyl acetate and lead citrate, ×15,500). (Reprinted with permission from Joshi VV et al: *Arch Pathol Lab Med* 110:100–106, 1986.)

ment of tumor cells with poorly stained or vacuolated cytoplasm and deceptively bland uniform nuclei into nests or cords by arborizing fibrovascular septa (Figures 13-13 and 13-14) (the details of morphologic features of CCSK are described below in the corresponding section). Foci of hematopoiesis and spicules of cartilage when present are helpful in distinguishing CCMN from CCSK (Figure 13-11). The distinction of CCMN from MRTK is based on the characteristic monomorphous cytologic features consisting of prominent single nucleolus and hyaline globules in the cytoplasm in the latter.[3]

Other Features. Other features of both CMN and CCMN are described here. Hypertension due to increased secretion of renin may occur. Cook et al[34] identified renin by immunoperoxidase method in the walls of blood vessels of the tumor and the entrapped renal cortex in seven of 12 cases of CMN. Renin has also been demonstrated in the tumor cells of CMN in two cases.[35] Hypercalcemia has been described in both CMN and CCMN.[36] The tumor is considered to be the source of high serum levels of parathormone observed in most of these patients since normalization of calcium levels is observed after surgical resection and no bony metastases were present in any of the cases. Prostaglandin E_2 secreted by the tumor has also been shown to be the cause of hypercalcemia.[37]

Higher counts of silver staining nucleolar organizing regions (Ag-NOR) which reflect proliferative activity were noted in the CCMN than in CMN by Guilland et al.[38] Molecular biologic studies in two cases of CMN revealed high level of expression of insulin-like growth factor II but unlike WT, expression of N-myc gene or Wilms' tumor suppressor gene (WT1) was absent.[39] Flow cytometric DNA analysis of cells obtained from paraffin-embedded tissue has shown euploidy in CMN and both euploidy and aneuploidy in CCMN.[26,40] Kovacs et al[41] demonstrated that the normocellular areas of a CMN had normal karyotype whereas the cellular area in the same tumor showed aneuploidy with 54 chromosomes. Schofield et al[42] performed fluorescence in situ hybridization by using probes to centromeric regions of chromosomes 7, 8, 9, 11, 12, 17, 18, and 20 and demonstrated trisomy and tetrasomy for chromosome 11 in seven of 10 cases of CCMN. Extra copies of chromosomes 7, 8, 12, 17, and 18 were also present in some of these tumors. In contrast, none of the CMN had chromosomal abnormalities.

Prognosis. We had reviewed 18 cases (including two of our own) in 1986 in order to characterize the pathologic features and biological behavior of CCMN.[17] Invasion of surrounding structures was present in three cases. One or more recurrences were observed in four cases in two of which there was fatal outcome. Pulmonary metastases were noted in two cases. The ages of these patients with aggressive behavior of their tumors were 1 day, 3 months, 4 months, 7 months, and 10 months. The tumors in all the cases showed predominant or diffuse hypercellularity with the exception of one case in which focal hypercellularity was present. High mitotic activity was also seen. In the editorial written by Beckwith and Weeks related to the aforementioned review, it was pointed out that 25–30% of the CMN specimens in infants less than 3 months of age registered with NWTS show high cellularity and other features associated with CCMN.[43] There was no recurrence noted following simple nephrectomy in any of these NWTS patients with the exception of the patient who was 1 day old at diagnosis (case 1 in the review published by us).[17,31]

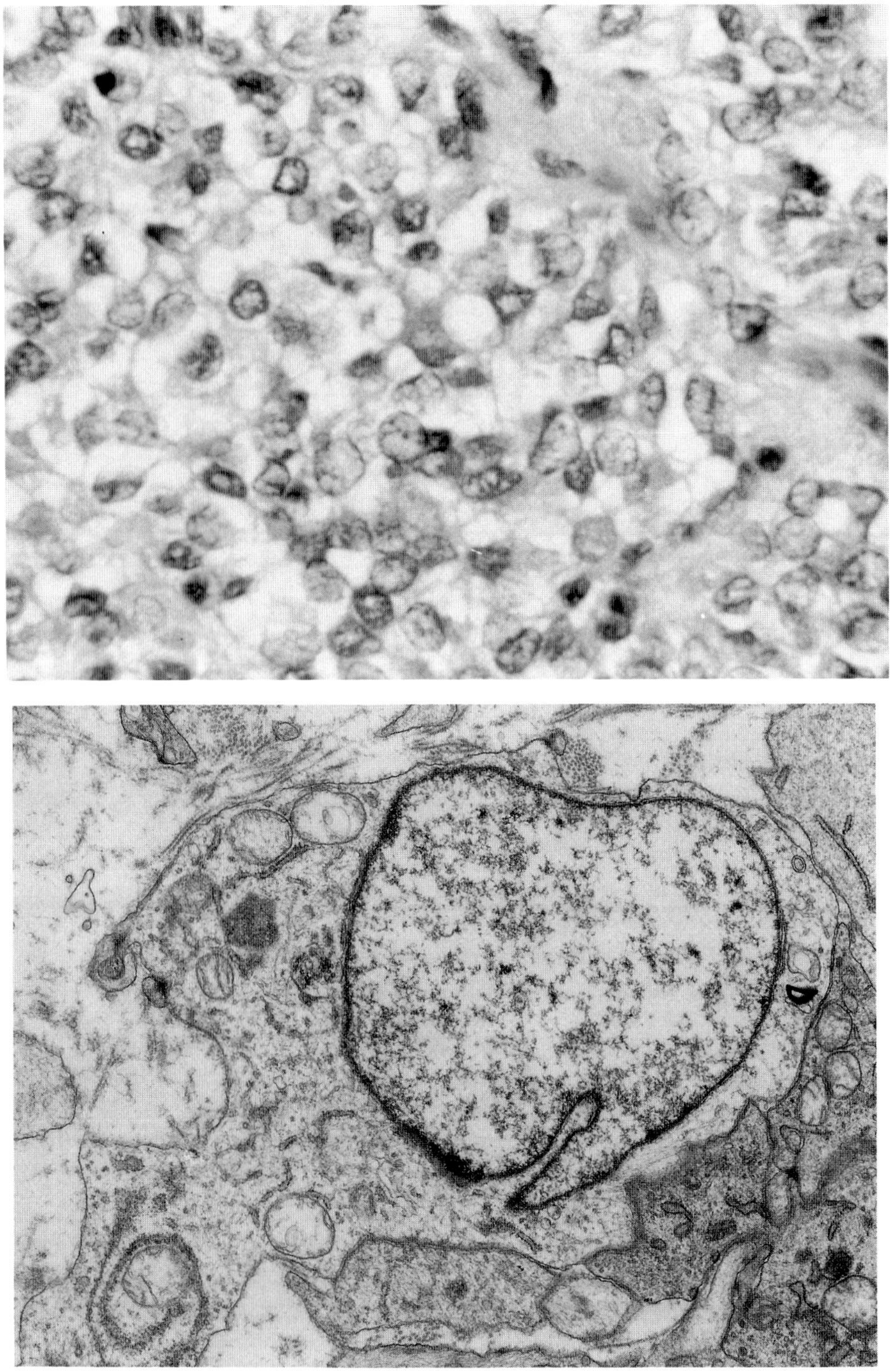

FIGURE 13-13. A: Clear cell sarcoma of kidney showing tumor cells with bland-appearing nuclei, clear or vacuolated cytoplasm, and indistinct outline (H&E, ×400). B: Electron micrograph showing electron-lucent nucleus and cytoplasm with few organelles in the cells of clear cell sarcoma of kidney (uranyl acetate and lead citrate, ×7,300). (Courtesy of Dr. Gary Mierau.)

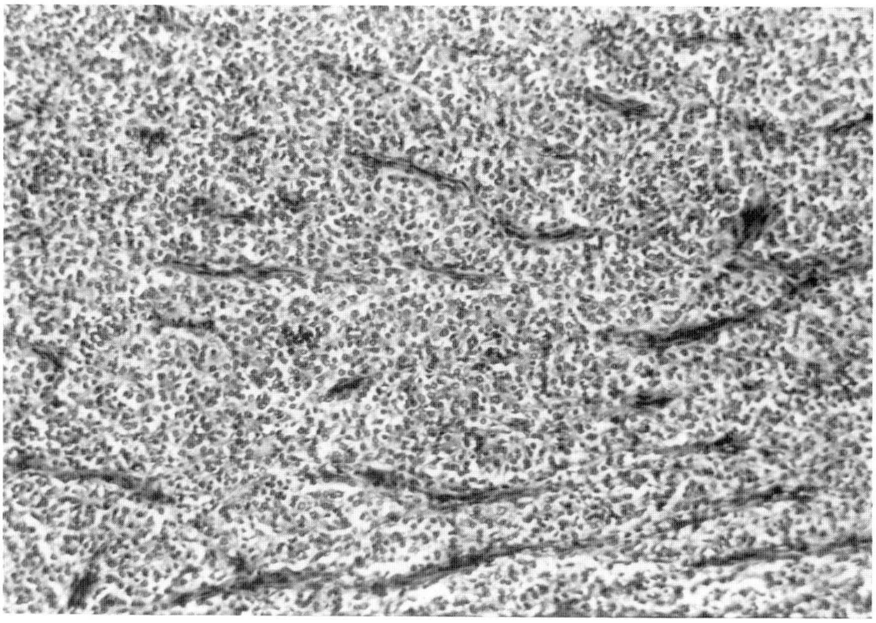

FIGURE 13-14. Classical pattern of clear cell sarcoma of kidney characterized by arrangement of cells into vaguely outlined groups bounded by fibrovascular septa. Note absence of clear cytoplasm (H&E, ×250).

Beckwith and Weeks therefore contended that the atypical features in a case of CMN should be of concern only if the patient is more than 3 months old[1,43] Subsequently three more series of CMN and CCMN have been published from North America.[26,44,45] Recurrence was noted in three of the 17 patients with CCMN reported by Chan et al.[44] These patients were 3 days, 52 months, and 10 months old. Chan and coworkers chose to resect the recurrent tumor surgically in all these cases but gave adjuvant therapy only in the two patients who were older than 3 months of age. All three patients were alive and without any disease at 11 years, 31 months, and 31 months after diagnosis. These investigators concurred with the recommendations of Beckwith and Weeks, that CCMN in an infant less than 3 months old requires only surgical resection, even if there is local recurrence after primary resection. Presence of tumor was noted at the resection margin of renal vein in one of the seven CCMN reported by Pettinato et al.[26] The patient, whose age is not indicated in the report, was given adjuvant chemotherapy. No evidence of recurrence was noted in any of their seven cases. Gormley et al[45] reviewed 38 cases of CCMN (35 reported in the literature and three from their institution). They divided the cases into two groups: those with recurrence (7 cases) and those without recurrence (31 cases). They carried out statistical analysis of various clinicopathologic features in these two groups and found that the only statistically significant variable suggesting recurrent disease was pathologically positive surgical margin. The presenting age was not predictive of recurrence. Recently a 14-month-old child with CCMN showing metastasis to lungs and heart was reported by Vujanic et al.[46]

From the review of cases of CCMN presented above, the following tentative conclusions are warranted: (1) CCMNs occur in both young and old infants but the tumors occurring in those younger than 3 months are not likely to show aggressive behavior (although aggressive behavior may be seen exceptionally in infants younger than 3 months). (2) Aggressive behavior is seen only in CCMN. Such behavior does not appear to occur in classical CMN. (3) Positive surgical margins are highly predictive of local recurrence. (4) Aggressive behavior may not be seen in all cases of CCMN. (5) Although most CCMNs are diffusely cellular, in some cases focal cellularity involving >25% of the tumor area may be present.[32,44] The tumors that show hypercellularity involving <25% of the tumor area and normocellularity in the remaining portions of the tumor may be tentatively categorized as combined CMN. The prognosis of the combined CMN is not known (see below).

Prediction of Aggressive Behavior in CCMN. Invasion of surrounding structures or presence of tumor at the resection margin or in the renal vein are clearly indicative of aggressive behavior. With the currently available data, it is not possible to delineate any gross or microscopic pathologic differences between those CCMN which show aggressive behavior and those which do not or between those CCMN which show local recurrence and those which metastasize. Such delineation must await a definitive and detailed analysis of a larger number of cases registered with the NWTS. It may be noted that CMN, CCMN, and CCSK may represent a continuum in terms of histogenesis and biologic behavior.

Therapy. A therapeutic approach to a patient with CCMN has not been agreed upon or standardized. The main concern is the aggressive behavior. There are two subgroups with reference to aggressive behavior: (1) aggressive behavior is evident at surgery, (2) it is not evident at surgery. In the first subgroup, aggressive behavior is evident in the form of adhesions to or invasion of surrounding structures (e.g., colon) or presence of tumor at the resection margins. Radical nephrectomy with resection of adherent structures is necessary in these cases. The question is whether adjuvant chemotherapy should be given following surgery in such cases. Chan et al[44] recommend that no adjuvant therapy is necessary in infants <3 months of age even if the surgical margins or perirenal connective tissues contained tumor. D'Angio in the proceedings of the Tumor Board of Children's Hospital of Philadelphia contends that no additional therapy is warranted in the 2-day-old infant under discussion in whom there was tumor at the resection margin.[47] According to Chan et al,[44] adjuvant therapy should be reserved for patients over 3 months of age who have grossly unresected tumors. On the other hand, Beckwith[1] recommends that if there is tumor at the resection margin, consideration should be given to adjuvant chemotherapy for any case of CMN regardless of degree of cellularity (and presumably regardless of age). The pathologist's role in determining the status of resection margins is thus very critical. In fact according to Gormley et al,[45] frozen sections are necessary at surgery to determine the status of resection margins.

In the second subgroup of CCMN in which the aggressive behavior is not evident at surgery and the margins of resection are free of tumor, data from the reviewed cases[17] indicates that there is a potential for subsequent aggressive behavior manifested mainly by local recurrence or rarely by metastasis. Unfortunately, the pathologic features of CCMN are not helpful in predicting aggressive behavior. The age of the patient appears to be a major determinant of the decision regarding further therapy. Beckwith and Weeks[43] are of the opinion that no further therapy is indicated in such cases if the age of the patient is <3 months. Whether postoperative adjuvant therapy should be given to infants >3 months of age or whether initially regular periodic follow-up by imaging techniques should be done followed by chemotherapy and/or surgery if local recurrence or metastasis occurs is not clear. In this regard, it should be noted that in a review of 18 cases of CCMN Joshi et al[17] found six patients in whom the tumor was completely resected and chemotherapy was prematurely discontinued or not given at all. In four of these six cases, there was recurrence and/or metastasis.

If a decision regarding adjuvant therapy is made, the details of adjuvant therapy are not agreed upon. Beckwith[1] recommends chemotherapeutic agents used for WT of FH (vincristine and actinomycin D) whereas Gormley et al[45] observed good response to "sarcomatous" chemotherapy (vincristine, cyclophosphamide, and doxorubicin in two cases of recurrent CCMN). Since CCMN is a mesenchymal tumor, it is logical that it responds to "sarcomatous" therapy. In a 5-month-old infant with unresectable CCMN reported by Stalens et al,[48] dramatic shrinkage of tumor with preoperative chemotherapy (vincristine, actinomycin D, and ifosfamide) made nearly complete surgical resection possible (microscopic residual tumor was suspected). The infant who was also given postoperative chemotherapy (cyclophosphamide replacing ifosfamide) was without evidence of disease 21 months from dignosis.

Combined CMN

This is a presumptive entity. In a number of cases of CMN, a few cellular areas involving usually <25% of the tumor are found. These tumors can be designated as mixed or combined CMN. Thus there were three cases of CMN, two of CCMN, and two of combined CMN in the series reported by Nadasdy et al.[25] In the series reported by Pettinato et al,[26] there were six cases of CMN, seven of CCMN, and three of combined CMN. The precise criterion for the diagnosis of combined CMN has not been delineated. We would like to suggest that tentatively the following criterion be used: A tumor in which there is focal high cellularity involving no more than 25% of the tumor and which otherwise shows the normocellularity seen in CMN should be designated as combined CMN. (CCMN has predominant areas of dense cellularity usually involving >90% of the tumor.) As mentioned above, differences in DNA content and karyotype have been demonstrated in the densely cellular (aneuploidy) versus normocellular areas (diploidy) of the combined CMN.[41] Immunoperoxidase staining for PCNA demonstrated positive staining in a larger proportion of nuclei in the densely cellular versus normocellular areas.[25] To the best of my knowledge, no atypical behavior has been reported thus far in any of the cases of combined CMN. However, it should be kept in mind that these tumors contain areas that, although small in size, have the same morphologic and probably biologic characteristics as CCMN. The determination of the precise significance of the combined pattern and whether atypical behavior occurs in these cases will have to await the detailed analysis of cases of CMN of all types registered with NWTS.

Clear Cell Sarcoma of Kidney (CCSK) (Undifferentiated Renal Sarcoma—URS)

CCSK is rare, constituting about 4% of all renal tumors in childhood (i.e., about 20 cases a year in the United States). In 1983 Beckwith[3] used the term CCSK which has since been widely used by him and other investigators. I have personally seen a number of cases of CCSK in which no clear cells were present. Beckwith and colleagues[2,49] indicate that they would prefer to replace the term CCSK by a more accurate term when the cell of origin of the tumor is identified. Marsden et al[50] and Morgan and Kidd[51] used the terms "bone metastasizing renal tumor of childhood" (BMRTC) and "undifferentiated sarcoma of the kidney" respectively. The primitive mesenchymal nature of the tumor has been amply demonstrated by ultrastructural and immunohistochemical studies.[49,52] Relationship of the tumor cells of CCSK to embryonal renal tissue is demonstrated by their latent epithelial nature which manifests in the cell lines derived from CCSK[53] and epithelial cell content in rare cases.[54] It has been suggested that CCSK may be at the extreme of the spectrum of mesenchymal renal tumors consisting of CMN, CCMN, and CCSK.[6] Thus, there is a considerable amount of evidence at this point which suggests that the tumor cells of CCSK are primitive mesenchymal cells and could be considered to be derived from nephrogenic mesenchyme. The term BMRTC is cumbersome and overemphasizes the propensity for skeletal metastases which have occurred only in 17% of NWTS cases of CCSK.[49] I would like to suggest that "undifferentiated renal sarcoma" (URS) should replace the term CCSK. This term, which includes references to the lack of differentiation, histogenetic relationship to renal tissue, and the mesenchymal nature of the tumor, is simple and unambiguous.

Gross and Histologic Features. CCSK is a unilateral tumor with spherical or irregular outline. The cut surface, which bulges, shows variegated appearance. There are fleshy areas with hemorrhage and necrosis and firm trabeculated areas. In tumors that produce abundant mucinous material, glistening appearance of the cut surface is observed.[55] Cysts, which are common, may involve large portions of the tumor in occasional cases. The interface with the surrounding kidney is well-demarcated but is irregular.[56] Histologically classical pattern and its variants are seen in the tumor (Figures 13-13 to 13-19). The surrounding uninvolved kidney rarely shows nephrogenic rests (3, 57).

Classical Pattern. The classical pattern consists of cells with poorly or faintly eosinophilic or vacuolated or clear cytoplasm having indistinct outline, oval to round uniform nuclei with finely granular chromatin, indistinct nucleoli, and a few mitotic figures. The cytoplasm is PAS-negative.[56] These cytologic features, which can be described as bland, are deceptive considering the malignant behavior of the tumor. The characteristic feature of the classical pattern is that the cells are divided into poorly to fairly outlined trabeculae, groups, cords, or columns by fibrovascular septa (Figures 13-14 and 13-15). The fibrovascular septa may not be prominent but are visualized after careful search. Reticulin stain is helpful in the recognition of this pattern (Figure 13-16A). As indicated above, many examples of CCSK may not contain clear cells and other investigators who have reported these tumors do not mention clear cells in their descriptions.[50,51] However, the pattern consisting of arrangement of tumor cells

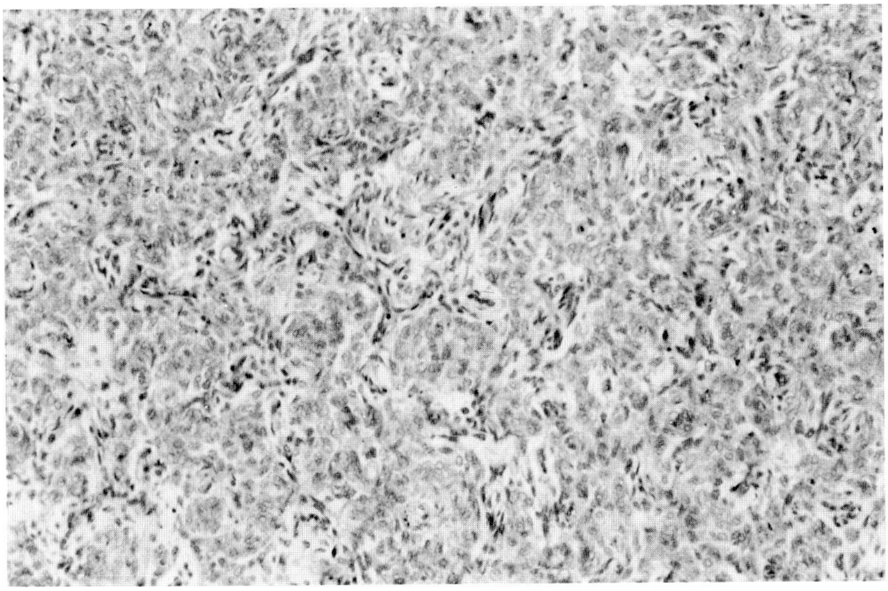

FIGURE 13-15A. Classical pattern of clear cell sarcoma of kidney characterized by groups of tumor cells without clear cytoplasm delineated by thin fibrovascular septa. Two types of cells, the "cord" cells and "septal" cells, can be seen. Note absence of clear cytoplasm in the tumor cells (H&E, ×250).

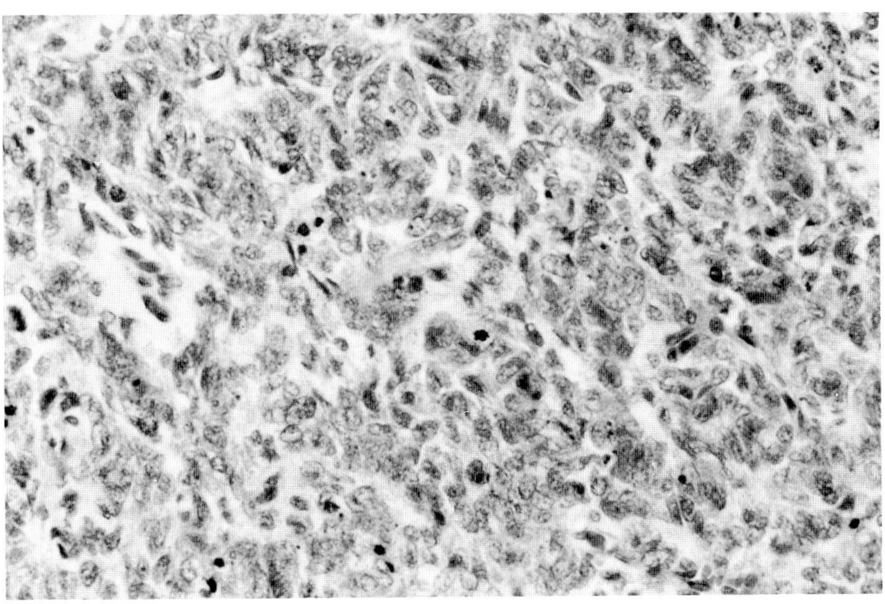

FIGURE 13-15B. Clear cell sarcoma of kidney showing tumor cells with nuclei containing finely granular chromatin, little cytoplasm, and vague outline. Occasional karyorrhectic cells with formation of nuclear dust and a mitotic figure are seen (H&E, ×400).

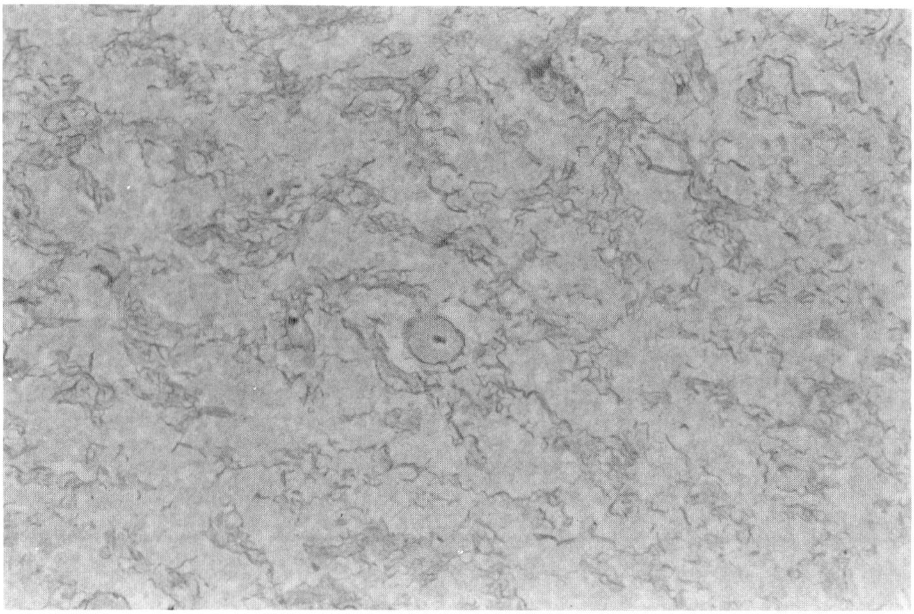

FIGURE 13-16A. Reticulin stain brings out the fibrovascular septa outlining groups of tumor cells in clear cell sarcoma of kidney (H&E, ×250).

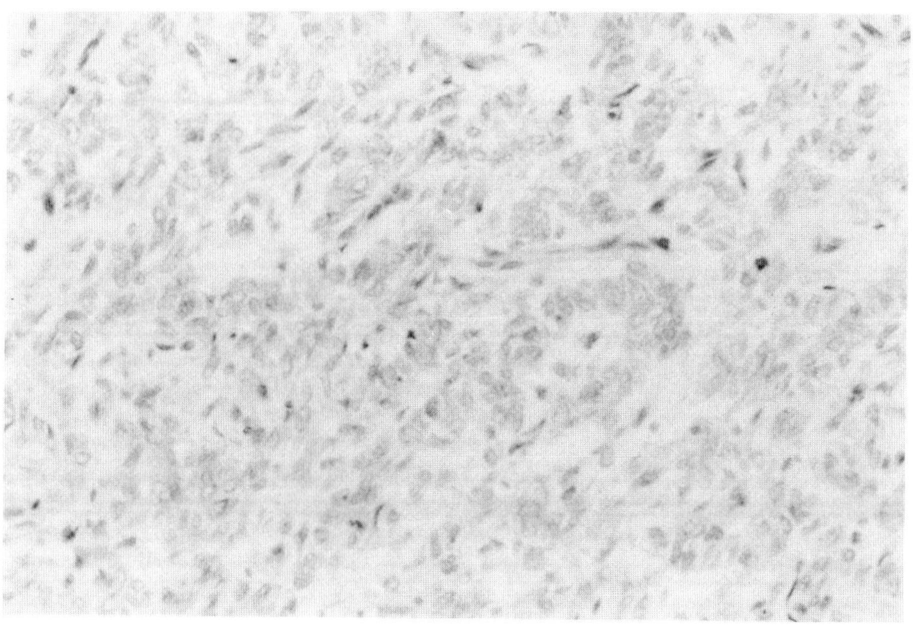

FIGURE 13-16B. Epithelioid trabecular pattern in clear cell sarcoma of kidney. This pattern may be mistaken for the epithelial pattern of Wilms' tumor by the uninitiated (H&E, ×400).

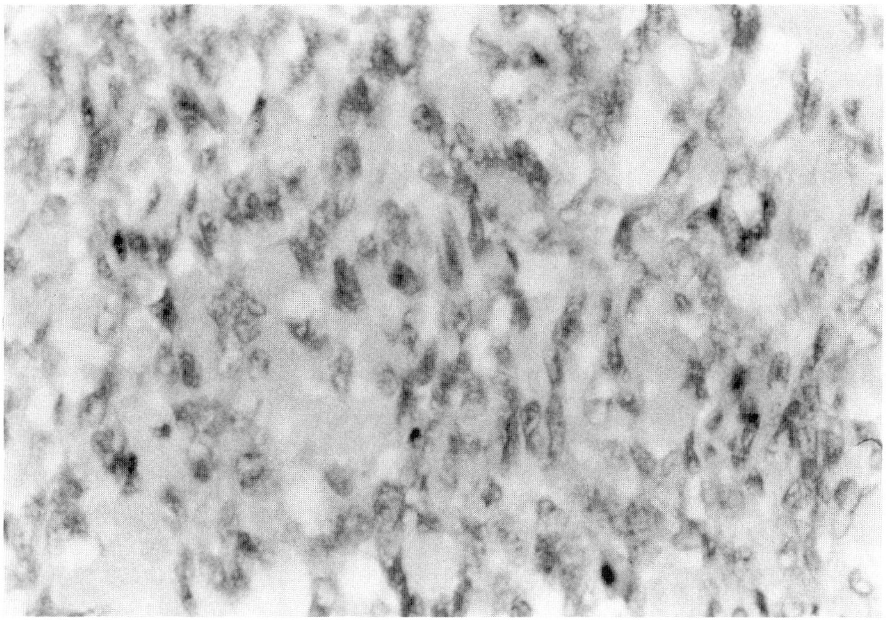

FIGURE 13-17A. Clear cell sarcoma of kidney showing focal stromal hyalinization isolating tumor cells into thin cords (H&E, ×400).

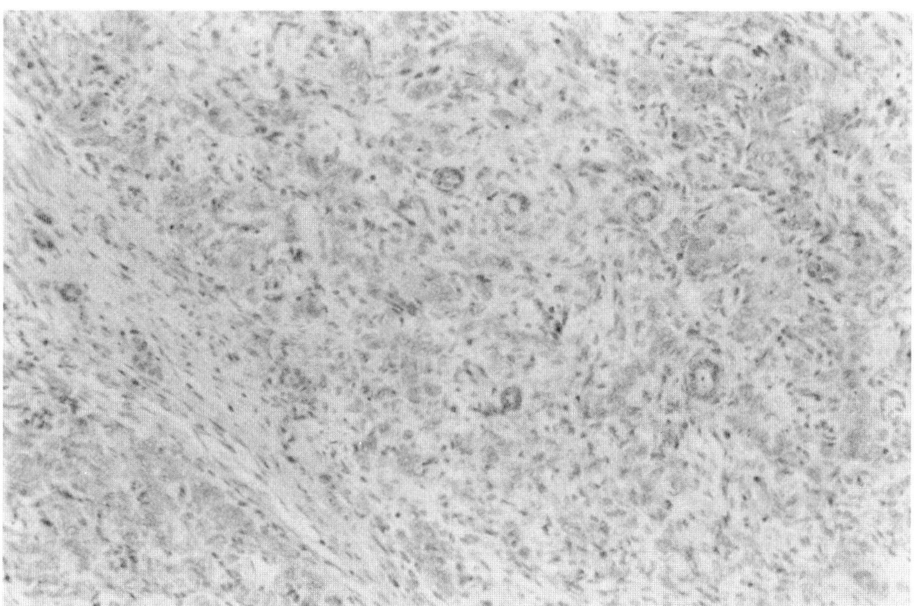

FIGURE 13-17B. Numerous small tubules and a focus of sclerosis are present (H&E, ×250).

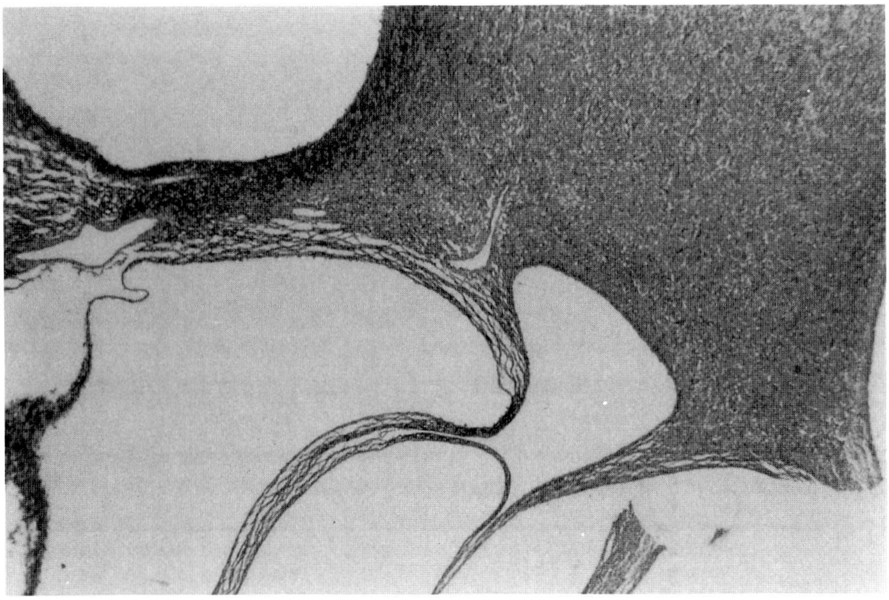

FIGURE 13-18. Clear cell sarcoma of kidney showing cystic pattern (H&E, ×40).

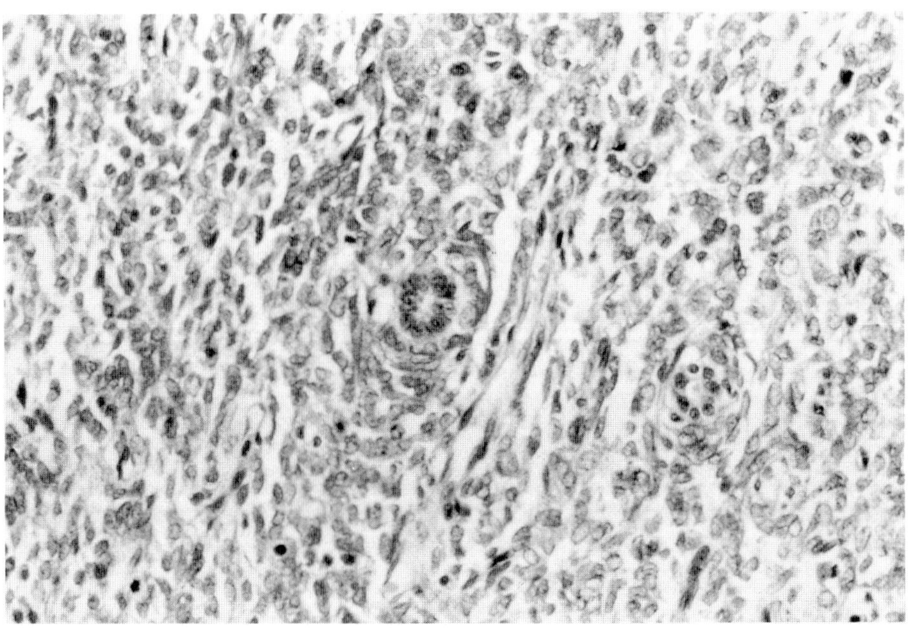

FIGURE 13-19. Clear cell sarcoma of kidney showing diffuse pattern with tubular structures. The fibrovascular septa are absent in this field (H&E, ×400).

into cords or columns surrounded by fibrovascular septa described above is consistently found and is of great diagnostic importance. Beckwith refers to the tumor cells comprising the cords as "cord cells" and the spindle cells of the fibrovascular septa as "septal cells."[57] Transition between cord cells and septal cells is seen frequently, which suggests that these two types of cells are different expressions of the same basic cell type. Tubular structures lined by cuboidal cells which may have hyperchromatic nuclei may be found particularly in the peripheral portion of the tumor.[50,57] These tubules are generally considered to be entrapped tubules but some of them may be neoplastic in nature. It is of interest to note in this regard that in one case of CCSK, polyhedral or columnar epithelial cells arranged in sheets were present.[54] The classical pattern described above is the only pattern in most of the cases. The tumors showing the variant patterns described below usually contain at least a few foci of the classical pattern. Furthermore, more than one variant pattern may be present in a given case.

Variant Patterns

1. *Epithelioid trabecular pattern.* The tumor cells are arranged in parallel ribbon-like bands alternating with the fibrovascular septa (Figure 13-16B). The ribbon-like bands may be mistaken for tubular structures and the tumor may be misdiagnosed as WT. Beckwith[3,57] cautions against the deceptive nature of this pattern which in his experience is most likely to be misinterpreted as the epithelial pattern of WT. In extremely rare cases the cord cells may in fact be arranged in a tubular pattern.[57]
2. *Fibrosis and stromal hyalinization.* The fibrovascular septa of CCSK are usually thin and short. In some cases, the septa may show fibroblastic, collagenous, and hyaline thickening which, when severe, can isolate small groups of tumor cells (Figure 13-17). The hyalinization may mimic osteoid. This pattern, which can also be seen in MRTK, was originally considered as a hyalinizing pattern in sarcomatous variants of WT.[3]
3. *Other patterns.* These include septal cell proliferation, neurilemoma-like pattern, myxoid pattern with or without cystic change, angiectatic pattern, and diffuse pattern (Figures 13-18 and 13-19). CCSK showing septal cell proliferation may be mistaken for CMN. In diffuse pattern the fibrovascular septa are absent or inconspicuous (Figure 13-19).

Immunohistochemical Features. Systematic studies in a series of a large number of cases are lacking. Of the various intermediate filaments, vimentin has been demonstrated in a few cases. Positive staining may also be seen for α_1-antichymotrypsin.[52,53,58] *Ulex europaeus* agglutinin accentuates the characteristic vascular pattern. Epithelial markers have been negative except in the tubular structures present in some cases. These studies are supportive of the mesenchymal nature of the tumor. However, it should be noted that negative staining is often obtained for a variety of markers including cytokeratin, vimentin, neuron-specific enolase, desmin, laminin, and neurofilament protein.

Ultrastructural Studies. Ultrastructural features have been described in a fairly large number of cases by a number of investigators.[6,49,50,55] The clear cell appearance in the hematoxylin and eosin–stained sections, when present is due to the presence of electron-lucent cytoplasm containing few organelles (Figure

13-13).[6] The vacuolated appearance of the tumor cells is considered to be due to enfolding of pale extracellular matrix by the tumor cell extensions.[49] However, in many cases, the cytoplasm presents a dense appearance due to abundant organelles and intermediate filaments. This ultrastructural appearance corresponds to the lack of clear appearance of the cytoplasm on light microscopy. Among the organelles, mitochondria and rough endoplasmic reticulin are most frequent. There are occasional primitive cell junctions. Thus, in contrast to the more differentiated mesenchymal cells of CMN, the cells of CCSK are primitive. The ultrastructural resemblance of the primitive cells of CCSK to those of the metanephric blastemal cap cells or mesangial cells has been pointed out by some authors.[49,50,59,60] In my opinion, the presence of ultrastructural features consisting of prominent endoplasmic reticulum in some of the cells, prominent intercellular matrix, and the overlap of ultrastructural features of CCSK and CCMN provides sufficiently strong indications of the primitive mesenchymal nature of the tumor cells. Such an interpretation also supports the proposed histogenesis of CCSK (and CMN and CCMN) from the derivatives of nephrogenic mesenchyme.

Differential Diagnosis. CCSK is the most frequently misdiagnosed renal tumor of childhood.[57] WT, CCMN, and MRTK need to be considered in the differential diagnosis. Blastemal WT, because of the prominent vascular pattern, may be confused with CCSK. The blastemal cells are more hyperchromatic, more densely packed, and tend to show mitotic karyorrhectic cells. Lobular pattern outlined by well-demarcated fibrovascular septa is present. On the other hand, CCSK showing a prominent epithelioid trabecular pattern may be mistaken for WT (Figure 13-16). In a few areas CCSK may show a pattern which appears to be diffuse to the inexperienced eye because the fibrovascular septa are not readily discernible. Rarely, the fibrovascular septa may be focally absent. If such an area contains tubules it can be mistaken for WT (Figure 13-19). CCSK showing prominent "septal" cell proliferation may be mistaken for CCMN. CCMN showing prominent vascular pattern or dilated ("angiectatic") blood vessels (Figure 13-10) may be diagnosed as CCSK. In such instances, the distinction between CCSK and CCMN is difficult. The more clearly appreciable mesenchymal nature of tumor cells on routine histology (fusiform to spindle-shaped cells and arrangement in vague or focally well-delineated fascicles) has helped me in the diagnosis of CCMN. MRTK may also be mistaken for CCSK particularly when the former shows a vascular pattern in which compact groups of tumor cells are surrounded by vascular septa and the tumor cells have fewer conspicuous nucleoli and cytoplasmic inclusions than usual. This vascular pattern in MRTK is referred to as CCSK-like pattern.[9] But in almost all cases of MRTK at least some foci exhibit the classical features consisting of a cellular tumor with diffusely arranged monotonous large round or oval tumor cells having prominent nucleoli and cytoplasmic inclusions. CCSK showing a prominent cystic change has only a small amount of solid tumor in the septa. The tumor tissue in the septa may be compressed thus obscuring the diagnostic pattern of CCSK (Figure 13-18). CCSK in such a specimen may be mistaken for cystic CMN or cystic CCMN. It should be emphasized that several sections of solid and cystic renal tumor should be available for examination. Such sampling of the tumor would reveal all the various patterns including the pattern considered as classical for a particular tumor type (CCSK, MRTK, etc.) represented by that particular case. The appropriate diagnosis will then be self-evident.

Beckwith[56] has listed the following clues to the diagnosis of CCSK: Various patterns seen in CCSK are variations of the same underlying pattern of cord cells arranged in groups bounded incompletely by fibrovascular septa. A CCSK-like pattern in an occasional focus in a tumor which otherwise shows presence of blastemal cells, skeletal muscle, or other features of WT can be discounted. At its periphery CCSK infiltrates the surrounding renal parenchyma separating individual tubules or glomeruli. The classical WT has a pushing margin with the presence of a tumor capsule. Blastemal WT which has an infiltrating margin usually isolates groups of tubules and glomeruli rather than individual renal structures as does CCSK. In WT, the nuclei of the tumor cells have coarse chromatin whereas the nuclei of the cells of CCSK exhibit finely granular dispersed chromatin. Nephrogenic rests are rare in kidneys with CCSK.

Other Features. In a study of seven cases of CCSK, Schmidt et al[61] have shown diploid DNA index in all cases. S-phase fraction and proliferation index were lower in CCSK than in MRTK and even typical WT. However, in one of these seven cases of CCSK, high values for these parameters were found (actual data for this case is not given separately). CCSK has been shown to express insulin-like growth factor II but not WT1 transcripts.[62] CCSK-like tumor has been described in extrarenal location and in an adult in rare instances.[63,64]

Cytologic Features. Cytologic features of CCSK in FNA biopsy specimens have been described by Akhtar et al[65] and Drut and Pomar.[66] The diagnosis of CCSK was confirmed by subsequent histopathologic examination in these cases. In the cytologic smears, the tumor cells which were arranged singly or in small loose clusters were polygonal, stellate, or spindle-shaped. In some cases the cells were monomorphic. The large round or oval nuclei contained evenly dispersed fine chromatin and inconspicuous nucleoli. Nuclear grooving may be present. None of these authors describe in detail, in the text or the legends of the illustrations, the appearance of the cytoplasm of tumor cells, but the illustrations included by Akhtar et al in their article[65] show moderate to abundant amounts of pale to somewhat densely staining cytoplasm. In none of the illustrations is vacuolated or clear cytoplasm seen. No mention of fibrovascular septa in the FNA smears is made in these articles, although the illustrations of histologic features of biopsy specimens show the septa. The cytologic features of CCSK are considered to be different from those of WT and MRTK (see below). Akhtar et al carried out ultrastructural examination of the FNA biopsy and noted the same ultrastructural features as described previously.[6,49] It appears to me that routine cytologic and ultrastructural features in a FNA biopsy specimen of CCSK, although sufficiently different from WT and MRTK to the experienced and "retrospective" eye, would be difficult to distinguish from those of CCMN. In my opinion, a tentative prospective diagnosis may be rendered on a FNA specimen.

Prognosis and Therapy. CCSK carried a poor prognosis in NWTS-1 and NWTS-2. The tumor showed a propensity to relapse and metastasis to the bones. The mortality rate was high. There was significant improvement in the prognosis

(75% survival at 4 years) with the addition of doxorubicin to actinomycin D and vincristine in NWTS-3.[11] This emphasizes the great practical importance of accurate pathologic diagnosis of CCSK.

Cytodifferentiated Mesenchymal Tumor (CMT)

This is a tentative entity. Only three cases have been described.[67,68] In all these cases prior to the detection of cytodifferentiated mesenchymal tumor (CMT), there was WT of one kidney which was treated by nephrectomy and chemotherapy. In each case, the CMT in the opposite kidney was detected metachronously after resection of the WT. CMT showed bland-appearing, moderately cellular areas composed of spindle-shaped or fusiform cells arranged in bundles. In addition, well-differentiated skeletal muscle was present (Figure 13-20). Foci of hematopoiesis and tubules were also seen. Some of the latter structures showed cystic dilatation in one of the cases. No blastemal or embryonal nephroblastic tissue was seen in any of the cases. CMN was considered in the differential diagnosis (Figures 13-4). It was ruled out because of the presence of skeletal muscle. On the basis of histologic features, CMT is considered to be a benign tumor and in each of the reported cases it was treated by partial nephrectomy.

Tumors Arising from Inducted Metanephric Blastema–Ureteric Bud Complex

Tumors Recapitulating Predominantly Derivatives of Inducted Metanephric Blastema

Nephrogenic Rests (NR) and Nephroblastomatosis (NBM). The landmark article on this subject was published by Bove and McAdams in 1976.[69] The

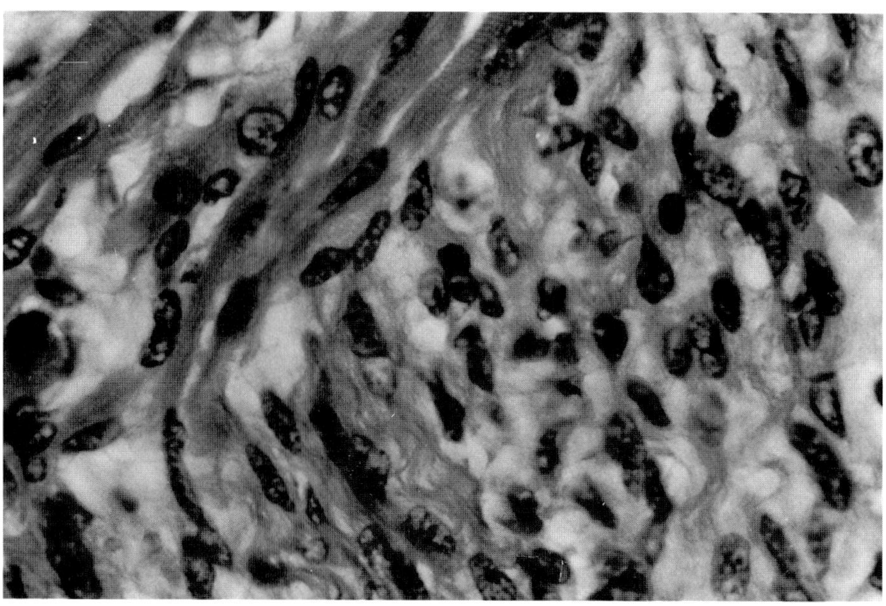

FIGURE 13-20. Cytodifferentiated mesenchymal tumor showing well-differentiated mature skeletal muscle cells (H&E, ×400).

terminology of these WT precursor lesions as used by them and other authors including Hou and Holman, who introduced the term "nephroblastomatosis" (NBM) in 1961, is complex.[70–73] Numerous terms, including "persistent nodular blastema," "in situ nephroblastoma," "sclerosing hamartoma," "Wilms' tumorlet," and "multifocal nephroblastomatosis" have been used to designate various subtypes of these lesions. Beckwith et al[4] in another landmark article on the subject have done much to clarify the complexity and confusion in the nomenclature by presenting new definitions, classification, and systematization which, in my opinion, have made the previous terminology obsolete. The following terminology and description of these lesions are according to the recommendations of Beckwith et al.[4]

Definitions. The generic term "nephrogenic rest" (NR) is defined as a focus of abnormally persistent nephrogenic cells, retaining cells that can be induced to form a WT. Two aspects of this definition are of importance. Abnormal persistence refers to persistence beyond 37 weeks' gestation until which time a bandlike subcapsular nephrogenic zone is normally present (Figure 13-8 of Chapter 10 Tumors in Children—General Aspects). The presence of abnormally large numbers of embryonal cells with or without immature tubular and glomerular structures in an immature kidney before 37 weeks' gestation will also have to be considered as NR. The potential of NR to give rise to full-fledged WT is also clearly indicated in the definition. NRs are seen in 99 and 94% of the cases of synchronous and metachronous bilateral WT respectively. NRs are also more frequent in the syndromes associated with high incidence of WT (hemihypertrophy, Beckwith-Wiedemann syndrome, aniridia, and Drash syndrome). The term "nephroblastomatosis" is defined by Beckwith et al[4] as the diffuse or multifocal presence of NRs or their recognized derivatives. Multicentric and bilateral WTs are also included in this definition since multifocal presence of NRs can be inferred in these cases.

Classification. There are two types of NRs based on their location with respect to the renal lobe and five subtypes of each type based on histologic features. The two types are perilobar NR (PLNR) situated at the periphery of the renal lobe, and intralobar NR (ILNR) situated randomly within the renal lobe. PLNRs are usually numerous. ILNR usually occurs singly. PLNRs have rounded margins. ILNR has irregular margins. NRs may be unifocal, multifocal, or diffuse. The former two are characterized by a focus or foci of blastemal and embryonal epithelial cells with or without other features described in Table 13-5. Diffuse NR is characterized by a continuous subcapsular band of such cells. The histologic features of the five subtypes seen in both PLNR and ILNR are summarized in Table 13-5 and illustrated in Figures 13-21 to 13-26. Blastemal cells are usually the predominant component in PLNR, whereas mesenchymal component (myxoid or fibrous tissue) is predominant in ILNR. The histologic subtypes outlined in Table 13-5 can also be considered as various stages in the development of NR (Figure 13-27). More than one developmental state, e.g., hyperplasia and sclerosis, may be present in the same NR (Table 13-5). The obsolescent NR may be subtle. Only a rare immature tubule or a microscopic cluster of blastemal cells may be present. Adequate number of sections of the uninvolved kidney and careful histologic examination for detection of PLNR and ILNR are essential. It should be noted that ILNR can occur in the wall of a calyx or in the tissues of the renal sinus.

TABLE 13-5 Histologic Features of Subtypes of Perilobar and Intralobar Nephrogenic Rests (NR)

Subtype of NR	Histologic features
Dormant NR	Oval or oblong outline, predominantly blastemal cells with rare mitoses.
Active/maturing NR	Oval or oblong outlines, predominantly differentiating epithelial and/or stromal cells with rare or absent blastemal cells.
Sclerosing NR[a]	Stromal hyalinization in dormant or active NR.
Involuting/obsolescent NR	Further stage of sclerosis with remaining rare tubular or glomerular structures.
Hyperplastic NR	Oval or oblong outline, larger than dormant or active NR, blastemal cells and embryonal epithelial cells lining tubular structures, sclerosis may be present focally, variable mitotic activity.
Adenomatous NR	Spherical nodular lesion arising in dormant, hyperplastic, or sclerosing rest (compressed rest at the periphery), composed of well-differentiated epithelial cells in papillary or tubular configuration, low or absent mitotic activity.
Nephroblastomatous NR[b]	Spherical nodular lesion arising in dormant, hyperplastic, or sclerosing rest (compressed rest at the periphery), compact aggregates of blastemal and embryonal epithelial cells, numerous mitotic figures as in Wilms' tumor. The term small or incipient or early Wilms' tumor may also be used to describe this lesion.
Cystic NR	Seen particularly in intralobar NR, cystic change occurs in the tubules of the NR or in tubules entrapped in the NR.

[a]Chemotherapy induces sclerosing changes with or without focal cystic change in the active and nephroblastomatous NRs.

[b]Histologic features of hyperplastic and nephroblastomatous NRs are similar. The distinction is made by the configuration of the lesion (oval or bandlike in hyperplastic vs nodular in nephroblastomatous NR) and by demonstrating the compressed portion of NR from which the nephroblastomatous NR arose.

Adapted from Beckwith et al: *Pediatr Pathol* 10:1–36, 1990.

Nephroblastomatosis (NBM). Four types are defined[4]: (1) Perilobar NBM: There are multiple PLNRs or a continuous subcapsular band of PLNR is present in this type (Figure 13-21). (2) Intralobar NBM: Multiple ILNRs are present. (3) Combined NBM: There are multiple PLNRs and ILNRs. (4) Universal NBM: The kidney is diffusely enlarged and is replaced by immature and disorganized nephrons.

Significance of NRs. NRs are of significance from both a theoretical and a practical point of view.[74] From a theoretical standpoint, NRs and WTs arising from them can be considered manifestations of first and second mutation, respectively, according to the two-hit theory of Knudson and Strong.[75] Therefore NRs are potential precursors of WTs. However, most NRs do not show progression to WTs. Therefore it can be inferred that the second mutation does not occur

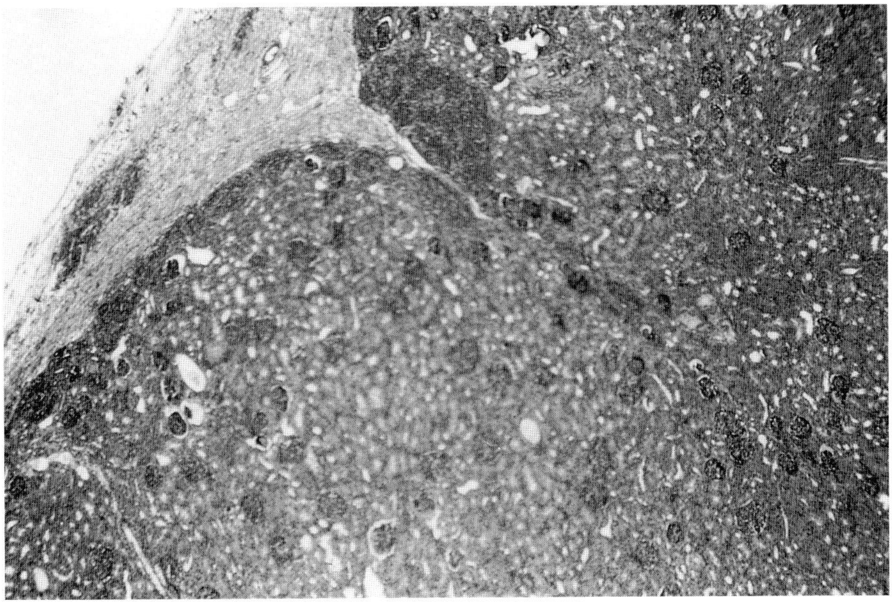

FIGURE 13-21. Diffuse perilobar nephrogenic rests characterized by continuous subcapsular band of mostly blastemal cells. Foci of hyperplasia are seen in the rest (H&E, ×40).

in most NRs and they remain dormant or involute. This also explains the far higher frequency of NRs than WTs in the general population. NRs are also bilateral. Therefore when NRs are detected in the kidney resected for unilateral WT, it is presumed that NRs are present in the opposite kidney. Since NRs are potential precursors of WT, there is a slightly increased risk of development of WT in the opposite kidney (4–5% and 1–2% respectively when ILNR and multiple PLNRs are detected in the kidney resected for unilateral WT). The risk of late recurrence is also apparently increased if there are NRs in the resected kidney. Thus NRs were present in the resected kidney in two of the five cases described by Kim et al[76] in which there was recurrence (pulmonary metastasis, local recurrence, tumor in opposite kidney) after more than 5 years of disease-free interval. Therefore a regular periodic follow-up about four times a year with imaging studies of these children is indicated. Another significant aspect of NRs is that these lesions may be histologic markers of heritable WT.

Nephrogenic Adenofibroma (NAF). Nephrogenic adenofibroma (NAF) occurs in children, adolescents, and young adults. It is a rare tumor; only five cases were detected among 7000 cases of various renal tumors recorded by the NWTS.[77] NAF is a poorly circumscribed tumor characterized by a predominant component of spindle-shaped cells admixed with a variable amount of metanephric blastema, papillary structures, psammoma bodies, and variably differentiated tubules. Nuclear atypia and mitosis are not seen. Occasional cysts lined by epithelium may be present. In three of five cases, in addition to the tumor with morphologic features described above there was a tumor with features of

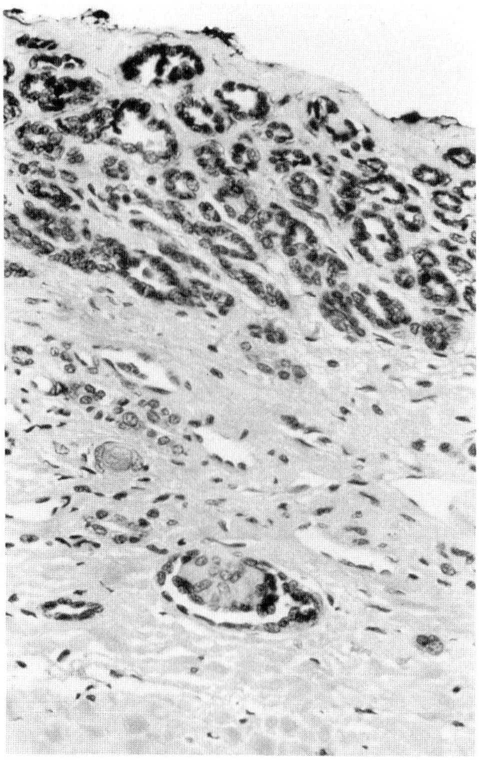

FIGURE 13-22. Sclerosis in an active and maturing perilobar nephrogenic rest (H&E, ×100).

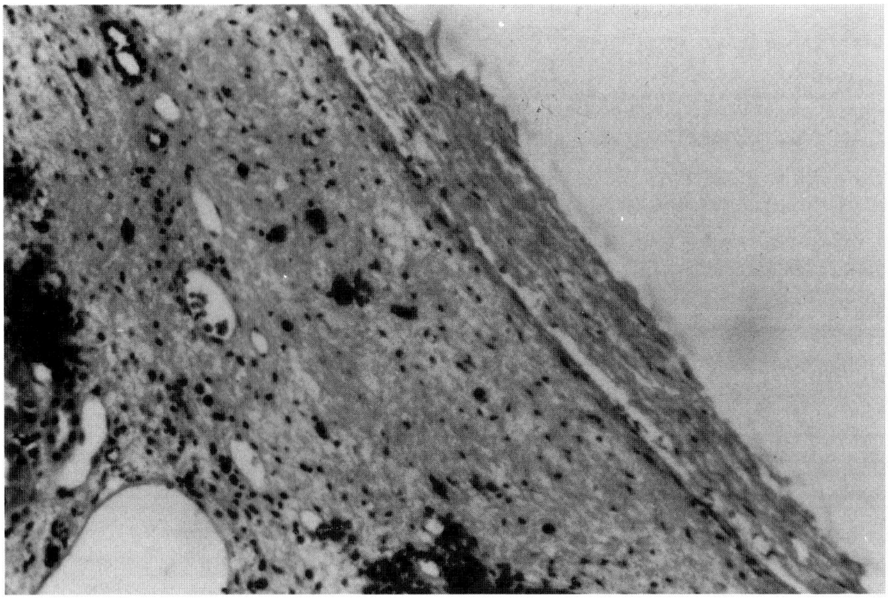

FIGURE 13-23A. Obsolescent perilobar nephrogenic rest showing collagenous fibrous tissue, with rare tubular structures and a few blood vessels (H&E, ×100).

collecting duct carcinoma (CDCA). CDCA was located near the renal hilum in continuity with NAF. Follow-up information was available in four patients who were disease-free from 1 to 2 years. The authors suggest and indeed imply by the choice of the name for the tumor that NAF has benign behavior. It appears to me that NAF that contains blastemal cells with or without a focus of CDCA would have a potential for aggressive behavior; therefore, these cases should be followed regularly for detecting possible relapse.

Wilms' Tumor (WT)

Incidence. The incidence of Wilms' tumor (WT) in the United States is 7 per million children (under age 16) per year (about 400 cases of WT every year). The incidence peaks at 2 to 3 years. Bilateral WT seen in about 5% of cases occurs at an earlier age than the unilateral WT. Fifteen to 20% of cases of WT are hereditary. Incidence of WT is lower in Japan, Asia, and Singapore than in Western countries.

Biological Markers and Paraneoplastic Syndromes. Erythropoietin, neuron-specific enolase, hyaluronic acid, hyaluronic acid–stimulating activity, and hyaluronidase are elevated in some patients with WT. The practical value of these biological markers for diagnosis of primary or recurrent WT needs to be evaluated.[78] Paraneoplastic syndromes such as hypertension, erythrocytosis, Cushing's syndrome due to ACTH production by WT, acquired von Willebrand's disease due to a factor secreted by WT leading to premature clearance of von Willebrand factor, and rarely hypercalcemia possibly due to parathormone

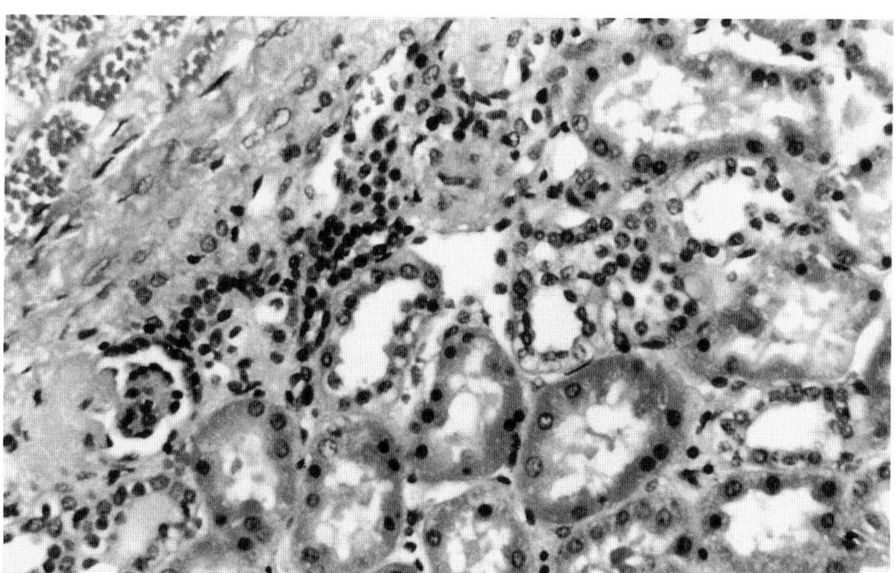

FIGURE 13-23B. Subtle obsolescent perilobar nephrogenic rest consisting of a few tubular structures (H&E, ×100).

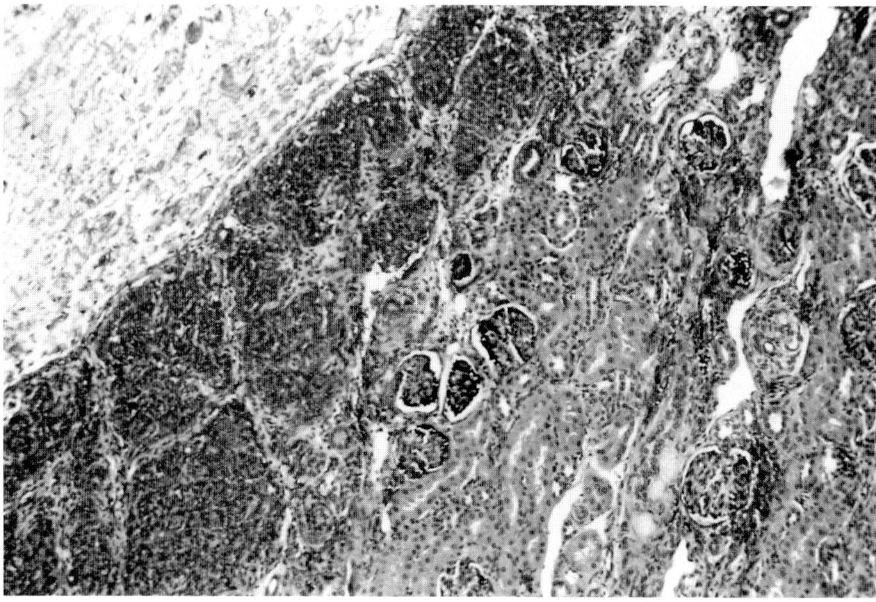

FIGURE 13-24. Hyperplastic perilobar nephrogenic rest composed of blastemal cells and immature tubular structures. The latter are not clearly visible (H&E, ×50).

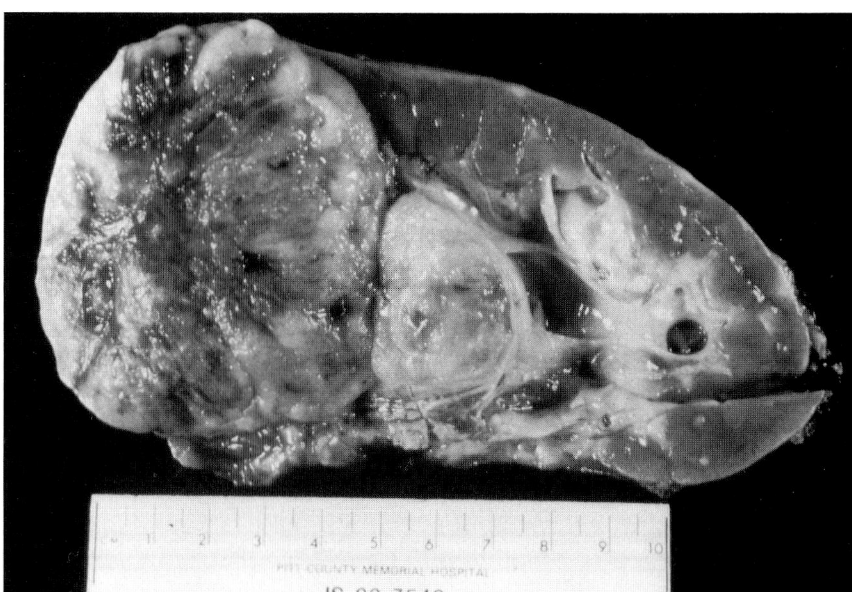

FIGURE 13-25. Gross photograph of nephrectomy specimen showing a multinodular Wilms' tumor, diffuse hyperplastic perilobar nephrogenic rests (seen as a strip of pale tissue at the periphery), and neoplastic perilobar and intralobar nephrogenic rests (seen as small pale spherical nodules).

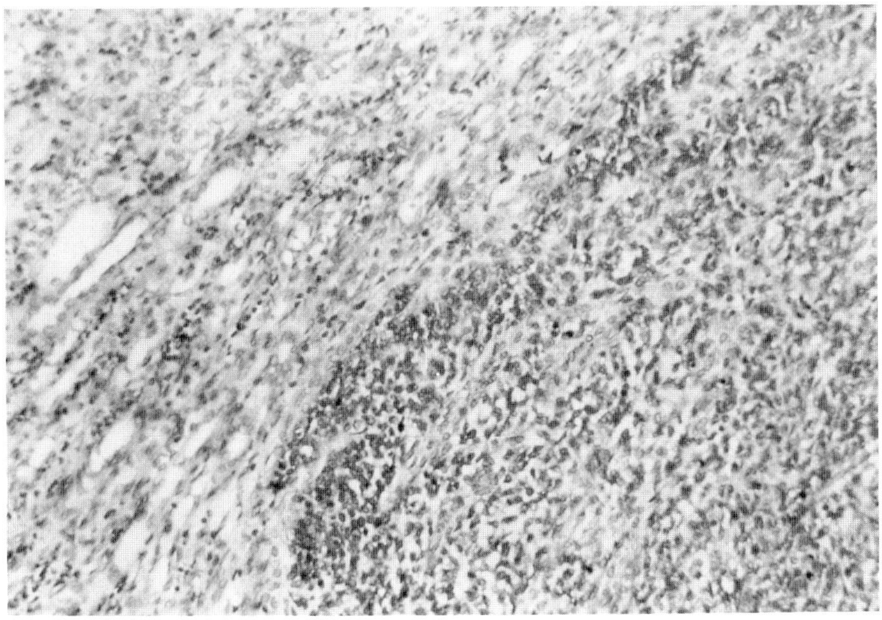

FIGURE 13-26. Nephroblastomatous intralobar nephrogenic rest with infiltrative but spherical border and predominant blastemal cells (H&E, ×250).

secretion have been reported in children with WT. The pathogenesis of hypertension is unclear. It may be related to secretion of renin by WT in some cases.

Gross Features of the Resected Tumor. The details of gross examination have been described above (Table 13-3 and Figures 13-2 and 13-3). Typically WT is a single, well-circumscribed, lobulated mass showing tan-gray appearance with or without foci of necrosis and hemorrhage on the cut surface (Figure 13-28A).[79] Multicentric tumors are likely to be seen in familial WT. Bilateral tumors are seen in about 5% of cases of WT. Pseudocysts due to hemorrhage and necrosis should be distinguished from true epithelial-lined cysts formed by dilated

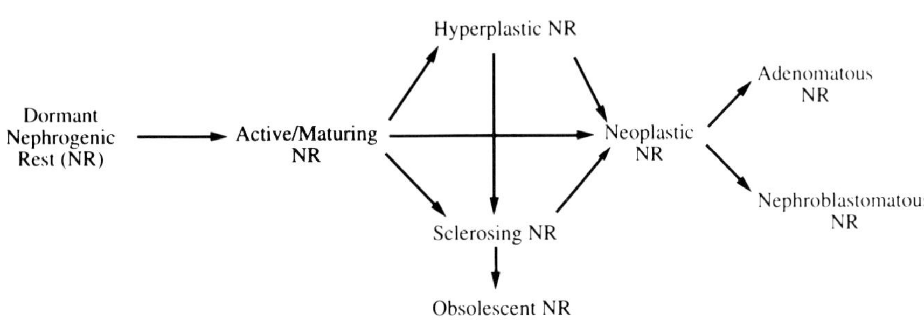

FIGURE 13-27. Diagrammatic representation of interrelationships between various histologic subtypes of nephrogenic rests. (Adapted from Beckwith JB et al: *Pediatr Pathol* 10:1–36, 1990.)

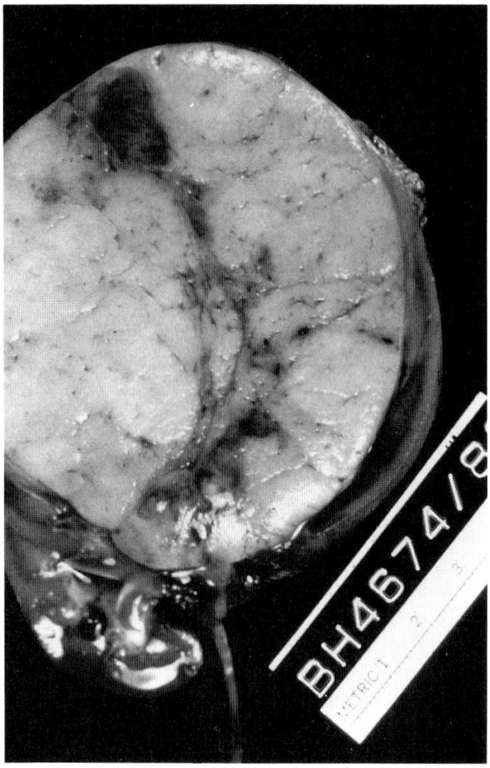

FIGURE 13-28A. Nephrectomy specimen of Wilms' tumor showing well-circumscribed fleshy tumor with small foci of hemorrhage and necrosis. Note the compression of renal sinus and surrounding kidney without invasion of these structures.

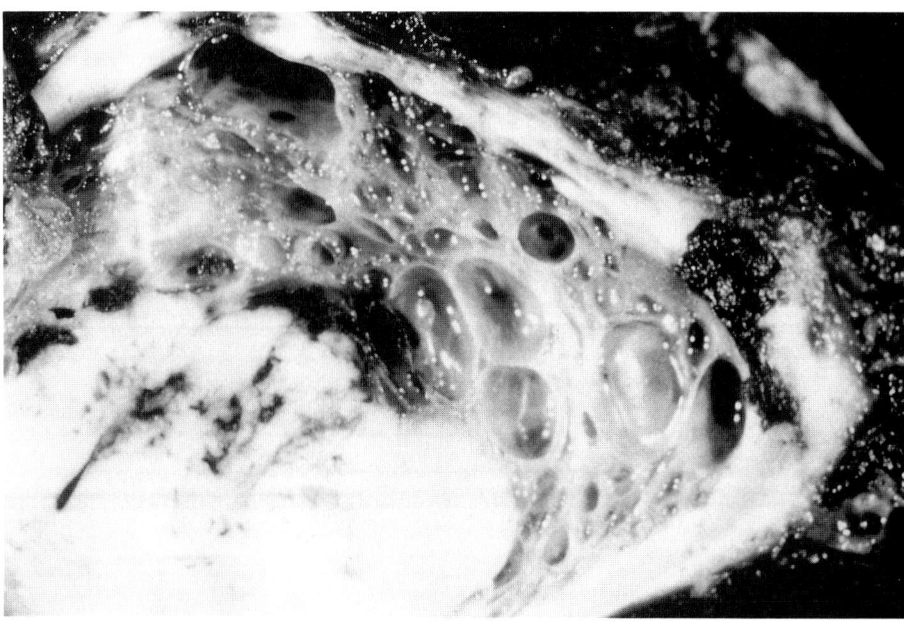

FIGURE 13-28B. True (epithelial-lined) cysts seen focally in an otherwise solid Wilms' tumor. (Reprinted with permission from Joshi VV, Beckwith JB: *Cancer* 64:466–479, 1989.)

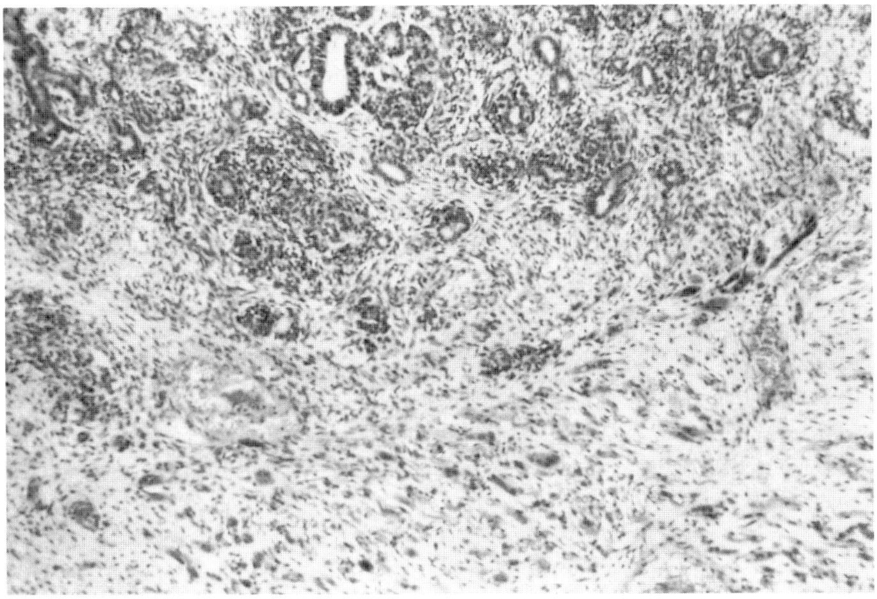

FIGURE 13-28C. Characteristic triphasic Wilms' tumor with undifferentiated and differentiating mesenchymal elements (skeletal muscle), blastemal cells, and epithelial (tubular) elements (H&E, ×100).

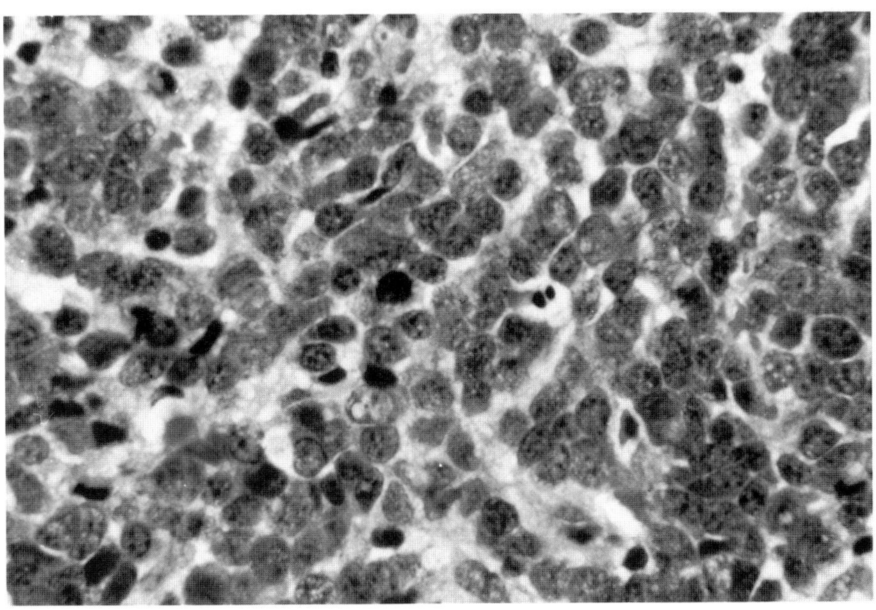

FIGURE 13-29. Blastemal cells of Wilms' tumor showing hyperchromatic nuclei with coarse chromatin pattern (H&E, ×400).

tubular structures (see the totally multicystic variant of WT, CPDN below) (Figure 13-28B). In rare cases, severe hemorrhage may occur into the tumor and it may rupture into the surrounding region. Calcification is extremely rare on gross (or microscopic) examination. However, radiologically calcification is present in about 9% of the cases. In some of these cases calcification may have been the result of therapy. The tumor may herniate into the renal pelvis or the ureter with hydronephrosis or may bulge into or invade the renal sinus or renal vein (Figure 13-3). Representative histologic sections should be taken and labeled as indicated in Table 13-3 and Figure 13-2.

Histologic Features. These can be considered as recapitulation of nephrogenesis and aberrant epithelial and/or mesenchymal differentiation. Histologic appearance of WT is characteristically described as triphasic (mesenchymal, blastemal, and epithelial elements) (Figure 13-28C). However, biphasic and monophasic WT are also seen. In most of the monophasic WTs rare small foci of some other elements (blastemal cells, tubules, etc.) which reveal the nephroblastic nature of the tumor are present. The mesenchymal elements include undifferentiated mesenchyme, striated and smooth muscle, fibroblasts, myxoid tissue, fat, cartilage, bone, elastic tissue, foci of hematopoietic cells, histiocytes, lymphoid cells, and vascular structures.[3] The skeletal muscle elements show varying degrees of differentiation extending from large round rhabdomyoblasts, strap-shaped cells, to fetal or well-differentiated rhabdomyocytes. The undifferentiated mesenchyme is not the product but the precursor of blastemal cells. Monophasic epithelial WT consists of mainly tubular structures.[80] Blastemal cells are small to large, round or oval, darkly staining cells with indiscernible cytoplasm. In blastemal cells the ratio of length of the nucleus to its width is <3, whereas in the cells of the mesenchymal elements the ratio is >3.[2] Blastemal cells are compactly arranged, and scattered individual tumor cells tend to show karyorrhexis. The nuclei are hyperchromatic and have a coarse chromatin pattern (Figure 13-29). Arrangement in nests surrounded by fibrovascular septa is seen. There may be palisading of cells at the periphery of these nests. Serpentine pattern characterized by anastomosing thin long cords of blastemal cells is also seen in some cases. Occasional tubular or rosette-like structures may be present within the blastemal foci (Figure 13-30). Rarely blastemal cells contain cytoplasmic inclusions. These details of the blastemal cell morphology are important from the point of view of distinguishing exclusively blastemal WT from the cellular CMN, CCSK, and MRTK. Eosinophilic granular cytoplasm, vacuolated cytoplasm, and hydropic clear cytoplasm may also be present in blastemal cells in some cases.[79,81] The unusual clear cell tumor of the kidney described by Glick et al[82] may represent clear cell adenoma of nephroblastic (metanephric) origin.[81] No blastemal cells were found in their case. It is not clear whether there was adequate histologic sampling of the tumor.

The epithelial elements consist of tubules resembling renal tubules or tubules lined by undifferentiated epithelium or a variety of epithelial cells (squamous, mucinous, urothelial, ciliated, columnar, and neuroendocrine cells). Neuroepithelium, neuroglia, and ganglion cells may also be seen. Monophasic fetal rhabdomyomatous WT has also been described.[83] These so-called monophasic tumors contain rare foci of other elements seen in classical

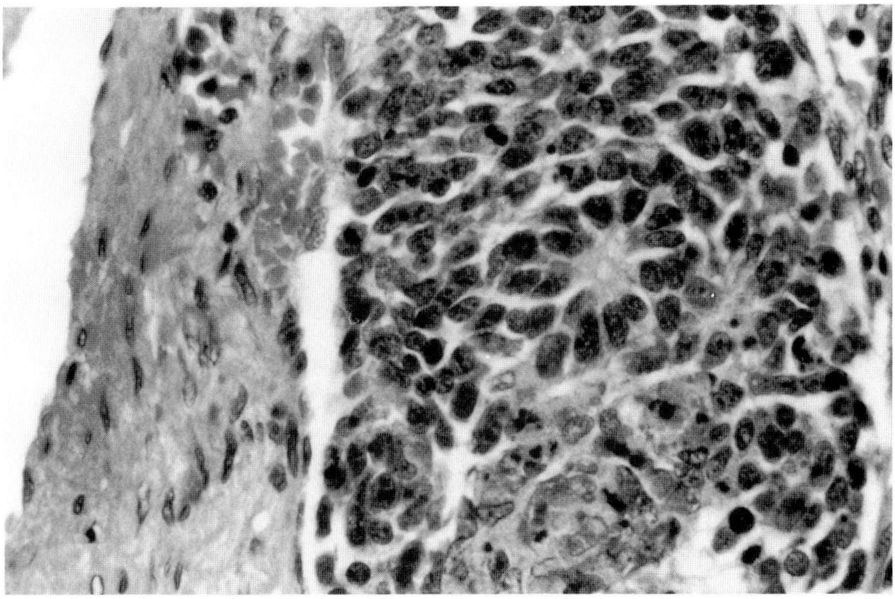

FIGURE 13-30. Blastemal cells of Wilms' tumor showing a Flexner rosette with central lumen (H&E, ×400).

triphasic WT. Thus rare tubules or glomeruloid structures or rare mesenchymal foci are seen in monophasic blastemal WT and occasional small foci of blastemal cells are present in fetal rhabdomyomatous variant of WT. In rare cases there is a prominent vascular component with severe hemorrhage into the tumor (Figure 13-31). Anaplasia is present in 5% of cases of WT (about 20 cases of anaplastic WT in the United States every year).

Prognostic Significance of Histologic Features. The only statistically significant and currently applicable morphologic features related to prognosis of WT are anaplasia and microsubstaging features.

In the landmark article based on the analysis of 427 NWTS cases published in 1978,[2] anaplasia of WT seen in about 5% of cases was shown to be a statistically significant histologic marker of poor prognosis in patients with stage II to stage IV WT (41% survival in anaplastic WT versus 91% survival in nonanaplastic WT). Anaplastic WTs are categorized as tumors showing unfavorable histology (UH). WT without anaplasia are categorized as tumors of favorable histology (FH). Anaplasia is rare in WT occurring in children <2 years of age. Criteria for anaplasia are as follows: (1) macronucleation characterized by at least threefold enlargement as compared with the nuclei of adjacent tumor cells, (2) hyperchromasia of the enlarged nuclei, and (3) markedly enlarged multipolar mitotic figures (Figure 13-32). Beckwith and colleagues emphasize that all three criteria must be present.[2,84] Anaplasia may be focal or diffuse. Focal anaplasia is defined as anaplasia found in <10% of high-power fields (usually ×400) of the histologic sections of WT.[2] There was no statistically significant difference between the survival in WT with focal and diffuse anaplasia.[84] In other words,

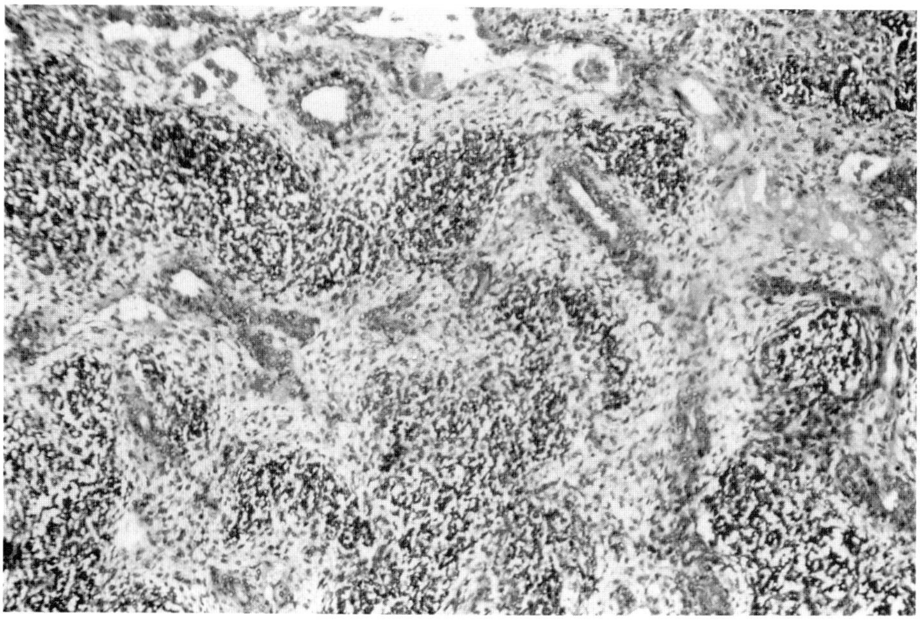

FIGURE 13-31. Wilms' tumor with blastemal cells, undifferentiated mesenchyme, and a prominent vascular component consisting of medium-sized blood vessels (H&E, ×100).

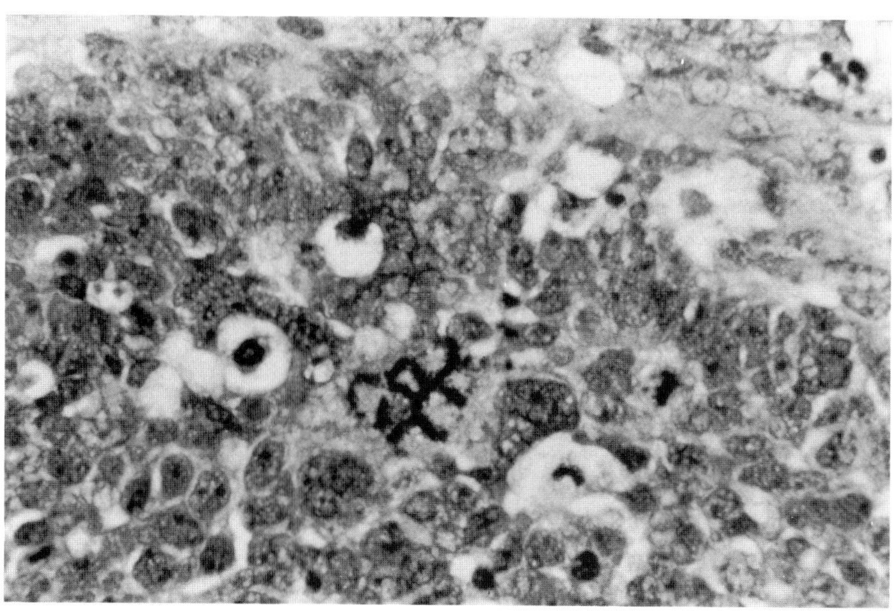

FIGURE 13-32. Anaplasia in Wilms' tumor characterized by macronucleation and a large multipolar mitotic figure (H&E, ×400).

both focal and diffuse anaplasia were associated with aggressive behavior. However, in a more recent analysis, focal anaplasia was not found to be associated with poor outcome.[85] In this preliminary report, focal anaplasia is defined as anaplasia occurring in a single focus or a few small closely placed foci (such as anaplasia occurring in histologic sections C5 and C8 in Figure 13-2). This new analysis requires clarification in a more detailed communication. Anaplasia can be seen in blastemal, mesenchymal, and epithelial elements of WT and in extrarenal sites such as renal sinus, metastatic tumor, tumor thrombus in renal vein or inferior vena cava, or extracapsular tumor extensions. It should be noted that anaplasia occurring in any of the cellular elements and any of the sites of stage II to IV WT is associated with significantly poor outcome but furthermore, anaplasia involving the blastemal elements and any of the extrarenal sites listed above is associated with a poorer outcome than anaplasia occurring in nonblastemal elements and confined to the intrarenal tumor.[84] In rare instances in which hyperchromasia and macronucleation are absent but convincing multipolar mitotic figures are present, diagnosis of anaplasia can be made.[84] Presence of moderate cytologic atypia (nuclear unrest) should alert the pathologist to the possibility of anaplasia although the latter is not found in all the cases showing nuclear unrest. Beckwith and Palmer[2] list the following features which may be confused with macronucleation and hyperchromasia: smudged nuclei, overlapping nuclei in thick sections, megakaryocytes, and calcification. True multipolar mitotic figures must be distinguished from "pseudomultipolar" mitotic figures resulting from incomplete separation of the nuclear material during the metaphase. Zuppan et al[84] indicate that each limb of the X- or Y-shaped true multipolar mitotic figure is of the same size as the entire limb of completely separated normal metaphase nucleus in the same or another section. In other words, the multipolar mitotic figures indicative of anaplasia are markedly enlarged as compared with the mitotic figures in nonanaplastic WT.

Pathologic Staging of WT. As indicated previously, stage of WT is determined at the time of diagnosis and at surgery. Details of the criteria for various stages are given in Table 13-2. Confirming or extending the clinical stage of WT is one of the most important objectives of pathologic study of the nephrectomy specimen since therapy is based on the stage (see the section on therapy below). A case of WT thought to be stage I may be converted to stage II if the completely excised tumor is found to extend beyond the renal capsule into the perirenal soft tissues on histologic examination of sections taken from the suspicious peripheral areas of the tumor (Figures 13-3 and 13-33). Similarly a stage II WT may be converted to stage III if tumor is found at the surgical resection margin or lymph node metastasis is found on histologic examination. Well-oriented and properly labeled sections from the inked peripheral and hilar margins of surgical resection are essential for demonstration of presence or absence of tumor at the margins. Presence of tumor at the margin of renal vein, if found, should be corroborated by consultation with the surgeon regarding the finding at surgery.

Metastasis to the lymph nodes may be obvious on examination at scanning power. If not, a careful histologic examination of each lymph node to detect micrometastasis is essential. Weeks et al[86] have described the following structures found in the nodal tissues, perinodal connective tissue, or the lymph node

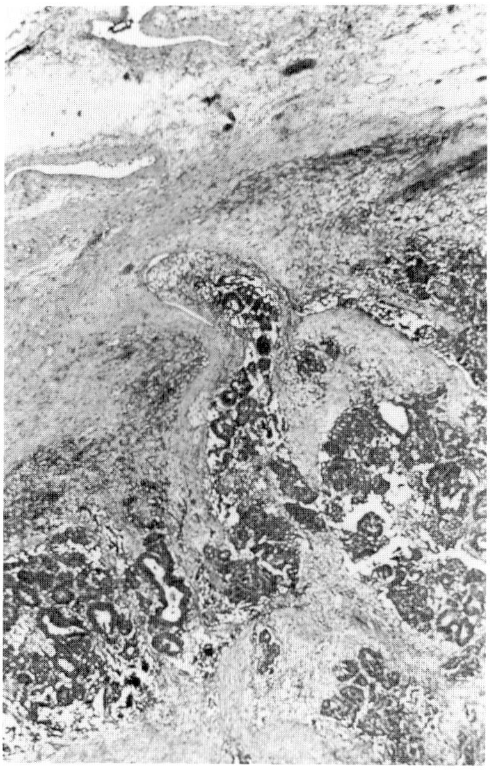

FIGURE 13-33. Photomicrograph of the bulge seen on the external surface shown in Figure 13-3A. Note the extension of the tumor into the perirenal fat (H&E, ×100).

itself which may be mistaken for lymph node metastasis: tubular structures lined by cytologically "benign" epithelial cells and embedded in Tamm-Horsfall protein, squamous epithelial cells admixed with keratin and histocytes, mesothelial inclusions, megakaryocytes, and venules lined by plump endothelial cells simulating epithelium-lined tubular structures. Portions of lymphoid follicles with germinal centers which are detached or protrude into the subcapsular sinus may also be mistaken for a metastasis.

Microsubstaging of Stage I WT. According to the criteria of NWTS, stage I WT with FH represents a WT which is confined to the kidney and is completely resected. With modern therapy, it is associated with over 90% survival. However, relapse does occur in a few patients with stage I FH WT. Weeks et al[87] studied histologic features in these tumors to determine their relationship to relapse (Table 13-6) (Figures 13-34 to 13-40). No relapses were observed in those cases in which all four histologic microsubstaging features were absent. One or more features were present in virtually all the 24 relapsed cases but also occurred in 46% of the 48 control cases without relapse. Therefore presence of one or more of these microsubstaging features was not of predictive value with respect to relapse, but absence of all four was predictive of absence of relapse.[87] The NWTS pathology checklist requires the data regarding microsubstaging features to be filled in by the institutional pathologist.

Histologic Features of "Perilobar" and "Intralobar" WT. Renal lobe consists of the medullary pyramid and its cortical mantle. The medullary portion of the lobe

TABLE 13-6 Features Evaluated for Microsubstaging of Favorable Histology Stage I Wilms' Tumor

Feature	Criteria	Comment
Capsular invasion	Presence of tumor in the outer half of tumor capsule which may be identifiable separately or may be fused with renal capsule.	Capsular penetration indicated by presence of tumor beyond renal capsule, i.e., in perirenal fat which is considered as a criterion of stage II, should be distinguished from capsular invasion seen in some stage I WT.
Inflammatory pseudocapsule	Presence of granulation tissue with or without inflammatory cells in the peripheral soft tissue at the surface of the tumor.	Inflammatory pseudocapsule may represent a reaction to contain the tumor which is attempting to invade the perirenal fat. This is the most significant of the four microsubstaging features.
Invasion of renal sinus	Presence of tumor in the soft tissues and blood vessels of the renal sinus which is the concavity on the medial aspect of the kidney containing pelvicalyceal system, connective tissue, blood vessels, lymphatics, and nerves.	Herniation of WT into the pelvicalyceal system or protrusion of WT into the renal sinus does not constitute renal sinus invasion. Renal sinus invasion beyond hilar plane (medial aspect of the sinus) is a criterion of stage II. Renal cortex lining the renal sinus does not have a capsule.
Intrarenal vessel involvement	Presence of tumor in the blood vessels and/or lymphatics within the renal parenchyma beyond the tumor indicated by: (a) distension of lumen by tumor, (b) adherence of tumor to inner aspect of the vessel wall, (c) tumor infiltration through the vessel wall, (d) formation of a thrombus containing tumor.	Vessels containing loose clusters of tumor cells in their lumen are not considered to be involved by tumor.

WT: Wilms' tumor.
Adapted from Weeks et al: *Cancer* 60:1204–1212, 1987.

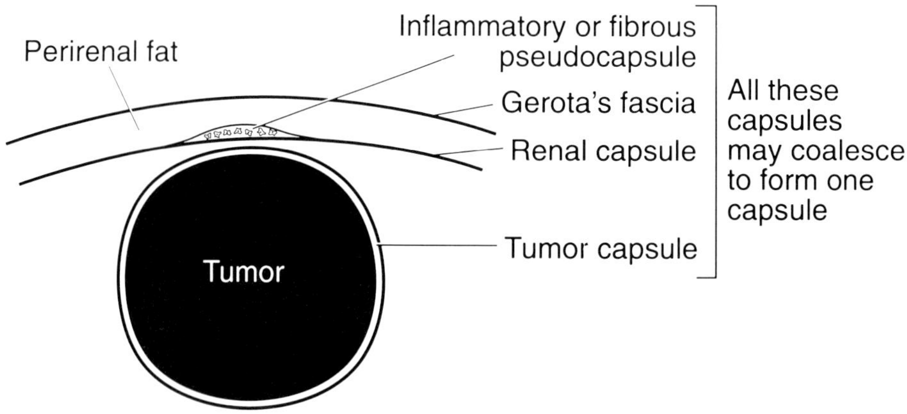

FIGURE 13-34. Diagrammatic representation of the various capsules which are seen in the nephrectomy specimen of Wilms' tumor.

develops first. About 12 generations of nephrons are added to the medulla to complete the lobar organization. The nephrons closest to the medulla are the oldest. Developmental disturbances occurring early and late in fetal life usually involve the medulla/deep cortex and periphery of the cortex respectively. Hence ILNR and PLNR are considered as early and late developmental disturbances respectively. Beckwith et al[4] have suggested "intralobar" and "perilobar" subtypes of WT based on these embryological considerations and concepts. Knudson also has suggested recently that WT may represent more than one genetic entity.[88] Thus "intralobar" WTs, occurring in association with ILNR, show recapitulation of early developmental stages of renal lobar development such as collecting ducts and ampullae and a prominent mesenchymal component. Heterologous elements such as skeletal muscle are more common in these tumors. (CN and CPDN are also considered to recapitulate the early stages of renal development.) In contrast, "perilobar" WTs occurring in association with PLNR show recapitulation of late stages of renal lobar development. These tumors contain predominant blastemal and epithelial elements with a small mesenchymal component and tend to contain more commonly tubular and glomeruloid structures. Many WTs cannot be readily categorized into perilobar and intralobar types and some overlap does occur.

Wilms' Tumorlet. This term was introduced by Bove and McAdams[69] to designate well-circumscribed WT composed of embryonal renal epithelial cells and measuring between 1 and 3.5 cm in diameter. Wilms' tumorlet is a lesion belonging to the spectrum of NBM. Beckwith et al[4] indicate that various lesions of NBM comprise a continuum and they prefer to use the terms "small," "incipient," or "early WT" to the term "Wilms' tumorlet."

Immunohistochemical Features. A number of investigators have studied the patterns of intermediate filaments and other markers in WT by using immunoperoxidase or immunofluorescence staining.[6,89–92] Blastemal cells generally show positive staining for both cytokeratin and vimentin. Mesenchymal cells are

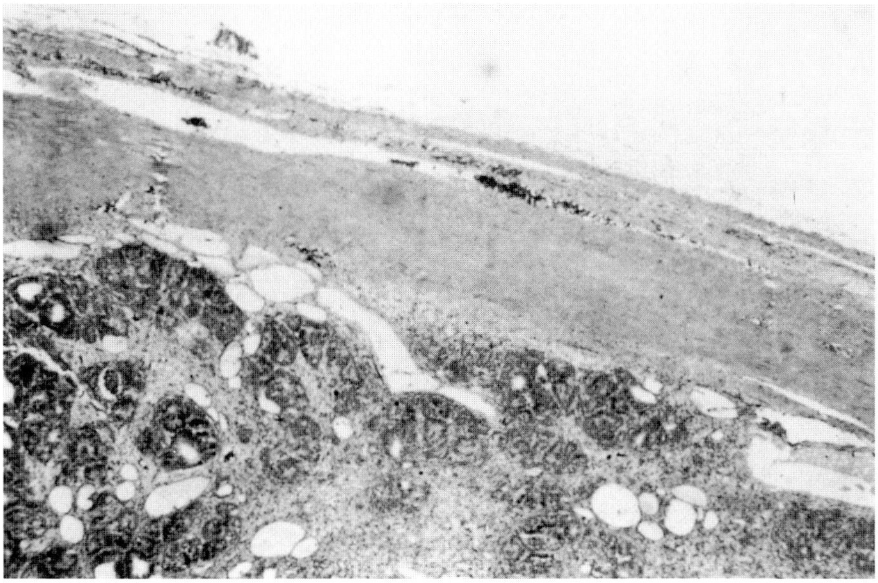

FIGURE 13-35A. Photomicrograph of Wilms' tumor showing the fusion of tumor capsule, renal capsule, and Gerota's fascia with effacement of perirenal fat. Demarcations between tumor capsule and renal capsule and between renal capsule and Gerota's fascia can be faintly discerned. The slit-like space between the different capsules is due to artifact (H&E, ×25).

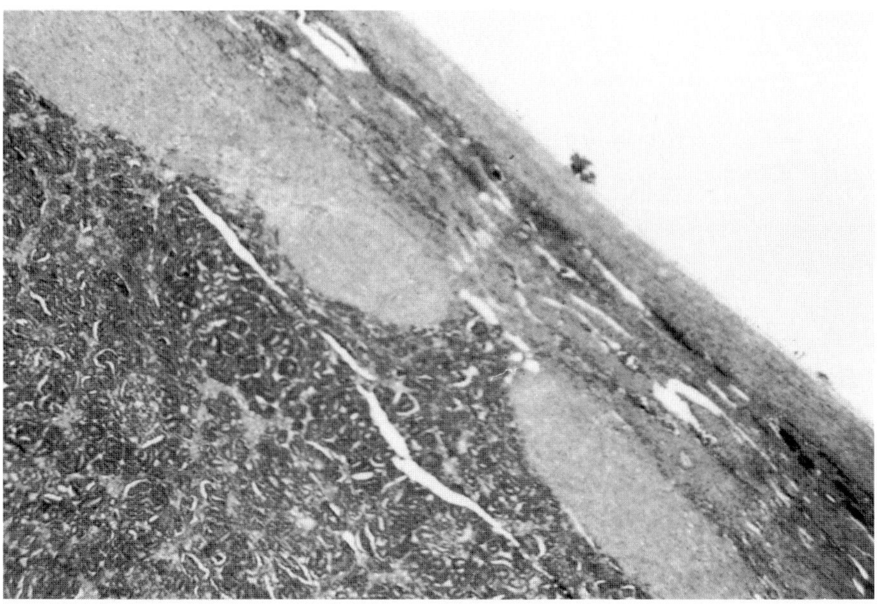

FIGURE 13-35B. Capsular invasion by Wilms' tumor up to the outer half of but not beyond the tumor capsule (H&E, ×25).

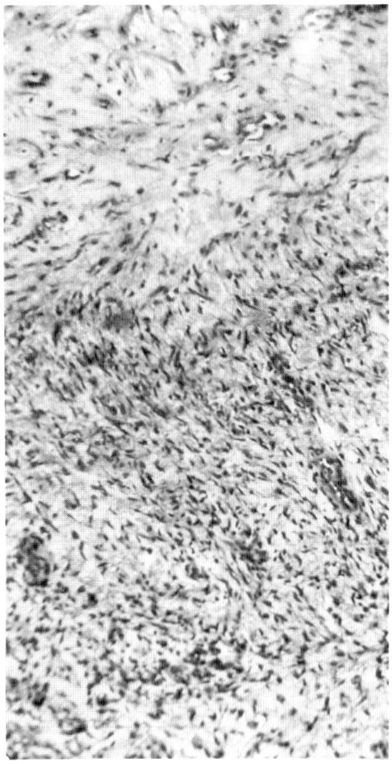

FIGURE 13-36. Inflammatory pseudocapsule in the perirenal soft tissue at the external surface of Wilms' tumor (H&E, ×100).

positive for vimentin and epithelial cells lining the tubules for cytokeratin alone.[89,90] Glomeruloid bodies usually stain for vimentin.[90] Cytoplasmic staining for neuron-specific enolase, S-100 protein and glial fibrillary acidic protein (GFAP) was demonstrated in the cytoplasm of blastemal and mesenchymal cells by Magee et al.[92] Neoplastic tubular analogues of proximal convoluted tubules and collecting ducts have been demonstrated by lectin histochemistry and immunohistochemistry.[93] The immunohistochemical markers are helpful in the distinction of predominantly blastemal WT from other small round cell tumors especially in a FNA biopsy. These markers would also be helpful in the histologic diagnosis of predominantly blastemal extrarenal WT or in FNA biopsy diagnosis of an abdominal tumor that was not suspected to be WT because the precise location could not be ascertained.

Ultrastructural Features. These have been reviewed by Mierau et al[6] and Schmidt et al.[94] The blastemal cells are polygonal in shape with large nuclei. The cytoplasm contains scanty organelles with numerous free ribosomes. There are well-developed desmosomes and flocculent material is seen surrounding the cells. Cilia are seen in larger numbers than in the cells of other childhood tumors (Figures 13-41 to 13-43).[6] Developing tubular structures may be discernible in the groups of blastemal cells. Kurtz has described what he considers an ultrastructural variant of WT in which the predominant blastemal cells contained abundant autophagolysosomes (Figure 13-44).[95] Glomeruloid bodies consist of epithelial cells; endothelial or mesangial cells are usually absent. The

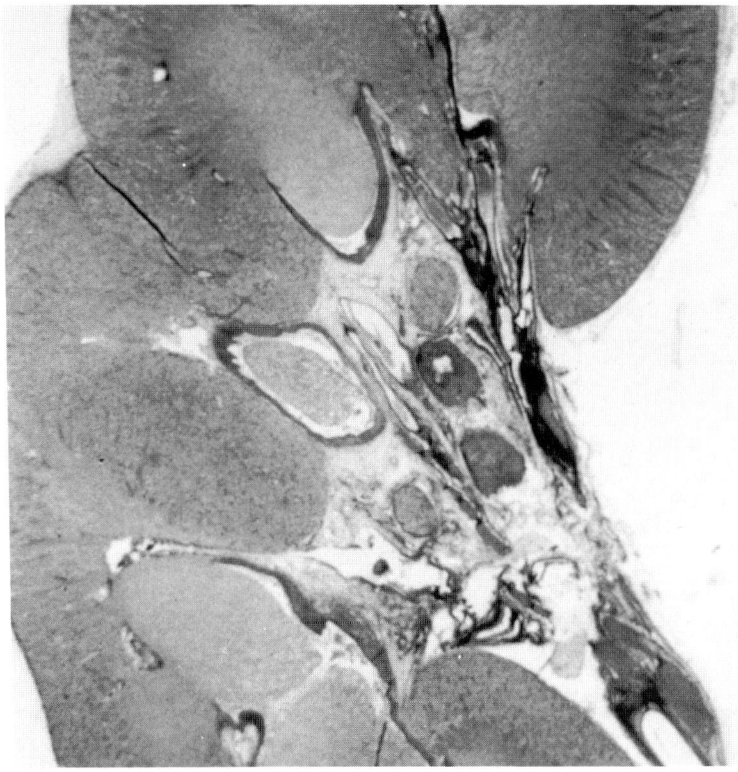

FIGURE 13-37. Whole mount of longitudinal section of the kidney to display the renal sinus outlined by the renal parenchyma on three sides and limited by renal hilus medially. The renal sinus contains pelvicalyceal system, blood vessels, lymphatic nerves, and soft tissue (H&E, ×1).

mesenchymal cells show flocculent coating, cilia, elongated nuclei, and varying amounts of rough endoplasmic reticulum.[91] Electron microscopic studies are not required for the diagnosis of most of the cases of WT. However, it is useful in the differential diagnosis of predominantly blastemal WT from CCSK, CCMN, or small round cell tumors of childhood. Electron microscopy is also helpful when only a FNA biopsy of a predominantly blastemal WT is available.

Cytologic Features. In most cases the preoperative diagnosis of WT is strongly suggested by the age of the patient and location of the tumor in the kidney. A nephrectomy is performed and the diagnosis is confirmed histologically. However, in some cases, the renal tumor may be inoperable, as demonstrated by findings on imaging procedures, or there may be clinical contraindication for major surgery—a situation more likely to arise in children in developing countries. Rarely, the precise location of the abdominal tumor may not be evident. A FNA biopsy may be indicated in such cases to establish a diagnosis so that appropriate therapy can be given to shrink the tumor for making it operable.

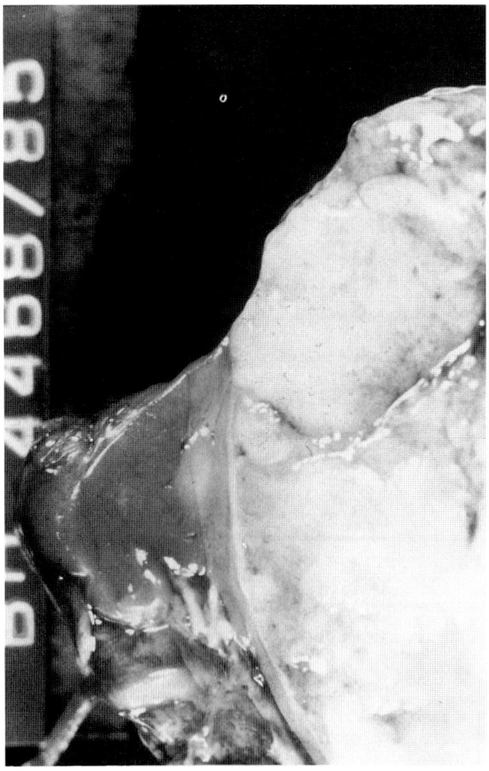

FIGURE 13-38. Nephrectomy specimen showing Wilms' tumor compressing but not invading the renal sinus.

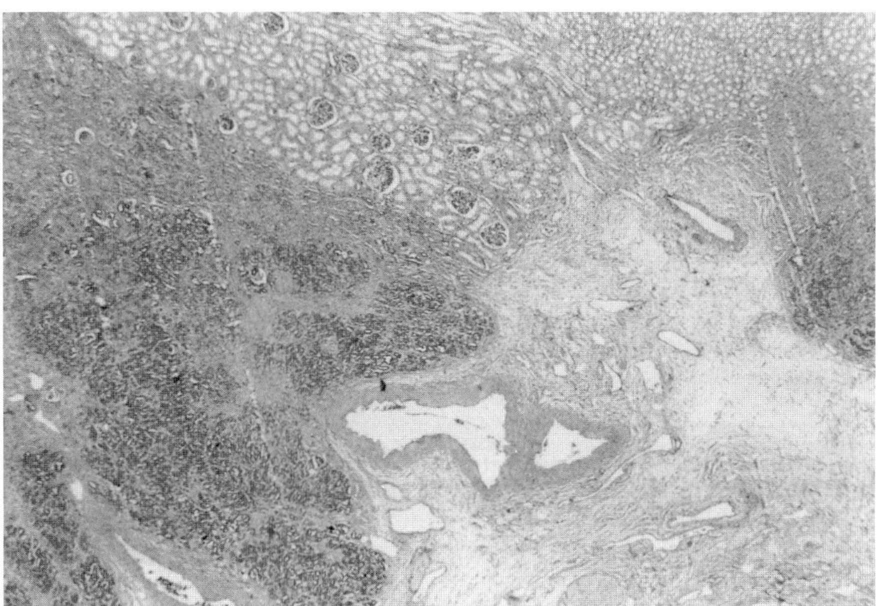

FIGURE 13-39. Invasion of renal sinus by Wilms' tumor. Note the proximity of the invading edge of the tumor to blood vessels and lymphatics (H&E, ×40).

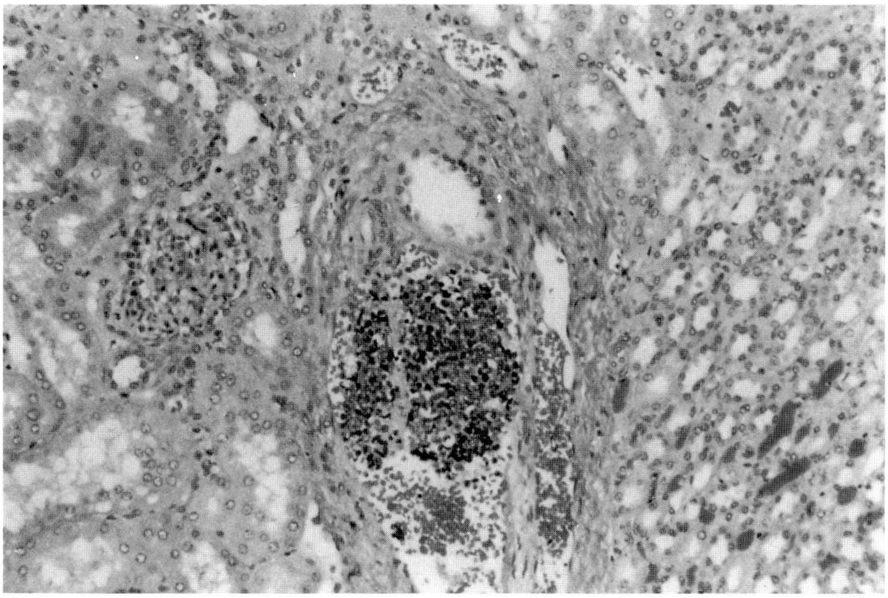

FIGURE 13-40. Involvement of a vein within the renal parenchyma but outside the Wilms' tumor. Note the distension of the vein by the tumor (H&E, ×100).

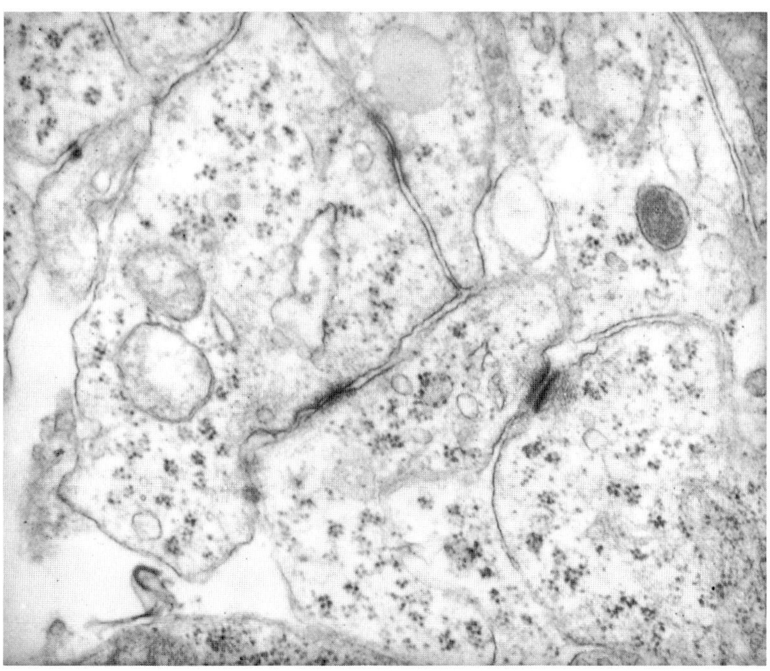

FIGURE 13-41. Electromicrographs of portions of blastemal cells of Wilms' tumor to show numerous free ribosomes and well-developed cell junctions (uranyl acetate and lead citrate, ×7,200).

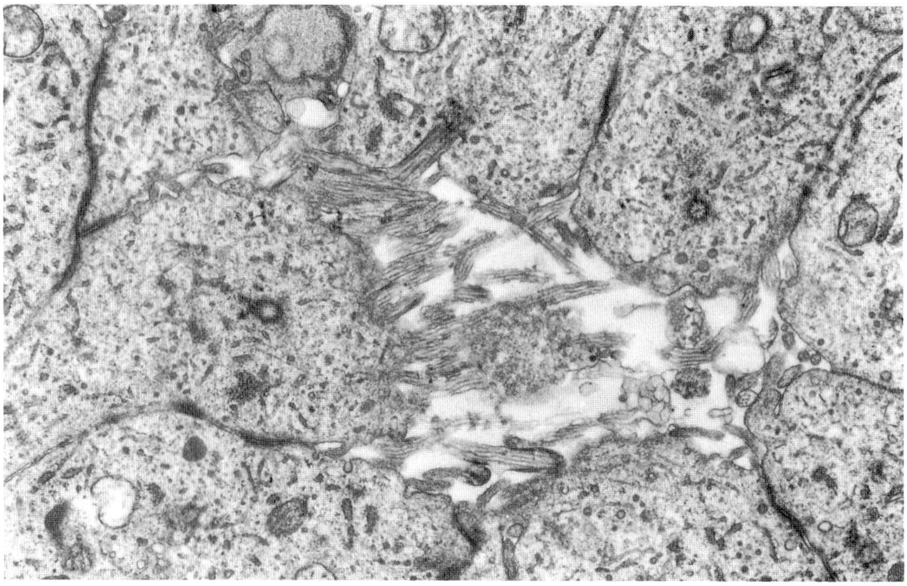

FIGURE 13-42. Cells of Wilms' tumor showing well-developed cilia (uranyl acetate and lead citrate, ×7,200).

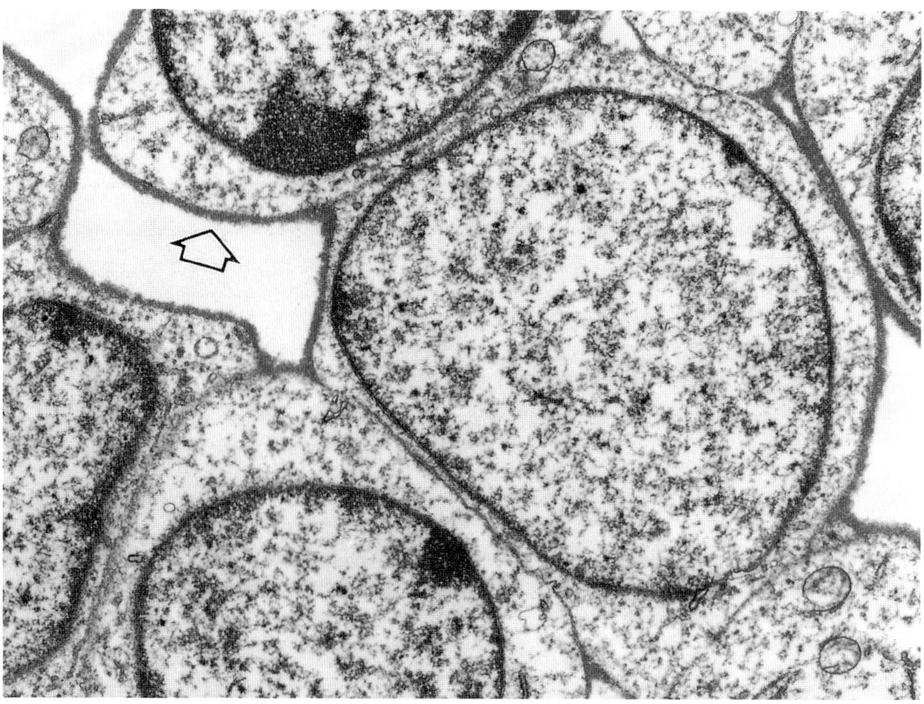

FIGURE 13-43. Blastemal cells of Wilms' tumor with characteristic coating of flocculent basement membrane–like material (*arrow*). Note the paucity of organelles (uranyl acetate and lead citrate, ×5,800). (Courtesy of Dr. Gary W. Mierau.)

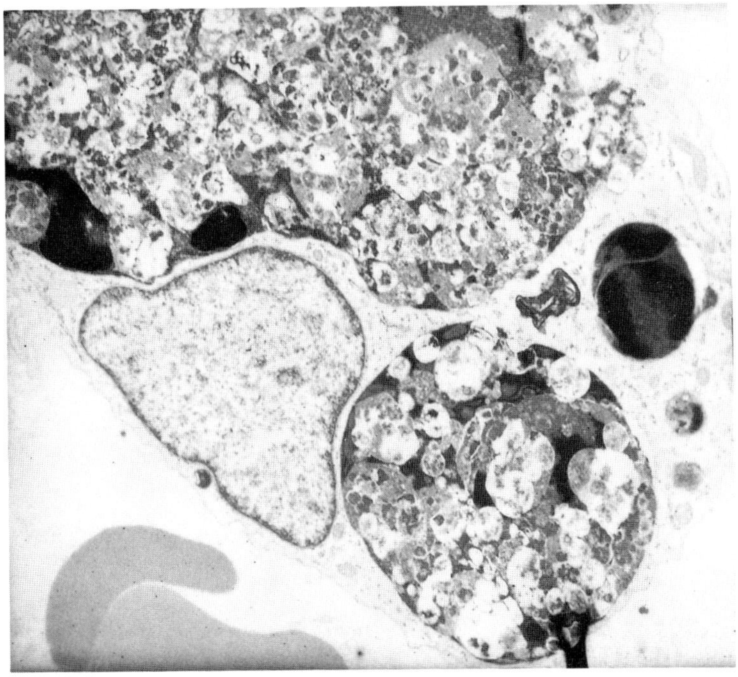

FIGURE 13-44. Blastemal cells of Wilms' tumor showing numerous autophagolysosomes containing amorphous material (uranyl acetate and lead citrate, ×1,400).

The NWTS guidelines regarding the effect of (FNA) biopsy on the staging of WT as outlined in Table 13-2 need to be modified at this time since there is no evidence that a FNA biopsy leads to tumor spillage. FNA biopsy may also be used for diagnosis of metastatic WT.

The FNA biopsy shows one or more of the following: blastemal cells, spindle-shaped mesenchymal cells, and tubular structures (Figures 13-45 to 13-47). Quijano and Drut describe finely dispersed chromatin pattern in the nuclei of blastemal cells.[96] On histologic examination, blastemal cells have coarse chromatin pattern, a feature which is of great importance in histologic differential diagnosis between blastemal WT and CCSK (Figures 13-15 and 13-29). Only blastemal cells or mesenchymal cells may be sampled by the FNA biopsy. Rosettes may be present in the blastemal cells (Figure 13-45). Differentiation from small round cell tumors of childhood and other renal tumors such as CCSK may be difficult in such cases. Immunohistochemical stains are helpful in this regard. Rarely blastemal rosettes of WT may show positive staining for neuron-specific enolase.[92,97] Histologic examination of the cell block from the FNA biopsy material, immunoperoxidase stains on the smears, and histologic sections and ultrastructural examination of the FNA biopsy material are helpful in making a diagnosis. Presence of flocculent basement membrane–like material, cilia, tight cell junctions, and autophagolysosomes are helpful ultrastructural features in the recognition of blastemal cells in the FNA biopsy of WT.

In the series of 10 cases described by Quijano and Drut,[96] anaplasia was found in three cases by histologic examination. In two of these cases anaplasia

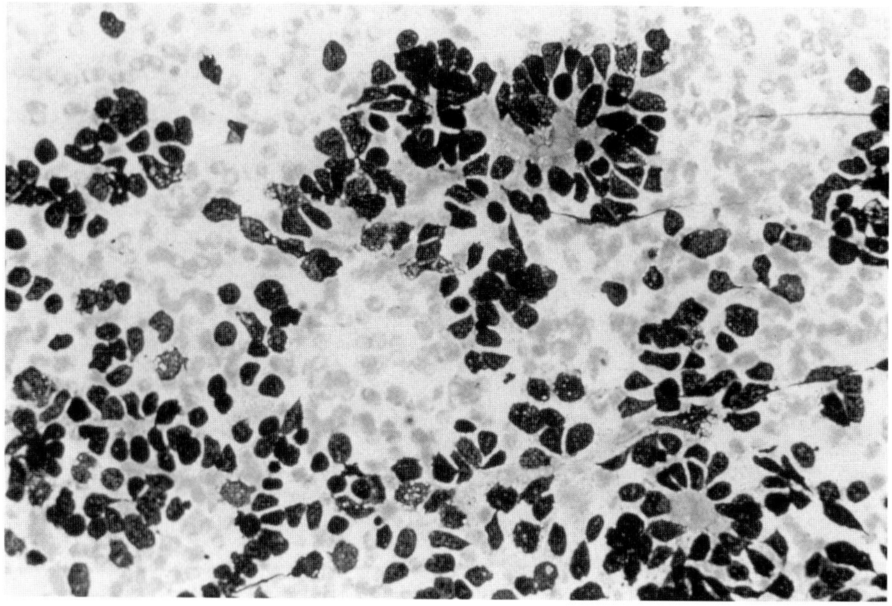

FIGURE 13-45. Smear from fine-needle aspiration biopsy of Wilms' tumor showing round tumor cells with large nuclei arranged singly, or in clusters. In one focus rosette-like arrangement is evident (Diff-Quik, ×400). (Courtesy of Dr. Jan F. Silverman.)

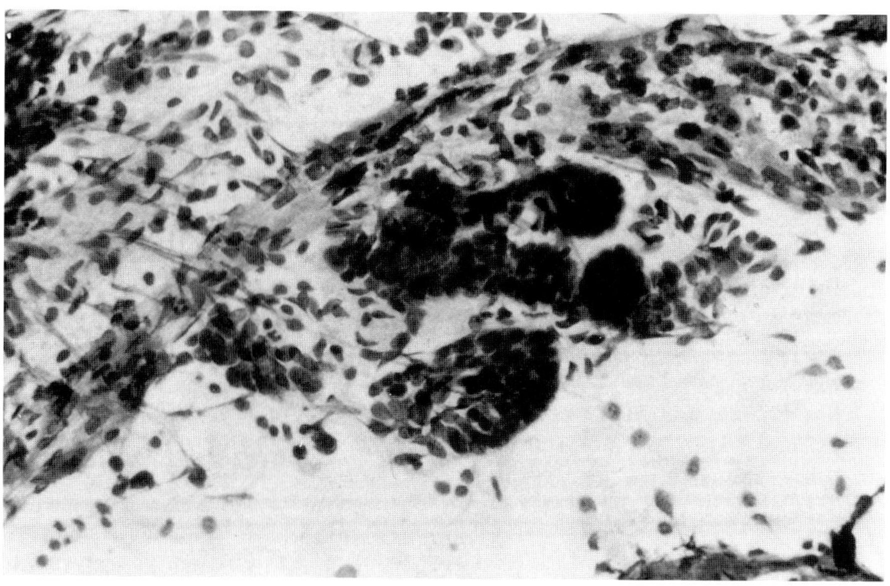

FIGURE 13-46. Smear from fine-needle aspiration biopsy of Wilms' tumor showing tubular arrangement of tumor cells. Note also the spindle-shaped cells of the mesenchymal component (Papanicolaou stain, ×250). (Courtesy of Dr. Jan F. Silverman.)

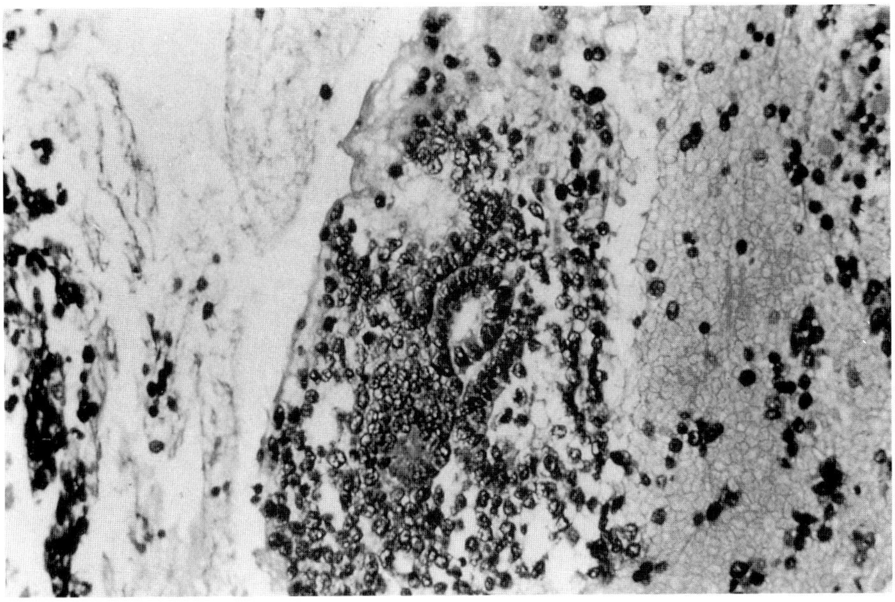

FIGURE 13-47. Cell block from fine-needle aspiration biopsy of Wilms' tumor showing blastemal cells and a tubule (H&E, ×250). (Courtesy of Dr. Jan F. Silverman.)

was detected in the FNA biopsy. Drut and Pollono[98] have also described anaplasia in FNA biopsy of WT. Thus anaplasia can be detected by FNA biopsy. However, its absence in the FNA biopsy smears or cell block does not rule out presence of anaplasia in the WT under investigation since the FNA biopsy represents a very small sample of the tumor.

Histologic Features of Treated WT. In a review of 83 NWTS cases with posttherapy resection of WT after an average interval of 10 weeks, Zuppan et al[99] have described the following features in tumors showing good response to therapy: coagulative necrosis, edematous or hyalinized connective tissue, foreign body granulomas around areas of necrosis, fibroblastic proliferation, mononuclear infiltration, old and recent hemorrhage, and thrombosis of blood vessels and small foci of residual tumor. The residual tumor was represented in some cases by isolated well-differentiated tubules set in a mature stroma. In the cases in which a large amount of viable tumor persists despite therapy, the findings are variable. There may be persistent blastemal elements, immature tubules, cystic change (sometimes resembling CPDN) and mature skeletal muscle, cartilage, and fatty tissue. In the NWTS series, comparison with the preoperative biopsy appeared to indicate that the blastemal component was the most sensitive. Extensive (>90%) necrosis of tumor, low mitotic activity, and good differentiation in the residual tumor were associated with better survival.

Anaplasia was found in nine of these 83 cases examined histologically after therapy. In two of these cases there was anaplasia in the preoperative biopsy. The disease-free survival in the tumors showing anaplasia was 55% as compared with 79% for nonanaplastic WT. These investigators ruled out the possibility of spurious production of anaplastic changes due to therapy. In some cses hyperchromatic enlarged nuclei were seen but multipolar mitotic figures were absent. Malignant fibrous histiocytoma-like changes may also be seen. It has been suggested that chemotherapy may induce epithelial differentiation and rhabdomyogenesis and radiation therapy may accelerate or induce nonepithelial differentiation.

WT in Adults. Babaian et al reviewed 167 cases of WT in adult patients.[100] Adult WT (AWT) is similar histologically to the childhood WT.[101] The median age in the series of 27 NWTS AWT cases was 24 years with the range extending from 16 to 74 years. Anaplasia was seen in one of the more recent cases of AWT reported in the literature.[102] Small cell carcinoma, non-Hodgkin's malignant lymphoma, sarcomatoid renal carcinoma, and sarcomas of the kidney should be distinguished from AWT.

Other Features. There are a few reports describing the chromosomal abnormalities and determination of DNA index (DI) in WT. Constitutional deletion of the band 11 p13 in WT patients with aniridia is well recognized.[103] Somatic deletion and rearrangements of the same region have also been identified in sporadic cases of WT.[104] Schmidt et al in a study of DI done on paraffin-embedded tumor material found a large number of aneuploid tumor DNA stemlines and high values of S-phase fractions and proliferation index in anaplastic WT and a moderate number of aneuploid tumor DNA stemlines and intermediate S-phase fractions and proliferation index for nonanaplastic WT.[61] In a study of 48 cases, Douglass et al demonstrated hyperdiploidy (DI $>$1.5) in nine of the 10 anaplastic WT whereas the DI in all the nonanaplastic WT was 1.05 to 1.39.[105] Anaplastic WT also showed numerous complex chromosomal translocations.

It is of interest to note that the tumor suppressor gene WT1 (see Chapter 10 Tumors in Children—General Aspects for definition and role of tumor suppressor genes) has been identified at chromosome 11p13.[106] Homozygous deletion of all or part of WT1 gene has been demonstrated in some cases of sporadic WT[107] and specific alterations of WT1 gene have been found in several sporadic and hereditary WTs.[108] These observations provide molecular evidence that inactivation of the tumor suppressor gene WT1 is involved in the pathogenesis of WT. In a recent preliminary communication, correlation between WT1 expression and histologic features of WT has been demonstrated.[109,110] Predominantly blastemal WTs expressed high levels of WT1, whereas predominantly mesenchymal WT or WT with heterologous differentiation had low level of expression.[109,110] There was inverse relationship between level of WT1 expression and degree of differentiation in WT, suggesting a relationship of WT1 to renal development. WT1 gene has been shown to play a role in the development of the genitourinary system. WT1 gene expression has been demonstrated in the condensed (nephrogenic) mesenchyme, renal vesicle, and glomerular epithelial cells.[111] WT2 has been identified recently and much work is being done concerning other WT genes.[112] Surgical pathologists can play a role in facilitating this work by providing appropriate specimens from *all* pathologic specimens of WT for molecular biologic studies and by exploring the correlation between genetic and morphologic features in their own laboratories. High level of N-myc gene expression in the absence of N-myc gene amplification and low level of C-myc gene expression have been demonstrated in WT. High level of N-myc expression is also present in human fetal kidneys.[113]

Differential Diagnosis of WT. In most of the cases, definitive diagnosis can be made by routine histologic methods, if an adequate number of sections are available. CCMN, CCSK, and small round cell tumors in children will have to be considered in the differential diagnosis of monophasic blastemal WT. This has been discussed in the sections on CCMN and CCSK and in Chapter 12 on small round cell tumors in children. Because of the prominence and diversity of heterotopic elements in certain cases of triphasic WT, renal teratoma may be considered in the differential diagnosis.[114] However, true renal teratomas are exceedingly rare. Beckwith has seen only one probable case among the 2600 NWTS specimens of renal tumors.[3] The main criterion for teratoma is the presence of some degree of organization in the cellular elements to form structures resembling bronchi, ventricles of the brain, gastrointestinal tract, cerebellum, etc. The diagnosis also depends upon the unequivocal intrarenal location of the tumor. Rhabdomyosarcoma (RMS) may have to be considered in the differential diagnosis of fetal rhabdomyomatous WT. The details of morphologic features of RMS are described in the chapter on small round cell tumors of children. Primary RMS of kidney is extremely rare.[115]

Prognostic Factors in WT. Besides anaplasia and the microsubstaging features, the following factors were related to relapse and metastasis of WT without demonstrable evidence of metastasis at diagnosis in NWTS-II[116]: microscopically confirmed regional lymph node metastasis, operative spillage of tumor, and tumor thrombus in renal vein with or without extension to inferior vena cava. Many of these factors are identified or confirmed by the pathologist. In the previous analysis of NWTS cases, age and specimen weight (>250 g) were found to be related to prognosis; however, in the analysis of NWTS II cases, the prognostic impact of age was explained by association of age with the other aforementioned prognostic factors. Specimen weight was no more a determinant of prognosis. In NWTS cases, the survival in FH stage I, II, III, and IV patients was 97, 92, 87, and 83% respectively and for UH stage I to III and stage IV patients 68 and 55% respectively.[11,117]

Renal Cell Carcinoma (RCC). Renal cell carcinoma (RCC) may be of two conceptual types: RCC occurring in association with WT[3] and RCC occurring by itself in older children and adults.[118] The latter is generally considered to arise from proximal tubules. RCC is rare in children, comprising <7% of the primary renal malignant tumors. Raney et al[119] and Lack et al[120] have described 20 and 17 children with RCC respectively. The mean age at diagnosis is about 11 years (range, 14 months to 19 years). Histologically the tumors are composed of clear or granular cells showing trabecular, tubular, or papillary pattern. Clear cell tumors are predominant. Sarcomatoid renal cell carcinoma apparently does not occur in children. Foci of RCC may be present in a WT, or RCC can occur following treatment of WT. Renal vascular invasion has been claimed to be the most important pathologic feature related to prognosis,[121] but this conclusion was not corroborated in a more recent series of RCC.[120] The overall prognosis in children with RCC (e.g., 80 to 100% survival in stage I) is similar to that of adults. The criteria for staging of RCC are as follows: tumor confined to the kidney (stage I), extension of tumor to perinephric fat but within Gerota's fascia (stage II), metastasis to regional lymph nodes or involvement of inferior vena cava (stage III), and metastasis to other organs (stage IV).

Tumors Recapitulating Predominantly Inducted Ureteric Bud

Cystic Nephroma or Multilocular Cyst of Kidney

Terminology. Multilocular cyst (MLC) of kidney and cystic nephroma (CN) are the two terms that have been used to describe renal tumors consisting of a well-demarcated multicystic mass with the cysts lined by epithelium and bounded by thin, mostly fibrous septa (see below for detailed criteria). We and others prefer the term CN[122,123] because the lesion under consideration is not of developmental origin but is a neoplastic lesion.

Pathologic Features. The revised criteria for the diagnosis of CN are as follows (Figures 13-48 and 13-49)[123]:

1. The lesion is composed entirely of cysts and their septa.
2. It forms a discrete mass, well-demarcated from the noncystic renal parenchyma.
3. The septa are the only solid portion of the tumor, conforming to the outlines of the cysts without solid expansile nodules.
4. The cysts are lined by flattened, cuboidal, or hobnail epithelium.

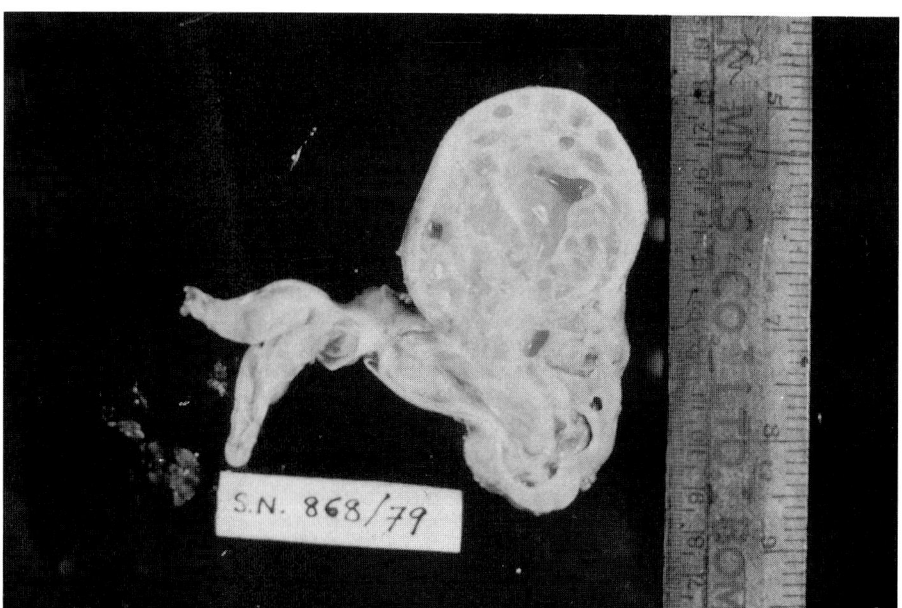

FIGURE 13-48. Cystic nephroma with herniation into the pelvicalyceal system and the ureter.

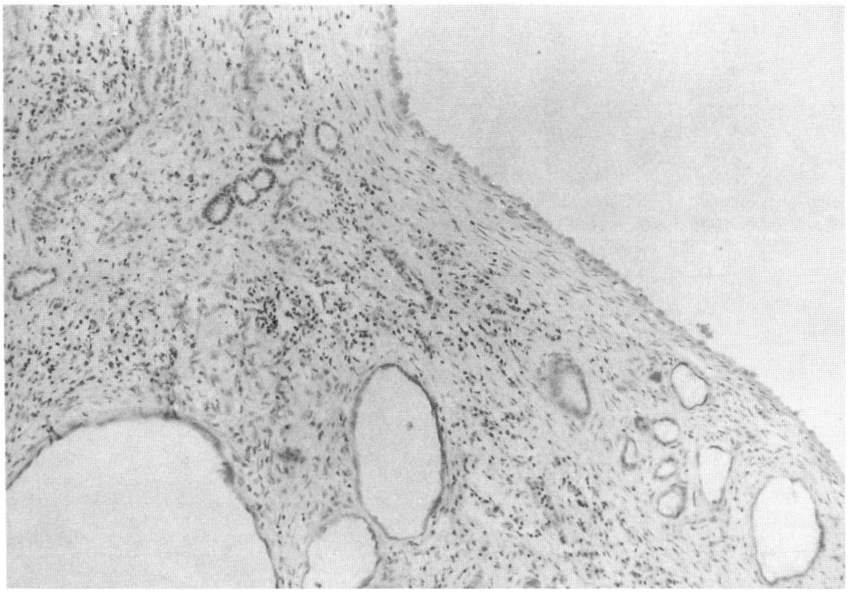

FIGURE 13-49A. Cystic nephroma showing cuboidal and hobnail epithelial lining and fibrous tissue with chronic inflammatory infiltrate and small tubular structures in the septa. The epithelial lining of one of the cysts is focally denuded (H&E, ×100). (Reprinted with permission from Joshi VV, Beckwith JB: *Cancer* 64:466–479, 1989.)

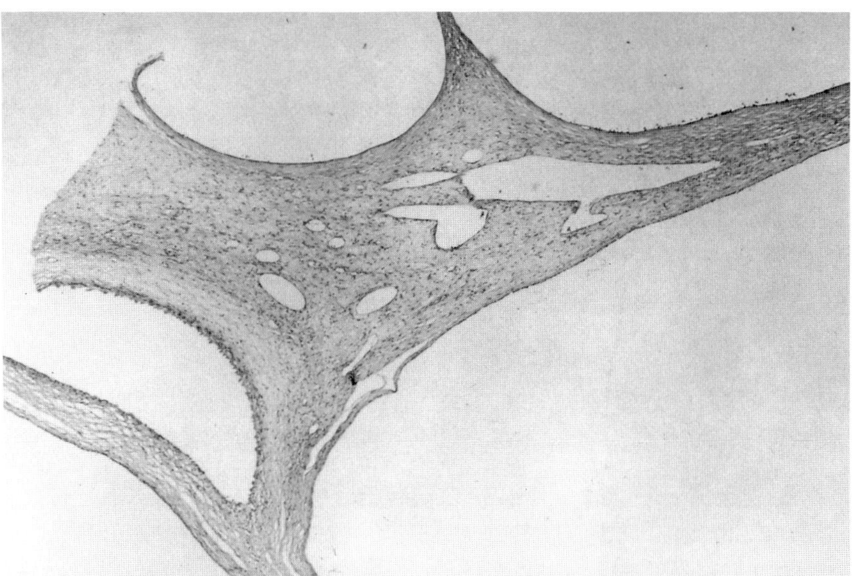

FIGURE 13-49B. Cystic nephroma with septa of varying width, all of which conform to the contours of the cysts. The septa are composed of fibrous tissue with a few blood vessels (H&E, ×40). (Reprinted with permission from Joshi VV, Beckwith JB: *Cancer* 64:466–479, 1989.)

5. The septa are composed of fibrous tissue in which well-differentiated tubules may be present.

Poorly differentiated tissues and blastemal cells are absent in the septa. Although not encountered in our series or in any of the cases reported in the literature, mature heterologous tissues such as skeletal muscle would be permissible in the septa of CN. Bilaterality and multifocality which is rare, would not exclude CN if all other features were consistent with that diagnosis.

Immunohistological and Ultrastructural Features. Positive staining for keratin and *Arachis hypogaea* (peanut) lectin is seen in the epithelial cells lining the cysts.[124] On electron microscopy the cells lining the cysts show features such as scanty short microvilli, tight junctions, scattered pinocytotic vesicles, cilia, and few cytoplasmic organelles.[6,125] These immunohistologic and ultrastructural features resemble those of the epithelial cells of distal convoluted tubules and collecting ducts of normal kidney.

Cytologic Features. The smears of the material from CN in a 3-year-old boy obtained by FNA biopsy showed epithelial cells arranged singly or in sheets.[126] The cells were monomorphic with a scant or large amount of cytoplasm. The latter probably represented the hobnail epithelium. The diagnosis of CN was confirmed by gross and microscopic examination of the resected specimen. In my opinion, it will not be possible to make a firm diagnosis of CN on FNA biopsy alone since such a biopsy may not sample the septal components. CPDN, which is distinguishable from CN solely on the basis of histologic features of the septa of the cysts, will thus not be diagnosed or ruled out by FNA biopsy. Nuclear atypia may be present in the cells of CN in adults.[127] The precise significance of this finding is not clear. However, it may represent early premalignant or incipient malignant change in the lining epithelium superimposed on a benign tumor like CN. In fact, microscopic foci or microscopic nodules with features of RCC have been described in rare cases of CN in adults.[127]

Solid Tumors Occurring in CN. There are also rare reports of full-fledged mural nodules of RCC in association with CN in adults.[128] Mural nodules of renal adenoma may also occur in association with CN. It is important to note that RCC with multiocular cystic change can be mistaken for RCC arising in a CN.[129]

Cystic Partially Differentiated Nephroblastoma (CPDN)

Terminology. CPDN is a rare tumor. We had found 18 cases up to 1977.[130] In subsequent reviews we reported 29 cases.[123,131] We recognize two types of CPDN: conventional type and papillonodular type. The pathologic features are as follows (Figures 13-50 to 13-53).

1. The lesion is composed entirely of cysts and their septa, and in some cases, papillonodular projections extending into the lumen from the septa.
2. It forms a discrete mass that is well-demarcated from the noncystic renal parenchyma.
3. The septa and the intraluminal papillonodules, when present, are the only solid portions of the tumor.
4. The papillonodules do not produce expansile solid areas in the septa.

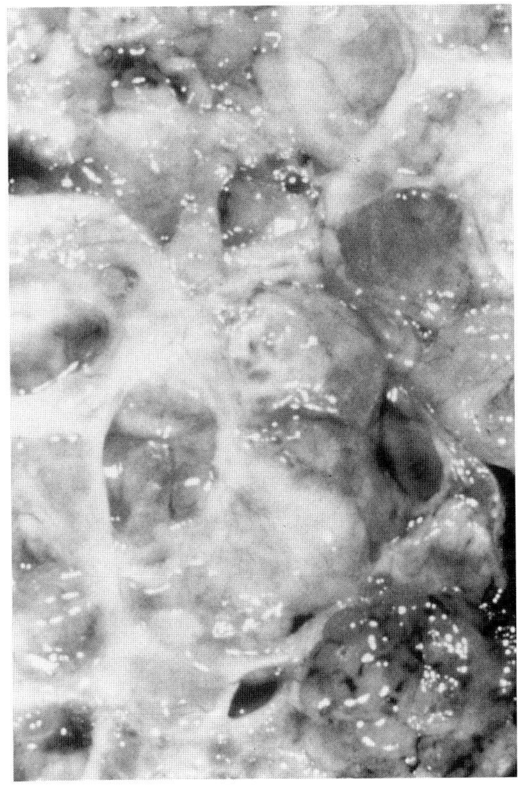

FIGURE 13-50. Gross photograph of cystic partially differentiated nephroblastoma of papillonodular type. Note the papillonodular projections into the lumens of the cysts. Other cysts are the same as the conventional type. (Reprinted with permission from Joshi VV, Beckwith JB: *Cancer* 64:466–479, 1989.)

5. The cysts are lined by flattened, cuboidal, or hobnail epithelium.
6. The septa and the papillonodules, when present, contain blastemal cells and variably differentiated glomeruli, tubules, mesenchyme, striated muscle, cartilage, fibrous tissue, and fat in various amounts and combinations.
7. The lesions composed of cysts without and with the grossly demonstrable intraluminal papillonodules extending from the septa are classified as the conventional and papillonodular type of CPDN, respectively.

Both types of CPDN are classified according to the amount of mature tissues in the septa (and papillonodules) into grade 1 ($>50\%$ mature tissues) and grade 2 ($<50\%$ mature tissues). In rare cases focal anaplasia is seen in the septal tumor tissue.[123]

Differential Diagnosis. The differential diagnosis between CN and CPDN hinges on the demonstration of blastemal cells and partially differentiated renal and aberrant elements in the septa of the cysts. The criteria for CN and CPDN are summarized in Figure 13-54. A rare, totally multicystic tumor of the kidney which should be considered in the differential diagnosis of CN is lymphangioma (LGA) of the kidney. It appears that most cases of LGA of the kidney (in children and adults) reported previously were in fact cases of CN. However, Anderson et al have reported recently a case of LGA of the kidney in a 76-year-old man in which the endothelial nature of the lining cells of the cysts was confirmed by

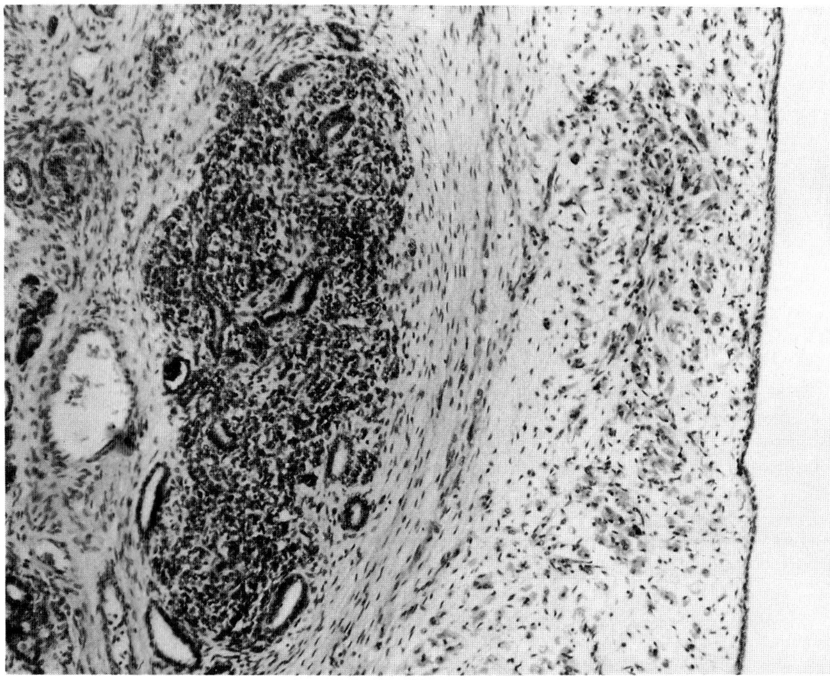

FIGURE 13-51. Septum of cystic partially differentiated nephroblastoma showing cuboidal epithelial lining. The septum contains blastemal cells, immature tubules, and skeletal muscle (H&E, ×250). (Reprinted with permission from Joshi VV, Beckwith JB: *Cancer* 64:466–479, 1989.)

immunocytochemical and electron microscopic studies.[132] The gross appearance of LGA of the kidney is similar to CN and conventional type CPDN. However, on histologic examination, the cells lining all the cysts are flat. No cuboidal or hobnail epithelial cells are present. The endothelial cells show positive reaction with the immunoperoxidase stain for factor VIII-related antigen and *Ulex europaeus* agglutinin and negative reaction for cytokeratin.

The rare "gray zone" lesions which are intermediate between CN and CPDN show poorly differentiated mesenchymal and/or epithelial elements but no blastemal elements in the septa (Figure 13-55). The "gray zone" lesions showing only immature mesenchymal elements should be distinguished from multicystic CCMN and CCSK. Lastly, solid WT may show foci of true cystic change or, rarely, a tumor that has the features of CPDN in most areas may show one or more expansile mural solid tumor nodules. Such lesions, which must be clearly distinguished from CPDN of conventional or papillonodular type, are characterized as solid WT with focal cystic change and multifocal change, respectively. It is not known whether foci of cystic change in an otherwise solid WT has any prognostic significance.

Therapy and Prognosis of CN and CPDN. CN is a fully differentiated benign neoplasm which requires partial or total nephrectomy, depending upon the size of the lesion, as a curative therapy. There are no reports of recurrences in CN with

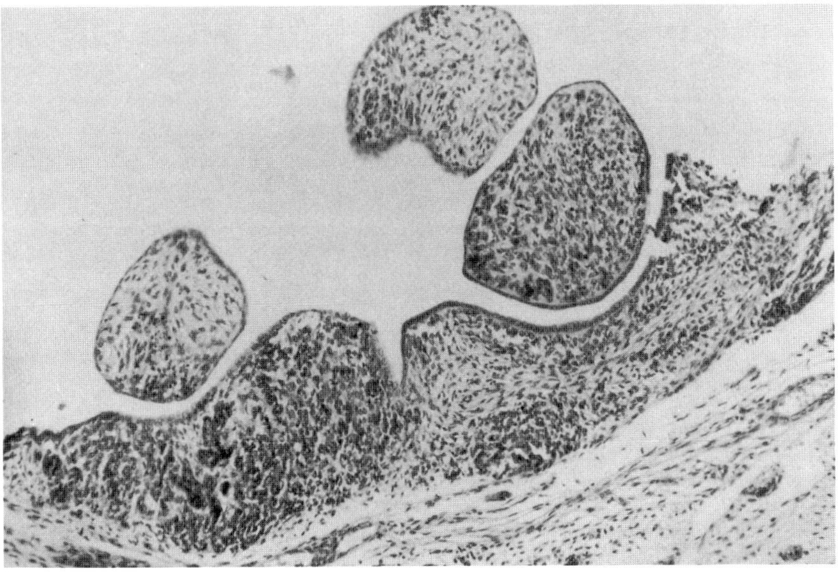

FIGURE 13-52. Microscopic papillonodular projections into the lumen of a cyst of cystic partially differentiated nephroblastoma. These are lined by epithelium continuous with the cyst lining and contain blastemal cells with immature mesenchyme. Clusters of small immature tubules are also present (H&E, ×40). (Reprinted with permission from Joshi VV, Beckwith JB: *Cancer* 64:466–479, 1989.)

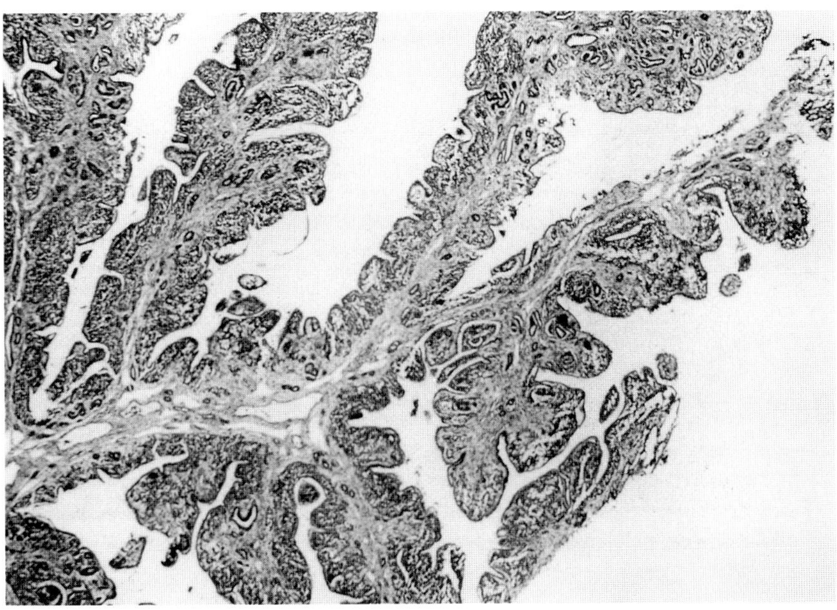

FIGURE 13-53. Intraluminal papillary projections in a cystic partially differentiated nephroblastoma of papillonodular type (H&E, ×40).

Multilocular Cystic Renal Tumor

Cystic Nephroma (CN)

1) Septa form the only solid component of the tumor.
2) No mural or luminal tumor nodules present.
3) There are no blastemal cells in the septa

Cystic Partially Differentiated Neproblastoma

Conventional Type

1) & 2) Same as in CN

3) Blastemal cells, immature and mature elements are present in septa

- Grade 1 — (Relatively mature subtype) > 50% mature elements
- Grade 2 — (Relatively immature subtype) < 50% mature elements

Papillonodular Type

1) Septa and luminal papillonodules of tumor form the only solid component
2) No mural tumor nodules are present
3) Blastemal cells, immature and mature elements are present in the septa and papillonodules

- Grade 1 — Same as conventional type
- Grade 2 — Same as conventional type

FIGURE 13-54. Criteria for diagnosis of cystic nephroma and cystic partially differentiated nephroblastoma.

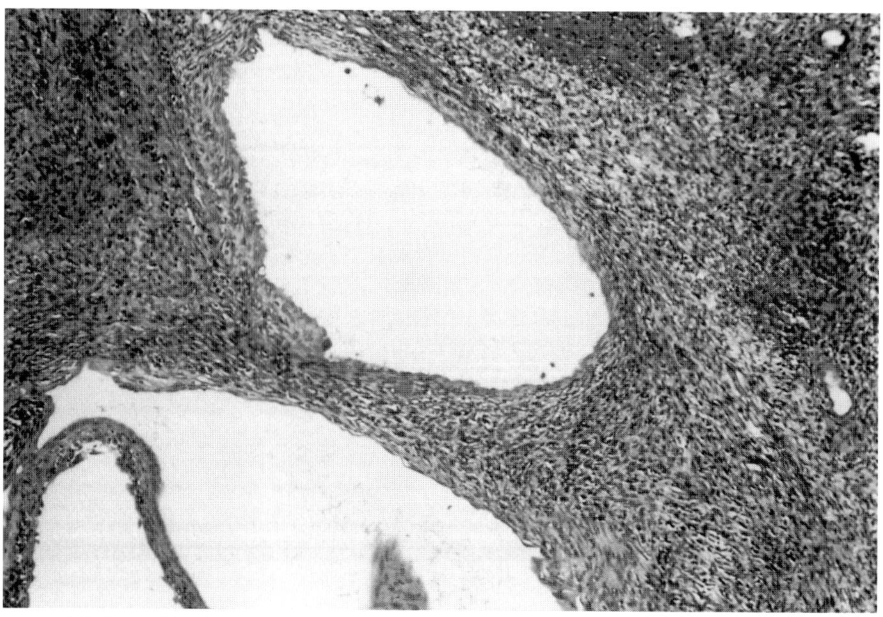

FIGURE 13-55. Totally multicystic renal tumor with hypercellular immature mesenchyme in the septa. No blastemal cells were present. Such lesions represent "gray zone" lesion between cystic nephroma and cystic partially differentiated nephroblastoma and are difficult to differentiate from cystic cellular variant of congenital mesoblastic nephroma or of clear cell sarcoma of the kidney (H&E, ×250).

the exception of one case in which there was recurrence attributable not to the aggressive behavior of the tumor but to unroofing of the lesion done at surgery.[133] Chemotherapy (vincristine and actinomycin D) and irradiation have been used in those cases which were designated as MLC (CN) but in fact were cases of CPDN. It should be noted that some authors use the same designation, viz., MLC for both CN and CPDN or CN for both CN and CPDN. However, we consider CN and CPDN to be distinctive lesions.

All the cases of CPDN except one reviewed by Joshi and Beckwith[123,131] were stage I. The exceptional case was categorized as stage II because there was rupture of capsule during surgery. The recommended curative therapy for CPDN of both types is simple nephrectomy. No recurrence has been reported in the cases of CPDN treated by nephrectomy alone with the exception of one case in the series reported by Joshi and Beckwith[123] in which there were two recurrences. Despite the recurrences, the patient was alive and well 4 years after surgery and appropriate therapy for the recurrences. In some patients with CPDN, chemotherapy and irradiation have been given but it appears that such additional therapy may not be required. However, in view of the presence of blastemal elements in the septa of the lesion, the potential for aggressive behavior in a rare case must be considered. Therefore, a regular periodic follow-up of patients and monitoring by imaging techniques after nephrectomy is advisable.

Tumors of Undetermined Histogenesis

Malignant Rhabdoid Tumor of Kidney (MRTK)

MRTK is the most highly malignant childhood renal tumor, with a mortality rate of 80% even with intensified therapy.[9] The age range was 3 months to 3.5 years with 75% cases occurring below 2 years of age. MRTK can also occur in older children. Male to female ratio was 2:1. MRTK accounts for 2% of renal tumors in children (about 10 cases/year in the United States). Extrarenal rhabdoid tumors (ERTs) in various sites (thymus, heart, liver, prostate, brain, pelvis, soft tissues, chest wall, extremities, paravertebral region, etc.) have also been recognized.[134–136] An interesting case of synchronous occurrence of malignant rhabdoid tumor arising in the pelvis and the right lung two decades after irradiation of both sites for WT has been reported.[137] The relationship between MRTK and ERT and the nature of ERT are controversial. Weeks et al[135] have suggested that "MRTK represents a histogenetic and clinical entity with considerable morphologic diversity and ERT will eventually emerge as a phenotypic concept encompassing a spectrum of histogenetic and clinical diversity."

Pathologic Features. These are described in detail in the series of 111 NWTS cases byWeeks et al.[9] MRTK tends to be a bulky tumor mass with soft, friable, and firm areas. The tumor–kidney interface is indistinct and the tumor is seen to infiltrate. Satellite nodules are frequently present. Weeks et al[9] describe the following classical pattern. There are diffuse sheets, cords, or nests of large oval to round monomorphic tumor cells which show characteristic single large owl-eye nucleolus, and abundant, usually eosinophilic but occasionally basophilic or amphophilic cytoplasm containing a large inclusion (Figure 13-56). Mitotic activity is prominent. The inclusion corresponds with whorled masses of vimentin as demonstrated by electron microscopy and immunohistology. The

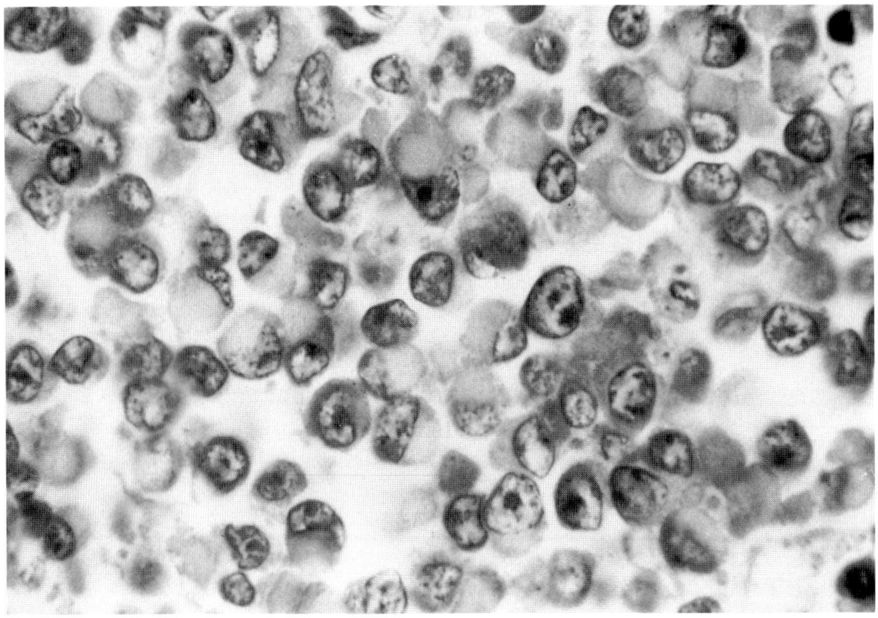

FIGURE 13-56. Malignant rhabdoid tumor of kidney composed of large oval or round cells with characteristic intracytoplasmic inclusions and prominent nucleoli (H&E, ×400). (Courtesy of Dr. J. Bruce Beckwith.)

number of cells showing the inclusions is variable. It must be emphasized that the prominent nucleolus must be demonstrated before a diagnosis of MRTK is made. In fact, the cytoplasmic inclusions may be rare, requiring intensive search, or exceptionally may even be absent in MRTK[9] (see discussion of neoplasms mimicking MRTK below). The cytoplasmic inclusion has a hyaline globular appearance and it shows variable positivity to periodic acid-Schiff stain (PAS) after diastase digestion. Cells without inclusions show faint PAS positivity. Occasionally, multiple small eosinophilic globular inclusions are seen in the tumor cells, particularly near the area of necrosis.[8] Reticulin is present around the individual cells and groups of cells. Vascularity of the stroma is not prominent. The tumor infiltrates the surrounding renal parenchyma with entrapment of tubules. In addition to this classical pattern, most cases of MRTK show one or more variant patterns summarized in Table 13-7. Embryonal renal elements are not seen in MRTK. However, entrapped medullary tubules may be present. These tubules may undergo cystic change. Capsular invasion, inflammatory pseudocapsule formation, intrarenal vascular invasion and renal pelvis involvement are frequently seen. Renal sinus invasion was present in all cases reviewed by Weeks et al.[9] Tubular arrangement of tumor cells may be seen in the medullary portion of the tumor. Nephrogenic rests are not present in the surrounding kidney. MRTK is unilateral. The cases with bilateral MRTK probably represent metastasis.

Immunohistological Features. MRTK shows positive staining for diverse

Table 13-7 Patterns[a] Seen in Malignant Rhabdoid Tumor of Kidney (MRTK)

Patterns	Features	Comment
Classical pattern	Large oval or round monomorphic cells with abundant eosinophilic cytoplasm, hyaline globular cytoplasmic inclusion, and large "owl-eye" nucleolus in the nucleus. Cells are arranged in sheets, cords, or nests. The inclusions are PAS-positive after diastase digestion. Prominent nucleoli are always present. Multiple small inclusions instead of a single large inclusion may be seen in the cytoplasms.	The following variations in classical pattern may be seen: cytoplasm may be basophilic or amphophilic; the cytoplasmic inclusions may be found only in a few cells after intensive search or may be absent in an exceptional case. The inclusion corresponds with a whorled mass of vimentin as demonstrated by electron microscopy and immunohistology (see text for details).
Sclerosing patterns	Fibrous stroma or hyaline stroma resembling osteoid or chondroid matrix with arrangement of cells in cords or nests or haphazard arrangement.	Most common variant pattern. This was considered originally as hyalinizing pattern in the "sarcomatous variant of Wilms' tumor."
Epithelioid patterns	Tumor cells arranged in trabeculae, sometimes in a PAS-positive mucoid matrix, glandlike or alveolar arrangement also seen.	The patttern resembles adenocarcinoma.
Lymphomatoid patterns	Noncohesive tumor cells arranged in sheets.	Scattered histiocytes containing pyknotic nuclei produce a "starry sky" pattern.
Histiocytoid patterns	Loosely arranged tumor cells with prominent nucleoli but inconspicuous cytoplasmic inclusions admixed with reactive multinucleated histiocytes and occasionally eosinophils.	The giant cells show features of histiocytes by electron microscopy.

(continued)

TABLE 13-7 Continued

Patterns	Features	Comment
Spindled patterns	Fascicles of spindle-shaped tumor cells admixed with stroma of the tumor.	Multinucleated histiocytes are frequently present. This pattern mimics congenital mesoblastic nephroma (CMN) or cellular variant of CMN depending upon cell density.
Myxoid patterns	Spindle-shaped tumor cells arranged in a loose "myxoid" matrix.	Cystic change related to expression of myxoid areas may occur.
Palisaded patterns	Spindle-shaped tumor cells showing palisading.	This pattern is rare. It resembles neurilemoma.
Hemangiopericytomatous patterns	Stroma with prominent vascularity resembling a hemangiopericytoma.	This pattern is uncommon.
CCSK[b]-like patterns	Vascular septa separating groups of tumor cells.	Cytoplasmic inclusions may be absent or inconspicuous. Dense chromatin and prominent nucleoli of tumor cells are helpful in the differential diagnosis between CCSK and MRTK.
Organoid patterns	Solid groups of tumor cells with fibrous septa almost completely encircling each group.	The pattern resembles that seen in a paraganglioma.
Multicystic patterns	Dilatation of "entrapped" tubules or degenerative change in the stroma produces multicystic pattern.	Some solid areas are always present. Therefore the multicystic MRTK can be distinguished from other totally multicystic tumors.

[a] One or more patterns in addition to the classical pattern described in the table are present in most of the tumors.

[b] CCSK: Clear cell sarcoma kidney.

Adapted from Weeks DA et al: *Am J Surg Pathol* 13:439–458, 1989.

markers. Thus low molecular weight cytokeratin, epithelial membrane antigen (EMA), vimentin, neuron-specific enolase (NSE), neurofilament protein, Leu 7 (HNK-1), myoglobin, desmin, and α_1-antichymotrypsin have been demonstrated in the tumor cells by various researchers.[9,10,138] Of these, vimentin, EMA, cytokeratin, and NSE are more frequently positive than others. The significance of the presence of such diverse markers in the histogenesis of MRTK has been discussed above. Weeks et al[9] have suggested that the nonspecific entrapment of antibodies in the filamentous inclusions of the cells of MRTK may explain some of the diverse results on immunohistochemical staining.

Ultrastructural Features. These have been described by Haas et al[8] and Mierau et al.[6,139] The salient ultrastructural features are the presence of concentric whorled masses of intermediate filaments (6 to 9 nm) in the paranuclear portion of the cytoplasm and prominent nucleolus (Figure 13-57). The masses of whorled filaments correspond to the cytoplasmic inclusions seen on light microscopy and their frequency is similarly variable. Elongated mass of 10-nm filaments can also be present. Other features include dilated endoplasmic reticulum, free tonofilament-like bundles, and occasional cell junctions.

Cytologic Features. There is a report of a single case of MRTK diagnosed initially by FNA biopsy and subsequently confirmed by histologic examination.[140] Large cells with vesicular nuclei, prominent nucleoli, and paranuclear cytoplasmic inclusions were seen in the smears of the FNA biopsy of a right kidney mass and of pleural effusion in the case reported by Drut.

Differential Diagnosis. The distinctive histologic features are the cytoplasmic inclusions and prominent nucleolus. Demonstrating the paranuclear mass of whorled filaments by electron microscopy is helpful. If only a small biopsy or only a few sections of the tumor are available and the cytoplasmic inclusions are rare, an intensive search may be required to find them or these

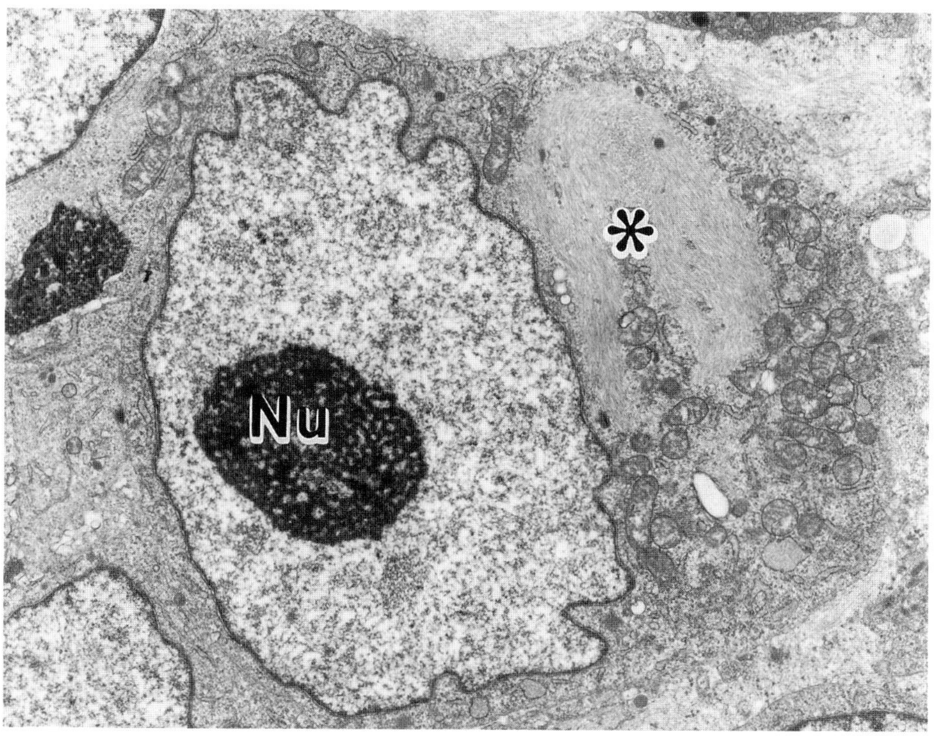

FIGURE 13-57. Electron micrograph showing a prominent nucleolus (Nu) and characteristic paranuclear intracytoplasmic whorled mass of intermediate filaments (*asterisk*) (uranyl acetate and lead citrate, ×4,500). (Courtesy of Dr. Gary Mierau.)

may not be seen at all. As mentioned previously, in one of the 111 NWTS cases, the cytoplasmic inclusions were not present. However, the case was considered as MRTK because other characteristic cytologic (particularly prominent nucleoli and general cell morphology) and clinical features were present.[49] The clinical profile consisting of young age of the child, male predominance, aggressive behavior (advanced stage at diagnosis), and association with embryonal tumors of the brain should also be taken into consideration. Weeks et al[141,142] have described various renal tumors in children (and to some extent in adults) which mimic MRTK because of presence of one or more "rhabdoid" features (cytoplasmic inclusions, abundant cytoplasm, and prominent nucleoli in medium-sized to large oval to round tumor cells). These include: WT with or without anaplasia, CCMN, RCC (including oncocytoma), CDCA, transitional cell carcinoma (age range, 15 to 51 years), rhabdomyosarcoma (RMS), malignant neuroepithelial tumors, and non-Hodgkin's lymphoma. The temptation to make a diagnosis of MRTK on the basis of the presence of cytoplasmic inclusions by light and/or electron microscopy or of prominent nucleoli in oval or round cells should be avoided. In the tumors mimicking MRTK, characteristic histologic, and/or ultrastructural and/or immunocytochemical features indicative of the correct diagnosis are always present at least focally when several sections are examined. In addition, the clinical profiles of these "pseudorhabdoid" tumors are different from that of MRTK. It should be noted that in some pseudorhabdoid tumors, whorled intermediate filaments are observed on electron microscopy. The opposite aspect of differential diagnosis of MRTK is that certain variant patterns seen focally or predominantly in a given case of MRTK mimic patterns seen in other renal tumors. For example, spindled pattern with spindle-shaped cells arranged in compact fascicles may be mistaken for the typical patterns seen in CMN or CCMN depending upon the cellularity. Similarly a vascular pattern with solid cords of tumor cells divided into lobules or cords resembles the classical pattern of CCSK. However, detailed examination of all the sections in these cases reveals the classical pattern enabling the diagnosis of MRTK.

Other Features. The association between MRTK and embryonal tumors of the brain was reported by Bonnin et al.[143] The brain tumors in the six cases described by these investigators included cerebellar medulloblastoma, pineoblastoma, and cerebral primitive neuroectodermal tumor. The brain tumor may be diagnosed before or after the diagnosis of MRTK. This association can be considered to be supportive of the theory of histogenesis of MRTK from primitive neuroectoderm. Cytogenetic studies have been done only in a few cases. In four of the six cases of MRTK studied by Douglass et al,[144] normal karyotype was present. In one case there was del(13)(q14). Occasional tetraploid cells were seen in another case. In a case reported by Hayashi et al,[145] del(11)(p13) has been described. It is of interest to note that in an established cell line from MRTK, t(11;22) (p15.5;q11.23) has been demonstrated.[146] None of the cases of MRTK reported by Kumar et al[147] and Schmidt et al[61] had aneuploidy when DNA analysis was done by flow cytometry. Laminin, fibronectin, and collagen type I and III have been demonstrated in MRTK by immunocytochemical studies.[24] Increased c-myc expression and expression of insulin-like growth factor-II have been described in a cell line derived from MRTK.[148]

Miscellaneous Tumors

These include collecting duct carcinoma,[149] juxtaglomerular cell tumor,[150] neuroblastoma,[151] primitive neuroectodermal tumor,[152] primary carcinoid tumor occurring by itself[153] or in a cystic teratoma of the kidney,[154] renal gastrinoma (with Zollinger-Eillison syndrome (Figures 13-58 and 13-59),[155] renal teratoma,[154,156] angiomyolipoma,[157] lymphangioma,[132] rhabdomyosarcoma, and unclassified sarcomas of the kidney.[115,142] These tumors are rare and some of them (e.g., collecting duct carcinomas, angiomyolipoma, carcinoid tumor) occur more commonly in adults.

COMMENT

Renal neoplasia in children is one of the most fascinating and challenging areas of pediatric surgical pathology. The detailed work published by Beckwith of the NWTS Pathology Center has placed the pediatric pathologist in a position of great responsibility of providing accurate diagnosis and a precise and comprehensive report since the prognosis assigned to and therapy chosen in an individual case will be determined by the diagnosis, histologic grouping, staging, and microsubstaging rendered by the pediatric pathologist. It should be a matter of great pride for pediatric pathologists that two of their own profession have made such fundamental contributions to the management of WT. Needless to say, I am referring to Dr. Sydney Farber who pioneered the chemotherapy of WT and Dr. Bruce Beckwith who discovered the two prognostic categories (FH and UH) of WT and the two highly malignant renal tumors, CCSK and MRTK, which require more aggressive therapy. Because of the fundamental and extensive contributions to the knowledge of pathology of WT made by Dr. Beckwith, I would like to suggest that the eponymic designation should now be modified to Wilms-Beckwith tumor.

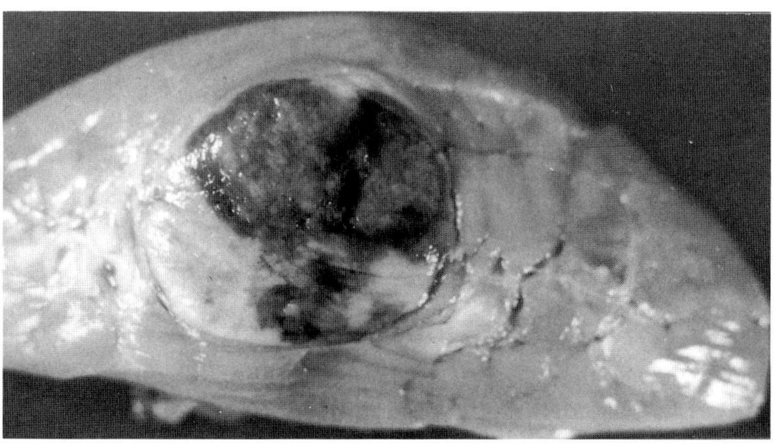

FIGURE 13-58. Gross photograph of renal gastrinoma. The mass was located in the hilum with compression of the surrounding renal parenchyma.

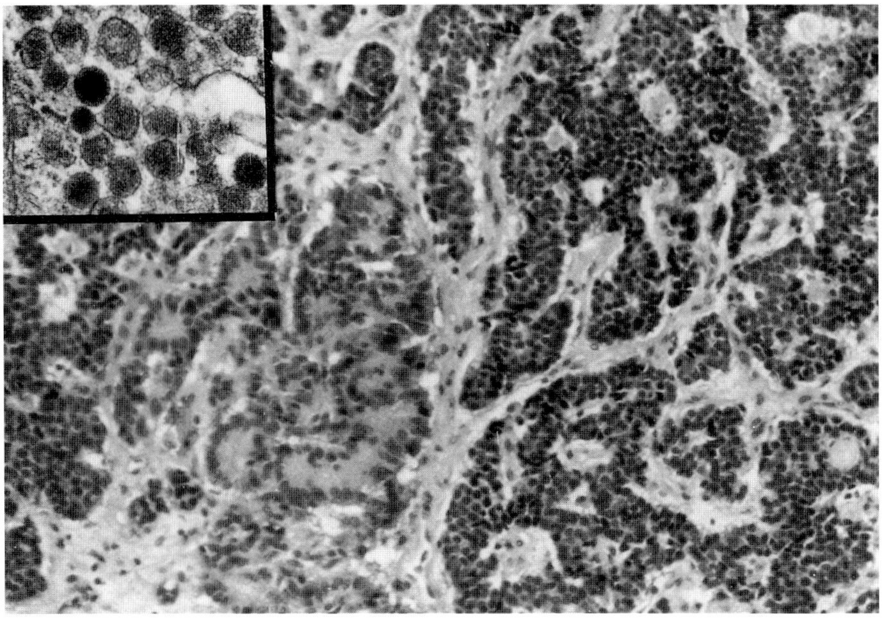

FIGURE 13-59. Renal gastrinoma characterized by medium-sized monomorphic tumor cells arranged in cords. In one area a glandular pattern is seen. The inset shows ultrastructural appearance of cytoplasmic granules in the tumor cells. Note that the granules are of variable electron density and are membrane-bound (H&E, ×100, inset: uranyl acetate and lead citrate, ×17,500). (Reprinted with permission from Joshi VV, et al: *Pediatr Pathol* 6:475–476, 1986.)

The challenges to pediatric pathologists include: (1) further refinement of the pathologic criteria of renal tumors, (2) more precise pathologic and "biologic" characterization of some of the poorly understood neoplasms such as CCMN, (3) determination of the histogenesis of CCSK and MRTK, and (4) further elucidation of the precise relationships of the various renal tumors of childhood to embryologic development of kidney and to one another.

REFERENCES

1. Beckwith JB: Wilms' tumor and other renal tumors of childhood: An update. *J Urol* 136:320–324, 1986.
2. Beckwith JB, Palmer NF: Histopathology and prognosis of Wilms' Tumor Study. *Cancer* 41:1937–1948, 1978.
3. Beckwith JB: Wilms' tumor and other renal tumors of childhood: A selective review from the National Wilms' Tumor Study Pathology Center. *Hum Pathol* 14:481–492, 1983.
4. Beckwith JB, Kiviat NB, Bonadio JF: Nephrogenic rests, nephroblastomatosis, and the pathogenesis of Wilms' tumor. *Pediatr Pathol* 10:1–36, 1990.
5. Ekblom P: Determination and differentiation of the nephron. *Med Biol* 59:139–160, 1981.

6. Mierau GW, Beckwith JB, Weeks DA: Ultrastructure and histogenesis of the renal tumors of childhood: An overview. *Ultrastruct Pathol* 11:313–333, 1987.
7. Gonzalez-Crussi F, Franklin WA: Embryologic considerations. In Gonzalez-Crussi F: *Wilms' Tumor (Nephroblastoma) and Related Renal Neoplasms of Childhood.* Boca Raton, FL, CRC Press, 1984, p 7–20.
8. Haas JE, Palmer NF, Weinberg AG, et al: Ultrastructure of malignant rhabdoid tumor of the kidney. A distinctive renal tumor of children. *Hum Pathol* 12:646–657, 1981.
9. Weeks DA, Beckwith JB, Mierau G, et al: Rhabdoid tumor of kidney: A report of 111 cases from the National Wilms' Tumor Study. *Am J Surg Pathol* 13:439–458, 1989.
10. Tsokos M, Kouraklis G, Chandra RS, et al: Malignant rhabdoid tumor of the kidney and soft tissues; Evidence for a diverse morphological and immunocytochemical phenotype. *Arch Pathol Lab Med* 113:115–120, 1989.
11. D'Angio GJ, Breslow N, Beckwith JB, et al: Treatment of Wilms' tumor. Results of the Third National Wilms' Tumor Study. *Cancer* 64:349–360, 1989.
12. D'Angio GJ, Breslow N, Beckwith JB, et al: Wilms' tumor (nephroblastoma, renal embryoma). In Pizzo PA, Poplack DG (eds): *Principles and Practice in Pediatric Oncology.* Philadelphia, J. B. Lippincott, 1989, p 583–586.
13. Beckwith JB: Pediatric renal neoplasia. In *Syllabus of the 13th Annual Aspen Conference on Pediatric Disease*, August 5–9, 1991, Aspen, CO.
14. Beckwith JB: Renal neoplasms in childhood. Sternberg SS (ed): *Diagnostic Surgical Pathology*, vol II. New York, Raven Press, 1989, p 1331–1353.
15. Bolande RP: Congenital mesoblastic nephroma in infancy. *Pediatrics* 40:272–278, 1967.
16. Bolande RP: Congenital mesoblastic nephroma in infancy. *Pediatr Pathol* 1:227–250, 1973.
17. Joshi VV, Kasznica J, Walters TR: Atypical mesoblastic nephroma. Pathologic characterization of potentially aggressive variant of conventional congenital mesoblastic nephroma. *Arch Pathol Lab Med* 110:100–106, 1986.
18. Howell CG, Othersen HB, Kiviat NE, et al: Therapy and outcome in 51 children with mesoblastic nephroma: A report of the National Wilms' Tumor Study. *J Pediatr Surg* 17:826–831, 1982.
19. Ganick DJ, Gilbert EF, Beckwith JB, et al: Congenital cystic mesoblastic nephroma. *Hum Pathol* 12:1039–1043, 1981.
20. Fernbach SK, Schlesinger AE, Gonzalez-Crussi F: Calcification and ossification in a congenital mesoblastic nephroma. *Urol Rad* 7:165–167, 1985.
21. Gonzalez-Crussi F, Sotelo-Avila C, Kidd JM: Mesenchymal renal tumors in infancy. *Hum Pathol* 12:78–85, 1981.
22. Bolande RP, Bernstein J, Libcke J: Tubulogenesis in mesoblastic nephroma. *Lab Invest* 58:2P, 1988.
23. Marsden HB, Newton WA: New look at mesoblastic nephroma. *J Clin Pathol* 39:508–513, 1986.
24. Kumar S, Carr T, Marsden HB, et al: Study of childhood renal tumours using antisera to fibronectin, laminin and epithelial membrane antigen. *J Clin Pathol* 39:51–57, 1986.
25. Nadasdy T, Roth J, Johnson DL, et al: Congenital mesoblastic nephroma: An immunohistochemical and lectin study. *Hum Pathol* 24:413–419, 1993.
26. Pettinato G, Manivel JC, Wick MR, et al: Classical and cellular (atypical) congenital mesoblastic nephroma. *Hum Pathol* 20:682–690, 1989.
27. Gonzalez-Crussi F: Variants and miscellaneous. In Gonzalez-Crussi F (ed): *Wilms' Tumor (Nephroblastoma) and Related Renal Neoplasms of Childhood.* Boca Raton, FL, CRC Press, 1984, p 77–118.
28. Favara BC, Johnson W, Ito J: Renal tumors in the neonatal period. *Cancer* 22:845–855, 1968.

29. Drut R: Cytologic characteristics of congenital mesoblastic nephroma in fine-needle aspiration cytology: A case report. *Diagn Cytopathol* 8:374–376, 1992.
30. Dey P, Srinivasan R, Nijhawan R, et al: Fine needle aspiration cytology of mesoblastic nephroma. A case report. *Acta Cytol* 36:404–406, 1992.
31. Joshi VV, Kay S, Milsten R, et al: Congenital mesoblastic nephroma of infancy: Report of a case with unusual behavior. *Am J Clin Pathol* 60:811–816, 1973.
32. Gonzalez-Crussi F, Sotelo-Avila C, Kidd JM: Malignant mesenchymal nephroma of infancy: Report of a case with pulmonary metastases. *Am J Surg Pathol* 4:185–190, 1980.
33. Sandstedt B, Delemarre JFM, Krul EJ, et al: Mesoblastic nephromas: A study of 29 tumors from SIOP nephroblastoma file. *Histopathology* 9:741–750, 1985.
34. Cook HT, Taylor GM, Malone P, et al: Renin in mesoblastic nephroma: An immunohistochemical study. *Hum Pathol* 19:1347–1351, 1988.
35. Lindop GBM, Lever AF: Anatomy of the renin-angiotensin system in the normal and pathological kidney. *Histopathology* 10:335–362, 1986.
36. Jayabose S, Igbal K, Neuman L, et al: Hypercalcemia in childhood renal tumors. *Cancer* 61:788–791, 1988.
37. Vido L, Carli M, Rizzoni G, et al: Congenital mesoblastic nephroma with hypercalcemia: Pathogenic role of prostaglandins. *Am J Pediatr Hematol Oncol* 8:149–152, 1986.
38. Guilland D, Bouvier R, Sonsino E, et al: Nucleolar organizing regions in congenital mesoblastic nephroma. *Pediatr Pathol* 12:811–821, 1992.
39. Tomlinson GE, Argyle JC, Velasco S, et al: Molecular characterization of congenital mesoblastic nephroma and its distinction from Wilms' tumor. *Cancer* 70:2358–2361, 1992.
40. Barrantes JC, Toyn C, Muir KR, et al: Congenital mesoblastic nephroma: Possible prognostic and management value of assessing DNA content. *J Clin Pathol* 44:317–320, 1991.
41. Kovacs G, Szucs S, Maschek H: Two chromosomally different cell populations in a partly cellular congenital mesoblastic nephroma. *Arch Pathol Lab Med* 111: 383–385, 1987.
42. Schofield DE, Yunis EJ, Fletcher JA: Chromosome aberrations in mesoblastic nephroma. *Am J Pathol* 143:714–724, 1993.
43. Beckwith JB, Weeks DA: Congenital mesoblastic nephroma. When should we worry? *Arch Pathol Lab Med* 110:98–99, 1986.
44. Chan HSL, Cheng MY, Mancer K, et al: Congenital mesoblastic nephroma: A clinicopathologic study of 17 cases representing the pathologic spectrum of the disease. *J Pediatr* 111:64–70, 1987.
45. Gormley TS, Skoog SJ, Jones RV, et al: Cellular congenital mesoblastic nephroma: What are the options? *J Urol* 142:479–483, 1989.
46. Vujanic GM, Delemarre JFM, Moeslichan S, et al: Mesoblastic nephroma metastatic to the lungs and heart: Another face of this peculiar lesion. Case report and review of the literature. *Pediatr Pathol* 13:143–153, 1993.
47. Walterhouse D: Proceedings of the Tumor Board of the Children's Hospital of Philadelphia: Mesoblastic nephroma. *Med Pediatr Oncol* 18:64–67, 1990.
48. Stalens JP, Gosseye S, Clapuyt P, et al: Preoperative chemotherapy of cellular congenital mesoblastic nephroma in a 5 month old infant. *Pediatr Hematol Oncol* 9:335–345, 1992.
49. Haas JE, Bonadio JF, Beckwith JB: Clear cell sarcoma of the kidney with emphasis on the ultrastructural features. *Cancer* 54:2978–2987, 1984.
50. Marsden HB, Lawler W, Kumar PM: Bone metastasizing renal tumor of childhood: Morphological and clinical features and differences from Wilms' tumor. *Cancer* 42:1922–1928, 1978.

51. Morgan E, Kidd JM: Undifferentiated sarcoma of the kidney: A tumor of childhood with histopathologic and clinical characteristics distinct from Wilms' tumor. *Cancer* 42:1916–1921, 1978.
52. Ogawa K, Nakashima Y, Yamabe H, et al: Clear cell sarcoma of the kidney: An immunohistochemical study. *Acta Pathol Jpn* 36:681–689, 1986.
53. Ishii E, Fujimoto J, Hara S, et al: Human sarcomatous Wilms' tumor lines: Evidence for epithelial differentiation in clear cell sarcoma of the kidney. *Cancer Res* 49:5392–5399, 1989.
54. Schmidt D, Harms D, Evers KG, et al: Bone metastasizing renal tumor (clear cell sarcoma) of childhood with epithelial elements. *Cancer* 56:609–613, 1985.
55. Sotelo-Avila C, Gonzalez-Crussi F, Sadowinski S, et al: Clear cell sarcoma of kidney: A clinicopathologic study of 21 patients with long term follow-up evaluation. *Hum Pathol* 16:1219–1230, 1986.
56. Beckwith JB: Syllabus of short course on pediatric renal tumors given at the annual meeting of U.S.-Canadian Academy of Pathology, New Orleans, March 1993.
57. Beckwith JB, Larson E: Case 7. Clear cell sarcoma of kidney. *Pediatr Pathol* 9:211–218, 1989.
58. Sibley RK, Wick M, Cherwitz D, et al: An immuno- and histochemical study of Wilms' tumor and its variants. *Lab Invest* 52:61A–62A, 1985.
59. Ito J, Johnson WW: Ultrastructure of Wilms' tumor: Epithelial cell. *J Natl Cancer Inst* 42:77–99, 1969.
60. Novak RW, Caces JN, Johnson WW: Sarcomatous renal tumor of childhood. An electron microscopic study. *Am J Clin Pathol* 73:622–625, 1980.
61. Schmidt D, Wiedemann B, Keil W, et al: Flow cytometric analysis of nephroblastomas and related neoplasms. *Cancer* 58:2494–2500, 1986.
62. Yun K: Clear cell sarcoma of kidney expresses insulin-like growth factor II but not WT1 transcripts. *Am J Pathol* 142:39–47, 1993.
63. Weeks DA, Malott RL, Zuppan C, et al: Primitive pelvic sarcoma resembling clear cell sarcoma of kidney. *Ultrastruct Pathol* 15:403–408, 1991.
64. Ogawa K, Nakashim Y, Kim YC, et al: Unusual renal sarcoma in a young adult: Its similarities to clear cell sarcoma of the kidney. *J Urol* 137:730–731, 1987.
65. Akhtar M, Ali MA, Sackey K, et al: Fine needle aspiration biopsy of clear cell sarcoma of the kidney: Light and electron microscopic features. *Diagn Cytopathol* 5:181–187, 1989.
66. Drut R, Pomar M: Cytologic characteristics of clear cell sarcoma of the kidney (CCSK) in fine needle aspiration biopsy (FNAB): A report of 4 cases. *Diagn Cytopathol* 7:611–614, 1991.
67. Hughson MD, Hennigar GR, Othersen HB: Cytodifferentiated renal tumors occurring with Wilms' tumors of the opposite kidneys. Report of two cases. *Am J Clin Pathol* 66:376–389, 1966.
68. Joshi VV, Meltzer MM, Amirtham D, et al: Sequential bilateral nephroblastic tumors of different cell types in an infant: Possible effect of chemotherapy versus de novo origin. *Cancer* 51:2209–2213, 1983.
69. Bove K, McAdams AJ: The nephroblastomatosis complex and its relationship to Wilms' tumor: A clinicopathologic treatise. *Perspect Pediatr Pathol* 3:185–223, 1976.
70. Hou LT, Holman RL: Bilateral nephroblastomatosis in a premature infant. *J Pathol Bacteriol* 82:249–255, 1961.
71. Machin GA: Persistent renal blastema (nephroblastomatosis) as a frequent precursor of Wilms' tumor; a pathological and clinical review. Part 1. Nephroblastomatosis in the context of embryology and genetics. *Am J Pediatr Hematol Oncol* 2:165–172, 1980.

72. Machin GA: Persistent renal blastema (nephroblastomatosis) as a frequent precursor of Wilms' tumor; a pathological and clinical review. Part 2. Significance of nephroblastomatosis in the genesis of Wilms' tumor. *Am J Pediatr Hematol Oncol* 2:253–261, 1980.
73. Machin GA: Persistent renal blastema (nephroblastomatosis) as a frequent precursor of Wilms' tumor; a pathological and clinical review. Part 3. Clinical aspects of nephroblastomatosis. *Am J Pediatr Hematol Oncol* 2:353–362, 1980.
74. Beckwith JB: Precursor lesions of Wilms' tumor: Clinical and biological implications. *Med Pediatr Oncol* 21:158–168, 1993.
75. Knudson AG, Strong LC: Mutation and cancer: A model for Wilms' tumor of the kidney. *J Natl Cancer Inst* 48:313–324, 1972.
76. Kim TH, Zaatari GS, Baum ES, et al: Recurrence of Wilms' tumor after apparent cure. *J Pediatr* 107:44–49, 1985.
77. Hennigar RA, Beckwith JB: Nephrogenic adenofibroma. A novel kidney tumor of young people. *Am J Surg Pathol* 16:325–334, 1992.
78. Coppes MJ: Serum biological markers and paraneoplastic syndromes in Wilms' tumor. *Med Pediatr Oncol* 21:213–221, 1993.
79. Gonzalez-Crussi F: The pathology of Wilms' tumor: In Gonzalez-Crussi F (ed): *Wilms' Tumor (Nephroblastoma) and Related Renal Neoplasms of Childhood*. Boca Raton, FL, CRC Press, 1984, p 178–206.
80. Chatten J: Epithelial differentiation in Wilms' tumor: A clinicopathologic appraisal. *Perspect Pediatr Pathol* 3:225–254, 1976.
81. Edwards O, Chatten J: Hydropic cell variant (clear cell variant) of Wilms' tumor. *Arch Pathol Lab Med* 109:956–958, 1985.
82. Glick AD, Tham KT, Leung NM, et al: Unusual clear cell tumor of the kidney in infancy. *Am J Surg Pathol* 5:581–585, 1981.
83. Wigger HJ: Fetal rhabdomyomatous nephroblastoma: A variant of Wilms' tumor. *Hum Pathol* 7:613–623, 1976.
84. Zuppan CW, Beckwith JB, Luckey DW: Anaplasia in unilateral Wilms' tumor: A report from the National Wilms' Tumor Study Pathology Center. *Hum Pathol* 19:1199–1209, 1988.
85. Faria P, Beckwith JB: A new definition of focal anaplasia (FA) in Wilms' tumor (WT) identifies cases with good outcome: A report from the National Wilms' Tumor Study. *Mod Pathol* 6:3P, 1993.
86. Weeks DA, Beckwith JB, Mierau GW: Benign nodal lesions mimicking metastases from pediatric renal neoplasms: A report from the National Wilms' Tumor Study Pathology Center. *Hum Pathol* 21:1239–1244, 1990.
87. Weeks DA, Beckwith JB, Luckey DW: Relapse-associated variables in Stage I favorable histology Wilms' tumor. A report from the National Wilms' Tumor Study. *Cancer* 60:1204–1212, 1987.
88. Knudson AG: Introduction to the genetics of primary renal tumors in children. *Med Pediatr Oncol* 21:193–198, 1993.
89. Denk H, Weybora W, Ratschek M, et al: Distribution of vimentin, cytokeratin, and desmosomal-plaque protein in human nephroblastoma as revealed by specific antibodies: Co-existence of cell groups of different degrees of epithelial differentiation. *Differentiation* 29:88–97, 1985.
90. Altmannsberger M, Osborn M, Schafer H, et al: Distinction of nephroblastomas from other childhood tumors using antibodies to intermediate filaments. *Virchows Arch B Cell Pathol* 45:113–124, 1984.
91. Droz D, Rousseau-Merck MF, Jaubert F, et al: Cell differentiation in Wilms' tumor (nephroblastoma): An immunohistochemical study. *Hum Pathol* 21:536–544, 1990.

92. Magee F, Mak RG, Taylor GP, et al: Neural differentiation in Wilms' tumor. *Hum Pathol* 18:33–37, 1987.
93. Hennigar RA, Spicer SA, Sens DA, et al: Histochemical evidence of tubule segmentation in a case of Wilms' tumor. *Am J Clin Pathol* 85:724–731, 1986.
94. Schmidt D, Dickersin GR, Vawter GF, et al: Wilms' tumor: A review of ultrastructure and histogenesis. *Pathobiol Ann* 12:281–300, 1982.
95. Kurtz SM: A unique ultrastructural variant of Wilms' tumor: Its possible histogenetic implications. *Am J Surg Pathol* 3:257–264, 1979.
96. Quijano G, Drut R: Cytologic characteristics of Wilms' tumors in fine needle aspirates: A study of ten cases. *Acta Cytol* 33:263–266, 1989.
97. Drut R: Neuron specific enolase positive rosettes in nephroblastoma: A possible diagnostic pitfall in aspiration cytology. *Diagn Cytopathol* 3:74–76, 1987.
98. Drut R, Pollono D: Anaplastic Wilms' tumor. Initial diagnosis by fine needle aspiration. *Acta Cytol* 31:774–776, 1987.
99. Zuppan CW, Beckwith JB, Weeks DA, et al: The effect of preoperative therapy on the histologic features of Wilms' tumor: An analysis of cases from the Third National Wilms' Tumor Study. *Cancer* 68:385–394, 1991.
100. Babaian RJ, Skinner DG, Waisman J: Wilms' tumor in the adult patient. Diagnosis, management and review of the world medical literature. *Cancer* 45:1713–1719, 1980.
101. Arrigo S, Beckwith JB, Sharples K, et al: Better survival after combined modality case for adults with Wilms' tumor: A report from the National Wilms' Tumor Study. *Cancer* 66:827–830, 1990.
102. Huser J, Grignon DJ, Ro JY, et al: Adult Wilms' tumor: A clinicopathologic study of 11 cases. *Mod Pathol* 3:321–326, 1990.
103. Riccardi VM, Hittner HM, Francke V, et al: The aniridia-Wilms' tumor association: The critical role of chromosome band 11p13. *Cancer Genet Cytogenet* 2:131–137, 1980.
104. Douglass EE, Wilimas JA, Green AA, et al: Abnormalities of chromosomes 1 and 11 in Wilms' tumor. *Cancer Genet Cytogenet* 14:331–338, 1985.
105. Douglass EC, Look AT, Webber B, et al: Hyperdiploidy and chromosomal rearrangements define the anaplastic variant of Wilms' tumor. *J Clin Oncol* 4:975–981, 1986.
106. Call KM, Glaser T, Ito CY, et al: Isolation and characterization of a zinc finger polypeptide gene at the human chromosome 11 Wilms' tumor locus. *Cell* 60:509–520, 1990.
107. Lewis WH, Yeger H, Bonetta L, et al: Homozygous deletion of a DNA marker from chromosome 11p13 in sporadic Wilms' tumor. *Genomics* 3:25–31, 1988.
108. Pelletier J, Bruening W, Li FP, et al: WT1 mutations contribute to abnormal genital system development and hereditary Wilms' tumor. *Nature* 353:431–434, 1991.
109. Tomlinson G, Timmons C, Miwa H, et al: WT1 expression in Wilms' tumor in relation to histopathology and therapy. *Med Pediatr Oncol* 21:230, 1993.
110. Gerald WL, Gramling S, Sens DA, et al: Expression of 11p13 Wilms' tumor gene, WT1, correlates with histologic category of Wilms' tumor. *Am J Pathol* 140:1031–1037, 1992.
111. Pritchard-Jones K, Fleming S, Davidson D, et al: The candidate Wilms' tumor gene is involved in genitourinary development. *Nature* 346:194–197, 1990.
112. Clericuzio CL, D'Angio GJ, Duncan M, et al: Summary and recommendations of the workshop held at the First International Conference on Molecular and Clinical Genetics of Childhood Renal Tumors, Albuquerque, NM, May 14–16, 1992. *Med Pediatr Oncol* 21:233–236, 1993.
113. Nisen PD, Zimmerman KA, Cotter SV, et al: Enhanced expression of the N-myc gene in Wilms' tumors. *Cancer Res* 46:6217–6222, 1986.

114. Variend S, Spicer RD, Mackinnon AE: Teratoid Wilms' tumor. *Cancer* 53:1936–1942, 1984.
115. Gonzalez-Crussi F, Baum ES: Renal sarcomas of childhood: A clinicopathologic and ultrastructural study. *Cancer* 51:898–912, 1983.
116. Breslow N, Churchill G, Beckwith JB, et al: Prognosis for Wilms' tumor patients with nonmetastatic disease at diagnosis—Results of the Second National Wilms' Tumor Study. *J Clin Oncol* 3:521–531, 1985.
117. National Wilms' Tumor Study Committee: Wilms' tumor—status report 1990. *J Clin Oncol* 9:877–887, 1991.
118. Wallace AC, Nairn RC: Renal tubular antigens in kidney tumors. *Cancer* 29:977–981, 1972.
119. Raney RB, Palmer N, Sutow WW, et al: Renal cell carcinoma in children. *Med Pediatr Oncol* 11:91–98, 1983.
120. Lack EE, Canady JE, Price EB: Renal cell carcinoma in childhood and adolescence. A clinical and pathologic study of 17 cases. *J Urol* 133:822–828, 1985.
121. Dehner LP, Leestma JE, Price EB: Renal cell carcinoma in children. A clinicopathologic study of 15 cases and review of literature. *J Pediatr* 76:358–368, 1970.
122. Gonzalez-Crussi F, Kidd JM, Hernandez RJ: Cystic nephroma: Morphologic spectrum and implications. *Urology* 20:88–93, 1982.
123. Joshi VV, Beckwith JB: Multilocular cyst of the kidney (cystic nephroma) and cystic partially differentiated nephroblastoma: Terminology and criteria for diagnosis. *Cancer* 64:466–479, 1989.
124. Davila RM, Kissane JM, Crouch EC: Multilocular renal cyst—immunohistochemical and lectin-binding study. *Am J Surg Pathol* 16:508–514, 1992.
125. Shimokama T, Watanabe T: Multilocular renal cyst—scanning and transmission electron microscopic observations. *Pathol Res Pract* 184:225–229, 1989.
126. Drut R: Cystic nephroma: Cytologic findings in fine-needle aspiration cytology. *Diagn Cytopathol* 8:593–595, 1992.
127. Taxy JB, Marshall FF: Multilocular renal cysts in adults. Possible relationship to renal adenocarcinoma. *Arch Pathol Lab Med* 107:633–637, 1983.
128. Sadlowski RW, Smey P, Williams J, et al: Adenocarcinoma in multilocular renal cyst. *Urology* 14:512–514, 1979.
129. Madewell JE, Goldman SM, Davis CJ, et al: Multilocular cystic nephroma: A radiographic-pathologic correlation of 58 patients. *Radiology* 146:309–321, 1983.
130. Joshi VV, Banerjee AK, Yadav K, et al: Cystic partially differentiated nephroblastoma: A clinicopathologic entity in the spectrum of infantile renal neoplasia. *Cancer* 40:789–795, 1977.
131. Joshi VV, Beckwith JB: Pathologic delineation of the papillonodular type of cystic partially differentiated nephroblastoma. *Cancer* 66:1568–1577, 1990.
132. Anderson C, Knibbs DR, Ludwig ME, et al: Lymphangioma of the kidney: A pathologic entity distinct from solitary multilocular cyst. *Hum Pathol* 23:465–468, 1992.
133. Gelles RA, Pataki KI, Finegold RA: Bilateral multilocular cysts with recurrence. *J Urol* 121:808–810, 1979.
134. Sotelo-Avila C, Gonzalez-Crussi F, deMello D, et al: Renal and extrarenal rhabdoid tumors in children: A clinicopathologic study of 14 patients. *Semin Diagn Pathol* 3:151–163, 1986.
135. Weeks DA, Beckwith JB, Mierau GW: Rhabdoid tumor: An entity or a phenotype? *Arch Pathol Lab Med* 113:113–114, 1989.
136. Berry PJ, Vujanic GM: Malignant rhabdoid tumor. *Histopathology* 20:189–193, 1992.
137. Litman DA, Bhuta S, Barsky SH: Synchronous occurrence of malignant rhabdoid

tumor two decades after Wilms' tumor irradiation. *Am J Surg Pathol* 17:729–737, 1993.
138. Vogel AM, Gown AM, Caughlan J, et al: Rhabdoid tumors of the kidney contain mesenchymal specific and epithelial specific intermediate filament proteins. *Lab Invest* 50:232–238, 1984.
139. Mierau GW, Weeks DA, Beckwith JB: Anaplastic Wilms' tumor and other clinically aggressive childhood renal neoplasms: Ultrastructural and immunocytochemical features. *Ultrastruct Pathol* 13:225–248, 1989.
140. Drut R: Malignant rhabdoid tumor of the kidney diagnosed by fine-needle aspiration cytology. *Diagn Cytopathol* 6:124–126, 1990.
141. Weeks DA, Beckwith JB, Mierau GW: "Pseudorhabdoid" tumors of kidney. *Lab Invest* 54:10P, 1986.
142. Weeks DA, Beckwith JB, Mierau GW, et al: Renal neoplasms mimicking rhabdoid tumor of kidney: A report from the National Wilms' Tumor Pathology Center. *Am J Surg Pathol* 15:1042–1054, 1991.
143. Bonnin JM, Rubinstein LJ, Palmer NF, et al: The association of embryonal tumors originating in the kidney and in the brain: A report of seven cases. *Cancer* 54:2137–2146, 1984.
144. Douglass EC, Valentine M, Rowe ST, et al: Malignant rhabdoid tumor: A highly malignant childhood tumor with minimal karyotypic changes. *Genes Chrom Cancer* 2:210–216, 1990.
145. Hayashi Y, Hanada R, Yamamoto K, et al: Cytogenetic studies on childhood solid tumors. *Proc Annu Meet Jpn Cancer Assoc* 44:177, 1985.
146. Ota S, Crabbe DCG, Tran TN, et al: Malignant rhabdoid tumor: A study with two established cell lines. *Cancer* 71:2862–2872, 1993.
147. Kumar S, Marsden HB, Cowan RA, et al: Prognostic relevance of DNA content in childhood renal tumors. *Br J Cancer* 59:291–295, 1989.
148. Gansler T, Gerald W, Anderson G, et al: Characterization of a cell line derived from rhabdoid tumor of kidney. *Hum Pathol* 22:259–266, 1991.
149. Kennedy SM, Merino MJ, Linehan WM, et al: Collecting duct carcinoma of the kidney. *Hum Pathol* 21:449–456, 1990.
150. Abbi RK, McVicar M, Teichberg S, et al: Pathological characterization of a renin-secreting juxtaglomerular cell tumor in a child and review of pediatric literature. *Pediatr Pathol* 13:443–451, 1993.
151. Shende A, Wind ES, Lanzkowsky P: Intrarenal neuroblastoma mimicking Wilms' tumor. *NY State J Med* 79:93, 1979.
152. Seemayer TA, Thelmo WL, Bolande RP, et al: Peripheral neuroectodermal tumors. *Persp Pediatr Pathol* 2:151–172, 1975.
153. Acconia A, Mirraco C, Mattei FM, et al: Primary carcinoid tumor of kidney. Light and electron microscopy, and immunohistochemical study. *Urology* 31:517–520, 1988.
154. Kojiro M, Ohishi H, Isobe H: Carcinoid tumor occurring in cystic teratoma of the kidney. A case report. *Cancer* 38:1636–1640, 1976.
155. Joshi VV, Nord KS, Hanna M: Case 3: Renal gastrinoma with Zollinger-Ellison syndrome. *Pediatr Pathol* 6:475–476, 1986.
156. Aubert J, Casamayou J, Denis P, et al: Intrarenal teratoma in a newborn child. *Europ Urol* 4:306–308, 1978.
157. Prie EB, Mostofi FK: Symptomatic angiomyolipoma of the kidney. *Cancer* 18:761–774, 1965.

INDEX

I